Minimally Invasive Shoulder and Elbow Surgery

Minimally Invasive Procedures in Orthopedic Surgery

Series Editors

Alexander R. Vaccaro
Rothman Institute
and
Thomas Jefferson University Hospital
Philadelphia, Pennsylvania, U.S.A.

Christopher M. Bono
Boston University Medical Center
Boston, Massachusetts, U.S.A.

1. Minimally Invasive Shoulder and Elbow Surgery, *edited by William N. Levine, Theodore A. Blaine, and Christopher S. Ahmad*

Minimally Invasive Shoulder and Elbow Surgery

Edited by

William N. Levine
Columbia Presbyterian Medical Center
New York, New York, U.S.A.

Theodore A. Blaine
Columbia Presbyterian Medical Center
New York, New York, U.S.A.

Christopher S. Ahmad
Columbia Presbyterian Medical Center
New York, New York, U.S.A.

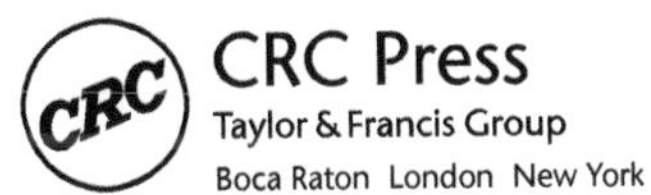

CRC Press
Taylor & Francis Group
Boca Raton London New York

CRC Press is an imprint of the
Taylor & Francis Group, an **informa** business

CRC Press
Taylor & Francis Group
6000 Broken Sound Parkway NW, Suite 300
Boca Raton, FL 33487-2742

First issued in paperback 2019

ISBN-13: 978-0-8493-7215-5 (hbk)
ISBN-13: 978-0-367-38948-2 (pbk)

Visit the Taylor & Francis Web site at
http://www.taylorandfrancis.com

and the CRC Press Web site at
http://www.crcpress.com

Preface

The management of shoulder and elbow pathology has changed more dramatically over the last decade than many other disciplines in medicine owing to the innovation of minimally invasive surgery. This spectrum of techniques has swept through orthopedic surgery, allowing surgeons to identify, manage, and treat their patients without requiring the large open incisions that could lead to postoperative difficulties. Fewer complications, shorter recovery periods, and the overall ease of treatment have all contributed to the success of these techniques.

This book was designed to provide the reader with the latest approaches in minimally invasive surgery as it applies to the shoulder and elbow. Our contributors are well-respected world leaders at the cutting edge of these procedures and its technology.

Minimally invasive shoulder surgery is covered in detail. This book discusses the basic setup and diagnostic arthroscopy before explaining, step by step, a multitude of procedures, including acromioplasty, distal clavicle resection, instability repair, glenoid debridement, and the treatment of cysts and inflammation, and provides a multi-chapter, in-depth look at rotator cuff repair.

Minimally invasive elbow surgery is also given detailed attention with several chapters devoted to both straightforward procedures, such as diagnostic arthroscopy and tennis elbow debridement, and procedures that only the most experienced arthroscopists should attempt, including managing cubital tunnel syndrome with arthroscopic medial epicondylectomy.

It is our hope that this book is embraced by the orthopedic surgery community as the definitive "how-to" guide on minimally invasive approaches to the shoulder and elbow.

William N. Levine
Theodore A. Blaine
Christopher S. Ahmad

Contents

Contributors

Jeffrey S. Abrams Princeton Orthopaedic & Rehabilitation Associates, Princeton, New Jersey, U.S.A.

Kenneth J. Accousti Department of Orthopedic Surgery, Mount Sinai Medical Center, New York, New York, U.S.A.

Robert Afra Department of Orthopedics, University of California, San Diego, California, U.S.A.

Christopher S. Ahmad Center for Shoulder, Elbow, and Sports Medicine, Department of Orthopedic Surgery, Columbia Presbyterian Medical Center, New York, New York, U.S.A.

Hari Ankem Center for Shoulder, Elbow, and Sports Medicine, Department of Orthopedic Surgery, Columbia Presbyterian Medical Center, New York, New York, U.S.A.

April D. Armstrong Department of Orthopedics and Rehabilitation, Penn State Milton S. Hershey Medical Center, Hershey, Pennsylvania, U.S.A.

Champ L. Baker, Jr. The Hughston Clinic and The Hughston Foundation, Inc., Columbus, Georgia, U.S.A.

F. Alan Barber Plano Orthopedic and Sports Medicine Center, Plano, Texas, U.S.A.

Shane A. Barwood Department of Orthopedic Surgery, The University of Calgary, Calgary, Alberta, Canada

John-Erik Bell Center for Shoulder, Elbow, and Sports Medicine, Department of Orthopedic Surgery, Columbia Presbyterian Medical Center, New York, New York, U.S.A.

Theodore A. Blaine Center for Shoulder, Elbow, and Sports Medicine, Department of Orthopedic Surgery, Columbia Presbyterian Medical Center, New York, New York, U.S.A.

Michael H. Boothby Plano Orthopedic and Sports Medicine Center, Plano, Texas, U.S.A.

Gabriel D. Brown Center for Shoulder, Elbow, and Sports Medicine, Department of Orthopedic Surgery, Columbia Presbyterian Medical Center, New York, New York, U.S.A.

Taylor D. Brown Mississippi Sports Medicine and Orthopedic Center, Jackson, Mississippi, U.S.A.

Stephen S. Burkhart The San Antonio Orthopedic Group, San Antonio, Texas, U.S.A.

Cordelia Carter Center for Shoulder, Elbow, and Sports Medicine, Department of Orthopedic Surgery, Columbia Presbyterian Medical Center, New York, New York, U.S.A.

Ryan Chen Department of Orthopedic Surgery, Washington University School of Medicine, Barnes-Jewish Hospital, St. Louis, Missouri, U.S.A.

A. Martin Clark, Jr. The CORE Institute, Sun City West, Arizona, U.S.A.

Brian J. Cole Departments of Orthopedics and Anatomy and Cell Biology and Division of Shoulder and Elbow Surgery, Department of Orthopedic Surgery, Rush University Medical Center, Rush Medical College, Chicago, Illinois, U.S.A.

Xavier A. Duralde Peachtree Orthopaedic Clinic, Emory University, Atlanta, Georgia, U.S.A.

Sara Edwards Center for Shoulder, Elbow, and Sports Medicine, Department of Orthopedic Surgery, Columbia Presbyterian Medical Center, New York, New York, U.S.A.

Neal S. ElAttrache Kerlan-Jobe Orthopedic Clinic and Department of Orthopedic Surgery, University of Southern California School of Medicine, Los Angeles, California, U.S.A.

Mitchell F. Fagelman Department of Orthopedic Surgery, University of Pennsylvania School of Medicine, Philadelphia, Pennsylvania, U.S.A.

Larry D. Field Upper Extremity Service, Mississippi Sports Medicine and Orthopedic Center, and Department of Orthopedic Surgery, University of Mississippi School of Medicine, Jackson, Mississippi, U.S.A.

Evan L. Flatow Department of Orthopedic Surgery, Mount Sinai Medical Center, New York, New York, U.S.A.

Michael Q. Freehill Sports and Orthopedic Specialists, Edina, Minnesota, U.S.A.

Leesa M. Galatz Department of Orthopedic Surgery, Washington University School of Medicine, Barnes-Jewish Hospital, St. Louis, Missouri, U.S.A.

Charles L. Getz Department of Orthopedic Surgery, University of Pennsylvania School of Medicine, Philadelphia, Pennsylvania, U.S.A.

Andreas H. Gomoll Department of Orthopedic Surgery, Brigham and Women's Hospital, Harvard Medical School, Boston, Massachusetts, U.S.A.

Eric H. Gordon Arkansas Specialty Orthopaedics, Little Rock, Arkansas, U.S.A.

David P. Huberty The San Antonio Orthopedic Group, San Antonio, Texas, U.S.A.

Kent Jackson Hospital for Special Surgery, New York, New York, U.S.A.

Jay D. Keener Department of Orthopedic Surgery, Washington University, St. Louis, Missouri, U.S.A.

Hyun-Min Kim Department of Orthopedic Surgery, Washington University School of Medicine, Barnes-Jewish Hospital, St. Louis, Missouri, U.S.A.

Christian Lattermann Department of Orthopedic Surgery, University of Kentucky, Lexington, Kentucky, and Midwest Orthopaedics at Rush, Rush University Hospital, Chicago, Illinois, U.S.A.

William N. Levine Center for Shoulder, Elbow, and Sports Medicine, Department of Orthopedic Surgery, Columbia Presbyterian Medical Center, New York, New York, U.S.A.

Ian K.Y. Lo Department of Orthopedic Surgery, The University of Calgary, Calgary, Alberta, Canada.

Emilio Lopez-Vidriero Center for Sports Medicine, Department of Orthopedic Surgery, University of Pittsburgh Medical Center, Pittsburgh, Pennsylvania, U.S.A.

R. Vaughan Massie The Hughston Clinic and The Hughston Foundation, Inc., Columbus, Georgia, U.S.A.

Augustus D. Mazzocca Department of Orthopedic Surgery, University of Connecticut Health Center, Farmington, Connecticut, U.S.A.

Peter J. Millett The Steadman-Hawkins Clinic, Vail, Colorado, U.S.A.

Anand M. Murthi Department of Orthopedics, The Shoulder and Elbow Service, University of Maryland School of Medicine, Baltimore, Maryland, U.S.A.

Gregory P. Nicholson Department of Orthopedic Surgery, Rush University Medical Center, Midwest Orthopaedics at Rush, Rush University Hospital, Chicago, Illinois, U.S.A.

John P. Peden Mississippi Sports Medicine and Orthopedic Center, Jackson, Mississippi, U.S.A.

Matthew L. Ramsey Department of Orthopedic Surgery, University of Pennsylvania School of Medicine, Philadelphia, Pennsylvania, U.S.A.

Herbert Resch Department of Traumatology and Sports Injuries, University Hospital of Salzburg, Salzburg, Austria

Mark W. Rodosky Department of Orthopedic Surgery, Division of Shoulder Surgery, University of Pittsburgh Sports Medicine, Pittsburgh, Pennsylvania, U.S.A.

Joaquin Sanchez-Sotelo Department of Orthopedic Surgery, Mayo Clinic Rochester, Rochester, Minnesota, U.S.A.

Felix H. Savoie Upper Extremity Service, Mississippi Sports Medicine and Orthopedic Center, and Department of Orthopedic Surgery, University of Mississippi School of Medicine, Jackson, Mississippi, U.S.A.

Jon K. Sekiya Center for Sports Medicine, Department of Orthopedic Surgery, University of Pittsburgh Medical Center, Pittsburgh, Pennsylvania, U.S.A.

Adam M. Smith Kentucky Sports Medicine Clinic, Lexington, Kentucky, U.S.A.

Stephen J. Snyder Southern California Orthopaedic Institute, Van Nuys, California, U.S.A.

Walter J. Song Department of Orthopedic Surgery, University of Connecticut Health Center, Farmington, Connecticut, U.S.A.

John W. Sperling Department of Orthopedics, Mayo Clinic, Rochester, Minnesota, U.S.A.

Jason A. Stein Department of Orthopedics, The Shoulder and Elbow Service, University of Maryland School of Medicine, Baltimore, Maryland, U.S.A.

Beth E. Shubin Stein Hospital for Special Surgery, New York, New York, U.S.A.

Scott P. Steinmann Department of Orthopedic Surgery, Mayo Clinic, Rochester, Minnesota, U.S.A.

Timothy J. Strigenz Department of Orthopedics and Rehabilitation, Penn State Milton S. Hershey Medical Center, Hershey, Pennsylvania, U.S.A.

Douglass E. Stull Department of Orthopedic Surgery, University of Pennsylvania School of Medicine, Philadelphia, Pennsylvania, U.S.A.

Robert Z. Tashjian Department of Orthopedic Surgery, Washington University School of Medicine, Barnes-Jewish Hospital, St. Louis, Missouri, U.S.A.

Mark Tauber Department of Traumatology and Sports Injuries, University Hospital of Salzburg, Salzburg, Austria

Ilya Voloshin Department of Orthopedics, University of Rochester Medical Center, Rochester, New York, U.S.A.

Gerald R. Williams, Jr. Department of Orthopedic Surgery, University of Pennsylvania School of Medicine, Philadelphia, Pennsylvania, U.S.A.

Ken Yamaguchi Department of Orthopedic Surgery, Washington University School of Medicine, Barnes-Jewish Hospital, St. Louis, Missouri, U.S.A.

1 Patient Positioning During Arthroscopic Shoulder Surgery

Ilya Voloshin
Department of Orthopedics, University of Rochester Medical Center, Rochester, New York, U.S.A.

Robert Afra
Department of Orthopedics, University of California, San Diego, California, U.S.A.

INTRODUCTION

The last decade has seen an exponential increase in the number of arthroscopic shoulder surgeries performed. The indications for shoulder arthroscopy continue to expand and the procedures are becoming more complex. With the widening indications, more surgical complications have been described (1). Given this robust growth in numbers of arthroscopic shoulder procedures, the surgeons must continue to master their efficiency and quality of surgical procedures. This efficiency, in part, derives from the operating room (OR) set up and proper patient positioning. The two most common positions utilized in shoulder arthroscopy are beach-chair and lateral decubitus positions. The surgeon's preference largely determines which position is used and for which procedures. Both positions have their advantages and disadvantages, requiring surgeon awareness to minimize risk and avoid complications. Regardless of the position chosen, prior to draping, the surgical team must take the time to fine-tune the patient's position. For both positions used for shoulder arthroscopy, this chapter describes setup technique, advantages and disadvantages for each position, complications, and senior author's (IV) rationale for position choice for different surgical procedures.

ANESTHESIA

A brachial plexus block is often utilized in conjunction with general endotracheal anesthesia. The reason for supplemental sedation is poor tolerance for lateral decubitus position by the completely awake patient for a prolonged period of time. This is due to some pressure points (especially, the axillary roll) that may irritate the patient if the procedure lasts beyond two hours. The use of a brachial plexus block should be discussed among the surgeon, anesthesiologist, and the patient, given the risks and potential complications. Although the procedural details are beyond the scope of this chapter, the two most common form of blocks for shoulder arthroscopy are the interscalene and supraclavicular. It is important for a surgeon to firmly appreciate the benefits and risks associated with each block. The block typically provides 8 to 18 hours of pain relief and motor paralysis, depending on the anesthetic cocktail delivered and the block quality.

LATERAL DECUBITUS POSITIONING

The lateral decubitus position with continuous arm traction applied is perhaps the most popular position because of its simple set up and low equipment cost (2).

Preparation of the Operating Room

Prior to the patient transferring from the gurney to the OR bed, it is important for a U-shaped bean bag (3 ft long size; 32 Vacupac, Olympic Medical Seattle, Washington, U.S.A.) and

Please refer to pages 8–12 for the figures in this chapter.

overlying sheet to be in proper position (Fig. 1). The U end of the bean bag should be cephalad so that the suction end is caudad (out of the way). The flaps should be positioned to avoid blocking adequate shoulder exposure. The base of the U is at the level of the scapula. Also, the suction should be anterior so that it is out of the surgeon's way. Make sure the beans are evenly distributed so that the position of the upper torso and the lower torso are adequately controlled. Deficiency of beans will lead to the body collapsing the bean bag once engaged. An overlying sheet is important because it protects the patient's skin from direct pressure of the bean bag, and it is an aid to position the patient. The authors use a nondisposable sheet to help levitate and reposition the patient to lateral decubitus. It is important not to drag the patient because this will lead to a shift in the bean bag position as it is dragged.

Initial Positioning

While supine on the OR table, general anesthesia is established. The authors prefer to have the endotracheal tube or laryngeal mask airway (LMA) secured to the contralateral side of the mouth, to decrease the risk of inadvertent extubation when removing drapes at the completion of surgery. The appropriate shoulder examination under anesthesia is performed.

The patient is placed into the lateral decubitus position with the aid of four people: anesthesiologist at the head, one person on the right, left, and foot of the bed. With the anesthesiologist's count, the patient is turned to the lateral decubitus position in two steps. First, the patient is suspended in the air using the overlying sheet. Then, the operative side is turned up. The person at the foot of the bed repositions to be able to insert an appropriate axillary roll, as the torso is elevated by the other three people. The roll should not be in the axilla per se, but at the U portion of the bean bag to support the thorax and prevent pressure on the dependent shoulder and axilla.

The primary surgeon controls the position of the anterior and posterior sand bag flaps, and the assistant surgeon controls the caudad end of the bean bag. The nurse applies suction to engage the bean bag. Ideally, the patient's torso should be tilted 20° posteriorly (Fig. 2). For a male patient, one must ensure that the genitals are not squeezed between the thighs or faced with excessive pressure against the bean bag. Padding should be placed to unload the fibular head of the bottom leg, to avoid a peroneal nerve palsy. Additional padding should protect the bottom ankle, elbow, and wrist. The anesthesiologist must provide adequate padding under the head to make sure that the neck is in neutral position, to avoid excessive strain on the brachial plexus (Fig. 3). Leg mechanical compression devices are placed to prevent deep venous thrombosis. A pillow is placed between the knees to relieve pressure on the hips (Fig. 4). A sheet is placed over the buttock and a safety strap is applied. The operating table is rotated 45° posteriorly, so the surgeon can approach the head. This allows the surgeon to access the anterior shoulder. The bottom arm is strapped to an arm board at 90° to 120° to the torso. The operative arm is suspended to allow adequate surgical prep, using tape, clamp, or IV pressure bag. A single U drape is placed in the axilla with the open end toward the head. Make sure the adherent flaps stick well to the skin so that the patient does not become wet and hypothermic from the arthroscopy fluid. A lower body bear hugger is applied to keep the torso and lower extremity warm. It is not activated until all sterile drapes are applied, so as not to compromise the sterile field. The double boom shoulder holder (Arthrex Three-Point Traction Tower) is attached at the caudad end of the anterior rail. The head of the boom is extended/rotated to sit 2- to 3-ft above the upper shoulder (Fig. 5).

Final Positioning and Preparation for Surgery

The surgical team should confirm whether perioperative antibiotics have been administered. Skin preparation is accomplished using the solution most preferred by the surgeon. The advantage of betadine is that it stains skin and missed spots are easily located. Some prefer Hibiclens (chlorhexadine), followed by alcohol scrub. Flammability is not an issue, since electrocautery is not used early in the case. In addition, the skin is less irritated than with betadine, and it does not need to be washed off at the end of the case. A drying towel is used along the field edge so that the adhesive on the sterile drapes will stick. A $\frac{3}{4}$ downsheet is placed caudad to the axilla. The gowned surgeon takes control of the forearm with a sterile towel. For surgical cases involving instability and superior labrum anterior-posterior (SLAP) lesions, the extremity is placed into the foam shoulder traction and rotation sleeve (StaR Sleeve, Arthrex Inc.; Naples, Florida, U.S.A.). So that there is adequate length for traction, it is important to place the foam deep into the axilla. The extremity is rotated so that the thumb is at the open side of the sleeve for the rotation to be controlled. Koban is used to wrap the arm and forearm for a snug fit. The distal end of the sleeve is secured to the bottom pulley with an S hook and suspended with 10 pounds for an average size extremity. The weight should be adjusted according to patient size and weight. The strap is opened and applied to the most proximal portion of the foam sleeve, near the axilla. Six to eight pounds are applied for traction to the second hook. Ideally, the arm is abducted 70° and forward flexed 15°. The strap is overwrapped with a second Koban (Fig. 6). The authors like to apply an impervious U drape below the axilla and the tails taken toward the head. A paper U drape is applied in a similar fashion. A paper U drape with fluid bag is based over the neck, and tails are taken toward the torso.

BEACH-CHAIR POSITION

For many surgeons, the beach chair is chosen because the shoulder is in position similar to open surgery and conversion to open surgery is easier (3). The beach-chair position is increasing in popularity since the advent of special arm and shoulder positioners, which facilitate the control of the arm and exposure to the posterior aspect of the shoulder.

Preparation of the Operating Room

The senior author (IV) has been using the T-max Shoulder Positioner and Spider Limb Positioner (Tenet Medical Engineering, Calgary, Alberta, Canada) for shoulder arthroscopy in the beach-chair position (Fig. 7). The Spider Limb Positioner allows excellent control, positional freedom, and ability to apply traction to the operative extremity.

The shoulder positioner needs to be safely secured to the OR table. Gel padding is used to avoid pressure points on patient's back. The arm positioner is attached to the shoulder positioner. A nitrogen hose from the arm positioner is connected to the nitrogen wall outlet set at 100psi.

Initial Positioning

The patient is initially in a supine position. Because patients tolerate the sitting position better than the lateral decubitus, beach-chair position allows the option of performing shoulder arthroscopy solely under the interscalene block without any supplemental sedation. This may be beneficial when a patient has a serious cardiopulmonary ailment. If additional sedation is desired, the patient is intubated in the supine position.

The shoulder positioner is raised, and the patient is flexed 80° at the waist. This brings the acromion parallel to the floor to facilitate access to the posterior portal (Fig. 8). The patient's head is secured on a padded head positioner. It is important to make sure that the neck is in neutral position (Fig. 9). The torso is secured by special side supports, to prevent shifting the patient during surgery when traction is applied (Fig. 10). The lower extremities are placed on a pillow with knees flexed, to protect the peroneal nerve and soft tissue. The contralateral arm is placed on an arm board with special attention paid to the padding for the ulnar nerve at the level of the cubital tunnel.

The operating table is rotated 45° posteriorly, so the surgeon has enough access to the posterior shoulder and does not feel cramped by the anesthesia equipment. The operative arm is suspended to allow adequate surgical prep, using tape, clamp, or IV pressure bag. A single U drape is placed in the axilla with the open end toward the head. Make sure the adherent flaps stick well to the skin so that the patient does not become wet and hypothermic from the arthroscopy fluid. A lower body bear hugger is applied to keep the torso and lower extremity warm. It is not activated until all sterile drapes are applied, so as not to compromise the sterile field.

Final Positioning and Preparation for Surgery

The operative extremity is prepped and a drying towel is used along the field edge, so that the adhesive on the sterile drapes sticks. Two sterile impervious U drapes are applied from below and above the shoulder creating a good seal to the skin. Two paper U drape are applied in a similar fashion. A paper U drape with fluid bag is based inferior to the axilla with tails taken toward the head. The gowned surgeon takes control of the forearm with a sterile towel. The extremity is placed into the special foam forearm cuff with metal bar (part of Spider Limb Positioner and shoulder stabilization kit) (Fig. 11). Koban is used to wrap the forearm for a snug fit. The Spider Limb Positioner is dressed with the special sterile limb positioner drape (part of the shoulder stabilization kit). The forearm sleeve is secured to the limb positioner, which allows motion and all three planes. At this point, the patient is positioned for the arthroscopic procedure with adequate access to all areas of the shoulder. If the decision is made to convert to an open procedure, it can be easily performed without the need to reposition the patient. Patient's flexion at the waist level can be easily adjusted without the need for redraping. Special attention must be paid to the neck and head position if patient is flexed or if extended at the waist level or intermittent traction is applied to the operative extremity during surgery.

DISCUSSION

Lateral Decubitus

Lateral decubitus position has several advantages. Access to the anterior, posterior, superior, and inferior labrum is easier in the lateral decubitus position compared to the beach-chair position (4). When performing shoulder arthroscopy for multidirectional instability, SLAP, or Bankart injury, visibility is improved with the lateral decubitus position.

Jerosch et al. (5), in a cadaveric study, determined that when performing an arthroscopic shoulder capsular release for adhesive capsulitis, the optimum position for the operative extremity is in the abducted, externally rotated position. This positioning mimics the lateral decubitus position. With the arm thus situated, the axillary nerve stays in its native position, while the glenohumeral capsule tightens. This increases the distance between the two structures, allowing the surgeon to release the inferior capsule more safely.

Hypotensive anesthesia improves visualization, allowing lower pump pressures to avoid excessive tissue distension. A potential advantage of the lateral decubitus position over the beach-chair position is a decreased risk of stroke. The cerebrum is in a dependent position, which decreases the risk of a cerebrovascular ischemic event during intraoperative hypotension. However, Palermo et al. (6) determined that patients with congestive heart failure were both subjectively and physiologically less tolerant of the lateral decubitus position, in comparison to the sitting position. When operating on patients with a history of heart failure, the surgeon must be cognizant of the fact that airway obstruction and lung diffusion impairment may become a clinical issue.

Several downsides to the lateral decubitus position exist. The risk of some of the complications can be minimized by surgical prudence. Other risks are inherent to the surgical position and must be dealt with as they arise.

According to Hoenecke et al. (4), conversion of the lateral decubitus position to an open approach could be more difficult than for the beach-chair position, especially for an anterior approach.

Various types of neurologic injuries have been described with the lateral decubitus position. Neurologic complications have included compression of the dorsal digital nerve of the thumb, peroneal nerve, ulnar nerve, and traction-induced trauma to the brachial plexus (7). According to Bigliani et al. (2), brachial plexus strain was the most common complication associated with the lateral decubitus position in the 1980s. The nerve injury usually resolved over a 6- to 12-week period.

Overstretching was the mechanism most commonly involved in neuropraxias that developed with shoulder arthroscopy in the lateral decubitus position. This was due to traction on the operative shoulder or lateral flexion of the neck. Klein et al. (8), in a cadaveric study, determined that, at a given flexion angle, increasing abduction of the operative shoulder leads to a decrease in the strain on the brachial plexus. At a given abduction angle, increasing flexion results in a decrease in the strain on the brachial plexus. At the extremes, however, visibility is thoroughly limited. As such, the authors proposed a balance between strain minimization and visibility maximization. They suggested such combinations of positions as 45° of forward flexion with 90° of abduction and 45° of forward flexion with 0° of abduction. The authors believed that repositioning during the case between these two positions would achieve a balance between adequate visibility and the least amount of strain on the brachial plexus. Pitman et al. (9) demonstrated, with somatosensory evoked potentials, that the incidence of subclinical neuropraxia is high in the shoulder operated on in the lateral decubitus position. The musculocutaneous nerve was the most vulnerable nerve; the injury usually occurred when the nerve enters the conjoint muscles. Others have proposed the head position to be the culprit. The angle between the head and shoulder is widened, as the head is placed into extension with lateral flexion to the contralateral side. Shaffer et al. (10) advocated use of no more than 10 pounds (4.5 kg) for arm traction, to decrease the risk of injury to the brachial plexus. However, no scientific evidence was offered to substantiate this weight. Berjano et al. (11) described three cases of ulnar nerve neuropraxia on the operative extremity, while the patients were in the lateral decubitus position. Symptoms resolved over a 12-week period. They attributed the neuropraxia to the way that the adhesive traction system was wrapped around the elbow. Traction on the extremities never exceeded 3 kg.

Pavlik et al. (12) described a shoulder arthroscopy case in the lateral decubitus position in which the patient developed a contralateral brachial plexus palsy. Ten pounds of traction were applied in the 45 min surgical case. The patient was found to have a C7-T1 palsy postoperatively. There was no mention of a brachial plexus block or placement of an axillary role. An x-ray of the neck revealed bilateral cervical ribs. In order to avoid a traction injury to the operative shoulder, the anesthesiologist, in this case, elevated the head slightly passed neutral to prevent stretch of the plexus; however, in effect, the contralateral brachial plexus was placed on stretch. They believed the head position, lack of an axillary role, in conjunction with the abnormal anatomy, resulted in stretching of the lower roots, leading to a palsy.

Gonzalez Della Valle et al. (13) measured the pressure under the inferior shoulder and chest wall, while using various devices as an "axillary role": 1 L lactated Ringer's bag in conjunction with a pillow under the head, a gel pad in conjunction with a pillow under the head, and a double inflatable pillow system, under the chest wall and head (Shoulder-Float, Trimline Medial Products; Branchburg, New Jersey, U.S.A.). They found the average pressure beneath the shoulder without any supporting device to be 64 mmHg, using the 1 L bag was 34 mmHg, using the gel pad was 27 mmHg, and using the inflatable pillow was 10 mmHg ($P < 0.001$). Additionally, a significantly positive correlation was found between body weight and pressure beneath the shoulder. The limiting factor in making clinical use of this data is that there is no threshold value of what pressure becomes clinically relevant. Of note, the inflatable pillows are easier to position, in that the patient's torso does not need to be elevated for the device to be placed.

Beach-Chair Position

According to Hoenecke et al. (4), using the beach-chair position during shoulder arthroscopy presents the anatomy in an "upright, anatomic" position. It minimizes spatial disorientation. More importantly, however, it is easier to convert to an open anterior procedure from the beach-chair position than from the lateral decubitus position. Yet, the most commonly mentioned reason surgeons choose to use the beach-chair position over the lateral decubitus position is most likely due to the lower incidence of nerve palsy.

According to Hoenecke (4), if traction is needed to facilitate visualization or space needed to perform surgery while shoulder arthroscopy is performed in the beach-chair position, one of two things is necessary. Either the assistant will be occupied applying traction, instead of helping the primary surgeon with the surgery; or a relatively expensive spatial positioning device is needed to provide traction for exposure of the subacromial or intra-articular space. As well, access to the axillary pouch and the posterior recess is difficult. Baechler et al. (14) acknowledged the difficulty of performing an arthroscopic SLAP repair, utilizing the beach-chair position. Depending on the lateral acromial morphology, the assistant surgeon may need to displace the humeral head inferiorly with longitudinal traction if the patient is in the beach-chair position. They concluded that if the surgeon determines preoperatively by the method they describe that the humeral head must be inferiorly displaced by greater than 25% of the humeral head diameter to achieve adequate arthroscopic access to the superior glenoid, they recommended the lateral decubitus position for that patient. However, modern limb positioners can apply intermittent traction without occupying the assistant surgeon and allow adequate access to the superior glenoid.

Several drawbacks to the beach-chair position have been described. When an open camera lens system is used during beach chair positioned shoulder arthroscopy, there is the potential for fogging of the arthroscopic lens as a result of the flow of irrigation down the scope when the camera is held in an "uphill" position from a posterior viewing portal (3).

Although many authors have discussed brachial plexus palsies after shoulder surgery in the lateral decubitus position, a few have described a neuropraxia in the beach-chair position. Mullins et al. (15) describe a hypoglossal nerve neuropraxia that developed after shoulder arthroscopy and open cuff repair with the patient in the beach-chair position. The nerve palsy was completely resolved by postoperative week eight. The complete vascular and neurologic work-up was negative. The authors offer two possible causes. Either the hypoglossal nerve was compressed by the endotracheal tube, or a change in the patient's head position during the case led to the nerve being compressed beneath the mandibular angle. A change in the head position is prone to occur during patient position changes, such as reclining the operative table or tilting it to one side or the other during the operative case. They suggest frequent checks to confirm proper head alignment and position. Interestingly, Cooper et al. (16) reported a case of a contralateral brachial plexus palsy while in the beach-chair position. This patient had an open shoulder procedure, while the contralateral arm was abducted to 90° and placed on an arm board. The patient developed a C5 and C6 root palsy. The authors believed it was due to prolonged stretching of the plexus.

Bhatti et al. (17) described a case in which the patient underwent a shoulder arthroscopy in the beach-chair position with postoperative loss of vision in one eye and significantly limited gaze in all directions. The neurologic and cardiovascular work-up was negative. The patient's vision returned to near normal over the ensuing two weeks. The authors reported intraoperative hypotension used to aid in visualization as a potential risk factor. The intraoperative blood pressure reading may have been falsely higher than the true pressure in this case, because the blood pressure cuff was placed around the ankle, which was in a dependent position. They believed the etiology of the visual loss and opthalmoplegia was an orbital or extraocular muscle ischemic process, suggesting the scattering of emboli and multiple vascular occlusions. Theoretically, because of the beach-chair position, the cerebral blood flow "fights" gravity. This "upright" position may become a risk factor of an ischemic insult during hypotensive surgery, especially in a patient with other known risk factors (i.e., obesity, high cholesterol level, hypertension, diabetes, hypercalcemia, and history of stroke or cardiovascular disease).

Modified "Hybrid" Position

Hoenecke et al. (4) introduced the La Jolla beach-chair position, which is a hybrid of the lateral decubitus and the traditional beach chair positions. The patient is placed on the OR table in the supine position and is propped up into a "lazy" lateral decubitus position at 45°, using a triangular foam pillow. The hips are flexed, the head elevated, and the foot dropped as with the traditional beach-chair position. A traction device is then used, as with a lateral decubitus position. They report on a case series of 50 patients with procedures varying from subacromial decompressions and rotator cuff repairs to SLAP and anterior instability repairs. Three cases were converted from an arthroscopic to an open procedure, and visualization was reportedly "excellent." They reported no complications with the surgical positioning. They felt they were able to benefit from the advantages of both traditional beach chair as well as lateral decubitus positioning. However, the predominant risk factor of the lateral decubitus position is due to the traction on the operative arm, that is, brachial plexus neuropraxia, it seems to us that this risk factor is not circumvented. As such, although Hoenecke et al. (4) believe that they have the advantage of both positions while using the La Jolla beach chair, the authors believe they also have the disadvantage of both positions while using the La Jolla beach-chair position.

SENIOR AUTHOR'S (IV) PREFERRED METHOD FOR POSITIONING

Beach-Chair Position

Senior author (IV) utilizes the beach-chair position for arthroscopic procedures involving rotator cuff repair and arthroscopic work in the subacromial space. The T-max Shoulder Positioner and Spider Limb Positioner are used. Even though this equipment is expensive, the advantages include the freedom to position and secure the limb in almost any location in space. This facilitates arthroscopic work during rotator cuff repair, especially with massive tears and subscapularis tears, where the shoulder may have to be fully internally rotated for visualization of the lesser tuberosity or fully externally rotated for visualization of the posterior aspect of the greater tuberosity. This can be done in the lateral decubitus position, but would certainly require an extra surgical assistant for holding the upper limb in desired position. Also, the beach-chair position can be easily converted to an open procedure. This is beneficial for chronic retracted subscapularis tears that may require extensive mobilization or when a pectoralis major transfer is contemplated. The hydraulic arm positioner also applies longitudinal traction when more space is needed in the subacromial space. The traction can subsequently be released once the necessary work is done. This intermittent application of traction allows the surgeon to apply considerable traction for a short period of time to perform necessary work without the risk of continuous traction that may result in brachial plexus injury.

Lateral Decubitus Position

The lateral decubitus position is used for arthroscopic SLAP repairs and arthroscopic procedures for shoulder instability, where access is needed to both the anterior, posterior, and inferior capsule (Fig. 12). In a beach-chair position, the humeral head hangs down and posterior secondary to gravity, making access to posterior capsule and axillary pouch more challenging. Whether the instability is anterior or posterior, it is important to mobilize the capsule in a south to north direction, reducing the volume of the inferior pouch and creating a shift similar to an open procedure. Having improved access to these areas in lateral decubitus position facilitates the ability to accomplish these tasks. Also, if a HAGL (humeral avulsion of the inferior glenohumeral ligament) lesion is identified, arthroscopic management would require adequate access to the axillary pouch for proper visualization.

In the arthroscopic SLAP repair, the lateral decubitus position is preferred because it allows the superior capsule and synovium to fall away form the superior labrum (Fig. 13). This provides for easier passage of sutures around the labrum and suture management. In a beach-chair position, the superior synovium and capsule tend to lie immediately on top of the superior labrum, secondary to gravitational forces. This makes arthroscopic suture passage more challenging. Also, access to posterior labrum, which is often required, is easier in lateral decubitus position. As described earlier, better visualization of posterior capsule and labrum leads to easier suture passage and management.

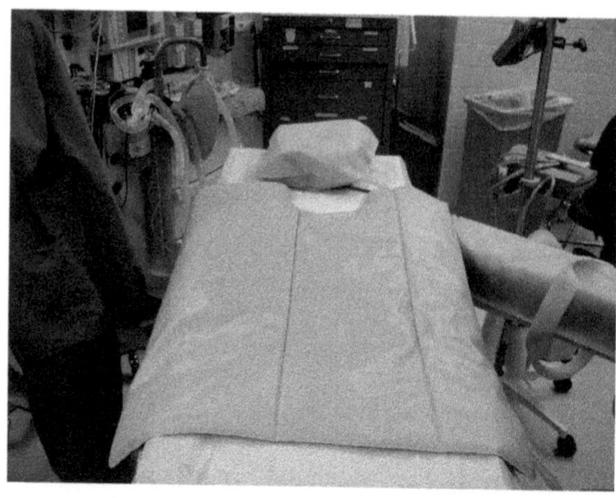

FIGURE 1 A U-shaped bean bag with U portion positioned cephalad.

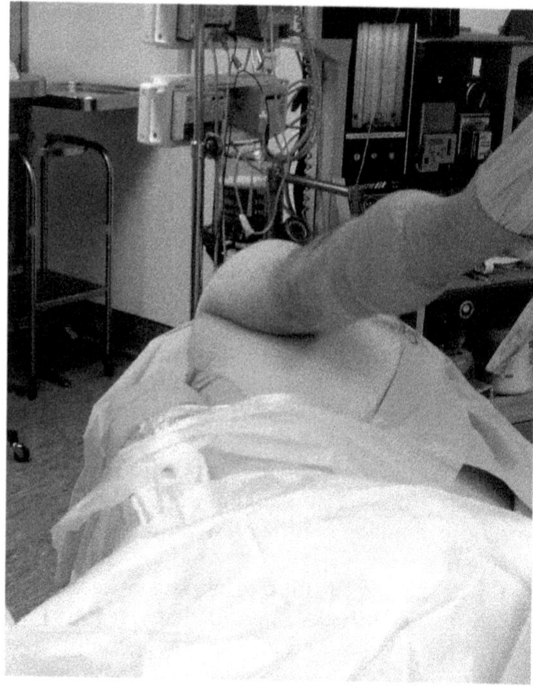

FIGURE 2 Torso should be tilted 20° posteriorly to keep glenoid parallel to the floor.

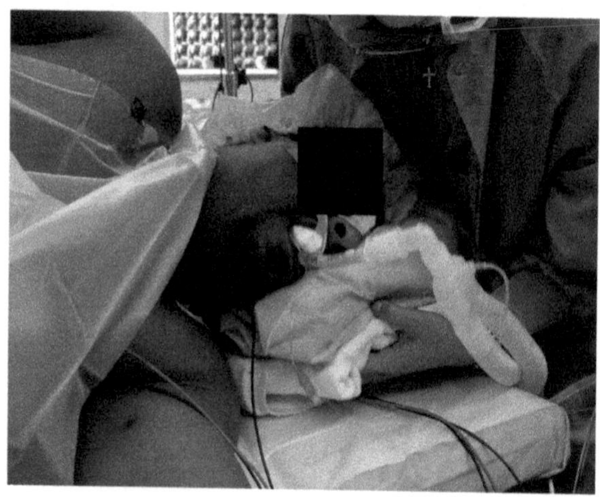

FIGURE 3 Adequate padding under the head keeps the head in neutral to avoid excessive strain on the brachial plexus.

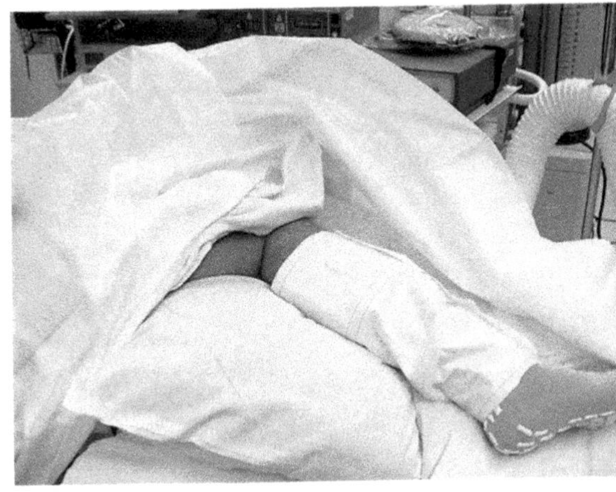

FIGURE 4 Pillows provide adequate padding for peroneal nerve on the bottom leg and take the tension off the hips. Sequential compression devices are placed on both calves.

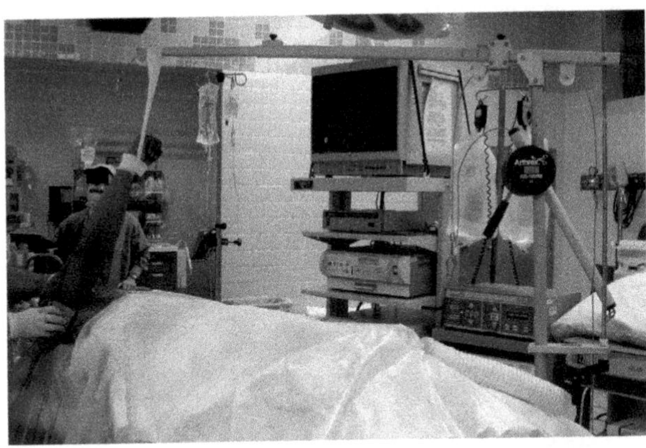

FIGURE 5 The double boom shoulder holder (Arthrex Three-Point Traction Tower) is positioned.

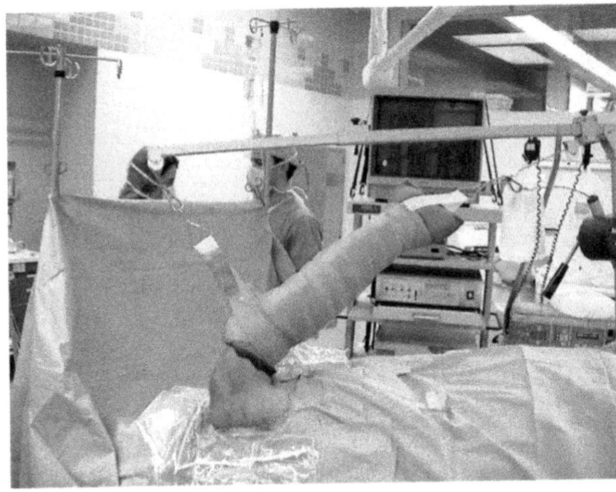

FIGURE 6 Final set up for lateral decubitus position.

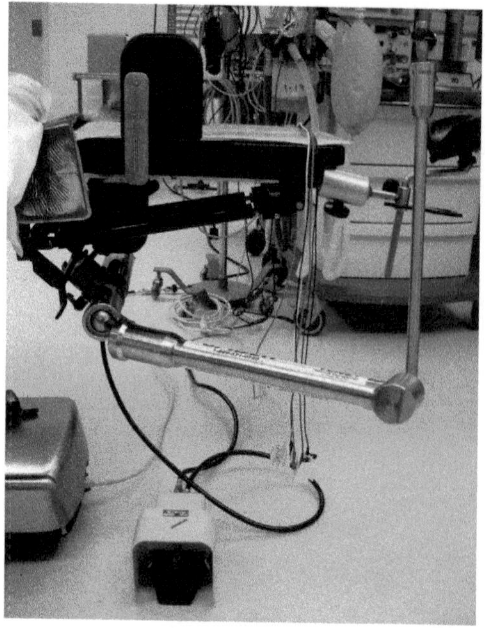

FIGURE 7 The T-max shoulder positioner and spider limb positioner.

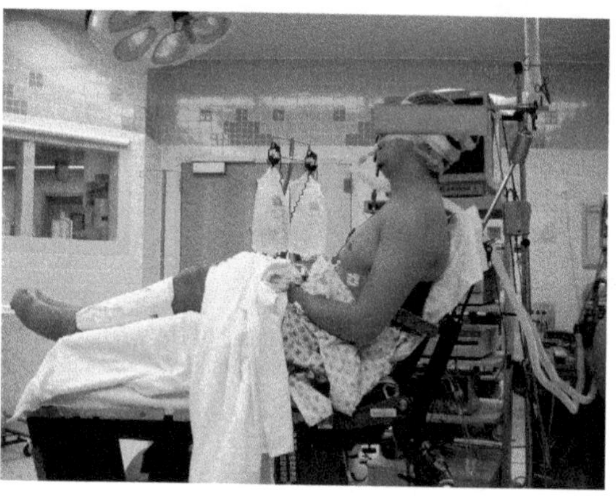

FIGURE 8 The patient is placed at 80° of flexion at the waist level.

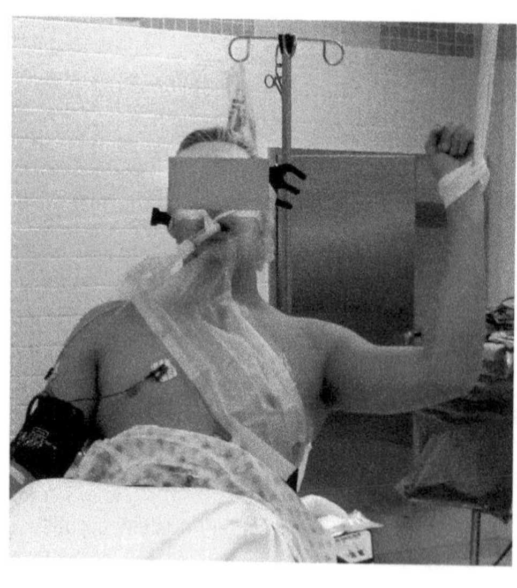

FIGURE 9 Head and neck are placed in neutral position.

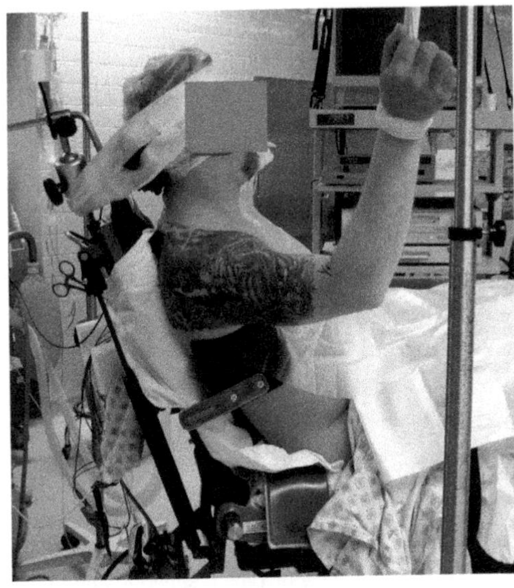

FIGURE 10 Side supports prevent shifting the patient during surgery.

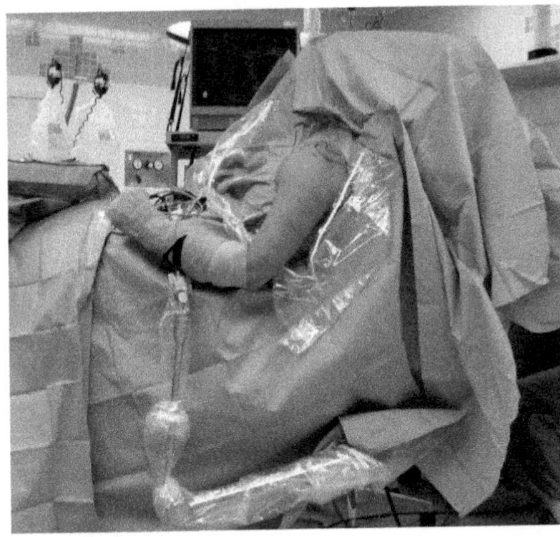

FIGURE 11 Final set up in beach-chair position.

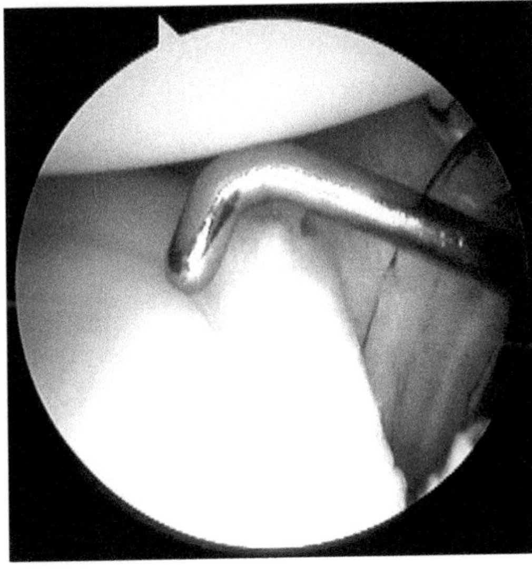

FIGURE 12 View of posterior-inferior labrum in lateral decubitus position.

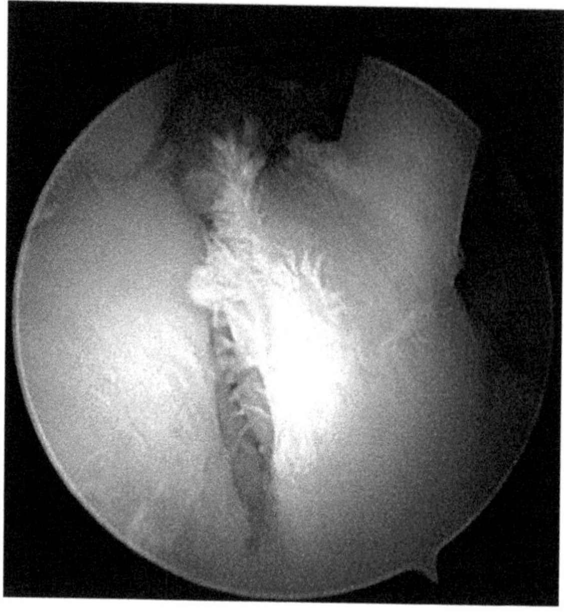

FIGURE 13 View of Type II superior labrum anterior-posterior lesion in the lateral decubitus position.

REFERENCES

1. Weber SC, Abrams JS, Nottage WM. Complications associated with arthroscopic shoulder surgery. Arthroscopy 2002; 18(2 suppl 1):88–95.
2. Bigliani LU, Flatow EL, Deliz ED. Complications of shoulder arthroscopy. Orthop Rev 1991; 20(9):743–751.
3. Skyhar MJ, Altchek DW, Warren RF, Wickiewicz TL, O'Brien SJ. Shoulder arthroscopy with the patient in the beach-chair position. Arthroscopy 1988; 4(4):256–259.
4. Hoenecke HR, Fronek J, Hardwick M. The modified beachchair position for arthroscopic shoulder surgery: the La Jolla beachchair. Arthroscopy 2004; 20(suppl 2):113–115.
5. Jerosch J, Filler TJ, Peuker ET. Which joint position puts the axillary nerve at lowest risk when performing arthroscopic capsular release in patients with adhesive capsulitis of the shoulder? Knee Surg Sports Traumatol Arthrosc 2002; 10(2):126–129.
6. Palermo P, Cattadori G, Bussotti M, Apostolo A, Contini M, Agostoni P. Lateral decubitus position generates discomfort and worsens lung function in chronic heart failure. Chest 2005; 128(3):1511–1516.
7. Rodeo SA, Forster RA, Weiland AJ. Neurological complications due to arthroscopy. J Bone Joint Surg Am 1993; 75(6):917–926.
8. Klein AH, France JC, Mutschler TA, Fu FH. Measurement of brachial plexus strain in arthroscopy of the shoulder. Arthroscopy 1987; 3(1):45–52.
9. Pitman MI, Nainzadeh N, Ergas E, Springer S. The use of somatosensory evoked potentials for detection of neuropraxia during shoulder arthroscopy. Arthroscopy 1988; 4(4):250–255.
10. Shaffer BS, Tibone JE. Arthroscopic shoulder instability surgery. Complications. Clin Sports Med 1999; 18(4):737–767.
11. Berjano P, Gonzalez BG, Olmedo JF, Perez-Espana LA, Munilla M. Complications in arthroscopic shoulder surgery. Arthroscopy 1998; 14(8):785–788.
12. Pavlik A, Ang KC, Bell SN. Contralateral brachial plexus neuropathy after arthroscopic shoulder surgery. Arthroscopy 2002; 18(6):658–659.
13. Gonzalez Della Valle A, Salonia-Ruzo P, Peterson MG, Salvadi EA, Sharrock NE. Inflatable pillows as axillary support devices during surgery performed in the lateral decubitus position under epidural anesthesia. Anesth Analg 2001; 93(5):1338–1343.
14. Baechler MF, Kim DH. Patient positioning for shoulder arthroscopy based on variability in lateral acromion morphology. Arthroscopy 2002; 18(5): 547–549.
15. Mullins RC, Drez D Jr, Cooper J. Hypoglossal nerve palsy after arthroscopy of the shoulder and open operation with the patient in the beach-chair position. A case report. J Bone Joint Surg Am 1992; 74(1):137–139.
16. Cooper DE, Jenkins RS, Bready L, Rock Wood CA Jr. The prevention of injuries of the brachial plexus secondary to malposition of the patient during surgery. Clin Orthop Relat Res 1988; 228:33–41.
17. Bhatti MT, Enneking FK. Visual loss and ophthalmoplegia after shoulder surgery. Anesth Analg 2003; 96(3):899–902, table of contents.

2 Diagnostic Shoulder Arthroscopy

Jason A. Stein and Anand M. Murthi
Department of Orthopedics, The Shoulder and Elbow Service, University of Maryland School of Medicine, Baltimore, Maryland, U.S.A.

INTRODUCTION

Diagnostic shoulder arthroscopy can be a simple and quick procedure. Each surgeon can develop his or her own order and method for performing the procedure, but it is paramount that a fast, efficient, and thorough examination be performed. Because of time limitations, surgeons must be able to quickly and accurately identify reparable pathologic abnormalities to ensure enough time to perform repairs. We find that a circular examination, starting with the articular surfaces and ending with the rotator cuff, is effective. This can be accomplished within minutes. A similar methodical approach is then used in the subacromial space.

ARTICULAR SURFACES

The articular surface of the glenoid and humeral head should be inspected at the beginning of the procedure. The articular surface of the humeral head is smooth and ovoid. The posterior lateral aspect of the humeral head is devoid of cartilage and is referred to as the *bare area*. This will be visualized later in the procedure. The glenoid is shaped like an inverted comma and has a normal indent in its anterior edge. A small circular area with very thin cartilage is present at the center of the glenoid and should not be mistaken for arthritis (Fig. 1).

SUPERIOR LABRUM

The superior labrum has received much attention in recent years. It usually is triangular in shape and blends with the insertion of the long head of the biceps tendon at the supraglenoid tubercle (Fig. 2). Anatomic studies describe two main types of superior labra. Sixty percent of the time, the labrum has a "central detachment": the labrum attaches at the periphery and is free centrally. In this case, normal hyaline cartilage covers the superior edge of the glenoid and it is normal to be able to insert a probe between the two. The labrum may appear mobile, but this is not abnormal. Forty percent of the time, the labrum is attached centrally and is therefore not mobile (1).

The superior labrum can become torn, causing pain and instability. These superior labral anterior to posterior (SLAP) tears occur in many varieties that can be categorized into four main types (some argue seven types) (2). Type I (Fig. 3) is simply fraying of the labrum, with an intact attachment. Type II (Fig. 4) is a detachment of the labrum from the glenoid. Type III is a bucket handle tear. Type IV is a bucket handle tear that extends into the biceps tendon (3).

ANTERIOR STRUCTURES

Simply move the camera up and over the humeral head, and the camera will present a view of the anterior structures (Fig. 5). The anterior superior labrum has a great deal of variation. In approximately 12% of shoulders, the labrum above the glenoid notch is absent. This is referred to as a *sublabral hole* and is a normal variant. In 1.5% of shoulders, the middle glenohumeral ligament (MGHL) is cordlike and inserts directly into the superior labrum. This leaves a hole, referred to as a *Buford complex* (4).

Please refer to pages 17–23 for the figures in this chapter.

The rotator interval is easily visualized. It is composed of the superior glenohumeral ligament (SGHL) (Fig. 6), the coracohumeral ligament (CHL) (Fig. 7), the joint capsule, the biceps tendon, and the superior portion of the MGHL. The SGHL is the primary restraint to inferior translation of the humeral head in adduction and medial translation of the biceps tendon. It originates from the supraglenoid tubercle and inserts just superior to the lesser tuberosity. It can be difficult to visualize and often is obscured by the synovium or the biceps tendon. It is present in approximately 94% to 100% of shoulders and can be visualized with the arm adducted and externally rotated.

The MGHL originates from the glenoid labrum below the SGHL and inserts just medial to the lesser tuberosity. It often crosses and blends into the subscapularis tendon. It is somewhat more variable and is present in only 85% of shoulders. The subscapularis tendon, which is anterior to the MGHL, is easily visualized, with its superior border making up the inferior aspect of the rotator interval. The entire tendon should be inspected, especially for partial superior tears, which often are discovered at its insertion into the lesser tuberosity (Fig. 8) (5).

INFERIOR STRUCTURES

Looking further down the anterior portion of the shoulder, the inferior glenohumeral ligament (IGHL) becomes visible (Fig. 9). This ligament really is a complex, composed of anterior (2 to 4 o'clock position) and posterior (7 to 9 o'clock position) bands, with an axillary pouch interposed. A great deal of variation exists: a distinct ligament is present in 72%, a capsular thickening is present in 21%, and nothing is present in 7% of shoulders. The ligament is best visualized by abducting the arm. The posterior band is more prominent with the arm internally rotated, and the anterior band is most visible with the arm externally rotated. The axillary pouch should be inspected (Fig. 10).

Bankart lesions can be visualized at this time (Fig. 11). They can represent avulsions of the labrum and/or the IGHL from the anterior inferior glenoid and can include a bony defect. The IGHL and/or labrum also can avulse from its glenoid attachment and heal along the medial glenoid neck. This is referred to as an *anterior ligamentous periosteal sleeve avulsion*. The axillary pouch can be lax and compose a larger than normal volume in patients with multidirectional instability, or it can be inflamed in adhesive capsulitis (Fig. 12). Occasionally, the IGHL can avulse from the humerus, and this is referred to as a *humeral avulsion of glenohumeral ligament* lesion. Posteriorly, the same pathologic abnormality can occur and often is referred to as a *posterior Bankart tear* (Fig. 13).

While examining the pouch, attention should be focused on the humeral head. Posteriorly, a "bare area" devoid of cartilage will be observed. This indicates the insertion area of the infraspinatus tendon and should not be mistaken for a Hill-Sachs lesion, which occurs more medially and is surrounded by cartilage.

POSTERIOR STRUCTURES

The posterior labrum can next be quickly inspected by bringing the arthroscope from the inferior pouch posteriorly (from inferior to superior) along the posterior margin of the glenohumeral joint (Fig. 14). The posterior labrum is variable in appearance, and sublabral holes often are present. The posterior labrum can be frayed and mobile.

LONG HEAD OF THE BICEPS

The long head of the biceps should be thoroughly inspected. First, its origin can be variable, as categorized by four different types: Type I (22%), posterior attachment; Type II (33%), small amount of anterior attachment; Type III (37%), equal posterior and anterior attachment; and Type IV (8%), mostly anterior attachment (6). The entire tendon should be examined for fraying and for inflammation. The portion of the tendon that lies inside the bicipital groove can be pulled into the joint and examined for pathologic abnormality (Figs. 15 and 16). Often, fraying (Fig. 17) or inflammation (Fig. 18) of the tendon is observed.

ROTATOR CUFF

Next, the intra-articular portion of the rotator cuff should be examined. This can be facilitated by abducting and externally rotating the arm to view the most anterior portions of the cuff. It often is necessary to lift the rotator cuff with the probe to fully visualize the insertion of the cuff into the greater tuberosity. The rotator cable also can be visualized. It is a thickening of the capsule that extends from the biceps to the insertion of the infraspinatus. This delineates the rotator crescent, the attachment of the infraspinatus and supraspinatus to the greater tuberosity. This is easily delineated because the vasculature of the cuff ends at the cable. The crescent appears avascular (Fig. 19). During this examination, attention must be paid to articular sided partial thickness rotator cuff tears, which may not be easily identified from the subacromial space (Fig. 20).

SUBACROMIAL SPACE

After the intra-articular portion of the diagnostic arthroscopy, attention turns to the subacromial space. The first structure that is apparent is the coracoacromial (CA) ligament (Fig. 21). This can be frayed (Fig. 22) or inflamed. It can be quadrangular (48%), Y-shaped (42%), or composed of a single band (8%) (7). Anteriorly, the ligament is separated from the deltoid, but posteriorly, the ligament can merge with the deltoid fascia. Subacromial impingement is tested by bringing the arm into forward elevation and internal rotation. In this position, the rotator cuff will abut the CA ligament (Fig. 23). After the bursal tissue is cleared, the extra-articular portion of the rotator cuff can be visualized along with its insertion into the greater tuberosity. Full-thickness and bursal sided partial thickness tears can be seen (Fig. 24).

The shape of the undersurface of the acromion is visualized and is categorized into three types: Type I, flat; Type II, curved; and Type III, hooked (8). Spurs can occur and usually are anterolateral, at the CA ligament insertion site (Fig. 25).

SUMMARY

Diagnostic arthroscopy can be a simple, quick, and efficient procedure. If performed systematically and methodically, in conjunction with a physical examination in the office and with the patient under anesthesia, all pertinent shoulder pathologic abnormalities can be identified and appropriately treated.

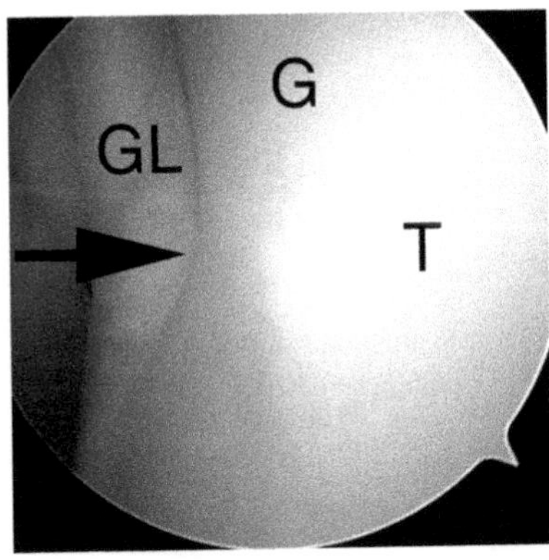

FIGURE 1 The glenoid (*G*) is shaped like an inverted comma. The *arrow* points to the indentation, which represents the fusion of its two ossific nuclei. The articular cartilage in the center of the glenoid (*T*) is very thin and should not be mistaken for arthritis. The glenoid labrum (*GL*) also is seen.

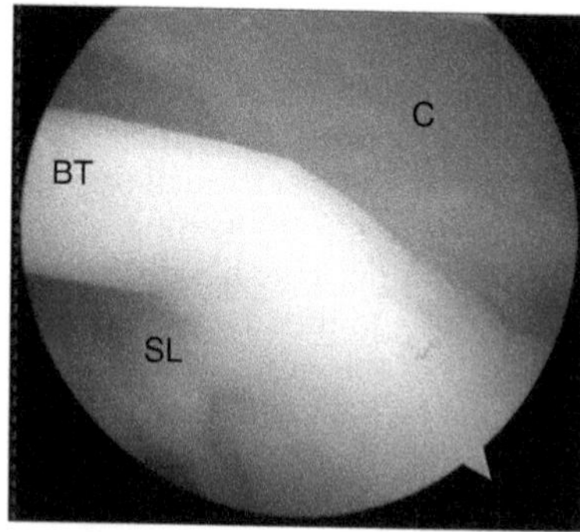

FIGURE 2 The superior labrum (*SL*) is peripherally attached in this patient. It blends with the insertion of the biceps tendon (*BT*). In this view, the capsular extension (*C*) can be seen over the glenoid.

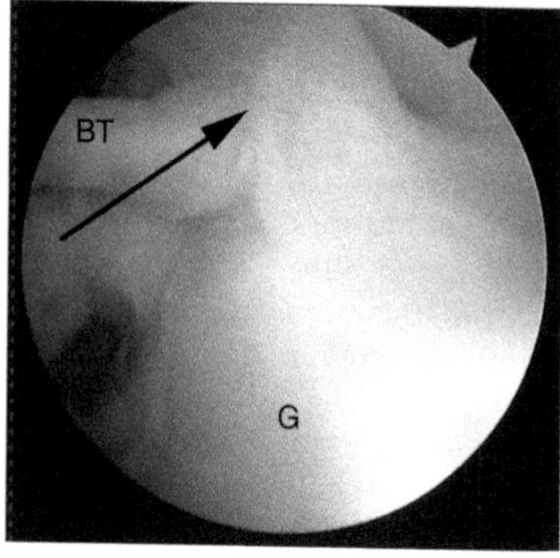

FIGURE 3 The *arrow* points to the superior labrum, which is frayed. This represents a Type I superior labral anterior to posterior lesion. The biceps tendon (*BT*) and glenoid (*G*) also can be seen in this view.

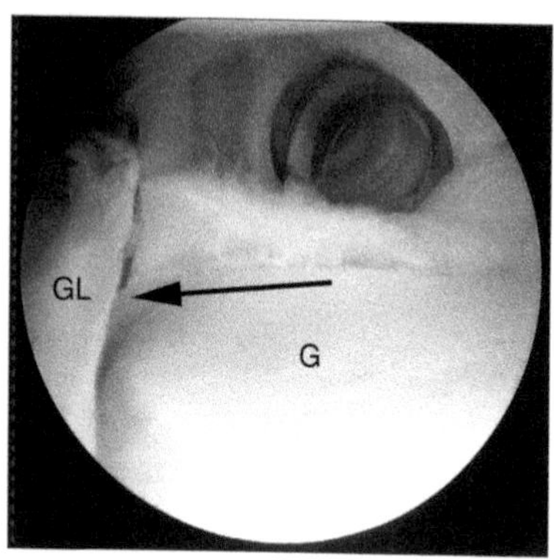

FIGURE 4 The *arrow* points to the area where the superior glenoid labrum (*GL*) has detached from the glenoid (*G*). This is a Type II superior labral anterior to posterior lesion.

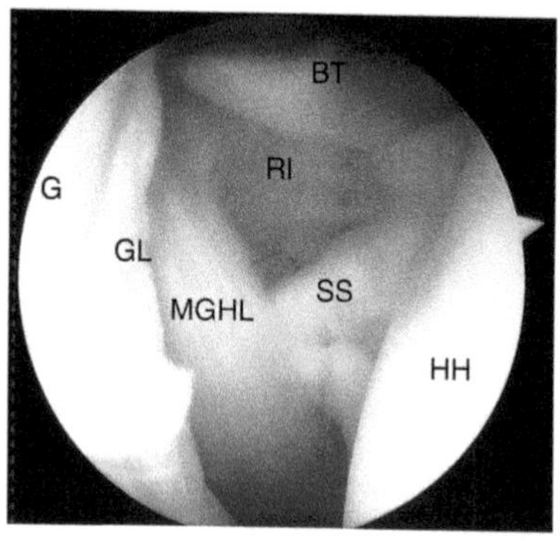

FIGURE 5 Viewed from posterior to anterior, the biceps tendon (*BT*), rotator interval (*RI*), middle glenohumeral ligament, subscapularis tendon (*SS*), and humeral head (*HH*) are clearly visualized. *Abbreviations*: G, glenoid; GL, glenoid labrum; MGHL, middle glenohumeral ligament.

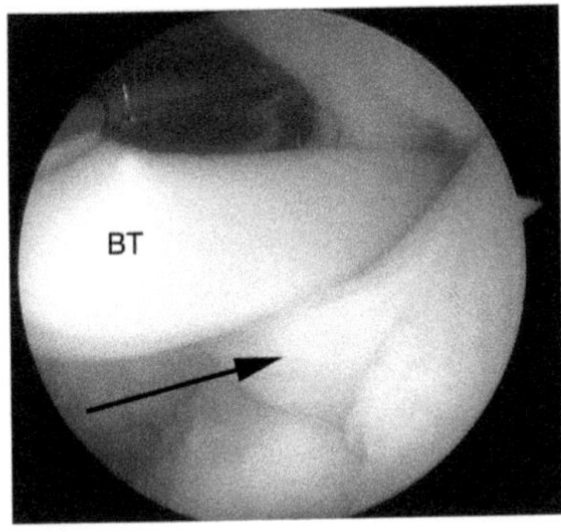

FIGURE 6 The *arrow* points to the superior glenohumeral ligament as it passes around the biceps tendon (*BT*).

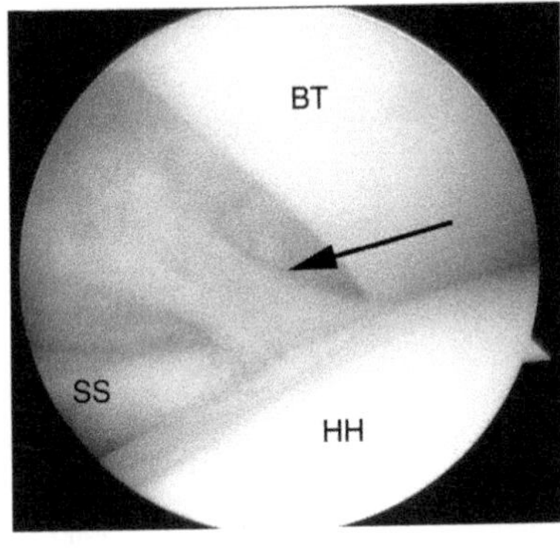

FIGURE 7 The *arrow* points to the deep band of the coracohumeral ligament. *Abbreviations*: BT, biceps tendon; HH, humeral head; SS, subscapularis tendon.

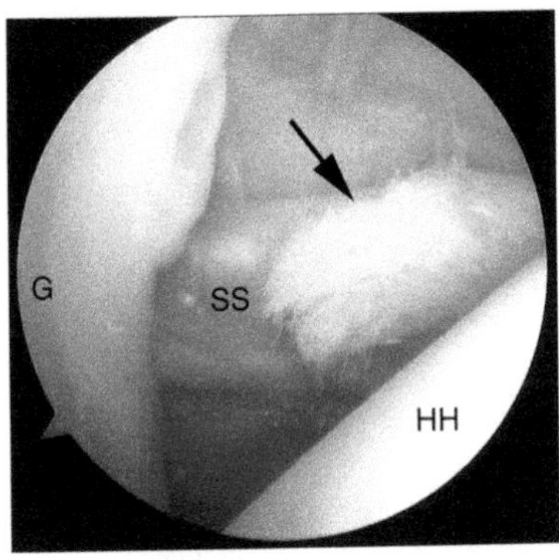

FIGURE 8 The *arrow* points to a partial thickness tear of the subscapularis tendon (*SS*). *Abbreviations*: G, glenoid; HH, humeral head.

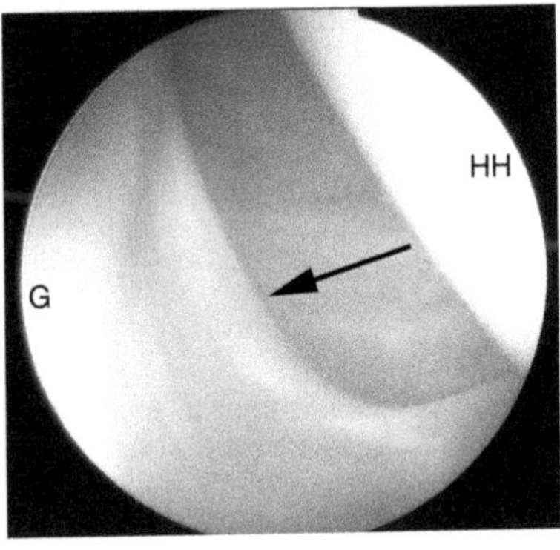

FIGURE 9 The *arrow* points to the inferior glenohumeral ligament. *Abbreviations*: G, glenoid; HH, humeral head.

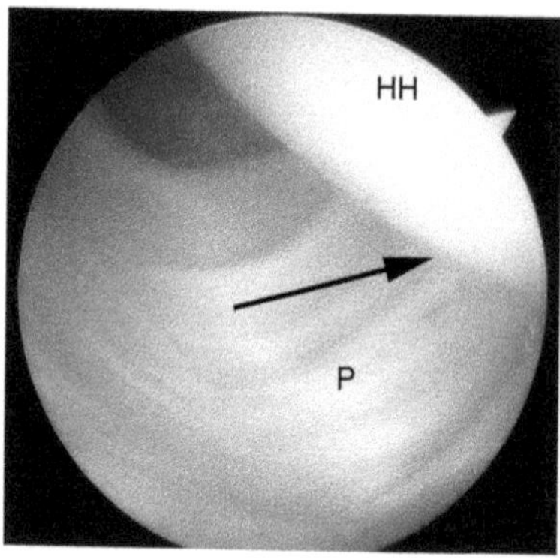

FIGURE 10 The axillary pouch (*P*) is shown. The *arrow* points to the insertion of the inferior glenohumeral ligament into the humeral head (*HH*).

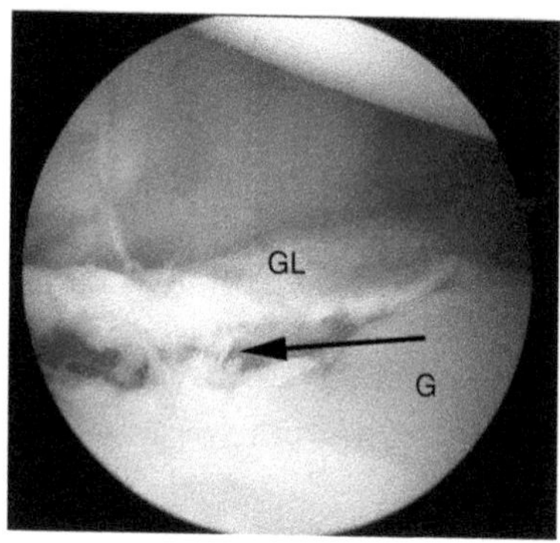

FIGURE 11 The *arrow* points to a Bankart lesion, which is the separation of the anterior inferior glenohumeral ligament and labrum from the glenoid rim. *Abbreviations*: G, glenoid; GL, glenoid labrum.

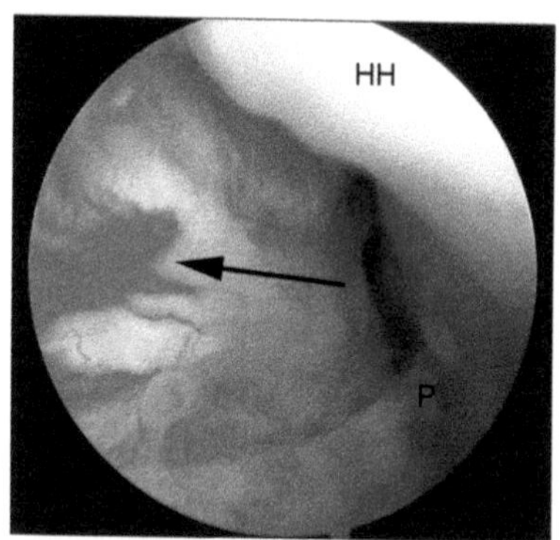

FIGURE 12 Axillary pouch (*P*) with adhesive capsulitis. The *arrow* points to inflamed synovium. *Abbreviation*: HH, humeral head.

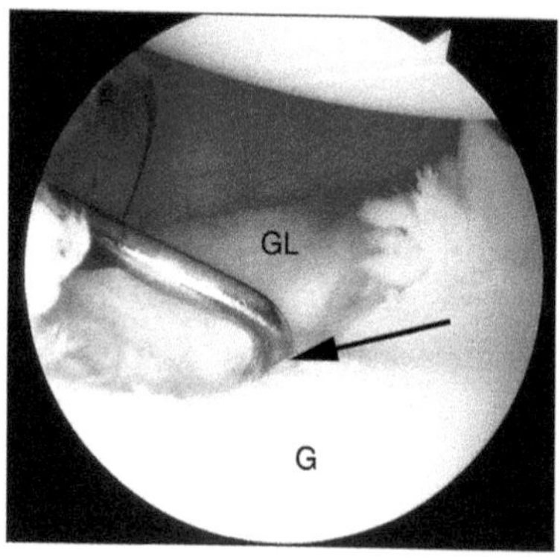

FIGURE 13 Posterior Bankart tear. This view is from anterior to posterior. The *arrow* is pointing to the area where the posterior labrum has torn off of the glenoid rim. *Abbreviations*: G, glenoid; GL, glenoid labrum.

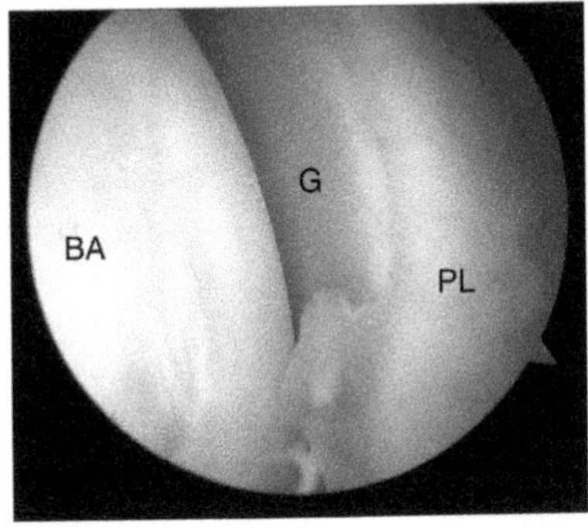

FIGURE 14 A posterior to anterior view shows the posterior labrum (*PL*) and the bare area of the humeral head (*BA*). *Abbreviation*: *G*, glenoid.

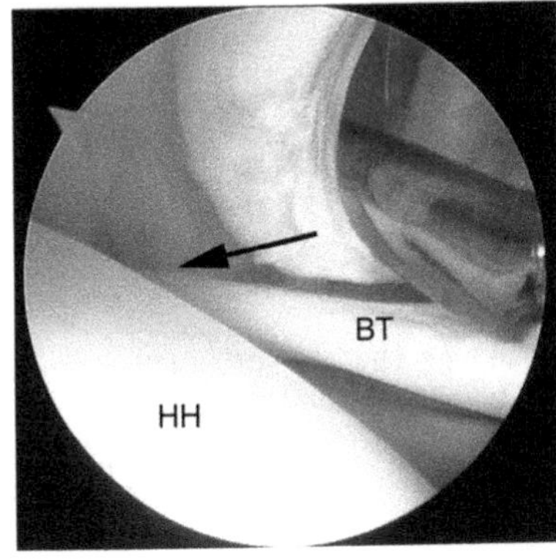

FIGURE 15 The *arrow* points to the extra-articular portion of the biceps tendon (*BT*) "pulled" into the joint. *Abbreviation*: HH, humeral head.

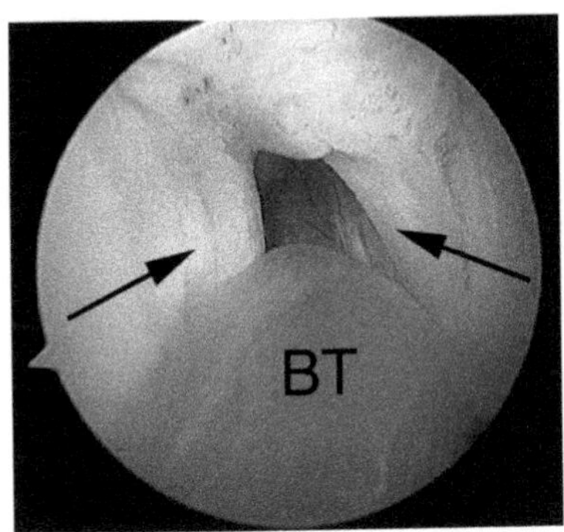

FIGURE 16 The exit of the biceps tendon (*BT*) through the rotator interval is shown. The superior bands of the coracohumeral (*arrows*) ligament are seen flanking the tendon.

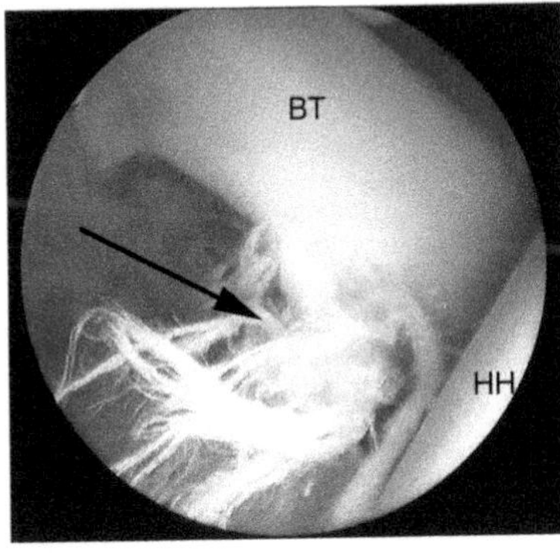

FIGURE 17 The *arrow* points to fraying of the biceps tendon (*BT*). *Abbreviation*: HH, humeral head.

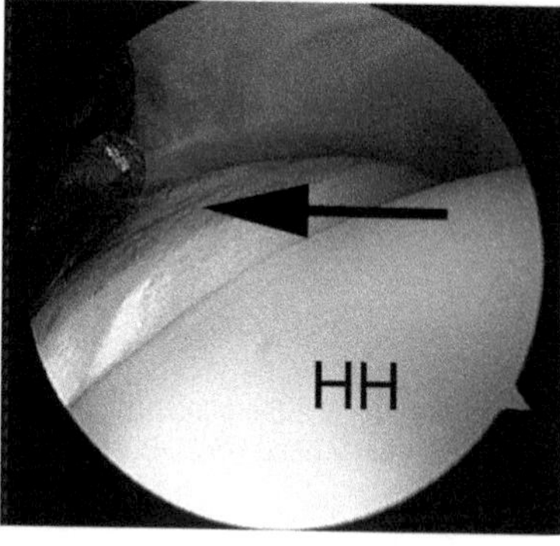

FIGURE 18 The *arrow* points to inflammation of the biceps tendon. *Abbreviation*: HH, humeral head.

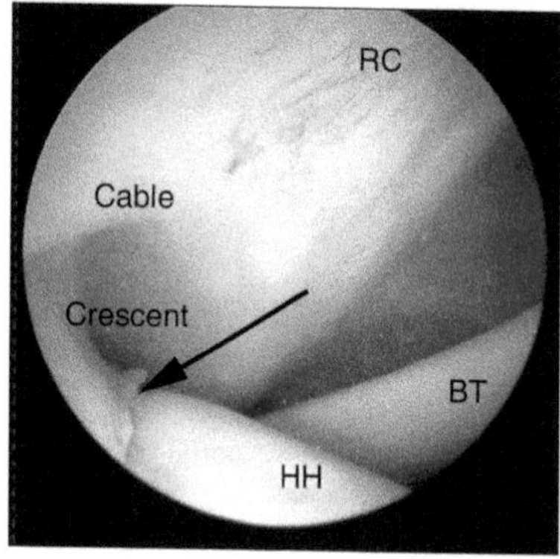

FIGURE 19 The articular side of the rotator cuff (*RC*) insertion is composed of two components. The vascular portions of the supraspinatus and infraspinatus end at the rotator cable and form a band. The cable then inserts into the greater tuberosity (*arrow*) through the rotator crescent. *Abbreviations*: BT, biceps tendon; HH, humeral head.

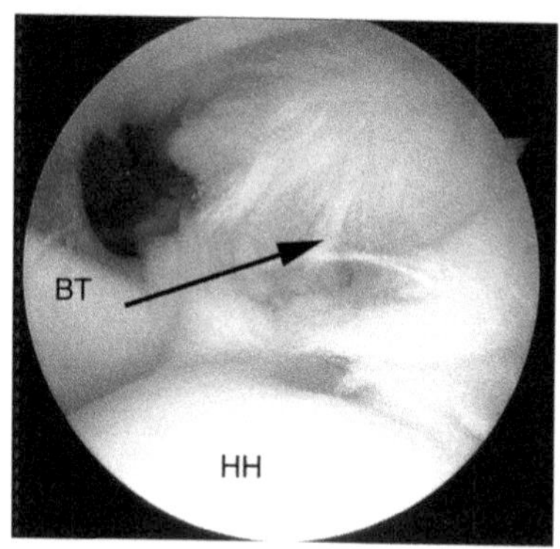

FIGURE 20 The *arrow* points to an articular sided partial thickness tear of the supraspinatus tendon. *Abbreviations*: BT, biceps tendon; HH, humeral head.

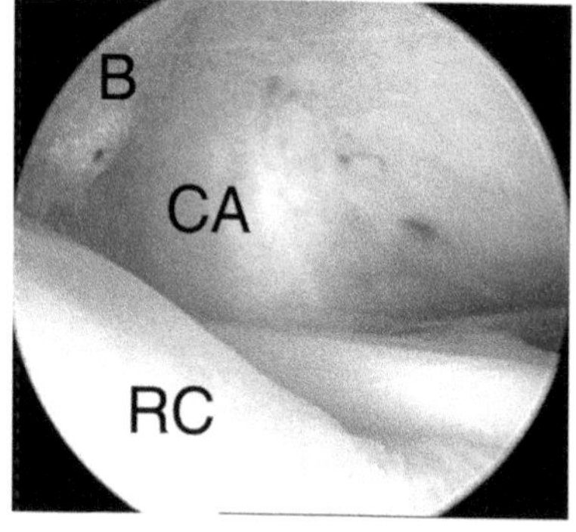

FIGURE 21 The coracoacromial (*CA*) ligament is the most anterior structure seen in the subacromial space. The rotator cuff (*RC*) and bursal tissue (*B*) also are seen in this picture.

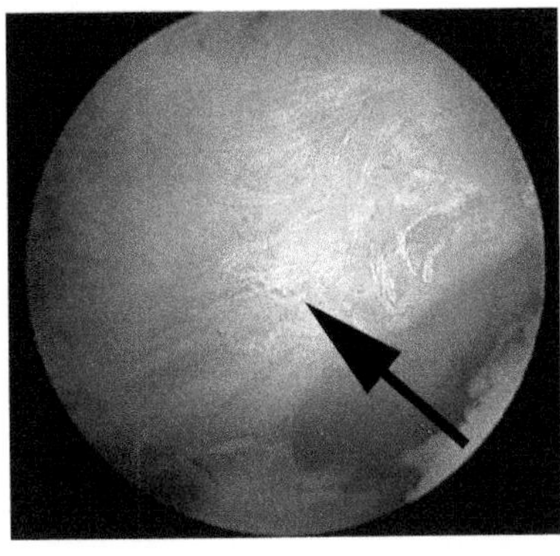

FIGURE 22 The *arrow* points to a thickened and frayed coracoacromial ligament.

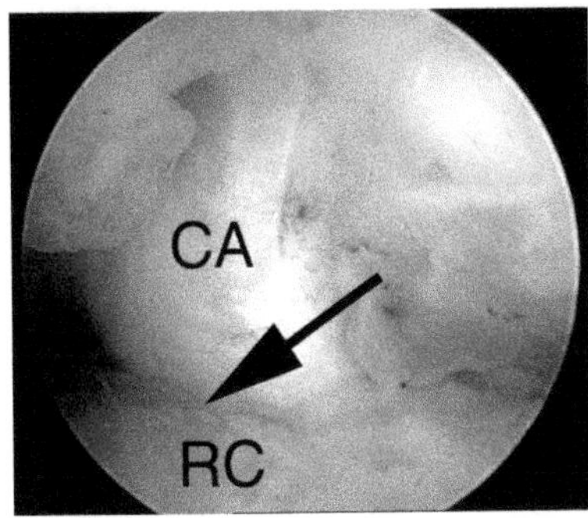

FIGURE 23 Subacromial impingement is tested by ranging the arm to determine whether the rotator cuff (*RC*) impacts the coracoacromial (*CA*) ligament. The *arrow* indicates the point of impact.

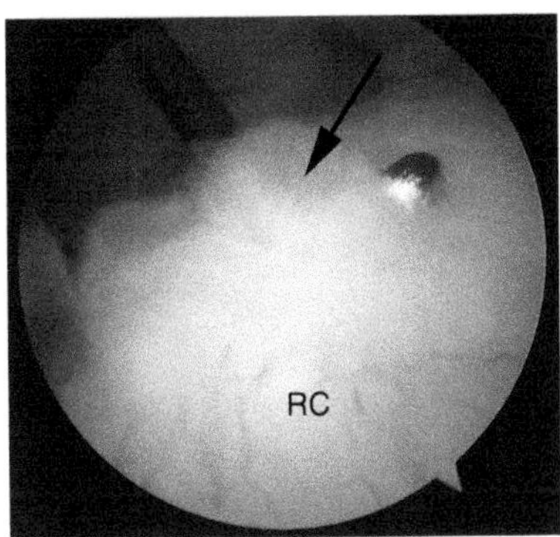

FIGURE 24 The *arrow* and probe indicate a bursal sided partial thickness rotator cuff tear. The remaining rotator cuff (*RC*) appears intact and well vascularized.

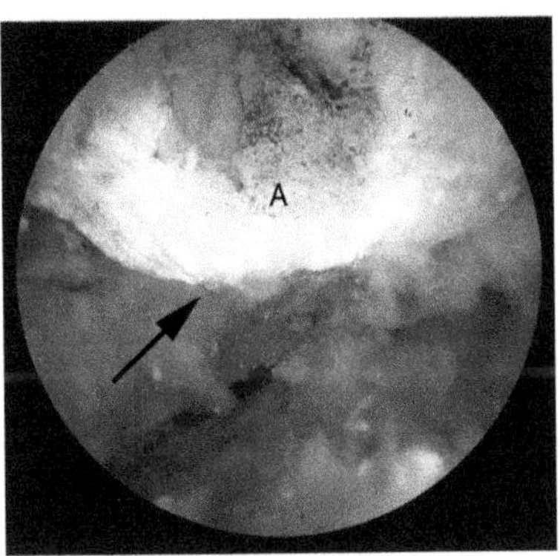

FIGURE 25 The *arrow* points to an acromial spur after the bursa and coracoacromial ligament have been removed during a subacromial decompression. *Abbreviation*: *A*, acromion.

REFERENCES

1. Detrisac DA, Johnson LL. Arthroscopic Shoulder Anatomy: Pathological and Surgical Implications. Thorofare: Slack 1986; 74.
2. Maffet MW, Gartsman GM, Moseley B. Superior labrum-biceps tendon complex lesions of the shoulder. Am J Sports Med 1995; 23(1):93–98.
3. Snyder SJ, Karzel RP, Del Pizzo W, et al. SLAP lesions of the shoulder. Arthroscopy 1990; 6(4):274–279.
4. Williams MM, Snyder SJ, Buford D Jr. The Buford complex: the "cord-like" middle glenohumeral ligament and absent anterosuperior labrum complex: a normal anatomic capsulolabral variant. Arthroscopy 1994; 10(3):241–247.
5. Steinbeck J, Liljenqvist U, Jerosch J. The anatomy of the glenohumeral ligamentous complex and its contribution to anterior shoulder stability. J Shoulder Elbow Surg 1998; 7(2):122–126.
6. Vangsness CT Jr, Jorgenson SS, Watson T, et al. The origin of the long head of the biceps from the scapula and glenoid labrum: an anatomical study of 100 shoulders. J Bone Joint Surg Br 1994; 76(6):951–954.
7. Holt EM, Allibone RO. Anatomic variants of the coracoacromial ligament. J Shoulder Elbow Surg 1995; 4(5):370–375.
8. Bigliani LU, Morrison D, April EW. The morphology of the acromion and its relationship to rotator cuff tears. Orthop Trans 1986; 10(216):228.

3 Knot Tying

Christian Lattermann
Department of Orthopedic Surgery, University of Kentucky, Lexington, Kentucky, and Midwest Orthopaedics at Rush, Rush University Hospital, Chicago, Illinois, U.S.A.

Gregory P. Nicholson
Department of Orthopedic Surgery, Rush University Medical Center, Midwest Orthopaedics at Rush, Rush University Hospital, Chicago, Illinois, U.S.A.

INTRODUCTION

Surgical knot tying has been a basic surgical skill for centuries. Over 1400 different knots have been described, most of which have their roots in fishing and sailing. Orthopedic knot tying used to be less of a technical difficulty then in other general surgery subspecialties; however, with the advent of minimally invasive techniques, arthroscopic surgery of the shoulder in particular, the need for simple but effective knot tying in tight spaces has become a crucial issue for the success of the surgical procedure. Particularly in the shoulder, the difficulty arises from the need to deliver an effective knot through soft tissue tunnels or cannulas over a distance. The knot cannot be tied until delivered through the soft tissues and has to be tied effectively with the use of finger extenders.

Despite the vast array of different knot options, there are only few knots that are suited for the use in arthroscopic surgeries. The knots have to meet two major criteria: (*i*) the knot must be easily tightened and locked once it has been delivered to the target tissue and (*ii*) the knot may not slide once it has been tied.

The major difficulty with arthroscopic knot tying arises out of the need to tie the knot across a distance through a soft tissue envelope. During the process of knot tying, the tension of the knot has to be maintained without incorporating distant tissues into the suture loop.

The purpose of this chapter is to provide the basic background of arthroscopic knot tying with basic steps that may reduce problems encountered during knot tying.

BASIC NOMENCLATURE/DEFINITIONS

Any suture passing through tissue will end up with two separate limbs. One limb will be held tight and serves as the *post* around which the knot will be tied. The other limb stays loose and will be looped around the post creating the knot. This limb is called the nonpost or wrapping suture. The post limb defines where the knot is going to be placed in the tissue since the thrown knot will glide along the postdown towards the tissue. Although the post and the nonpost can be arbitrarily chosen by the surgeon, it is important to consider the placement of the final knot. For labral repairs or superior labral, anterior-posterior (SLAP) repairs, for example, one would not like to have the knot sit directly on the glenoid surface but rather on the labral surface where the knot is less likely to interfere with joint mechanics. It is therefore important to choose the suture limb penetrating the labrum (or farthest from the joint) as the post in order to guide the knot down onto the labral surface away from the glenoid cartilage. In rotator cuff repair fixation, the post is the limb that passes through the tendon.

Furthermore, it is important for knot security to understand the concept of *switching the post*. When switching the post, the surgeon alternates the post for each successive loop. Another important concept is that of *tying alternating over and underhanded knots*. This refers to the

---

Please refer to pages 31–32 for the figures in this chapter.

direction in which the loop passes around the post and refers to the free suture limb passing over or under the post when the knot is thrown.

BASIC KNOTS

Arthroscopic surgeons encounter two basic suture configurations that require fundamentally different knot-tying techniques. The suture from an anchor that has been passed through soft tissue can either be sliding free through the tissue or eyelet of the anchor or it can be tethered at the anchor or within the tissue itself. If the suture is sliding free, the surgeon has the option to either tie a sliding or a nonsliding knot. If the suture is tethered, only a nonsliding knot can be tied. Since any suture can end up being tethered at the anchor eyelet or inside the tissue, the surgeon is well-advised to have at least one sliding and one nonsliding knot in his armament.

Sliding Knots

Sliding knots can only be used with sutures that are free gliding through soft tissues and/or the suture anchor eyelet. Before a sliding knot is utilized, it is imperative that the free passage of both suture limbs is verified.

The basic principle of a sliding knot is that the knot is assembled entirely outside the cannula or joint around the post limb of the suture. The knot typically is dressed and tightened around the post. Once the knot is dressed, it slides down the post limb by pulling on the post limb until the sliding knot sits directly on top of the soft tissue. Sliding knots have a better ability to maintain their tension than nonsliding knots, and are therefore preferentially used in situations where tissue needs to be tied under tension. Multiple different sliding knots have been described, such as the "Duncan loop" (1), the "Tennessee Slider," the "Roeder" (2), the "SMC" (3), the "Weston" (4) knot, and others (5). At this point we will not describe these knots individually. At the end of this chapter we will describe our preferred sliding knot. Any of the aforementioned sliding knots will be appropriate if tied correctly. It is therefore important for the arthroscopic surgeon to be able to tie at least one of these knots well and reproducibly.

Sliding knots can further be subdivided into locking and nonlocking knots. A nonlocking sliding knot can be delivered to the tissue and can be initially tensioned. It will, however, not maintain its initial tension unless it is secured by alternating half hitches that need to be tied subsequently. An example of a nonlocking sliding knot is the "Duncan loop."

Locking sliding knots have the advantage that they can be delivered to the tissue and can be tensioned in situ without having to add additional half hitches for knot security. The sequence to allow for the knot locking involves usually a reversal of the post such that the loop captures the post. Once this maneuver has been performed, the knot cannot be tightened further. Also, the knot will loose some of its initial tension due to the fact that the post/nonpost reversal will allow the knot to fold back onto itself and therefore increase the size of the initial suture loop minimally.

A third group of knots are sliding knots that can only be advanced in one direction along the post. These so called *ratchet knots* have the advantage of a sliding knot that locks once the soft tissue pressure acts against it. These knots, however, still require a set of alternating half hitches for adequate knot security. An example of the ratchet knot is "Nicky's knot" (6) or the "Giant knot" (7).

Nonsliding Knots

If the suture limbs do not readily pass through the tissue or suture anchor, a nonsliding knot has to be used. Nonsliding knots are tied outside the cannula as single over or underhanded loops and then sequentially passed through the cannula to the tissue. The difficulty with these knots is that they have to be tensioned carefully at the tissue and the tension has to be maintained while the next loop is being passed down through the cannula. One example of a nonsliding knot is the simple "square knot." It is the most difficult knot to tie arthroscopically, since it requires equal tension on both limbs to prevent the knot from converting into a stack of half hitches that will not maintain its tension. It is therefore rarely used. Another example of a nonsliding knot is the "Revo knot" (8).

Knot and Loop Security

The two basic principles in knot tying are knot and loop security. Loop security can be defined as the ability of the suture loop holding the tissue to maintain the initial tension and length as the knot is tied and tightened. Loop security is obviously greatest when the knot is initially tightened, and it is important not to loose loop security during the process of completing the knot. Loop security can be influenced by the mechanical property of the suture used and by the initial tension that was applied while tightening the knot.

Knot security can be defined as the ability of the knot to withstand slippage and hold its initial tension. It is important to understand that loop security and knot security play their role together. If the knot is not secure, the loop will not be able to stay secure. If the loop is not tensioned securely initially, the knot will not create soft tissue fixation alone.

Biomechanical experiments on knot security have shown that there is a significant difference between different suture materials in terms of their knot security. Loutzenheiser et al. (9) showed that braided sutures (Ethibond) had 10% to 50% greater holding strengths and 50% less knot slippage than nonbraided (PDS) knots. His groups also showed that complex knots (Duncan loop and Revo knot) were 50% stronger than the overhand throw knot when tied with a braided suture. Burkhart et al. (10) found that nonbraided sutures may provide better knot security when tied on nonalternating posts; however, Loutzenheiser could show clearly that half hitches along alternating posts have a much higher knot security than half hitches along the same post (9). The overall strength that a knot may need to withstand is not known. However, Burkhart could show that cyclic loading of suture repairs leads to failure through the suture-soft tissue junction, and not necessarily through the knot or the loop. The cyclic loading therefore may not have such a great impact on the loop and knot security. It is estimated that that sudden loading through muscular contracture may stress the individual suture up to 60 N (10). According to Loutzenheiser, the alternating posts with a braided suture would technically be able to withstand this force as would the Duncan loop tied with PDS (9). These forces can be lowered by utilizing double-armed anchors and distributing more than one suture per centimeter. In this case, the maximum load can be reduced to approximately 37 N (10). All tested knot configurations were able to withstand this load without knot slippage or loss of loop security.

SUTURE MANAGEMENT

Suture Material

A vast variety of suture material is available to the orthopedic surgeon. Principally, suture material can be divided according to its absorbability, whether they are braided or monofilament and if they are reinforced through ultrabraiding (MaxBraid, Arthrotek, Warsaw, Indiana, U.S.A.) or additional core material such as kevlar (Fiberwire, Arthrex, Naples, Florida, U.S.A.).

Most arthroscopic surgeons prefer nonresorbable sutures for their repairs since absorbable sutures, either braided (i.e., Panacryl, Ethicon, Somerville, New Jersey, U.S.A.) or monofilament [Polydioxanone (PDS)], have a lower tensile strength and are designed to loose strength over time. While this is a desired property for soft tissue repairs near the skin or in muscle, it may not be desirable for tendon or cartilage to bone repairs.

Nonabsorbable sutures have been popular among arthroscopic surgeons for their high initial tensile strength. The most popular suture material has traditionally been braided polyester. The use of #2 polyester sutures (i.e., Ethibond, Ethicon, Somerville, New Jersey, U.S.A.) used to be the standard suture used for rotator cuff repairs and labral refixation. Recently, reinforced braided polyester sutures have been introduced that provide significantly higher tensile strengths and are close to "unbreakable" during the knot-tying process. These suture materials are reinforced by an ultrabraiding process (MaxBraid, Arthrotek) or by coweaving of metallic filaments such as kevlar (Fiberwire, Arthrex, Naples, Florida, U.S.A.).

Suture material has its main impact during the process of knot tying. This is where its handling characteristics can play a crucial role. While monofilament sutures are stiffer, more ductile, and tend to slide better, they also have a memory and recoil making maintenance of knot security difficult. Braided suture material generally is less stiff, leads to more friction during the knot-tying process and is more pliable, making maintenance of knot security easier, although it may be slightly more difficult to slide the knot into place.

The newer "unbreakable" sutures are not all the same. MaxBraid is a braided polyethylene suture with a hollow core. It has enhanced lubiricity, meaning it slides very well while tying knots. Because the core is hollow, as the knot is tied, the suture material deforms. This enhances knot security and prevents loss of loop security. The number of throws needed to create a "locked" secure knot is not increased. This is different and better than the characteristics of the most popular Kevlar core "unbreakable" suture, which does not deform, has high lubricity, but requires potentially more half hitches to prevent slippage and create the necessary knot security.

The ultimate tensile strength of braided polyester sutures exceeds the required force that has been calculated to act on a single suture in a rotator cuff repair (10). Hence, many surgeons continue to use just simple braided polyester sutures for their repairs because they feel that the suture has slightly less friction than the new reinforced polyester sutures and therefore may be easier to tie. Others prefer the security that the reinforced polyester sutures provide during the knot-tying process and will accept the slightly higher friction. Ultimately, it depends on the individual surgeons' preference which suture material is used. As a general rule, one should know the advantages and disadvantages of the suture material used, in order to anticipate problems during the knot-tying process.

Suture anchor eyelet design also affects knot tying. Early metallic anchors had edges on the eyelets that could fatigue and wear suture material. This led to suture breakage during the knot-tying process. Repetitive cycling the suture material through the eyelet was shown to weaken the suture material. This led to redesign of eyelets with smoother edges. The nonmetallic anchors (plastic and bio-absorbable) evolved with more suture friendly eyelets. Suture eyelet orientation is important to consider, depending upon what type of repair, and what type to stitch configuration is being used. In general, the surgeon should try to align the eyelet so that it is facing the direction the suture is traveling to and through the tissue and will be tied. This will prevent kinking at the anchor eyelet, allow suture sliding, and allow the loop to be tightened efficiently.

Arthroscopic Cannulas

As a general rule, cannula placement is the single most critical aspect of knot tying and anchor placement in shoulder surgery. It is not the goal of this chapter to explain the different concepts of cannula placement for the different procedures since this will be done in great detail in the Chapters 8, 9, 11, 20, 22, and 23. However, there are some general aspects about arthroscopic cannulas that would be addressed at this stage. The arthroscopic cannula is designed to help with the knot delivery, increase knot-tying visualization, and help avoid tanglement of sutures during the knot-tying process. Arthroscopic cannulas can generally be divided into clear and not clear cannulas. Not clear cannulas are usually of smaller diameter (5–6 mm) and are designed to be primarily outflow cannulas for fluid management, they usually accommodate a small shaver blade or an arthroscopic probe, they are not designed to accommodate larger instruments or knot tying. Larger cannulas (6–8.25 mm) that are designed for larger instruments and knot tying are usually clear cannulas. These cannulas improve visualization of the suture material inside as well as outside the joint. This helps to avoid tangles. Many larger cannulas have threads that prevent dislodgement during knot tying or anchor placement process. In order for cannulas to help during the knot-tying process, they have to be delivered in a straight line to the area of interest. This can be challenging in muscular or large individuals, and extra long arthroscopic cannulas should be available.

Use of a Knot Pusher

Once the knot has been tied, it has to be advanced into the joint. This generally requires a knot pusher. If a sliding knot is utilized, the knot pusher is placed on the post limb of the suture in order to gently push the assembled sliding knot down the post to its destination. This does generally not require much pressure since the sliding knot is simultaneously pulled down the post. Once the knot is delivered to the tissue, the knot pusher should be used to tightly position the knot on the tissue with gentle pressure. This process ensures initial knot and loop security.

The knot pusher is used differently when half hitches are tied. During the process of tying half hitches, the surgeon alternates over and underhanded half hitches and also switches posts in order to provide excellent knot security. Since the half hitch is a loose loop tied around the post, several problems can arise during the process of pushing the half hitch along the post. The pusher can easily be pushed passed the knot and simply not deliver the knot down the post at all. If an overhand loop is thrown around the post and knot pusher is advanced along the post it will lead to a "jerky" advancement and requires alternating tension on the post and nonpost that can lead to fraying of the suture and eventual breakage. Chan and Burkhart advised the arthroscopic surgeon to utilize the knot pusher to "pull" an overhand loop of the nonpost limb down the post limb. This is done by having the knot pusher on the nonpost limb and leading the half hitch down the post limb. Thus, the knot pusher "pulls" the half hitch behind it into the joint and then tightens the throw with the "past pointing" position. This will lead to a smooth delivery of the half hitch, avoiding suture fraying. Once the knot has been delivered to the tissue, it can either be past-pointed to 180° or the tension can be switched from the post to the nonpost flipping the knot and thus allow for tying of half hitches around alternating posts without the need to move the knot pusher to the nonpost limb (11).

There are different types of knot pushers available. Single-looped knot pushers can be either straight barreled with a small oblique opening at the tip through which the suture is passed or they can be shaped like a small shoe with a ring at the end through which the suture is passed. Any of the single-hole knot pushers can be utilized to tie any sliding or nonsliding knot proficiently. A thumb hole is an accepted feature that all knot pushers incorporate. Double diameter knot pushers have been introduced in order to help with the initial loop security while the knot is being finished. The inner diameter knot pusher will hold the knot in place while the securing half hitch is advanced by the outer diameter pusher. This is an excellent tool to improve initial loop security.

OUR TECHNIQUE

At a minimum, at least one sliding and one nonsliding knot or knot arrangement should be mastered by the arthroscopist. In the following, the preferred sliding knot as well as preferred nonsliding knot are described, followed by some tips and tricks that may be helpful.

Our Preferred Sliding Knot

In the author's practice, "Nicky's knot" is utilized (taut line hitch) (6). This is a sliding "ratchet" knot that has an excellent initial locking ability while being a nonlocked sliding knot. After the suture is passed through the tissue, both suture limbs are brought out the same cannula. The post limb is confirmed and a suture manipulator/grasper is run down the limb to confirm that there are no tangles. Then the ability of the suture to slide through the tissue and the anchor is confirmed. The post limb is shortened. A right-handed tie starts with an overhand half hitch around the post, but the hitch is not tightened around the post, preserving the hitch loop. Then the free suture is passed overhand again around the post, but through the same half hitch loop formed by the first throw. A third overhand half hitch is now thrown, but through its own hitch loop and behind the previous two throws on the post (Figs. 1A–C, Figs. 2–3). The knot is lightly dressed. The knot pusher is placed on the post limb. The knot is easily advanced in only one direction by pulling on the post. The post limb is pulled, "pulling" the knot into the joint with the knot pusher "chasing" the knot but not pushing it. Once the knot is down onto the tissue, the knot pusher pushes the knot down while still pulling on the post limb. Once the Nicky knot is set, it will stay, but loop security can be enhanced by now tensioning the loop limb to "lock" the knot. This then allows the surgeon to secure the knot completely with three individual half hitches. Then the knot is secured with three alternating half hitches, also alternating the post. It is a fast, easy knot to tie. It has excellent loop and knot security characteristic and can be used in almost every repair application in shoulder surgery where a sliding knot is appropriate (Figs. 4 and 5).

Our Preferred Nonsliding Knot

Five alternating half hitches switching the post twice are utilized. This knot is also called the "Revo knot" (8). The initial two half hitches are tied over handed down the same post. Even though it is a nonsliding knot, there is usually the ability to tension and tighten the knot by pulling on the nonpost limb, as the throws are brought down and past pointing is done to tighten them. The third half hitch is an underhand throw down the same post. The fourth hitch is again an overhand hitch down the same post. Then the post is switched and alternated with the finishing two half hitches. Thus, the first four throws are down the same post and can be thought of as: hitch A, A, B, A. This nonsliding knot can be tensioned easily due to the initial two half hitches that are thrown in the same direction. Loop security can be maintained easily.

TIPS/TRICKS

Finally, a couple of little details that can help tremendously during the knot-tying process are pointed out. By far the most frustrating and frequent problem during the process of knot tying is tanglement of sutures. In order to avoid tanglement, one should try to place the cannula directly over the area that is going to be tied. The cannula should not come out of the joint during this process since it may re-enter through a different pass and the suture may be caught in soft tissues that will be incorporated into the knot before it has reached its destination. In addition, it is advisable to only store the suture limbs of the suture being tied in the working cannula. All other sutures should be stored in a different portal. Suture should ideally pass straight through the tissue that is going to be tied together. When using anchors, the eyelet should be facing the direction of suture travel to and through the tissue. This helps prevent that the suture does not get kinked in the eyelet. This may create false loop security (the loop is not actually as tight as it looks). Suture abrasion at the eyelet is minimized with proper eyelet orientation. Finally, one should always run a knot pusher down the individual suture limbs in order to assure that there is no tangle inside the cannula. Free passage of the knot pusher down the post limb will assure this. Follow the knot with eyes (and the arthroscope). If the knot is tied and it appears to be tangled, it is important not to tighten the knot down, since at this stage it may still be reversed or untangled using a hooked probe. If a knot is tied down and appears loose, one may try to untangle the knot with a hooked probe. If all fails, it is better to remove the suture and start over.

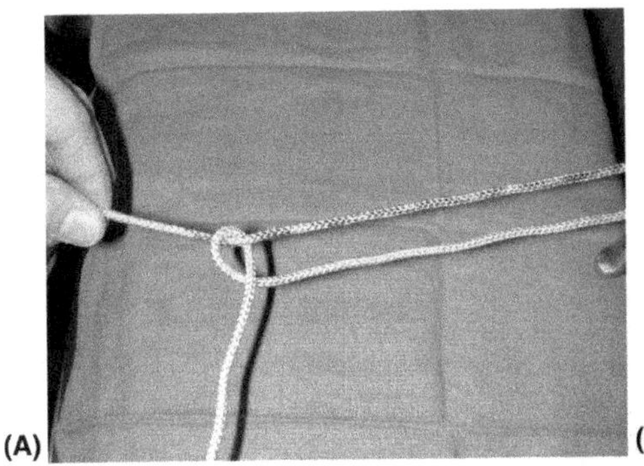

(A)

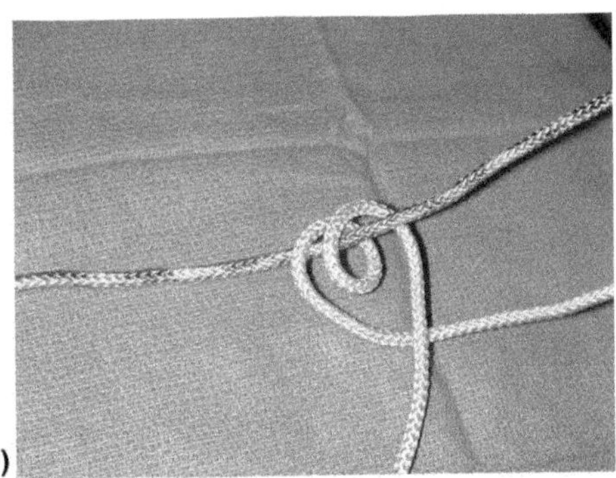

(B)

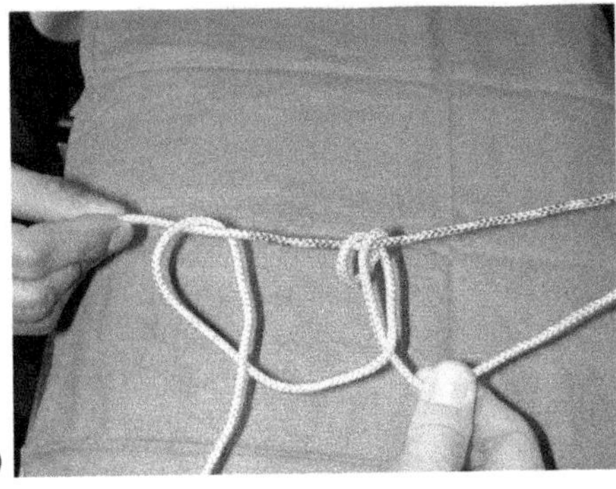

(C)

FIGURE 1 (**A**) Nicky knot 1st overhand throw: To tie Nicky's knot (taut-lint hitch), a sliding locking knot, the post limb is shortened (stippled limb). The loop limb (plain limb) is past in an overhand hitch. (**B**) Nicky knot 2nd overhand throw: The loop limb is passed again in an overhand throw around the post limb, but passed through the same suture loop formed by the first throw. (**C**) Nicky knot 3rd overhand behind in separate loop: The loop limb is now passed as a third overhand throw around the post, but through a separate suture loop behind the first two throws.

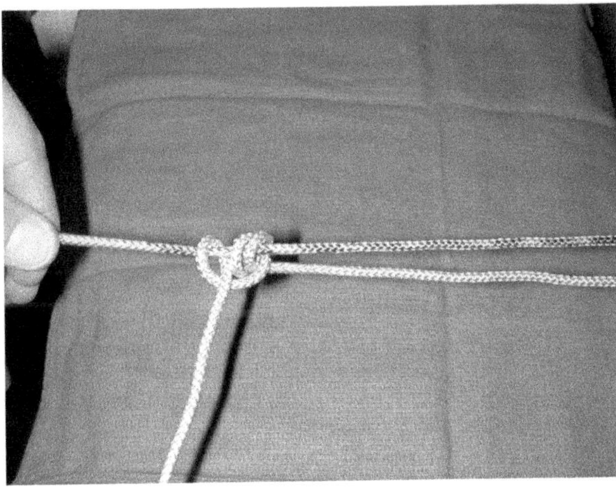

FIGURE 2 Nicky dressed ready to slide: The knot is *lightly* dressed and the loop limb left free. The knot will pulled into the joint by pulling on the post limb. A knot pusher is placed on the post limb and "chases" the knot into the joint.

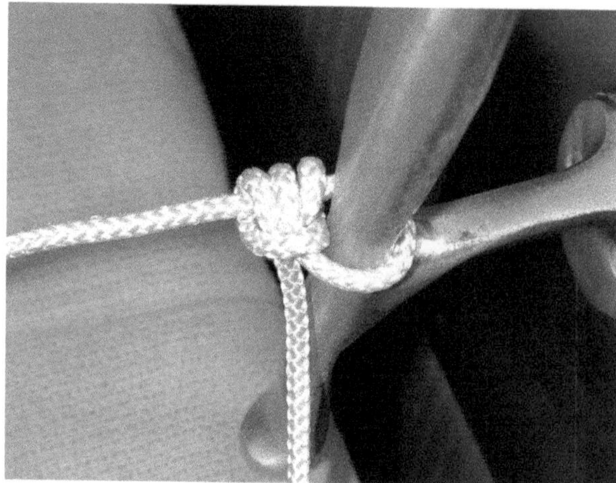

FIGURE 3 Nicky tight closure: When the Nicky knot is pulled into the joint, it will tighten around the soft tissue with excellent loop security. The ratchet character of the knot will not allow it to slide backwards.

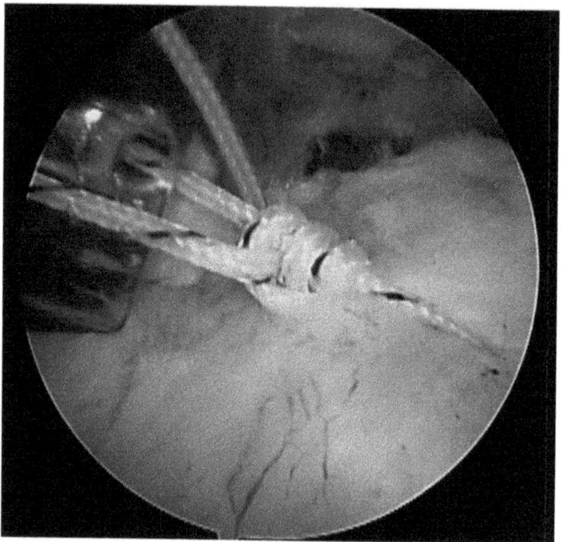

FIGURE 4 Nicky knot L RCR onto cuff: A sliding, locking knot almost down to the rotator cuff in a left shoulder. Note the knot pusher just behind the knot. When the knot gets down onto the cuff, the knot pusher will push the knot down, the post limb will be pulled and the loop limb can be tensioned to "lock" the knot even more securely.

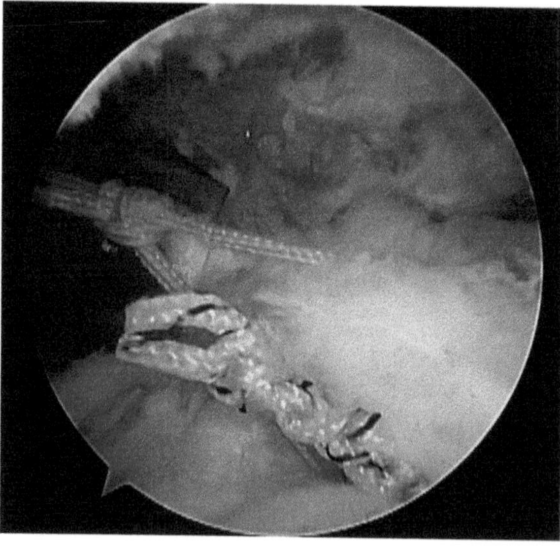

FIGURE 5 Nicky knot coming down cannula: A second Nicky knot is seen being pulled down the clear cannula in this left arthroscopic rotator cuff repair. Note the knot configuration and that it "travels" down the post limb onto the soft tissues. The knot is secured with three alternating half hitches with alternating posts.

REFERENCES

1. Wolf EM. Arthroscopic capsulolabral repair using suture anchors. Orthop Clin North Am 1993; 24(1):59–69.
2. Mishra DK, Cannon WD Jr, Lukas DJ, et al. Elongation of arthroscopically tied knots. Am J Sports Med 1997; 25:113–117.
3. Sharp HT, Dorsey JH, Choven JD, et al. A simple modification to add strength to the Roeder knot. J Am Assoc Gynecol Laparosc 1996; 3:305–307.
4. Kim SH, Ha KI. The SMC knot—a new slip knot with locking mechanism. Arthroscopy 2000; 16: 563–565.
5. Weston PV. A new clinch knot. Obstet Gynecol 1991; 78:144–147.
6. DeBeer JF, VanRooyen K, Boezaart AP. Nicky's knot—a new slip knot for arthroscopic surgery. Arthroscopy 1998; 14:109–110.
7. Fleega BA, Sokkar SH. The giant knot: a new one way self locking secured arthroscopic slip knot. Arthrsocopy 1999; 15:451–452.
8. Snyder SJ. Technique of arthroscopic rotator cuff repair using implantable 4-mm revo suture anchors, suture shuttle relays and no.2 non-absorbable mattress sutures. Orthop Clin North Am 1997; 28:267–275.
9. Loutzenheiser TD, Harryman DT II, Ziegler DW, et al. Optimizing arthroscopic knots using braided or monofilament suture. Arthroscopy 1998; 14:57–65.
10. Burkhart SS, Wirth MA, Simonick M, et al. Loop security as a determinant of tissue fixation security. Arthroscopy 1998; 14:773–776.
11. Chan KC, Burkhart SS. How to switch posts without rethreading when tying half hitches. Arthroscopy 1999; 15:444–450.

4 Suture Anchor Update

F. Alan Barber and Michael H. Boothby
Plano Orthopedic and Sports Medicine Center, Plano, Texas, U.S.A.

INTRODUCTION

With the increasing popularity of arthroscopic and minimally invasive surgery throughout medicine, the need for appropriate surgical implants that complement new surgical techniques has become obvious. The earliest arthroscopic interventions were confined to the observation and debridement of pathologic lesions. Later, arthroscopic surgeons developed techniques that included both repair and fixation of tissue rather than simply removal. Broadening the surgical options in arthroscopy required the development of devices aimed to accomplish this soft tissue fixation. These efforts to expand the proven surgical options lead to the development of a wide range of devices known as suture anchors.

Arthroscopic implants are made from a variety of metal and biodegradable materials. These implants include suture anchors, meniscal repair devices, soft tissue (tendon and ligament) fixation devices, as well as, adjuncts for articular cartilage repair (1). As minimally invasive surgeries have become more prevalent, the new implants have been applied to many different joints and in a variety of different specialties (2–5). Although in arthroscopic surgery, suture anchors are most commonly used in the shoulder, these anchors also find applications elsewhere in the body (knee, wrist, foot, and ankle), as well as in open orthopedic procedures (6–8).

The number and variety of suture anchors available on the market today is remarkable. The impetus to develop more stable, less invasive devices has generated the creation of a broad range of implants. Issues such as anchor size, number used, shape, composition, and insertion techniques are some of the factors surrounding a surgeon's selection of a particular suture anchor. Recently, biodegradable suture anchors have become more popular than metal anchors. This requires the surgeon to fully understand the characteristics of these biodegradable materials and their strength loss, suture interface characteristics, and degradation profiles. The goal of this chapter is to describe the current types, characteristics, improvements, benefits, and uses of suture anchors.

SUTURE ANCHOR HISTORY

Historically the attachment of bone to a soft tissue such as ligament and tendon was accomplished by creating bone tunnels and passing suture through the bone. The bone tunnels were created by awls or drills and suture was passed through the tunnels and tied over a bone bridge, which attached the soft tissue to bone. Although quite successful, this technique was not amenable to minimally invasive, arthroscopic procedures. With momentum growing to perform increasingly less invasive surgery, Mitek provided the first generation suture anchor, which was called the G1 anchor (9). This anchor looked similar to a fishhook, and allowed the arthroscopic surgeon to attach a suture to the bone without the use of a bone tunnel (Fig. 1).

The Statak anchor was developed about the same time as the Mitek G1 and was a "screw-in" design. The original Statak anchor, designed by Marlowe Goble, had a suture securely fixed in the center of a screw anchor (Fig. 2). Many other anchoring devices have followed the development of these first anchors, and today there are dozens of different screw and nonscrew designs. The common thread, however, is that while designs differ and the insertion techniques vary, they all are designed to accomplish the same task: attaching a suture to the bone.

Please refer to pages 44–48 for the figures in this chapter.

SUTURE ANCHOR BIOLOGY AND BIOMECHANICS

The biology and biomechanics of suture anchors are important to understand because one type of anchor may be more appropriate than another for a particular application. The biology of soft tissue healing is well established and undergoes three phases: inflammation, repair, and remodeling (10). Gaps between bone and soft tissue are initially filled by inflammatory cells, gradually organized, and are invaded by a vascular supply that removes debris and aids collagen forming cells in closing the gap. This process occurs over a period of weeks and is necessary to understand since it determines how quickly a surgical repair can tolerate stress (10). If the fixation of soft tissue to bone is inadequate, the tissue will gap, healing will not occur, and the repair will fail. For successful results a surgeon must make decisions that correctly match the biomechanics and material properties of a suture anchor with its intended task such that it holds the tissue securely in place while soft tissue healing occurs.

The choice between metal or biodegradable suture anchors illustrates the need for surgeons to understand some of the biomechanical properties of various implants (11). Biodegradable suture anchors that contain a higher percentage of polyglycolic acid (PGA) are hydrolyzed and dissolve more rapidly when inserted into bone than anchors made of various stereoisomers of poly-lactic acid (PLA), which dissolve more slowly (10). The rate of degradation of an implant is important because it directly correlates to implant strength over time and may affect the overall success of a repair. For many of the biodegradable devices on the market today, the exact rate of degradation and length of time for complete absorption have not been clinically determined. More investigation in this area may help to clarify an optimum time to degradation for bioabsorbable anchors.

In general, when discussing the biomechanics of suture anchors one must consider the interfaces of the implant with the soft tissue, the implant with the suture, and the implant with the bone (10). Only when all these factors are considered can one appreciate the true complexity of suture anchor design and use.

SUTURE ANCHOR CRITERIA

The evaluation of a suture anchor must consider several components. The fundamental characteristics of a good anchor are that it must (*i*) fix the suture to the bone, (*ii*) not pull out of the bone, (*iii*) permit an easy surgical technique including the ability for arthroscopic knot tying, and (*iv*) to prevent the cause of long-term morbidity. Other desirable features include biocompatibility, adequate strength, easy insertion, and the ability to allow early rehabilitation. While suture anchors have many advantages over conventional bone tunnels, they do require special instrumentation that is specific for each anchor. Other disadvantages of anchors include cost, the learning curve for their use, and placement of a retained foreign material. For convenience, useful lists of specifications for common nonabsorbable and absorbable anchor implants are presented in Table 1 and Table 2.

A thorough evaluation of suture anchors must consider such issues as anchor size, the number and size of suture an anchor can accommodate, the suture type, the anchor material, the anchor type, the anchor insertion technique, and modes of anchor failure.

Anchor Size

Suture anchors currently come in a wide assortment of sizes. Size can be considered both in terms of major diameter (the outside measurement of the anchor) and minor diameter (size of the anchor core). Anchors range from small to large with differences in the size of suture they accommodate and load to failure strength. In selecting the appropriate anchor size, it is important to consider the application. Small anchors are appropriate in many hand surgery cases while larger anchors may be more appropriate in the shoulder or in areas of poor bone quality. Rotator cuff repairs are probably the most common shoulder application for suture anchors. Because of the osteoporotic nature of the humeral head, screw anchors with deep threads function better for this application than smaller anchors with less ability to grip porotic bone. Since multiple sutures are currently being used for cuff repairs and considering

TABLE 1 Common Nonbiodegradable Suture Anchors

Company	Anchor	Sizes	Material	Sutures
Arthrex	Corkscrew	3.5, 5.0, 6.5 mm	Titanium	2 (#2)
Arthrex	Fastak	2.8 mm	Titanium	1 (#2)
Arthrex	Parachute	5.0 mm screw, 6.5 mm PLLA button	Titanium and PLLA	N/A (#4 suture attaches button to screw)
ArthroCare	Magnum	3.2 × 7 mm	Steel	1 (#2)
Arthrotek	Ti screw	3.0, 5.0 mm	Titanium	2 (#2)
Mitek	G2	2.4 mm	Nickel titanium	#2
Mitek	Superanchor	2.9 mm	Nickel titanium	#5
Mitek	Rotator cuff	2.9 mm	Nickel titanium	#2
Mitek	MiniMitek	2.1 mm drill	Nickel titanium	#0
Mitek	MicroMitek	1.3 mm	Nickel titanium	#3–0
Mitek	Fastin 3, 4, 5.2	3.0, 4.0, 5.2 mm	Titanium	1 (#2)
Mitek	Fastin RC		Titanium	2 (#2)
Mitek	ROC EZ	2.3, 2.8, 3.5 mm	Polyethylene	1 (#2)
Mitek	Tacit 2.0	1.7 mm drill	Titanium	#2–0
Mitek	Knotless	2.9 mm	Titanium	1 (#1)
Linvatec	Revo	4 mm	Titanium	1 (#2)
Linvatec	MiniRevo	2.7 mm	Titanium	1 (#2)
Linvatec	SuperRevo	5.0 mm	Titanium	2 (#2)
Linvatec	Ultrafix RC	3.2 mm hole	Stainless steel	2 (#2)
Linvatec	Ultrafix MiniMite	2.4 mm hole	Stainless steel	1 (#2)
Linvatec	Ultrafix microMite	1.8 mm hole	Stainless steel	1 (#2–0)
Multitak	Titanium anchor	3 × 6 mm, 1.8 × 3.7 mm	Titanium	1 (#2), 1(#2–0)
Smith & Nephew	MiniTac	2.0 mm	Titanium	2 (#3–0)
Smith & Nephew	Twinfix Ti	2.0, 2.8, 3.5, 5.0	Titanium	2.8 has #1; 3.5 has 2 (#2); 5.0 has 2 (#2)
Smith & Nephew	Twinfix Ti 4.0, 6.5	4.0, 6.5 mm	Titanium	Large eyelet allows for multiple sutures
Stryker endoscopy	Mainstay (Zip)	2.7, 3.5, 4.5 mm	Titanium	2.7 has #0; 3.5 has #2; 4.5 has 2 (#2) or 1(#5)
Stryker endoscopy	Cuff anchor	5.0 mm	Titanium	2 (#2)
Stryker endoscopy	Glenoid anchor	3.0 mm	Titanium	1 (#2)
USS sports medicine	Herculon	2.5, 3.5, 4.5, 5.5, 7.4 mm	Titanium	#0, #1, #2, 2 (#2)
Zimmer	Statak	2.5, 3.5, 5.0, 5.2 mm	Tivanium alloy	1 (#2)

Abbreviations: PGA, polyglycolic acid; PLLA, poly L-lactic acid.

the increased popularity of double row fixation, anchors with larger eyelets that can accommodate two and three sutures have advantages over smaller anchors. In contrast, Bankart, superior labrum (SLAP) and biceps tendon repairs require anchor insertion into denser bone. In these applications, and especially with anchors used in the glenoid rim, smaller anchors have fewer tendencies to cut through and damage the articular cartilage. Since a #2 suture is the largest suture commonly chosen for these areas, the anchor chosen here does not need to accept several #5 sutures. The anchor should fit securely in the glenoid without either breaking out during insertion or being so small that it does not gain adequate purchase.

Suture Size

The size of the suture in a suture anchor is related to the repair strength and thus influences anchor selection. In addressing shoulder instability, multiple points of fixation in the glenoid using #2 suture exceed the suture strength requirements for Bankart repair. The tensile strength of a doubled #2 Ethibond suture is approximately thirty pounds. Newer suture materials (the so-called super sutures) make previous concerns about suture size and strength less of an issue. The use of ultra high molecular weight polyethylene (UHMWPE) in sutures means that suture breakage either during insertion or with cyclic loading is less likely. On the other hand, concerns about loop security and whether tying a sliding knot will weaken the biodegradable anchor's suture eyelet increase.

TABLE 2 Common Biodegradable Suture Anchors

Company	Anchor	Sizes	Material	Sutures
Arthrex	BioCorkscrew	5.0, 6.5	PDLLA	2 (#2)
Arthrex	Bio-Fastak	3.0	PDLLA	1 (#2)
Arthrex	Bio-SutureTak	3.0	PDLLA	1 (#2)
Arthrex	TissueTak	3.0	PDLLA	N/A
Arthrotek	LactoScrew	3.5, 5.5 mm	PLLA (82%)/ PGA (18%)	N/A
Arthrotek	Lactosorb anchor	5.5 mm	PGA/PLLA	2 (#2)
Arthrotek	Bio-Phase	2 mm, 3 mm	PGA/PLLA	2 mm #1; 3 mm #2
Linvatec	Duet anchor	6.0 OD, 3.3 mm CD	PD(4%)L(96%)LA or PLLA	2(#2)
Linvatec	Bioanchor	3.5 mm OD/2.1 mm CD	PLLA	1 (#2)
Linvatec	Biotwist	2.9 mm	PLLA	N/A
Linvatec	Ultrasorb	3.5 mm	PLLA	2 (#2)
Mitek	Bioknotless	2.9 mm	PLLA	#2-0
Mitek	BioROC EZ	2.8 mm and 3.5 mm	PLLA	1 (#2)
Mitek	CuffTack	4.5 mm body, 8.9 mm wings	PLLA	N/A
Mitek	ConTack	3.5 mm	PLLA body, PDLLA washer	N/A
Mitek	Panalok	3.5 mm	PLLA	1 (#2)
Mitek	Panalok RC	3.5 mm	PLLA	1 (#2)
Regeneration technologies	AlloAnchor RC	5 mm	Allograft cortical bone	2 (#2)
Smith & Nephew	Phoenix 5.0	4.85 mm OD, 3.1 mm CD	Allograft	2(#2)
Smith & Nephew	Twinfix PMR	5.0 mm OD, 3.2 mm CD	Polyacetyl	2(#2)
Smith & Nephew	Twinfix AB	5.0 mm OD, 3.2 mm CD	PLLA	2 (#2)
Smith & Nephew	RotorloC	4.5 mm drill	PLLA	2 (#2)
Smith & Nephew	Suretac 6.0, 8.0	3.4 mm, 3.7 mm	PGA-TMC	N/A
Smith & Nephew	Suretac II/spikes	3.4 mm	PGA-TMC	N/A
Smith & Nephew	TAG Wedge 3.7	3.7 mm	PGA-TMC	1 (#2)
Smith & Nephew	TAG Rod II	3.7 mm	PGA-TMC	1 (#2)
USS sports medicine	PolySorb 2, 3	2.2, 3.2 mm	PGA/PLLA	1 (#2)
Zimmer	BioStatak	2.5 CD, 5.0 OD	PLLA	1 (#2)

Abbreviations: PGA, polyglycolic acid; PLLA, poly dextro levo lactide acid.

Suture Number

Most newly developed suture anchors have eyelets that allow multiple sutures to be used per device. Anchors, which have eyelets allowing the use of two or more sutures, have clear advantages in rotator cuff surgery where the amount of tension on a repair is high. Using multiply loaded anchors is not advantageous in Bankart repairs, where more points of bony fixation provide statistically better strength in the anterior shoulder. At least two anchors are needed to exceed the strength of the anterior shoulder capsule and ligaments (12). Additionally, anterior-inferior translation with the shoulder in 90 degrees abduction is statistically reduced by the use of three separate fixation points when compared to two fixation points (13). Using smaller anchors allows more fixation points in the glenoid rim.

Suture Material

Suture material is another factor important in a surgeon's choice of suture anchor. Both absorbable and nonabsorbable sutures are used for various repairs. A commonly used nonabsorbable suture in the shoulder is Ethibond. Ethibond is a braided polyester suture coated with polybutylate providing improved arthroscopic knot tying with greater suture loop and knot security. An example of an absorbable suture is the monofilament polydioxanone (PDS) suture, which is easy to work with using only suture hooks and punches because of its "memory." PDS, however, retains only 40% of its implantation strength six weeks after

TABLE 3 Suture Loads-to-Failure

Suture	Number tests	Mean force (N)	SD (N)	Mean pounds
FiberWire #5	10	482.7	22.9	112.2
MagnumWire #2	10	303.1	28.3	70.5
Force Fiber #2	13	288.5	22.0	67.0
Ultrabraid #2 (white)	10	279.6	19.2	65.0
Ultrabraid #2 (Cobraid)	10	264.5	21.0	61.5
Maxbraid PE #2	9	256.1	14.5	59.6
Herculine #2	11	249.7	21.6	58.0
Orthocord #2[a]	10	197.9	19.4	46.0
Ethibond #5	20	193.1	13.6	44.9
FiberWire #2	20	187.9	12.2	43.7
Ethibond #2	12	91.7	5.4	21.3
FiberWire #2-0	10	81.6	5.1	19.0

[a]denotes a partially biodegradable suture.

surgery, and will dissolve nine weeks after implantation (14). Other absorbable suture materials are available including Panacryl, which offer different rates of suture degradation.

Newly developed so-called "super sutures" are now available which have dramatically increased the loads to failure. FiberWire (Arthrex, Naples, Floride, U.S.A.) was the first super suture. It consists of an UHMWPE multifilament core with a braided polyester coating. The non-braided core resists elongation and is protected by the polyester jacket (15,16). Other super sutures are made with Dyneema Purity (DSM Dyneema, Netherlands), a suture material made from UHMWPE. Orthocord is a new suture made from a combination of the UHMWPE and PDS. The orthocord suture is different from other super sutures because it consists of a PDS core with a UHMWPE sleeve and is coated with polyglactin 910 for better suture handling characteristics. This combination is designed to create a low profile suture after the PDS component has dissolved, while retaining strength from the outer sleeve of UHMWPE. Most of the new suture constructs are available in the traditional #2 size. Samples of common "super sutures" are compared in (Table 3) (15,16). Although the ultimate strength and composition of the new suture materials vary, it is important to remember that the mean load to failure for all the tested "super sutures" far exceed the presumed requirements for secure tendon to bone fixation.

Anchor Material

Although both metal and biodegradable suture anchors exist, the trend has been toward the increased development and implantation of bioabsorbable fixation. Many implanted anchors, however, are still metal and provide both strength and ease of insertion. These anchors are easily evaluated radiographically and since most are titanium, will not complicate postoperative imaging. Metal anchors continue to outperform their bioabsorbable counterparts in ultimate load to failure, even though both constructs typically can far exceed the requirements for soft tissue to bone repair. Although biodegradable anchors have lower failure loads and are slightly more complicated to insert, they are typically stronger than the sutures for which they are matched. The less-abrasive eyelet of the biodegradable anchor is less likely to damage and fray a suture, which could ultimately lead to suture anchor failure. Biodegradable suture anchors offer several other apparent advantages: easier revision, less obstructed imaging, eventual anchor absorption, and use with pediatric applications—not possible with nonbiodegradable materials. The biodegradable nature of the implant allows for the anchor to do its job and then disappear. The radio-transparent quality of the implant facilitates postoperative imaging studies including magnetic resonance imaging (MRI) (17). Because the anchor can be drilled out at a later date if it has not been completely absorbed, revision surgery is simplified and concerns about an infected implant are reduced (18). Concern regarding anchor migration leading to articular cartilage damage is also reduced with a biodegradable anchor (19).

Chemically, bioabsorbable anchors are made of several different polymers. PGA and poly L-lactic acid (PLLA) are polymers that comprise the majority of absorbable anchors. The differences in rates of degradation of PLLA and PGA affect the strength of various suture anchors over time. An example of a hybrid anchor composed of both PLA and PGA is the Panalock anchor (DePuy-Mitek), which is believed to retain 90% of its original implantation strength at nine months from surgery (20).

Of the several different bioabsorbable polymers used in suture anchors, each polymer has been shown to exhibit slightly different behavior. Purified nonreinforced PLLA has been shown to be well tolerated over time in vivo in the interference fixation screws (21). Biodegradable tacks for anterior shoulder stabilization are reported to achieve good results as well (22). Biodegradable suture anchors composed of other materials have been found to be successful in open Bankart procedures (23,24).

Some complications have been reported using PGA implants (25–27). Restricted postoperative shoulder motion (44%) and a hyper inflammatory response (20%) requiring additional surgery have both been reported (28). This was not reported in open anterior shoulder stabilizing procedures using PGA/TMC anchors. There is speculation that the lack of such a response may be due to smaller volume of material and a decreased surface area (29). The authors of the study suggest that the methyl group in the polymer's composition may protect carbonyl carbons from tissue depolymerization (30).

PLLA material can require up to four years to reabsorb completely (14). Problems reported with PLLA implants seem to be mostly mechanical. Loosening of an investigational PLLA tack device has been reported but without evidence of bone lysis, inflammation, or synovitis. The mechanical symptoms caused by the PLLA tack completely resolved after implant removal (31).

Complications are certainly not restricted to biodegradable implants. Cases of late infection have been reported with nonabsorbable anchors (18). Metal anchors may be the cause of several complications (19), including anchor migration resulting in articular cartilage damage (18,32).

One asset of biodegradable anchors is that revision surgery can be less problematic than with metal anchors. At revision, if another anchor needs to be placed into the same footprint of a biodegradable anchor, a drill is simply used to clear a new track for insertion of the anchor. There are very few metal anchors with instrumentation that permit the surgeon to "unscrew" and remove a previously placed anchor. Metal nonscrew anchors typically cannot be easily removed once inserted.

Anchor Type

While there are several different types of anchors on the market, all can be grouped into either a screw or nonscrew type design (33,34). Nonscrew devices can be further subdivided into those that require sutures to attach the tendon to bone, and those that do not require sutures and instead use the device itself to attach the tendon to bone. Screw anchors are typically very efficient with excellent failure-load statistics that usually outperform the tack or pronged design (35). Screw anchors have eyelets that can hold a variety of suture types and sizes, allow for suture substitution, and permit tying slipknots. The nonscrew anchors have many different designs that include expanding anchors, toggle anchors, push-in anchors, and wedges (36). The nonscrew designs also allow the tying of sliding knots, although some nonscrew anchors do not permit suture substitution.

Some screw type suture anchors have instruments that allow removal via "unscrewing" of the anchor. Tack like anchors, conversely, do not allow for removal after insertion unless they are removed by drilling out of a biodegradable or plastic anchor. The nonscrew anchors require a hole to be drilled or punched to allow anchor insertion. After drilling out a nonscrew anchor a large bony deficit can be encountered, especially in osteoporotic bone. The screw anchors typically create their own hole which is no larger than the minor diameter of the screw.

Insertion Technique

Insertion technique is paramount when discussing a thorough evaluation of suture anchors. Several technical points must be considered including the steps and equipment needed to place the anchor in the bone. Does a hole need to be made to accept the anchor, and if so, does it need to be tapped? How is the anchor released from the insertion device, and once inserted, how are the sutures brought through the various portals? The surgeon should have a strategy for suture management, how to pass sutures through the tendon, and where to tie a secure arthroscopic knot.

There are various techniques for passing the suture through the tissue (tendon or ligament) and these techniques have implications for anchor selection. These include the "anchor first" method, in which the anchor is placed securely in the bone and then the associated suture passed through the soft tissue. With the "suture first" technique, the suture is initially passed through the soft tissue and then threaded onto an anchor, which is subsequently placed in the bone. Finally, in the "trans-tissue" technique, a threaded anchor and suture are passed simultaneously through the tissue during insertion. The "suture first" technique precludes the use of any screw-type suture anchor. The "trans-tissue" technique requires an anchor with a sharp enough tip to pass through the tissue with the associated suture. The "anchor first" technique is applicable to both screw and nonscrew type anchors.

The insertion angle of a suture anchor is also critical. While the concept of the "Deadman" angle is clearly valid, its direct application in the humeral head does not provide the best insertion angle for secured fixation of the rotator cuff. When considering the anatomy of an osteoporotic humeral head, placing the anchor at a 45° angle puts the tip of the implant in the central cavity of the humerus, which has few trabeculae. Using a more acute angle is desirable since it yields better bony fixation for the implant. Suture anchors that are inserted on the greater tuberosity should enter at an oblique angle to catch the denser subcortical bone.

COMMON MODES OF FAILURE

Pull Out

Pull out is a term used to describe a failure of the suture anchor in the bone. Pull out can occur in both nonscrew and screw anchor designs, but is much more common in push-in designs because of the lack of threads. The osteoporotic bone of the elderly shoulder increases the risk of anchor pull out. Pull out is less likely in an area with good cortical bone stock such as the glenoid or elbow. Forces on the suture can toggle the anchor and create a trough in the bone; loosening the implant and permitting anchor pull out. If the angle of insertion of an anchor is too large (>45°), the anchor can be inserted into poor bone stock and not into the dense subchondral bone, again leading to a higher likelihood of anchor pull out. Metal anchors are historically stronger than their biodegradable counterparts when tested for pull out strength, but both constructs exceed the estimated force required for rotator cuff repair or anterior stabilization procedures.

Suture Lacerates Tendon

The suture–tendon interface is the weakest link in a soft tissue repair to bone (37). This is even more likely with the newer super sutures and the increased load-to-failure strength of the newer suture anchors. The concern is that the suture passed through the tendon can cut tendon fibers either with cyclic loading in the postoperative period or during surgery when a sliding knot "runs" the more abrasive super suture through the tissue.

Eyelet Breakage

While metal eyelets may damage sutures, abrasive sutures may damage softer biodegradable eyelets. Cyclic loading super sutures in the postoperative period or suture movement while tying sliding knots may cut through a biodegradable anchor eyelet. Eyelets are usually a molded part of the anchor, but some designs use a separate piece of suture for an eyelet (Arthrex anchors). Eyelet "crowding" may have some influence. While some eyelets contain one suture, others have multiple sutures in the same eyelet. From an anchor security standpoint, it may be better for multiple sutures to be threaded through separate eyelets. By doing so, if one eyelet breaks the entire construct will not be jeopardized.

Suture Breakage

With the use of super sutures and newer arthroscopic instrumentation, the risk of breaking while tying an undamaged suture is relatively low. If the suture is frayed, however, the risk of suture breakage increases dramatically. Sutures can be damaged upon insertion and knot tying, inadvertent clamping of the suture in the area where the knot will ultimately lie, using damaged arthroscopic instruments, or nicking the coating of the suture in any other manner thus weakening even a super suture and resulting in suture breakage during knot tying. Anchors placed deep into bone with eyelets within the anchor also have the possibility of suture damage by the suture rubbing against the edge of the bony hole into which the anchor was placed.

CURRENT ANCHOR DEVELOPMENTS

Competition in the suture anchor industry has resulted in newer, more effective designs, and has led to changes in the suture anchor models available. A review of currently available anchors reveals some trends. Most of the newly released anchors provide two sutures. The suture material options include both the conventional braided polyester and the newer high strength super sutures. The addition of two sutures to the anchor is handled by either enlarging the existing eyelet or providing two separate suture eyelets. Both screw anchors and nonscrew anchors are still being developed, but the most commonly chosen material is biodegradable. PLLA suture anchors predominate.

The following list (in alphabetical order by manufacturer name) is by no means comprehensive and is not meant to serve as a recommendation of one anchor over another. Instead, these suture anchors are cataloged in an effort to offer the reader a better understanding of some of the anchors available.

Arthrex (Naples, Florida, U.S.A.)

Bio-Corkscrew

This is one of the anchors made from a copolymer of lactic acid (dextro and levo forms). This poly dextro (4%) levo (96%) lactide acid (PDLLA) material has a more rapid degradation than the standard PLLA. The eyelet is not made from a polymer but from #4 braided polyester (or #2 Fiberwire) suture loop that is molded into the anchor body to create a unique suture eyelet that results in less suture-eyelet abrasion when tying the attached sutures. The load to failure strength of the anchor in cancellous bone is good. The Bio-Corkscrew is available with two braided polyester #2 sutures (one green and one white), with two solid color #2 FiberWire sutures, or with two #2 TigerTail (FiberWire with stripes) sutures. The anchor comes in two sizes: 5.0 and 6.5 mm (Fig. 3).

Bio-Corkscrew Fully Threaded

The Bio-Corkscrew fully threaded (FT) is a 5.5 mm diameter bioabsorbable PLLA-suture anchor designed to be inserted flush with the cortical bone surface to maximize fixation strength and anchor stability (Fig. 4). The Bio-Corkscrew FT has a #2 FiberWire eyelet recessed into the body of the anchor to reduce suture abrasion at the eyelet during knot tying. It comes preloaded with two #2 FiberWire sutures (one solid blue; one white with black TigerTail suture).

Corkscrew II

This is the original titanium anchor revised to have two individual suture eyelets and is suitable for rotator cuff repair (Fig. 5). It carries two sutures (either #2 FiberWire or braided polyester). The anchor threads are widely spaced to work in cancellous bone, and the anchor is 5 mm in diameter. The anchor insertion shaft has a vertical laser mark on the distal part to indicate the suture eyelet orientation.

Arthrocare (Sunnyvale, California, U.S.A.)

Magnum Knotless Fixation Implant

This is a metal anchor with a single #2 braided polyester suture (Fig. 6). It is inserted into the bone and, when deployed, the toggle opens to fix the anchor in the bone. It has a very high load-to-failure strength. The anchor's internal mechanism provides guaranteed and reversible tension to allow adjustments to the single suture.

Depuy-Mitek (Norwood, Massachusetts, U.S.A.)

Spiralok

This is a screw anchor with dual eyelets and two sutures (Fig. 7). There are two separate suture eyelets on an eyelet shaft, which are oriented at 90° to each other. The anchor is made from PLLA and has a blue color. The sutures available include braided polyester, Orthocord (composed of PDS and UHMW polyester), and Panacryl (an absorbable suture). It is available in 5.0 and 6.5 mm sizes.

Fastin RC

This is a metal screw-in anchor that holds two sutures through dual eyelets (Fig. 8). This anchor is 5.0 mm in diameter and because of the strength provided by its metal composition has a small central core with deep screw threads, which allow a very good load-to-failure strength and good fixation in the bone of the humeral head. The sutures available include #2 braided polyester, Orthocord (partially biodegradable), and Panacryl (a fully biodegradable suture).

Linvatec (Largo, Florida, U.S.A.)

Impact

This is an impaction, nonscrew anchor that is white in color and made from self reinforced PDLLA (SR-PDLLA) (Fig. 9). It has two separate eyelets placed parallel to one another in the shaft of the anchor, which maintain the ability to tie sliding knots. The proximal suture (white) must be tied first. It is 3.5 mm in diameter and 10.5 mm long. The sutures available are #2 braided polyester and #2 Herculine (the Linvatec version of Dynema).

Duet

In contrast to the Impact anchor, the Duet (Fig. 10) is a screw-in anchor made from the same SR-PD(4)L(96)LA as the Impact anchor. It holds two #2 Herculine or #2 braided polyester sutures through two separate eyelets that are located in an eyelet shaft located above the screw threads. It is 6.0 mm in major diameter, 3.3 mm minor diameter, and 16.5 mm long.

Super Revo

This is a conventional titanium screw-in anchor that has been modified with a widened eyelet to hold two #2 Herculine or two #2 braided polyester sutures (Fig. 11). These sutures share the same eyelet and if sliding knots are desired, careful attention should be given to eyelet position when anchor insertion is complete so that one suture does not bind the other during knot tying. The anchor is 5.0 mm in diameter. A three-suture version called the "ThreeVo anchor" is also available.

Smith and Nephew Endoscopy (Andover, Massachusetts, U.S.A.)

BioRaptor

This is a nonscrew push-in anchor with a ribbed design (Fig. 12). It is white in color, biodegradable (made of PLLA), and holds two #2 braided polyester sutures. It also comes with either one or two #2 Ultrabraid (Dynema–UHMW polyethylene) sutures. These sutures pass through a single eyelet that is positioned in the mid portion of the anchor, thus avoiding a superior stump above the ribs. It is smaller (3.7 mm) in diameter and this may limit its suitability for rotator cuff repair.

TwinFix AB

This screw-in anchor is white in color and made of PLLA (Fig. 13). It accommodates two sutures through dual eyelets that are located toward the upper portion of the screw and not in a post at the top of the anchor. The sutures are made of #2 braided polyester. It comes in 5.0 and 6.5 mm diameters.

TwinFix Ti

This titanium screw-in anchor come preloaded with two #2 braided polyester sutures, or two #2 Ultrabraid sutures (one white; and one stripped called "cobraid") (Fig. 14). Ultrabraid is the Smith & Nephew Endoscopy (S&N) version of Dynema suture. The anchor is available in 5.0 and 6.5 mm diameters.

TwinFix Quick T

This anchor provides a single-step trans-tendon tissue repair method that uses a prettied knot behind a "T" bar made of nonabsorbable polymer (plastic) (Fig. 15). The screw portion of the anchor is the TwinFix Ti titanium screw and is available with both 3.5 and 5.0 mm diameters. The "T" portion measures 10 mm × 1.5 mm and has four spikes that are 0.1 mm in length. A single #2 braided polyester suture is attached to the anchor and the second eyelet is empty. The prettied knot is advanced by a single lumen knot pusher to hold the tissue against the bone.

Stryker Endoscopy (San Jose, California, U.S.A.)

BioZip

This suture anchor is a white screw-in anchor that accommodates two #2 braided polyester or two #2 ForceFiber (Stryker version of Dynema) sutures through two separate suture channel (Figs. 16A, B) These channels are located on opposite sides of the central shaft of the suture anchor. The anchor is made of PLLA and comes in 5.0 and 6.5 mm sizes.

CONCLUSIONS

This chapter has discussed the history and current concepts surrounding the use of suture anchors for soft tissue to bone fixation. A comprehensive discussion of suture anchors is difficult since the indications for using anchors in various applications is continuously evolving. Trends do exist, however, and show that the newest anchors are more likely to be biodegradable, multiple loaded with super sutures, and incorporate a screw design. The technological advances in anchor and suture design coupled with improvements in instrumentation continue to provide more secure soft tissue to bone fixation in both the shoulder and elbow.

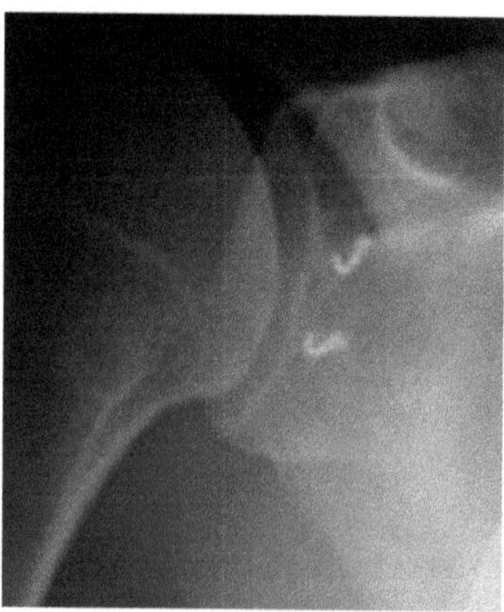

FIGURE 1 The first generation suture anchor which was called the G1 anchor.

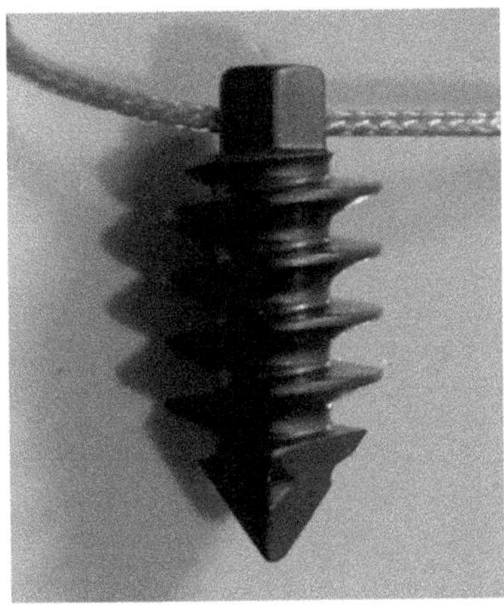

FIGURE 2 The original screw anchor was the Statak anchor.

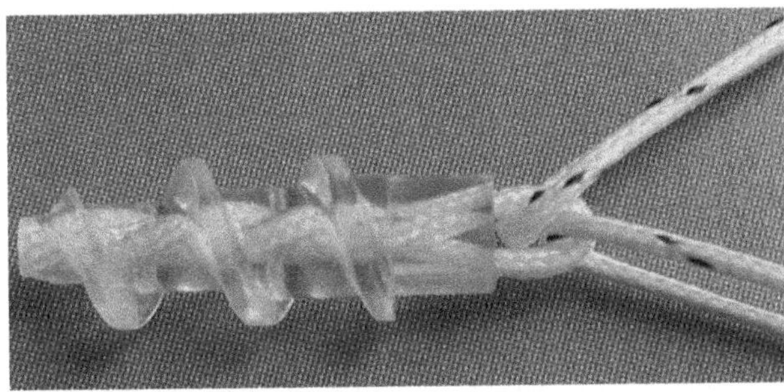

FIGURE 3 The Bio-Corkscrew is available with two braided sutures and comes in 5.0 and 6.5 mm sizes.

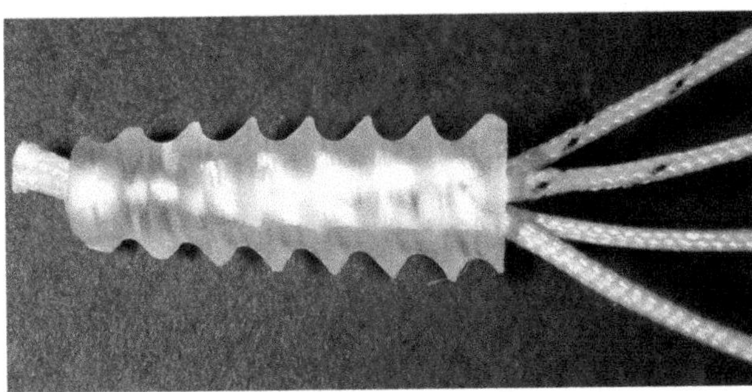

FIGURE 4 The Bio-Corkscrew fully threaded is a 5.5 mm diameter bioabsorbable poly L-lactic acid suture anchor designed to be inserted flush with the cortical bone surface to maximize fixation strength and anchor stability.

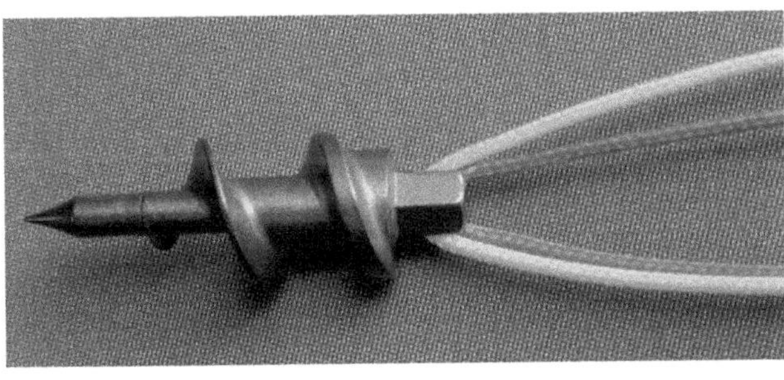

FIGURE 5 The Corkscrew II is a titanium anchor with two sutures.

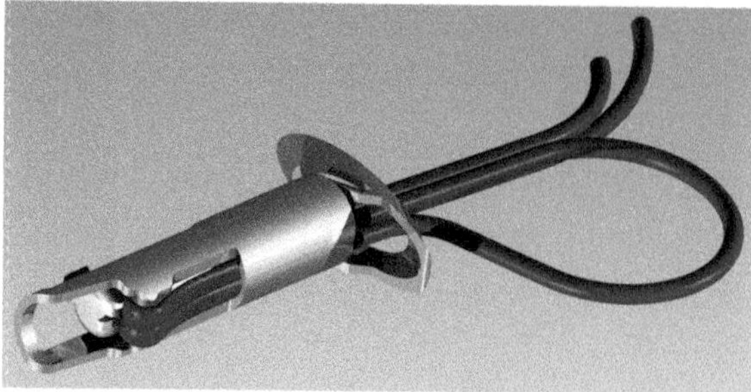

FIGURE 6 The Magnum knotless fixation implant is a metal anchor with a single #2 braided polyester suture.

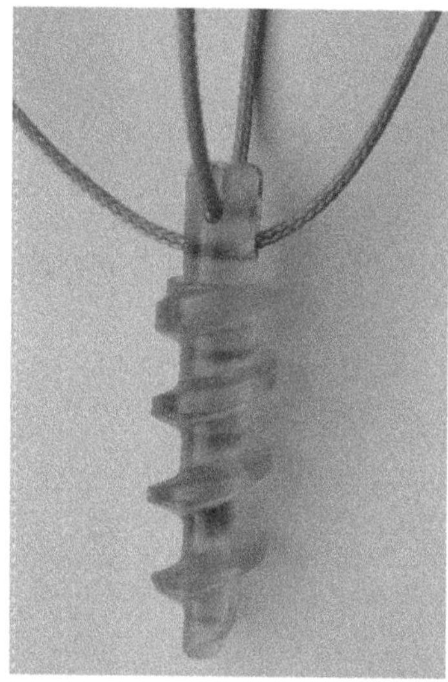

FIGURE 7 The SpiraLok is a poly L-lactic acid screw anchor with dual eyelets oriented at 90° to each other for two sutures.

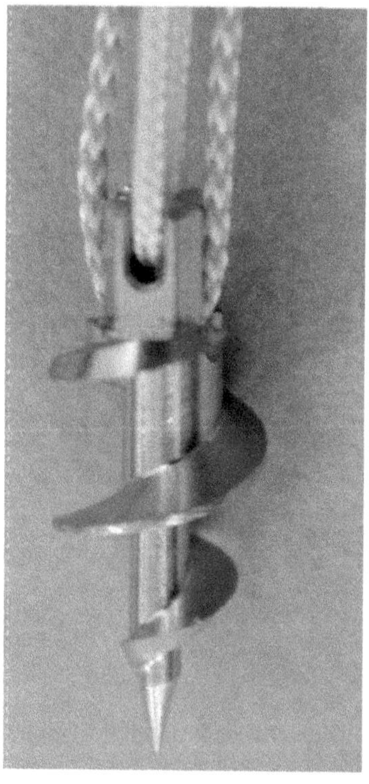

FIGURE 8 The Fastin RC is a metal screw-in anchor that holds two sutures through dual eyelets.

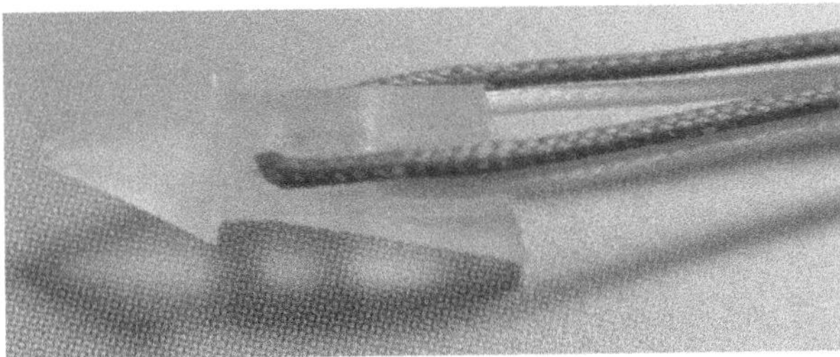

FIGURE 9 The impact anchor is an impaction, nonscrew anchor that is white in color and made from self reinforced poly L-lactic acid.

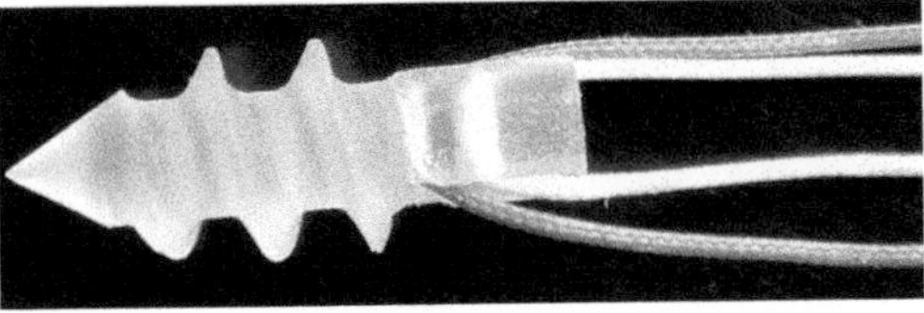

FIGURE 10 The duet anchor is a screw-in anchor made from SR-PD(4)L(96)LA and holds two sutures through two separate eyelets.

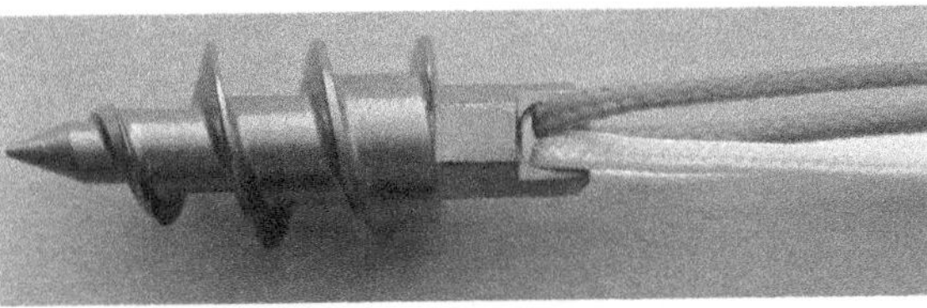

FIGURE 11 The super revo anchor is a conventional titanium screw-in anchor that has been modified with a widened eyelet to hold two #2 sutures.

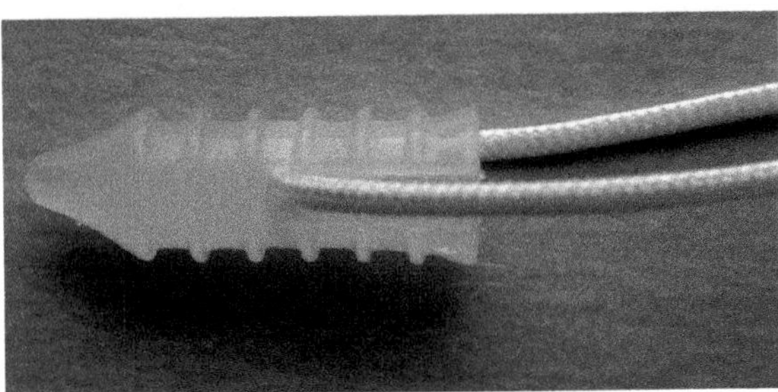

FIGURE 12 The BioRaptor is a nonscrew poly L-lactic acid push-in anchor with a ribbed design and holds two #2 sutures.

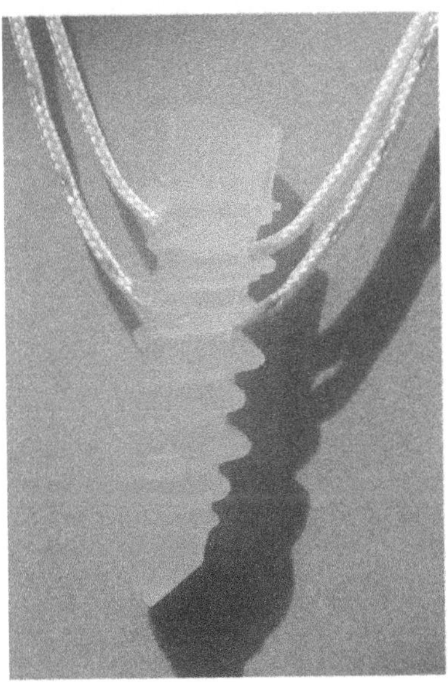

FIGURE 13 The TwinFix AB is a poly L-lactic acid screw-in anchor with two sutures through dual eyelets located toward the upper portion of the screw.

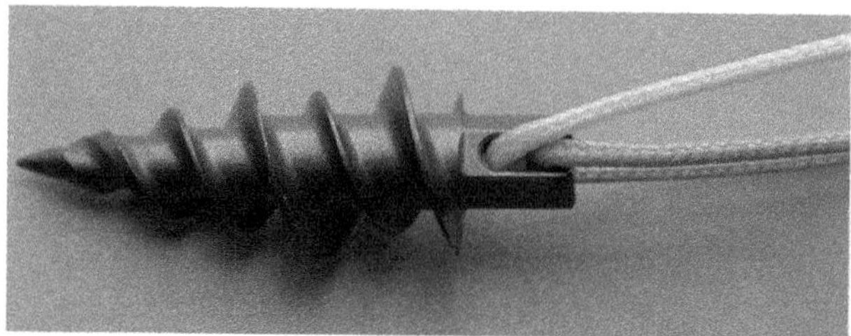

FIGURE 14 The TwinFix Ti is a titanium screw-in anchor preloaded with two sutures.

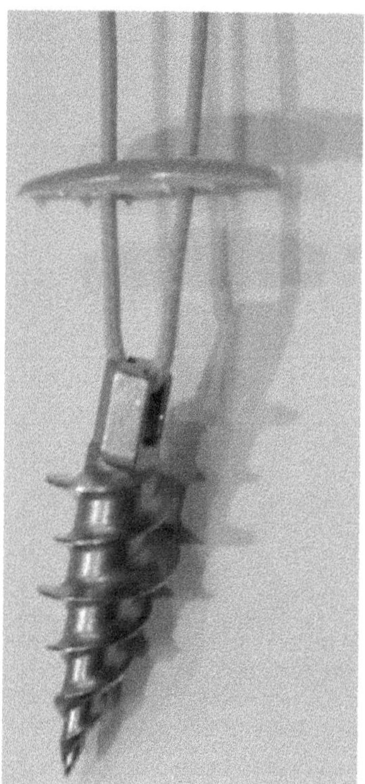

FIGURE 15 The TwinFix Quick T is a screw anchor inserted by a trans-tendon tissue repair method that uses a prettied knot behind a "T" bar made of nonabsorbable polymer.

(A)
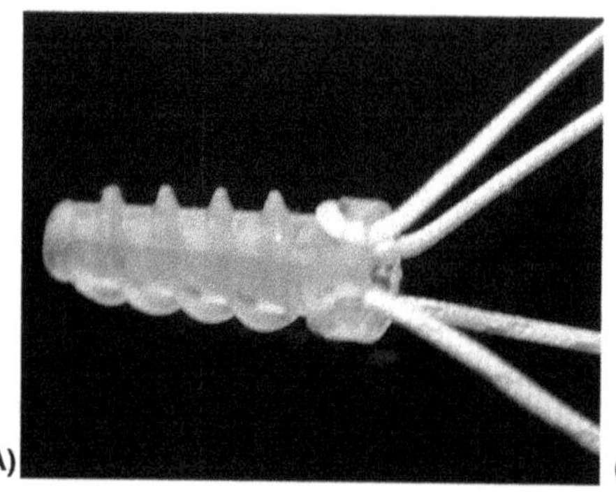

(B)
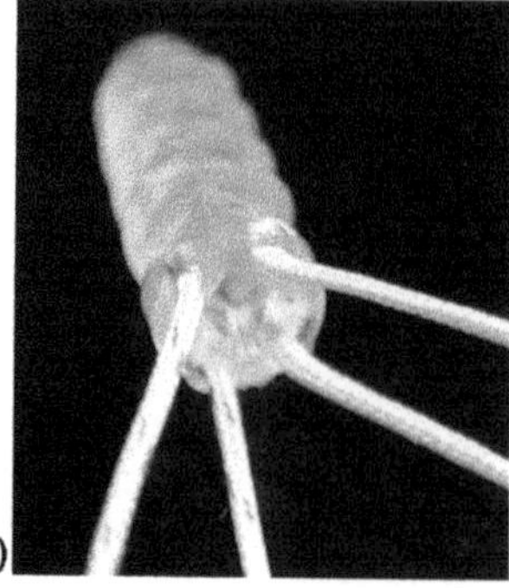

FIGURE 16 The BioZip is a screw-in anchor that accommodates two #2 sutures through two separate suture channels located on opposite sides of the central shaft of the anchor.

REFERENCES

1. Petsche TS, Selesnick H, Rochman A. Arthroscopic meniscus repair with bioabsorbable arrows. Arthroscopy 2002; 18:246–253.
2. Dawson DM, Julsrud ME, Erdmann BB, Jacobs PM, Ringstrom JB. Modified Kidner procedure utilizing a Mitek bone anchor. J Foot Ankle Surg 1998; 37:115–121.
3. DeRowe A, Gunther E, Fibbi A, et al. Tongue-base suspension with a soft tissue-to-bone anchor for obstructive sleep apnea: preliminary clinical results of a new minimally invasive technique. Otolaryngol Head Neck Surg 2000; 122:100–103.
4. Hallock GG. The Mitek mini GII anchor introduced for tendon reinsertion in the hand. Ann Plast Surg 1994; 33:211–213.
5. Klutke JJ, Bullock A, Klutke CG. Comparison of anchors used in anti-incontinence surgery. Urology 1998; 52:979–981.
6. Pederson B, Wertheimer SJ, Tesoro D, Coraci M. Mitek anchor system: a new technique for tenodesis and ligamentous repair of the foot and ankle. J Foot Surg 1991; 30:48–51.
7. Rehak DC, Sotereanos DG, Bowman MW, Herndon JH. The Mitek bone anchor: application to the hand, wrist and elbow. J Hand Surg [Am] 1994; 19:853–860.
8. Rinehart GC. Mandibulomaxillary fixation with bone anchors and quick-release ligatures. J Craniofac Surg 1998; 9:215–221.
9. Schenck RC Jr, Kaar TK, Wirth MA, Rockwood CA. Complications of metallic suture anchors in shoulder surgery. Arthroscopy 1999; 15:559.
10. McFarland EG, Park HB, Keyurapan E, Gill HS, Selhi HS. Suture anchors and tacks for shoulder surgery, part1: biology and biomechanics. Am J Sports Med 2005; 33:1918–1923.
11. Barber FA. Biology and clinical experience of absorbable materials in ACL fixation. Tech Orthop 1999; 14:34–42.
12. McEleney ET, Donovan MJ, Shea KP, Nowak MD. Initial failure strength of open and arthroscopic Bankart repairs. Arthroscopy 1995; 11:426–431.
13. Black KP, Schneider DJ, Yu JR, Jacobs CR. Biomechanics of the Bankart repair: the relationship between glenohumeral translation and labral fixation site. Am J Sports Med 1999; 27:339–344.
14. Barber FA, Herbert M. Suture anchors—update 1999. Arthroscopy 1999; 15:719–725.
15. Barber FA, Herbert MA, Richards DP. Sutures and suture anchors: update 2003. Arthroscopy 2003; 19:985–990.
16. Barber FA, Herbert MA, Coons DA, Boothby MH. Sutures and suture anchors-update 2006. Arthroscopy 2006; 22:1063–1069.
17. Gaenslen ES, Satterlee CC, Hinson GW. Magnetic resonance imaging for evaluation of failed repairs of the rotator cuff. J Bone Joint Surg 1996; 78-A:1391–1396.
18. Ticker JB, Lippe RJ, Barkin DE, Carroll MP. Infected suture anchors in the shoulder. Arthroscopy 1996; 12:613–615.
19. Tamai K, Sawazaki Y, Hara I. Efficacy and pitfalls of the Statak soft-tissue attachment device for the Bankart repair. J Shoulder Elbow Surg 1993; 2:216–220.
20. Schneeberger AG, von Roll A, Kalberer F, Jacob HAC, Gerber C. Mechanical strength of arthroscopic rotator cuff repair techniques: an in vitro study. J Bone Joint Surg Am 2002; 84-A:2152–2160.
21. Barber FA, Elrod BF, McGuire DA, Paulos LE. Bioscrew fixation of patellar tendon autografts. Biomaterials 2000; 21:2623–2629.
22. Arciero RA, Taylor DC, Snyder RJ, Uhorchak JM. Arthroscopic bioabsorbable tack stabilization of initial anterior shoulder dislocations: a preliminary report. Arthroscopy 1995; 11:410–417.
23. Barber FA, Snyder SJ, Abrams JS, Fanelli GC, Savoie FH III. Biodegradable suture anchors: preliminary clinical results. Arthroscopy 1998; 14:449.
24. Warme WJ, Arciero RA, Savoie FH III, Uhorchak JM, Walton M. Nonabsorbable versus absorbable suture anchors for open Bankart repair. A prospective, randomized comparison. Am J Sports Med 1999; 27:742–746.
25. Cheng JC, Wolf EM, Chapman JE, Johnston JO. Pigmented villonodular synovitis of the shoulder after anterior capsulolabral reconstruction. Arthroscopy 1997; 13:257–261.
26. Bostman OM. Intense granulomatous inflammatory lesion associated with absorbable internal fixation devices made of polyglycolide in ankle fractures. Clin Orthop 1992; 278:178–199.
27. Edwards DJ, Hoy G, Saies AD, Hayes MG. Adverse reactions to an absorbable shoulder fixation device. J Shoulder Elbow Surg 1994; 3:230–233.
28. Bennett WF. Bioabsorbable soft tissue fasteners: failure mode an exaggerated inflammatory response? Arthroscopy 1998; 14:449–450.
29. Messer TM, Cummins CA, Ahn J, Kelikian AS. Outcome of the modified Brostrom procedure for chronic lateral ankle instability using suture anchors. Foot Ankle Int 2000; 21:996–1003.
30. Hollinger JO, Battistone GC. Biodegradable bone repair materials: synthetic polymers and ceramics. Clin Orthop 1986; 207:290–305.
31. Berg EE, Oglesby JW. Loosening of a biodegradable shoulder staple. J Shoulder Elbow Surg 1996; 5:76–78.

32. Ekelund A. Cartilage injuries in the shoulder joint caused by migration of suture anchors or mini screw. J Shoulder Elbow Surg 1998; 7:537–539.
33. Barber FA, Herbert MA, Click JN. Suture anchor strength revisited. Arthroscopy 1996; 12:32–38.
34. Barber FA, Herbert M, Click JN. Internal fixation strength of suture anchors—update 1997. Arthroscopy 1997; 13:355–362.
35. Abboud JA, Bozentka DJ, Soslowsky LJ, Beredijiklian PK. Effect of implant design on the cyclic loading properties of mini suture anchors in carpal bone. J Hand Surg [Am] 2002; 27:43–48.
36. Kuwada GT. Use of the ROC anchor in foot and ankle surgery. A retrospective study. J Am Podiatr Med Assoc 1999; 89:247–250.
37. Cluett J, Milne AD, Yang D, Morris SF. Repair of central slip avulsions using Mitek Micro Arc bone anchors. An in vitro biomechanical assessment. J Hand Surg [Br] 1999; 24:679–682.

5 Arthroscopic Acromioplasty

Xavier A. Duralde
Peachtree Orthopaedic Clinic, Emory University, Atlanta, Georgia, U.S.A.

INTRODUCTION

Subacromial decompression as described by Neer (1) has proven to be a safe and effective treatment for subacromial impingement syndrome (2). He recommended removal of the anterior edge and undersurface of the anterior one-third of the acromion, release of the coracoacromial ligament, excision of hypertrophic bursa, and removal of overhanging osteophytes from the acromioclavicular joint. Multiple series in the literature have demonstrated successful management of impingement syndrome utilizing Neer's open acromioplasty (2,3). In 1987 Ellman (4) was the first to describe an arthroscopic technique of acromioplasty. Gartsman (5) demonstrated in an anatomical study that arthroscopic techniques were equivalent to open surgery in achieving adequate bony decompression as described by Neer. Later clinical studies have demonstrated the reliability of arthroscopic acromioplasty for the treatment of impingement syndrome (6,7). Recent comparison studies of open versus arthroscopic acromioplasty have shown these two procedures to be equivalent in success (8,9).

Arthroscopic acromioplasty offers multiple advantages over open techniques including adequate visualization of associated glenohumeral joint pathology. Multiple sources of shoulder pain such as superior labral tears, partial thickness articular-sided rotator cuff tears, and biceps tendon lesions often remain undetected by MRI and open techniques in the face of an intact rotator cuff may result in missed and untreated pathology in the shoulder. Arthroscopic decompression decreases the chances of deltoid origin injury and is associated with greater comfort in the first month following the surgery compared to open techniques. It does, however, require specialized equipment and a significant learning curve. Poor results have been associated both with inadequate resections (3,10) and with excessive resection, which may lead to acromial fracture (11). Arthroscopic techniques generally do not afford visual and tactile feedback associated with open surgery that allows the surgeon to be confident that an adequate subacromial decompression has been accomplished.

The goal of arthroscopic acromioplasty is to reliably reproduce the decompression obtained through open techniques. This requires adequate visualization in the subacromial space and recognition of abnormal pathology. The desired amount of bony resection must be determined through preoperative radiographic studies and intraoperative observations. Both overresection and underresection of bone must be avoided, as each has been associated with failure of the procedure. The deltoid origin must be protected through cautious exposure of the acromial edge without detachment of the deltoid origin and acromioclavicular joint pathology must be clearly visualized and treated at the time of surgery. Hypertrophic bursa must be removed.

PREOPERATIVE EVALUATION

Preoperative evaluation requires a careful history and physical examination as well as radiographic evaluation of the shoulder. The typical patient presenting with subacromial impingement syndrome is over the age of 40 with insidious onset of symptoms. Night pain and pain with overhead activities are common. Physical examination should include a near normal range of motion, tenderness at the greater tuberosity, and a positive arc of pain at 90°, suggestive of pain due to contact between the greater tuberosity and acromion. Very often subacromial crepitus is appreciated and impingement signs typically are positive.

Please refer to pages 57–59 for the figures in this chapter.

Radiographic evaluation is useful in identifying acromial morphology, subacromial spurs, and acromioclavicular (AC) joint spurs. An impingement series includes an anteroposterior (AP) of the shoulder joint with the humerus in external rotation, a supraspinatus outlet view (12), a 30° caudal tilt view (13), and an axillary lateral view. The AP view with the humerus in external rotation allows visualization of excrescences on the undersurface of the acromion as well as the greater tuberosity. The supraspinatus outlet view allows clear visualization of acromial shape and slope, as well as demonstrating subacromial spur formation. The 30° caudal tilt view often demonstrates spur formation, which may not be well seen on the outlet view but does allow clear visualization of that portion of the acromion that extends beyond the anterior cortex of the clavicle. The axillary lateral view will allow identification of an unfused os acromiale and is also sensitive for glenohumeral joint osteoarthritis. MRI is extremely helpful in identifying soft tissue pathology in the shoulder, including the presence of rotator cuff tears associated with more advanced stages of subacromial impingement.

INDICATIONS

The indications for arthroscopic subacromial decompression in the absence of a full thickness rotator cuff tear is the failure of a conservative treatment program to achieve adequate symptom relief over a reasonable period. The length of appropriate rehabilitation is generally felt to be between three and six months. The majority of patients presenting with outlet impingement will respond to a course of conservative management and not require surgery. A temporary response to a subacromial Xylocaine injection test, as described by Neer, is an excellent prognostic indicator for success with subacromial decompression (14). In addition, bony morphology typically associated with outlet impingement, such as a Type II or III acromion described by Bigliani (15), subacromial spurs, or acromioclavicular joint spurs helps support the diagnosis of impingement. The AC joint and biceps are variably involved and routine treatment of these areas is not recommended unless pathology is encountered.

PEARLS AND PITFALLS

Acromioplasty is not performed in all cases of rotator cuff pathology. In a massive, irreparable rotator cuff tear, the coracoacromial arch is preserved to prevent anterosuperior escape.

CONTRAINDICATIONS

It is important for the surgeon to remember that, not all anterior shoulder pain is due to impingement and that not all rotator cuff inflammation is due to outlet impingement. Intrinsic causes of inflammation such as muscle weakness, overuse, and degenerative tendinopathy contribute to impingement syndrome and are often successfully treated with a structured rehabilitation program designed to reduce inflammation, regain flexibility, and reestablish balanced muscle strength about the shoulder. Younger patients with subtle glenohumeral instability may present with signs of rotator cuff inflammation.

Subacromial decompression in this patient group has had a high-failure rate because their primary cause of cuff inflammation is instability and not impingement against the subacromial arch (16). Other diagnoses that can mimic rotator cuff inflammation such as adhesive capsulitis, osteoarthritis, calcific tendonitis, and cervical spondylosis must be excluded prior to embarking on arthroscopic acromioplasty.

SPECIFIC INSTRUMENTS

Part of the success of arthroscopic acromioplasty depends on the availability of adequate equipment. A standard 30° arthroscope is used for the procedure. Inflow can be achieved either with gravity or a pump. Four, three liter saline bags hung at 8′ in height generally produce an adequate pressure gradient. A 5.5 mm full radius resector is helpful in debridement of the subacromial bursa as well as the rotator cuff if necessary. A 5.5 mm flat burr allows for smooth contouring of the undersurface of the acromion. These larger shavers and burrs fit easily into the shoulder and are more efficient than smaller instruments. One milliliter of 1:1000 epinephrine solution is placed in each of the first four bags of irrigation fluid. This results in a mixture of 1 mg/300,000 cc of saline solution. This is adequate to achieve hemostasis, and epinephrine in subsequent bags is unnecessary. Excessive use of epinephrine may result in hypertension and a paradoxical increase in bleeding during surgery.

SURGICAL TECHNIQUE

The patient is placed in the beachchair position with adequate exposure to both the anterior and posterior aspects of the shoulder. A neurosurgical headrest is beneficial to increase exposure to the posterior and superior shoulder. The technique described will be a modification of the "cutting block" technique (17). A combination anesthetic using interscalene block and general anesthesia is preferred both for pre-emptive analgesia and postoperative-pain management. Three portals are required for arthroscopic acromioplasty (Fig. 1). The posterior portal is placed at the "soft spot" posteriorly approximately 2 cm inferior and medial to the posterolateral corner of the acromion. The anterior portal is placed in the skin lines between the palpable corocoid and anterior edge of the acromion. The midlateral portal is placed 3 cm inferior to the lateral border of the acromion in line with the clavicle. The portals are infiltrated with one quarter percent Marcaine with epinephrine for hemostasis. The posterior portal is not included in the field of the interscalene block and injection of this portal also aids with post-operative analgesia.

The glenohumeral joint is localized via the posterior portal with a spinal needle and is filled with 40 cc of saline solution. Insufflation allows insertion of the scope cannula to proceed more easily and atraumatically. The 30° arthroscope is then inserted into the glenohumeral joint via the posterior portal. An anterior portal is established using an outside-in technique with a spinal needle. This spinal needle should pass directly through the center of the rotator interval anteriorly bordered by the subscapularis inferiorly and the anterior border of the supraspinatus superiorly. An 8 mm working cannula is then placed into the glenohumeral joint via the anterior portal. The diagnostic arthroscopy of the glenohumeral joint is then undertaken and glenohumeral pathology is addressed accordingly.

The arthroscope is now redirected via the posterior portal into the subacromial space. The cannula and trocar are used to sweep the subacromial space free of bursal adhesions and are then pushed through the deltoid muscle and out through the anterior portal (Fig. 2A). Next, an inflow cannula is placed over the arthroscopic cannula and is directed back into the subacromial space in this fashion (Fig. 2B). This guarantees that the inflow cannula is placed directly into the subacromial space adjacent to the arthroscope and allows reliable insufflation of the subacromial bursa to facilitate the beginning of the subacromial surgery. A large inflow cannula increases hydrostatic pressure in the subacromial space and is more effective than inflow through the scope cannula in maintaining hemostasis during shaving. A mid-lateral portal is then established as described earlier. Placement of this portal very close to the acromion will not allow the surgeon to drop his hand and aim the instruments up at the acromion. An 8 mm working cannula is then passed from the mid-lateral portal into the subacromial space. The surgeon should push perpendicular to the deltoid initially to assure that the cannula passes through the deltoid muscle. Upon reaching the bone, the surgeon should redirect the cannula superiorly and slightly anteriorly into the subacromial space. This will often result in a sudden loss of visualization in the subacromial space, as bursal tissues are pushed in front of the arthroscope.

The first step in subacromial decompression is the bursectomy. Patients with chronic impingement syndrome will typically demonstrate a hypertrophic bursa in the subacromial space (18,19). Although the role of the subacromial bursa is controversial, it has been shown to have a high concentration of inflammatory mediators and free nerve endings and does require debridement. Bursectomy is an important component of the procedure to allow visualization of both the acromion as well as the rotator cuff tendons.

Several technical errors are common at the beginning of subacromial bursoscopy. The surgeon can pass the working cannula into the subcutaneous tissues superior to the acromion. This is especially true if the patient is obese. It is therefore critical to assure that the cannula penetrates the deltoid before pointing it superiorly. Secondly, a common tendency is to push the arthroscope too far anteriorly so that it lies directly against the anterior deltoid, obscuring visualization. Thirdly, the full radius resector or ablation device is typically placed too far medially. This medial area posterior to the AC joint is very vascular and shaving here will result in a "red out" immediately, thereby, further delaying the subacromial surgery. Shaving and ablation should be performed only under direct visualization to avoid these problems. If the surgeon cannot visualize his working instrument, a "chopsticks" maneuver may be of benefit. The full radius resector can be touched to the superior surface of the scope cannula. The resector can then be moved anteriorly across the scope cannula until it is placed immediately in front of the scope. Bursectomy can then be started.

The bursa is relatively avascular in the midportion of the acromion and the lateral gutter. There are three areas of the subacromial space that have a tendency to bleed during surgery. Shaving of tissues in these areas should be done with great caution or should be done with an ablation device, which can be used to cauterize bleeders when they are encountered. The first area of bleeders is the deltoid muscle, which is encountered at the margins of the acromion during coracoacromial (CA)-ligament excision. The second is the acromial branch of the thoracoacromial artery, which will be encountered when taking down the coracoacromial ligament from the anterior acromion. The third area of increased vascularity is found in the fatty tissues, which lie just inferior and posterior to the acromioclavicular joint. It is critical that the lateral gutter between the lateral aspect of the greater tuberosity and the deltoid be cleared of bursal adhesions. Care should be taken to avoid the axillary nerve on the undersurface of the deltoid in this area.

After adequate bursectomy the coracoacromial ligament can be resected from its insertion on the undersurface and anterior surface of the acromion. The surgeon should keep in mind that the coracoacromial ligament has a complex anatomy and inserts along the entire undersurface of an acromion to its lateral edge. At first, the surgeon should palpate the undersurface of the acromion with the ablation device and begin the resection of the coracoacromial ligament in this area. The ablation device can then be moved in the circumferential fashion away from the central area of the acromion until its edges are encountered. It is critical to expose the entire acromion so that the bone can be evenly resected during acromioplasty. Although deltoid fibers should not be released from the acromion, they should be clearly visible to assure that the acromion has been completely exposed. When reaching the anterior portion of the acromion the surgeon should point the ablation device at the bone and avoid ablating into the deltoid muscle, as this will lead to bleeding and possible damage to the muscle origin itself. The coracoacromial ligament should be released completely from its attachment on the anterior surface of the acromion and the acromial branch of the thoracoacromial artery should be cauterized at this point in time.

The coracoacromial ligament does blend into the inferior portion of the acromioclavicular joint capsule, and this inferior portion of the capsule should be ablated as well in order to expose spurs on the undersurface of the acromion at this joint, and associated spurs on the inferior portion of the distal clavicle.

Learning to deal with bleeding in the subacromial space is a critical skill necessary for shoulder arthroscopy. The surgeon should first remember the three most common sources of bleeding and determine which is the most likely at that point of the procedure. The status of the inflow and fluid bags is checked. The outflow on the scope cannula can be opened to allow an exit for the blood. The direction from which the bleeding is occuring can be observed, and the scope and ablation probe are both moved to that location. These steps are usually successful in controlling the bleeding.

Viewing direction of the arthroscope for optimal visualization varies from case to case. Often the camera is best directed pointing medially or inferiorly. The surgeon must drop his hand to allow adequate visualization of the acromion from the posterior portal. Following ablation of the coracoacromial ligament from the undersurface of the acromion, charred ligamentous tissue will remain, which will hinder the bony portion of the procedure. A full radius resector should therefore be inserted via the midlateral portal to shave any soft tissue adherent to the undersurface of the acromion. The shaver can be run in one direction rather than in an oscillating fashion, as it will be working against an unyielding surface. In patients with soft bone, the surgeon should avoid making ruts or grooves in the bone, which will distort the anatomy.

AUTHOR'S TECHNIQUE

The patient is now adequately prepared for acromioplasty. The amount of bone removed in acromioplasty is variable depending on the preoperative acromial morphology, but usually requires only a few millimeters of anterior acromion. The anterior-inferior portion of the acromion in prior biomechanical studies has been shown to be the only site where the supraspinatus tendon consistently contacts with arm elevation (20). The amount of bone to be resected is determined based on preoperative X-rays, intraoperative observations, and surgeon preference. One technique involves drawing a line across the anterior cortex of the clavicle on the 30° caudal tilt view. The bone on the acromion anterior to this line may be resected (Fig. 3). On the outlet view, a straight line can be drawn along the posterior inferior cortex of the acromion. The bone inferior to this on the anterior acromion should be resected to convert the acromion into a Type I acromion (Fig. 4). In patients with a long Type II curved acromion, care should be taken to avoid excessive resection of the bone, as this can result in damage to the deltoid origin. Care should be taken especially in the cases of smaller women in whom the thickness of the acromion averages approximately 8 mm as excessive resection can result in damage to the deltoid. During arthroscopy, the hooked portion of the acromion can be visualized while viewing from the posterior portal. The 5.5 mm burr serves as an excellent gauge to the amount of resection to be performed. A line can be drawn from medial to lateral using the 5.5 mm burr to mark the limits of acromioplasty (Fig. 5A). While viewing from the posterior portal, the 5.5 mm burr is inserted through the midlateral portal and the resection is carried out in a lateral to medial direction. The burr is passed straight anteriorly across the previously marked line from posterior to anterior and proceeds in this fashion in a lateral to medial direction until the entire hooked portion of the bone has been resected (Fig. 5B and C). To assure that an even resection has been performed, no cancellous bone should be visible anterior to the marked line while viewing from the posterior portal. The surgeon should avoid scooping the bone on the undersurface of the acromion, which would create an "inverted spoon" configuration to the acromion. This can result in continued impingement along the rim of the acromion and will excessively weaken the central portion of the acromion without benefit to the patient. For this reason, the burr must be passed in a straight line from the marked portion of the acromion anteriorly to create a flat surface. Great care should be taken to protect the deltoid origin during this procedure. When bone removal is performed from "inside out," the periosteum of the acromion and adjacent deltoid origin can be visualized as a white line of tissue attached to the anterior acromion. Preservation of this tissue insures preservation of the deltoid origin. Once a few millimeters of acromion have been removed in this location and a smooth transition to the middle and posterior acromion is established, no further bony resection is required. The lateral edge of the acromion is now planed back to the level of the midlateral portal, creating a gentle, rounded edge at the anterolateral acromion and creating a smooth transition with the posterior acromion.

The "cutting block" technique is now utilized to remove the central ridge in the acromion and complete the acromioplasty. The arthroscope is placed in the midlateral portal, with the camera pointing posteriorly parallel to the acromion, and the burr is placed in the posterior portal. At this point, the surgeon will observe a transition point between the posterior acromion and the resected portion of the anterior acromion (Fig. 6). This ridge in the acromion can then be smoothed in a similar fashion by passing the burr from posterior to anterior while sweeping from medial to lateral. The flat posterior undersurface of the acromion is used as a cutting block to guide the burr forward. This technique is not fool proof and caution should be exercised to avoid excessive bone resection. Also at this point, the surgeon can clearly visualize spurs on the acromion at the acromioclavicular joint, which can be easily resected with the burr in the posterior portal while viewing from the midlateral portal. Once the cortical shell has been removed from the acromion, the underlying cancellous bone may be soft and easily excised. In order to smooth the surface of the acromion, the surgeon can run the burr in a reverse direction to buff the undersurface of the acromion. If a large clavicular spur is noted once the acromioplasty has been performed, this can be resected in a similar fashion with the scope in the midlateral portal and the burr in the posterior portal. The undersurface of the clavicle is beveled flush with the undersurface of the acromion. Finally, the scope is placed back in the posterior portal and the acromioplasty is visualized. Any rough edges or grooves on the undersurface of the acromion can be smoothed using a rasp, which fits easily in the midlateral portal and can be used to further buff the undersurface of the acromion (Fig. 7). If the surgeon is unsure as to the adequacy of the acromioplasty, the anterior portal can be enlarged slightly and a finger can be passed through the portal to palpate the undersurface of the acromion. This is especially helpful early in the learning curve on performing arthrosopic acromioplasty (10).

CLOSURE

The subacromial space should be irrigated copiously and suctioned of all bony debris to avoid heterotopic bone formation (8), and any bleeders noted at this time should be further cauterized with a thermal ablation device. Portals are closed using 4.0 absorbable inverted subcutaneous sutures followed by steristrips. A dry, sterile dressing is then placed over this and the patient's arm is placed in a well-padded sling.

POSTOPERATIVE REHABILITATION

In cases of arthroscopic subacromial decompression without soft tissue reconstruction, such as rotator cuff repair, sling immobilization is used outdoors only for the first two weeks following surgery. Active-assisted forward elevation, external rotation, and internal rotation exercises are begun immediately within the limits of comfort. Pain modalities such as ice are used for pain and edema control in the early postoperative period. Arthroscopic wounds are generally kept clean and dry for three days following surgery at which point showering is allowed. The patient is limited to light activities of daily living for the first six weeks and strenuous activities are avoided. Isometric strengthening exercises and light resistive exercises for the rotator cuff and deltoid are initiated at six week following surgery. Patients generally advance to vigorous resistive exercises by twelve weeks following surgery. Activities are liberalized as symptoms recede, generally between three and six months following surgery.

SUMMARY

Arthroscopic acromioplasty can reliably duplicate the bony decompression achieved through open techniques while protecting the deltoid origin and allowing visualization of associated glenohumeral joint pathology. Arthroscopic techniques result in decreased pain in the early postoperative period, but require significant technical skill to allow adequate decompression. This procedure is not indicated for other diagnoses causing anterior shoulder pain especially instability, as bony contact between the coracoacromial arch and greater tuberosity is not the cause of pain in these patients. Careful patient selection, preoperative planning, and arthroscopic surgical technique lead to reliably good results in patients with subacromial impingement syndrome.

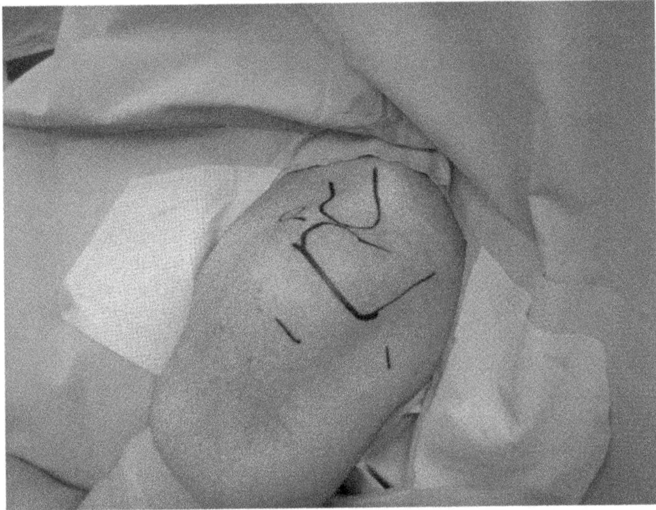

FIGURE 1 The beach-chair position allows easy access to the front and back of the shoulder and allows easy conversion to open techniques. Portals for arthroscopic anterior acromioplasty include the anterior, posterior, and midlateral portals as shown.

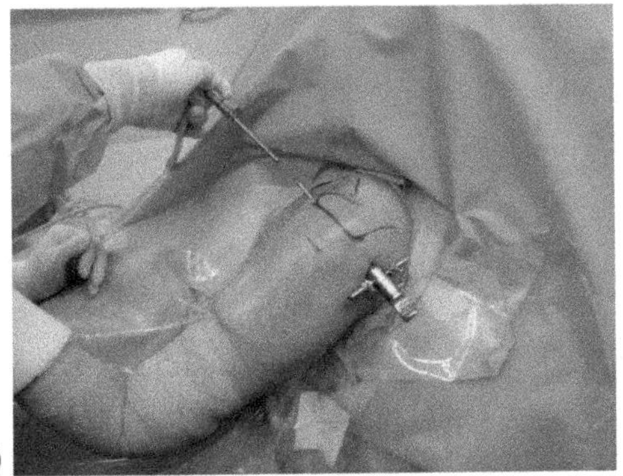

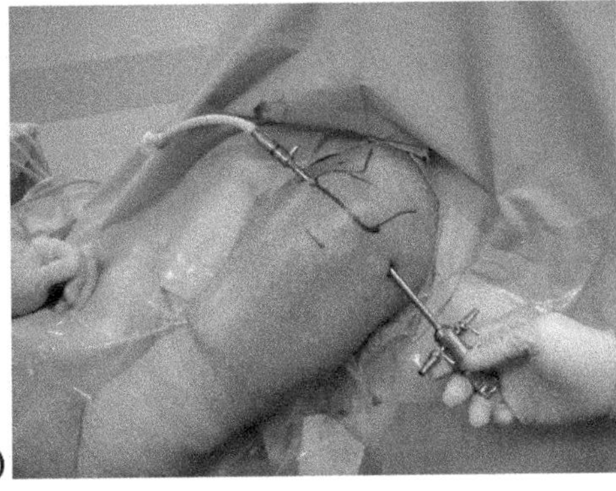

FIGURE 2 (**A**) The arthroscopic cannula is passed from the posterior portal across the subacromial space and out the anterior portal. This will be used to place the inflow cannula directly into the subacromial space. (**B**) The inflow cannula follows the arthroscopic cannula back into the subacromial space, guaranteeing placement of the inflow cannula into the subacromial bursa.

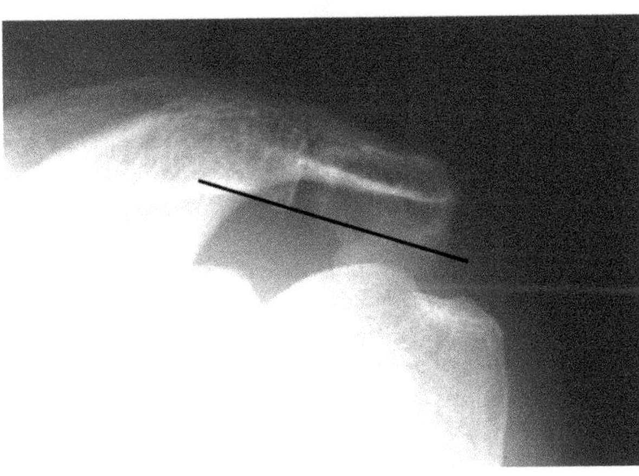

FIGURE 3 The 30° caudal tilt view allows clear visualization of any portion of the acromion, which extends anterior to the clavicle. This portion should be resected at the time of acromioplasty.

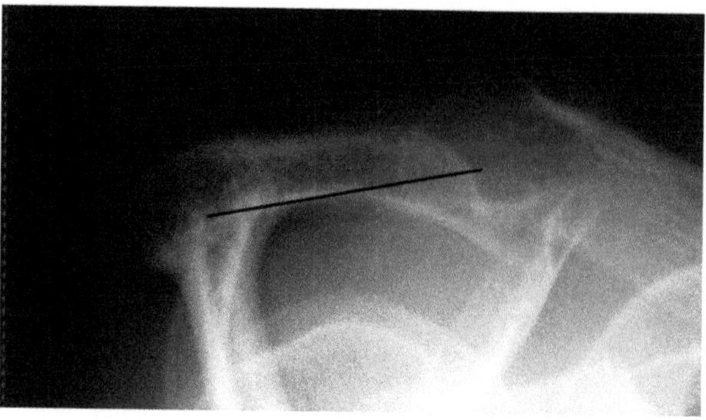

FIGURE 4 The supraspinatus outlet view allows clear visualization of acromial morphology and associated subacromial spurs. The area of resection includes the acromion and spur inferior to the line.

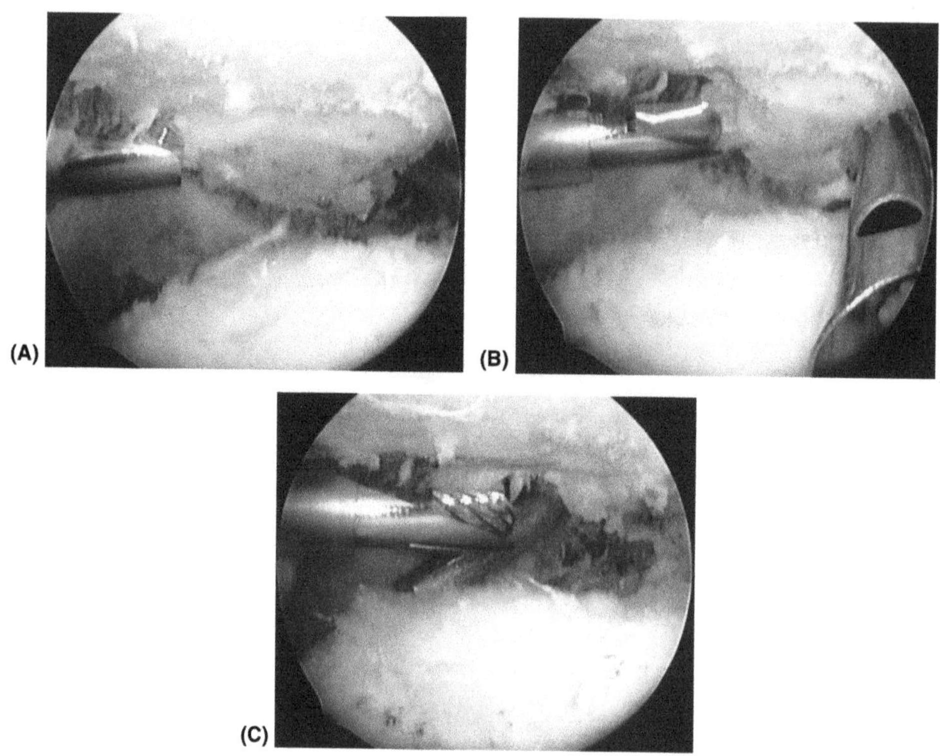

FIGURE 5 (**A**) A line is drawn across the anterior acromion designating the portion of the anterior acromion that is to be resected. This technique avoids a loss of orientation and allows the surgeon to keep track of exactly the amount of acromion removed. The amount of resection is determined both by preoperative X-ray evaluation and intraoperative observations. (**B**) The burr has progressed from lateral to medial halfway across the acromion flattening the acromion from the marked line forward. (**C**) The anterior acromial overhang has been resected.

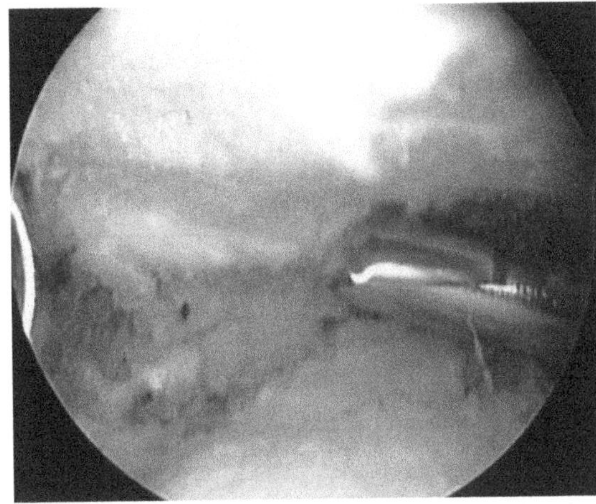

FIGURE 6 The cutting block technique is now used with the scope in the mid lateral portal and the burr in the posterior portal. A ridge is clearly visible between the native acromion posteriorly and the resected portion of the acromion anteriorly.

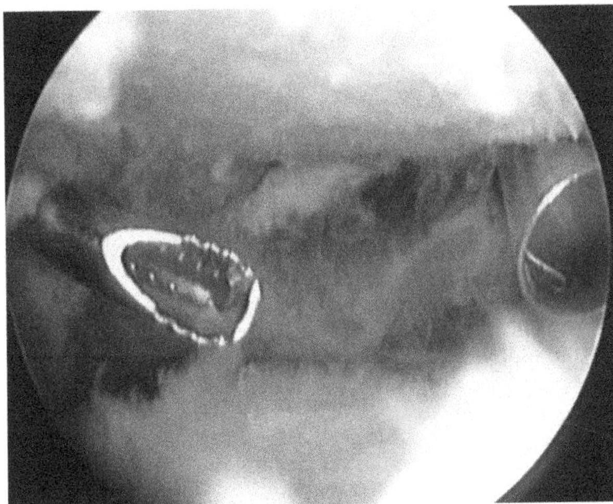

FIGURE 7 The final appearance of the acromion following acromioplasty. A smooth, flat surface is noted superior to the rotator cuff.

REFERENCES

1. Neer CS II. Anterior acromioplasty for the chronic impingement syndrome in the shoulder. A preliminary report. J Bone Joint Surg 1972; 54A:41–50.
2. Neer CS II. Impingement lesions. Clin Orthop 1983; 173:70–77.
3. Rockwood CA Jr, Lyons FR. Shoulder impingement syndrome: diagnosis, radiographic evaluation, and treatment with a modified neer acromioplasty. J Bone Joint Surg 1993; 75A:409–424.
4. Ellman H. Arthroscopic subacromial decompression: analysis of one to three year results. Arthroscopy 1987; 3:173–181.
5. Gartsman GM, Blair ME Jr, Noble PC, et al. Arthroscopic subacromial decompression. An anatomical study. Am J Sports Med 1988; 16:48–50.
6. Gartsman GM. Arthroscopic acromioplasty for lesions of the rotator cuff. J Bone Joint Surg 1990; 72A:169–180.
7. Altchek DW, Warren RF, Wickiewicz TL, et al. Arthroscopic acromioplasty. J Bone Joint Surg 1990; 72A(8):1198–1207.
8. Lazarus MD, Chansky HA, Misra S, et al. Comparison of open and arthroscopic subacromial decompression. J Shoulder Elbow Surg 1994; 3:1–11.
9. Husby T, Haugstvedt JR, Brandt M, et al. Open vs. arthroscopic subacromial decompression: a prospective, randomized study of 34 patients followed for 8 years. Acta Orthop Scand 2003; 74(4):408–414.
10. Hawkins RJ, Plancher KD, Saddemi SR, et al. Arthroscopic subacromial decompression. J Shoulder Elbow Surg 2001; 10(3):225–230.
11. Matthews LS, Burkhead WZ, Gordon S, et al. Acromial fracture: a complication of arthroscopic subacromial decompression. J Shoulder Elbow Surg 1994; 3:256–261.
12. Neer CS II, Poppen NK. Supraspinatus outlet. Orthop Trans 1987; 11:234.
13. Ono K, Yamamuro T, Rockwood CA. Use of a thirty-degree caudal tilt radiograph in the shoulder impingement syndrome. J Shoulder Elbow Surg 1992; 1:246–252.
14. Lim JT, Acornley A, Dodenhoff RM. Recovery after arthroscopic subacromial decompression: prognostic value of the subacromial injection test. Arthroscopy 2005; 21(6):680–683.
15. Bigliani LU, Morrison DS, April EW. The Morphology of the acromion and its relationship to rotator cuff tears. Orthop Trans 1986; 10:228.
16. Jobe FW, Kvitne RS, Giangarra CE. Shoulder pain in the overhand or throwing athlete. The relationship of anterior instability and rotator cuff impingement. Orthop Rev 1989; 8:963–975.
17. Sampson TG, Nisbet JK, Glick JM. Precision acromioplasty in arthroscopic subacromial decompression of the shoulder. Arthroscopy 1991; 7:301–307.
18. Blaine TA, Kim YS, et al. The molecular pathophysiology of subacromial bursitis in rotator cuff disease. J Shoulder Elbow Surg 2005; (1 suppl S):84S–89S.
19. Voloshin I, Gelinas J, et al. Proinflammatory cytokines and metalloproteases are expressed in the subacromial bursa in patients with rotator cuff disease. Arthroscopy 2005; 21(9):1076.
20. Flatow EL, Soslowsky LJ, et al. Excursion of the rotator cuff under the acromion. Patterns of subacromial contact. Am J Sports Med 1994; 22(6):779–788.

6 Arthroscopic Distal Clavicle Resection

Jay D. Keener
Department of Orthopedic Surgery, Washington University, St. Louis, Missouri, U.S.A.

BACKGROUND

The acromioclavicular (AC) joint is a common source of shoulder pain. Both post-traumatic and primary degenerative conditions are frequently encountered. Primary degenerative changes of the AC joint are common in the aging population and, often, well tolerated. These changes are often seen in conjunction with other shoulder pathology, including impingement syndrome and rotator cuff disease. Distal clavicle excision has long been effective in the management of a variety of painful conditions involving the AC joint. Open distal clavicle excision was first described by Gurd and Mumford, separately, in 1941 (1,2). Since first described, open distal clavicle resection performed, alone, or in conjunction with other reconstructive procedures, has proven reliable in the management of degenerative AC joint disorders.

Advances in arthroscopic equipment and surgical techniques allow effective, minimally invasive management of AC joint disorders. Arthroscopic distal clavicle excision has gained popularity since first described in the late 1980s and early 1990s. Outcomes of arthroscopic distal clavicle excision have compared favorably with open treatment. Advantages of arthroscopic resection include preservation of AC joint ligaments and deltotrapezial fascia, quicker recovery, improved cosmesis, and the ability to perform concomitant arthroscopic subacromial procedures. This chapter will review the pertinent anatomy and biomechanics of the AC joint and highlight the surgical indications and techniques of both indirect and direct arthroscopic distal clavicle excision.

ANATOMY AND BIOMECHANICS

The AC joint is a diarthrodial joint surrounded by a thin capsule. The articular surface of the convex distal clavicle articulates with the medial facet of the acromion, both of which are covered with hyaline cartilage at a young age. By the third decade, the articular hyaline cartilage becomes fibrocartilagenous (3). The articular surfaces of the clavicle and acromion at the level of the joint are relatively flat. A thin fibrocartilagenous disc of variable anatomy exists within the joint. Attrition of this disc is a natural process and related primarily to age. Degeneration of the articular disc is generally felt to start in the second decade of life (4). The angle and relationship of the articular surface of the distal clavicle to the acromial facet is variable (5). In the coronal plane, the shape of the distal clavicle can range from straight vertical to an angulation of 50°, superolateral to inferomedial. The flatter the angle of inclination the more the clavicle appears to override the acromial facet. Urist (6) has shown, radiographically, that the clavicle overrides the acromion to some degree in approximately 50% of individuals. Variability in the morphology of the articular surfaces is also seen, to a lesser degree, in the sagittal plane. The capsule of the AC joint is reinforced on all sides by the AC joint ligaments. The superior aspect of the AC joint is supported by the strong fascia of the deltoid and trapezius muscles. The AC joint is innervated by branches of the suprascapular, axillary and lateral pectoral nerves.

The AC joint is subjected to tremendous physical stresses. The articular surfaces are small in comparison to the forces transmitted across the joint creating high contact pressures at the articular surfaces (7). The weight of the relaxed upper extremity is supported by the AC and coracoclavicular ligaments. Cadaveric studies have isolated the primary function of the AC ligaments. At physiologic loads, the AC ligaments are the primary restraint to both

Please refer to pages 68–73 for the figures in this chapter.

anteroposterior translation of the clavicle and inferior displacement of the acromion (8). Klimkiewicz et al. (9) have demonstrated that the posterior and superior AC ligaments are the primary restraint to posterior displacement of the clavicle. Resistance to posterior translation of the clavicle is important clinically to prevent abutment of the posterolateral aspect of the clavicle against the spine of the scapula. The inferior AC ligament is the primary restraint to anterior translation of the clavicle (10). Sectioning of the AC joint capsule and ligaments results in significant anteroposterior translation but minimal instability in the coronal plane (6,8).

The coracoclavicular ligaments are comprised of the stout conoid and trapezoid ligaments. Both ligament pass from the base of the coracoid to the inferior surface of the clavicle. The coracoclavicular ligaments provide vertical stability to the AC joint. The conoid ligament is medial in location and conical in shape and provides the greatest resistance to superior migration of the clavicle. The trapezoid ligament is lateral to the conoid and broader in shape. Because of the oblique orientation of the trapezoid ligament, it provides the primary restraint to lateral displacement of the clavicle in relation to the acromion (compression forces) (8). Due to their vertical orientation, the coracoclavicular ligaments provide minimal restraint to anteroposterior translation. The AC joint is further supported superiorly by the thick fascia of the deltoid and trapezius muscles. Separation of the AC joint results in inferior displacement of the acromion and superior prominence of the lateral clavicle and requires disruption of both the AC ligaments and the coracoclavicular ligaments (6,11).

The clavicle rotates about its long axis as much as 50° with full elevation of the shoulder (12). The majority of rotation occurs at the sternoclavicular joint. The amount of AC joint motion that occurs with elevation of the shoulder is debated. Between 5° to 8° and 20° of motion is thought to occur at the AC joint with full shoulder elevation (12,13). Motion at the AC joint is mitigated by the synchronous movement of the scapula and clavicle that occurs with elevation of the shoulder.

PATHOLOGY

Pathology at the AC joint is common. Both traumatic and primary degenerative processes frequently afflict the AC joint. Traumatic injuries involving the AC joint can result from both direct and indirect trauma. Direct trauma is more common, usually resulting from of a forceful load to the point of the shoulder such as a fall from a bicycle or a forceful tackle (13). The energy of the impact is transmitted from the weight of the body through the clavicle to the AC joint. The magnitude of ligamentous injury is proportional to the position of the extremity and the energy of the collision. The force initially disrupts the AC ligaments. If the energy is sufficient, the coracoclavicular ligaments and the deltotrapezial fascia are disrupted. Trauma to the AC joint can predispose to secondary degenerative changes. Post-traumatic degenerative arthritis has been well described, following less severe grade I and II AC joint separations (14,15). Injuries that result in fractures of the lateral clavicle and injury to the AC joint ligaments can also result in post-traumatic AC joint arthritis.

The AC joint undergoes significant age-related changes (4). The joint space gradually narrows with advancing age (16). Osteolysis of the distal clavicle is a unique condition caused by repetitive stress to the AC joint (17,18). These activities create subchondral stress fractures in the distal clavicle, followed by a hypervascular response (19). As the condition advances, bone is resorbed obscuring the cortical margin of the distal clavicle. Often, the radiographic AC joint space will be widened and the boney detail of the distal clavicle diminished (20). This condition most commonly afflicts weightlifters and is a common cause of AC joint pain in young males. Other conditions can affect the AC joint, including rheumatoid arthritis, crystal induced arthritis (gout and pseudogout), septic arthritis, and hyperparathyroidism. Cystic destruction of the AC joint can accompany massive rotator cuff tears and cuff tear arthropathy. Primary musculoskeletal tumors can occasionally afflict the distal clavicle and therefore must be considered as a part of the differential diagnosis of AC joint pain.

CLINICAL EXAMINATION AND SURGICAL INDICATIONS

Physical Examination

Physical examination of the AC joint is generally straightforward, although frequently AC joint pain will present in the context of other shoulder disorders, such as rotator cuff disease.

Pain from the AC joint is usually experienced local to the joint. Injection of an irritant into the normal AC joint generally produces localized pain with radiation into the anterolateral neck, the trapezial region and down the anterolateral arm (21). Because the AC joint is fairly subcutaneous, palpation reproduces pain local to the joint. Hypertrophic osteophytes on the superior aspect of the joint are easily palpable. Crepitation may be appreciated with palpation during active range of motion (AROM) of the shoulder. Usually range of motion (ROM) of the shoulder is unrestricted, but pain can be experienced with end ranges of elevation. Stability of the distal clavicle is determined by assessing the degree of horizontal and inferior mobility of the distal clavicle in relation to the acromion. Pain with cross body adduction, which is localized to the AC joint, is the hallmark examination findings. Chronopoulos et al. (22) retrospectively assessed the accuracy of three common physical examination tests in detecting pathology of the AC joint: the cross arm adduction stress test, the AC joint resisted extension test, and the active compression test (O'Brien's test). The cross body adduction stress test had the greatest sensitivity (72%), and the active compression test had the greatest specificity (95%). All three tests had good negative predictive value (>94%), but poor positive predictive value (<30%). The authors showed that a combination of the three tests increased the diagnostic value for detecting AC joint pathology. Relief of pain following injection of local anesthetic into the AC joint is confirmatory of symptomatic AC joint pathology (23).

Radiographic Evaluation

Radiographic AC joint degeneration is common and must be interpreted in the context of patient symptoms and physical examination findings. Primary osteoarthritis of the AC joint is common radiographically, however, frequently asymptomatic (24–26). One study showed radiographic AC joint osteoarthritis in 54% to 57% of elderly patients (26). DePalma (27) noted degenerative changes in the majority of AC joint specimens obtained from patients following their fourth decade of life. Radiographic findings include narrowing of the joint space, subchondral sclerosis, osteophyte formation on the superior and inferior aspect of the clavicle as well as periarticular cyst formation. Inferior clavicular osteophytes can be a source of extrinsic impingement to the rotator cuff tendons (28,29). Because of the high prevalence of asymptomatic degenerative changes, treatment should be based on clinical symptoms rather than radiographic changes alone.

The standard shoulder series include an anteroposterior (AP) of the shoulder, true AP, outlet and axillary views. The AP view usually provides the best imaging of the AC joint, but the boney anatomy can be obscured by overpenetration and overlap of the scapular spine (Fig. 1). Joint space narrowing, sclerosis and osteophyte, and cyst formation are commonly seen with AC joint degeneration. The axillary view will identify anteroposterior displacement of the clavicle and the presence of an os acromiale. The Zanca view allows optimal visualization of the AC joint. This view is a modified AP view of the shoulder with the beam angulated 15° cephalad with 50% of the standard glenohumeral radiation dose (30). Subtle reactive changes within the lateral aspect of the clavicle are best appreciated with the Zanca view.

Advanced imaging is rarely indicated for the evaluation of the AC joint. Reactive edema within the clavicle on magnetic resonance imaging (MRI) is often seen in patients with symptomatic AC joint arthritis and distal clavicle osteolysis (31). However, the presence of edema in the distal clavicle does not always correlate with symptoms. Positive MRI findings are not diagnostic of AC joint pathology in the context of a normal physical examination. One recent study demonstrated increased T2 signal within the distal clavicle in 12.5% of shoulder MRI examinations, irregardless of diagnosis (32). Another study showed 82% of asymptomatic shoulders had arthritic changes of the AC joint on MRI, including two-thirds of those under the age of 30 years (33). Nonetheless, one recent study did demonstrate an association between edema on both side of the AC joint on MRI examination with the presence of clinical AC arthritis (34). Furthermore, MRI allows thorough assessment of the rotator cuff tendons, which can be irritated by inferior projecting osteophytes from a degenerative AC joint.

Surgical Indications/Contraindications

For patients with isolated AC joint pain, a single AC joint steroid injection is usually performed, followed by a three- to six-month trial of rest, activity modification, and physical therapy, if warranted. Stability of the AC joint must be carefully assessed, especially in those with a history of trauma, as distal clavicle instability may lead to persistence of symptoms postoperatively. A significant percentage of AC joint pathology is seen in association with rotator cuff disease, and a significant percentage of middle-aged patients with rotator cuff disease will have radiographic degeneration of the AC joint that is not symptomatic. Careful clinical evaluation and differential injections will identify those patients who should undergo distal clavicle excision in conjunction with subacromial decompression and/or rotator cuff repair.

The primary indication for distal clavicle excision is pain localized to the AC joint that has failed conservative treatment. The decision to perform the procedure arthroscopically is most dependent on surgeon preference. However, the presence of a large superior osteophyte may compel some surgeons to perform distal clavicle excision through an open approach. Arthroscopic resection has the advantages of preservation of the stabilizing soft tissues (the superior AC joint ligaments and deltotrapezial fascia), less postoperative pain, and quicker recovery time compared to open distal clavicle resection. The indirect (bursal) arthroscopic distal clavicle resection is favored when concomitant subacromial procedures are indicated—subacromial decompression and acromioplasty and/or rotator cuff repair. Direct (superior) arthroscopic distal clavicle excision should be reserved for patients with isolated AC joint pathology. This technique is technically difficult and usually requires the use of small joint arthroscopic equipment. Proponents of the direct arthroscopic resection cite preservation of the AC joint ligaments as a significant advantage of this technique. The presence of os acromiale (mesacromion type or larger) is a relative contraindication for concomitant subacromial decompression and AC joint resection as the os fragment may be rendered unstable and become symptomatic.

SURGICAL TECHNIQUE

Indirect (Bursal) Approach

Equipment:

1. A 4.0 mm, 30° arthroscope lens.
2. Arthroscopic fluid pump system—epinephrine can be added to the arthroscopic fluid to improve hemostasis and visualization. A 1 to 2 cc of 1:1000 concentration of epinephrine is added to each of 3 L of fluid.
3. A 7.0 or 7.5 mm working cannula.
4. Arthroscopic electrocautery wand.
5. A 4.5 mm arthroscopic shaver.
6. A 5.5 mm round or oval arthroscopic burr.

Surgery is performed in the beach chair position with the operative arm prepped free (Fig. 2). An arm holder is used both for positioning of the extremity and to provide inferior traction to the shoulder. The bony anatomy is outlined with a marking pen. Landmarks include the acromion, clavicle, AC joint, spine of the scapula, and the coracoid process. The portal incisions are marked as well: posterior, lateral subacromial, and anterior portals (Fig. 3). The lateral portal is made two fingerbreadths lateral to the acromial edge in line with the posterior aspect of the AC joint. The anterior portal is shifted slightly superior to the standard anterior portal 1.5 to 2 cm inferior to the anterior edge of the AC joint in line with the lateral edge of the coracoid. This position allows the direct access to the anterior aspect of the AC joint needed for bone removal. The subacromial space is then infiltrated with 20 cc of 0.5% marcaine with epinephrine to promote hemostasis. The skin in the region of the portal incisions is then injected with 1% lidocaine with epinephrine. If medically permissible, mean arterial blood pressure is maintained near 70 mmHg.

The skin incision for the posterior portal is made in the "soft spot" of the shoulder, generally 2 cm inferior and medial to the posterolateral edge of the acromion. The arthroscope is introduced into the glenohumeral joint. An anterior working portal is localized through the prior designated anterosuperior incision with a spinal needle. The needle is angled inferiorly and medially to enter the glenohumeral joint within the rotator interval below the biceps tendon and above the subscapularis tendon. Diagnostic arthroscopic evaluation then commences in the usual fashion. Careful inspection of the biceps tendon, superior labrum, and rotator cuff insertions is performed, as pathology with these structures can mimic or coexist with AC joint pathology.

Prior to entering the subacromial space, inferior traction is placed on the humeral head through the arm holder. The subacromial space is then swept with the cannula and blunt trocar of the arthroscope to develop the planes between the rotator cuff and acromion and the humeral head and deep deltoid fascia. Often, inferior projecting osteophytes from the anterior acromion and the clavicle can be felt with the tip of the trochar. This sweep enhances initial visualization within the subacromial space. The arthroscope is introduced into the subacromial space anteriorly. The pump pressure must be closely monitored and is generally set between 30 and 40 mmHg. This pressure range is usually adequate to maintain hemostasis while preventing early tissue edema, which can occur with higher pump pressures. The lateral subacromial portal incision is localized with a spinal needle. With the scope in the anterior aspect of the subacromial space, the needle is triangulated to the camera tip entering the skin approximately two fingerbreadths lateral to the acromion in line with the posterior aspect of the AC joint. The needle should enter the subacromial space at a flat angle. If the lateral portal is placed too superior, fluid extravasation and tissue edema will displace the portal further superiorly making bone resection difficult.

The subacromial space is cleared of bursal tissue with a shaver and cautery device through the lateral portal exposing the rotator cuff tendons inferiorly and acromion superiorly. The fatty and more vascular bursal tissue adjacent to the AC joint is best removed with the cautery device (Fig. 4). If indicated, soft tissue is removed from the anterior acromion and a subacromial decompression is performed. Removal of excess bone from the undersurface of the anterior and medial facet of the acromion improves exposure to the bursal side of the AC joint (Fig. 5). The inferior AC joint capsule and adjacent soft tissue are removed to expose the distal clavicle (Figs. 6 and 7). A spinal needle is introduced into the subacromial space through the anterior portal at the anterior aspect of the AC joint (Fig. 8). An 11 blade is introduced through this portal to release the anterior AC joint capsule (Fig. 9). The anterior portal should be localized parallel to the AC joint. Using electrocautery, the distal clavicle is further cleared of soft tissue. Manual pressure can be applied to the clavicle to improve exposure to the peripheral soft tissues. Access to the posterior aspect of the clavicle is more difficult, and the fatty tissue in this region is very vascular.

The arthroscope is then transferred to the lateral portal, improving visualization of the distal clavicle. A 7.0 to 7.5 mm cannula can be placed in the anterior portal to tamponade soft tissue bleeding, if needed. Using the anterior portal, a 5.5 mm burr is used to resect the anterior aspect of the distal clavicle, initially (Fig. 10). The width of the burr is used to judge the amount of boney resection. Generally, 5 to 6 mm of clavicle is removed creating 8 mm or more of space between the distal clavicle and the medial acromion. Resection of the clavicle proceeds in an anterior to posterior and inferior to superior direction (Fig. 11). Manual pressure can be applied to the clavicle to improve visualization of the superior bone. Care is taken to protect the superior AC joint capsule to prevent horizontal instability of the clavicle. The most common errors made during resection include inadequate resection of the posterior and superior aspect of the clavicle. The arthroscope should be placed in the anterior portal to confirm adequate and even resection of the clavicle (Fig. 12). The subacromial space is lavaged of all bony debris. The portal incisions are closed with suture.

Direct (Superior) Approach

Equipment:

1. A 2.7 mm, 30° arthroscope lens.
2. Arthroscopic fluid pump system—epinephrine can be added to the arthroscopic fluid to improve hemostasis and visualization. A 1 to 2 cc of 1:1000 concentration of epinephrine is added to each of 3 L of fluid.
3. Arthroscopic cautery wand.
4. A 2.0 mm arthroscopic shaver.
5. A 2.0 or 3.5 mm arthroscopic burr.
6. Arthroscopic rasp.

The patient is placed in the modified beach chair position with the arm draped free. The bony anatomy of the shoulder is carefully outlined with a marking pen. The anterior and posterior AC joint boundaries can be precisely localized with 22 gauge needles (Fig. 13). The anterosuperior and posterosuperior portals are marked 0.75 cm anterior and posterior to the AC joint, respectively. To improve hemostasis, the AC joint is injected with 0.5% marcaine with epinephrine. The skin in the regions of the portal incisions is infiltrated with 1% lidocaine with epinephrine.

The skin and AC joint capsule are then incised posteriorly and anteriorly with an 11 blade. A 2.7 mm arthroscope is placed in the posterior aspect of the AC joint. The pump pressure is set at 30 to 40 mmHg. A small cautery wand is initially introduced into the anterior portal to obtain hemostasis. The meniscal remnant is removed and soft tissues are cleared with cautery or a small shaver. The distal clavicle is exposed with subperiosteal elevation of the anterior, inferior, and superior capsule with electrocautery. Exposure of the peripheral cortical margins of the clavicle is needed to ensure resection of all cortical ridges of bone. Care is taken to preserve the integrity of the superior and inferior AC joint ligaments to maintain horizontal stability of the clavicle.

With the arthroscope in the posterior portal, bony resection is initiated at the anterior aspect of the clavicle (Fig. 14). The width of the burr is used to judge the amount of boney resection. Generally, 5 to 6 mm of clavicle is resected. Once the joint space has been enlarged, a larger burr can be used for more efficient resection of bone. Boney resection proceeds from an anterior to posterior manner. The arthroscope is then positioned through the anterior portal. Once the joint space has been enlarged, a 4.0 mm arthroscope can be used for enhanced visualization and higher fluid flow. The posterior aspect of the clavicle is exposed circumferentially in a subperiosteal manner. The posterior clavicle is then removed in line with the resected anterior clavicle.

Adequate resection of bone is necessary for a successful outcome. Retained cortical ridges of bone must be avoided with the direct type of arthroscopic distal clavicle resection. Elevation of the AC capsule from the periphery of the clavicle enhances visualization of the peripheral cortical bone. Final beveling of the bone can be performed with a rasp to minimize risk of damage to the surrounding soft tissues. Boney debris is lavaged from the joint. The portals are closed with suture.

POSTOPERATIVE MANAGEMENT

The operative arm is supported with a sling for comfort. The patient is instructed with pendulum exercises and elbow, wrist, and hand range of motion activities until the first postoperative visit. Sutures are removed and the sling is discontinued 7 to 10 days following surgery. From one to four weeks, range of motion is increased as tolerated advancing from passive to active assisted and active motion. Terminal elevation and horizontal adduction of the shoulder is avoided for the first month. At four weeks following surgery, stretching into terminal ranges of motion is initiated with the goal of restoring full shoulder range of motion by six to eight weeks. At six weeks, gentle rotator cuff strengthening is initiated and advanced as tolerated. Isometrics are used initially and followed by progressive resisted isotonic strengthening. The rotator cuff, deltoid, and scapular stabilizer muscles are targeted. By 12 weeks, full function and strength of the shoulder should be restored.

OUTCOMES

The outcomes of arthroscopic distal clavicle excision have compared favorably with open resection. Most patients experience a significant reduction in pain and improvement in function as measured by validated outcome scores. Both indirect and direct arthroscopic procedures produce reliable clinical results so long as an adequate amount of bone is resected and stability of the AC joint is maintained.

Snyder et al. (35) reported the results of 50 patients, following indirect arthroscopic distal clavicle excision at an average of two years follow-up. The mean age of the patients was 42 years. An average of 14.8 mm of bone was resected. The authors reported 94% good to excellent results as measured by the University of California Los Angeles (UCLA) shoulder score. There were no intraoperative complications. Gartsman (36) reviewed the results of 20 out of 26 patients two years following arthroscopic distal clavicle excision. He reported subjective improvement in 85% of patients and noted three clinical failures that were successfully treated with a revision open resection. Zawadsky et al. (37) reviewed the results of arthroscopic distal clavicle excision in 37 patients (41 shoulders) with isolated distal clavicle osteolysis. The average age of the patients was 39 years. At an average follow-up of six years, 38 shoulders were considered to have an excellent result. Three failures occurred, all of which had a traumatic etiology. Auge and Fischer (19) successfully treated 10 weightlifters with distal clavicle osteolysis with arthroscopic distal clavicle excision. The authors noted rapid return to sport and weightlifting and no clinical failures at 18 months follow-up.

Successful clinical results have also been reported following arthroscopic distal clavicle excision combined with subacromial decompression and acromioplasty. Kay et al. (38) retrospectively reviewed the results of 20 patients, following arthroscopic subacromial decompression and distal clavicle excision. Outcome scales reported in the patients included the UCLA shoulder score and Constant scores. All patients were reported to have an excellent outcome at an average of the six years postsurgery. The average UCLA score was 29.8, and the average Constant score was 98.5. There were no complications. Twenty-five percent of patients were noted to have calcifications at the distal clavicle radiographically, but were asymptomatic. Martin et al. (39) retrospectively reviewed the outcomes of arthroscopic subacromial decompression and acromioplasty with distal clavicle excision in 31 patients (32 shoulders) with a mean age of 36 years. An average of 9 mm of distal clavicle was resected. At an average follow-up of 4 year and 10 months, all patients were satisfied with their result. Twenty-six patients reported no pain, and seven shoulders had mild pain with strenuous or sporting activities. Isokinetic strength testing showed restoration of full shoulder strength. Twenty-two of 25 patients who participated in sporting activities were able to return to their prior level of activity. Levine et al. (40) reviewed the results of 24 selected patients, following arthroscopic subacromial decompression and distal clavicle excision from a bursal approach. The average duration of follow-up was 32 months. Bone resection was minimal (average 5.4 mm). Twenty-one patients were noted to have a good or excellent result and there were three clinical failures. The average pain score decreased from 4.3 to 1.8.

Flatow et al. (41) reported good clinical results, following arthroscopic distal clavicle excision from the superior (direct) approach. Forty-one patients were treated with this technique and the results were reported at a mean of 31 months following surgery. Ninety-three percent of patients with AC joint osteoarthritis (OA) or distal clavicle osteolysis had satisfactory results compared with 58 percent of those with a previous grade II AC joint separation or distal clavicle hypermobility. Residual symptoms were felt to be related to residual distal clavicle hypermobility. The amount of bone resected did not correlate with the outcome as long as a smooth, even resection was performed.

In a recent series of 66 shoulders where the direct (superior) approach (42 shoulders) was compared to the indirect (bursal) approach (24 shoulders), Levine et al. found that the indirect approach yielded slightly superior results with fewer complications than the bursal approach. Though not statistically significant, American Shoulder and Elbow Surgeons (ASES) scores averaged 94 in the indirect group and 90 in the direct group. Two patients in the direct group required reoperation for AC instability and two patients for recurrent symptoms compared to no reoperations in the indirect group. While these results support successful use of either technique, the study suggests that the superior ligaments may be more at risk with the superior approach and should be carefully preserved if this approach is used (42).

COMPLICATIONS

The most common postoperative complication of arthroscopic distal clavicle excision is persistent shoulder pain. The etiology of residual pain is likely multifactorial and can include diagnostic error, inadequate resection of bone, AC joint instability, and residual shoulder weakness (43). Diagnostic error can be avoided with careful history, physical examination, and radiographs. Selective AC joint injections are very helpful to confirm clinical suspicion of AC joint mediated pain and should be performed in cases where the clinical picture is uncertain.

Persistent AC joint pain following a traumatic event should alert the clinician to the possibility of subtle AC joint instability. Instability of the AC joint following distal clavicle excision may lead to persistent pain postoperatively (7,41,44,45). Blazar et al. (46) retrospectively examined horizontal AC joint mobility in a group of patients, following distal clavicle excision. The average increase in horizontal motion of the clavicle was 5.5 mm compared to the contralateral shoulder. The authors correlated the magnitude of translation to the visual analog pain score, but not to the amount of resected bone. The combination of iatrogenic instability and pre-existing AC joint hypermobility places patients with low-grade AC joint separations at risk for residual AC joint instability, following distal clavicle excision. Miller et al. (47) showed no difference in posterior translation of the clavicle, following direct and indirect arthroscopic distal clavicle resection (5 mm of bone resection) in a cadaveric study.

Pathology of the superior labrum can mimic the symptoms of AC joint pain. Suspicion of SLAP tears should be entertained in younger patients, throwing athletes and in those with a history of trauma to the shoulder. Berg et al. (48) reported the findings of repeat shoulder arthroscopy in 20 patients, following distal clavicle resection. Fifteen patients were found to have SLAP lesions missed at the index procedure. These patients were young (age 37 years) and the majority had a traumatic onset of shoulder pain.

Residual AC joint pain can follow an inadequate resection of bone. The concern for uneven resection or retained ridges of bone is greater with arthroscopic surgery compared to open distal clavicle resection. With the evolution of arthroscopic technique, most surgeons have advocated less resection of bone (4–6 mm) with good clinical results (19,40,41,49). Combined with the residual AC joint space and the smoothed surface of the acromial facet, 4 to 6 mm of resected clavicle usually results in 8 to 10 mm of distance between the clavicle and the acromion. Two studies have shown in separate cadaveric models that 5 mm of clavicle resection is adequate to prevent residual contact between the clavicle and the acromion (50,51). An even, parallel line of resection is likely more important than the amount of bone removed. The most common error is retained bone at the posterior and superior aspects of the clavicle.

Heterotopic ossification can occur, following distal clavicle excision. The presence of heterotopic bone formation is generally well tolerated, although one study reported the results of 20 revision procedures for the removal of extensive heterotopic bone in the subacromial space and AC joint regions, following both open and arthroscopic distal clavicle excision (52). Many series that use radiographic evaluation as an outcome tool note the presence of heterotopic bone in a minority of patients (35,38,39). The incidence of postoperative heterotopic bone has ranged from 3.2% to 25% (38,52). Risk factors may include chronic obstructive pulmonary disease, prior trauma, and/or spondyloarthropathies.

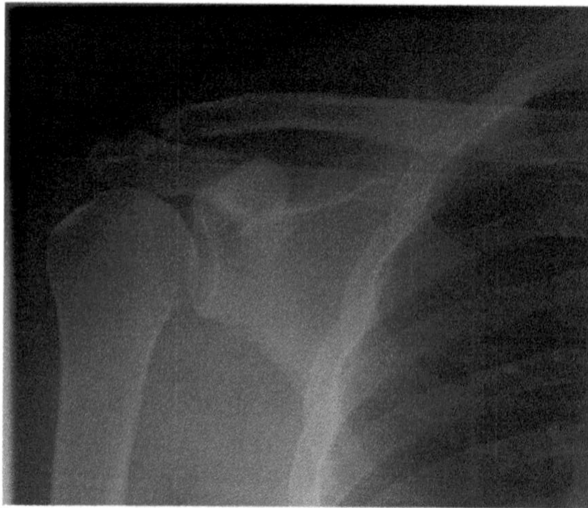

FIGURE 1 An AP radiograph of the shoulder. This patient is a 33-year-old weightlifter with right shoulder pain. Radiographs show distal clavicle osteolysis. Note the presence of subchondral cysts and localized osteopenia within the lateral clavicle.

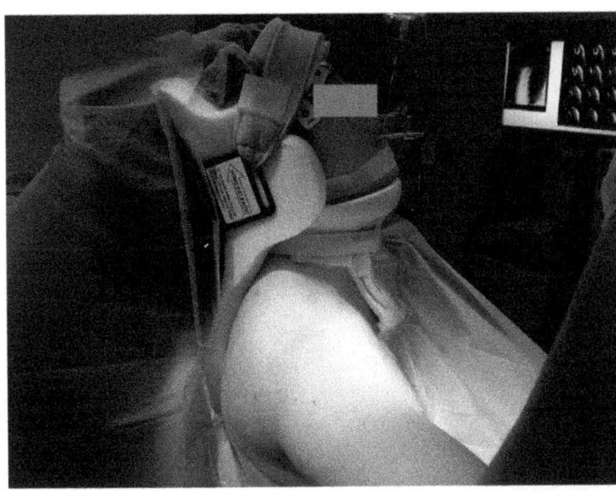

FIGURE 2 Modified beach chair position. The cervical spine is stabilized with a cervical collar. The shoulder is positioned in a manner allowing exposure to the entire shoulder, including the acromioclavicular joint.

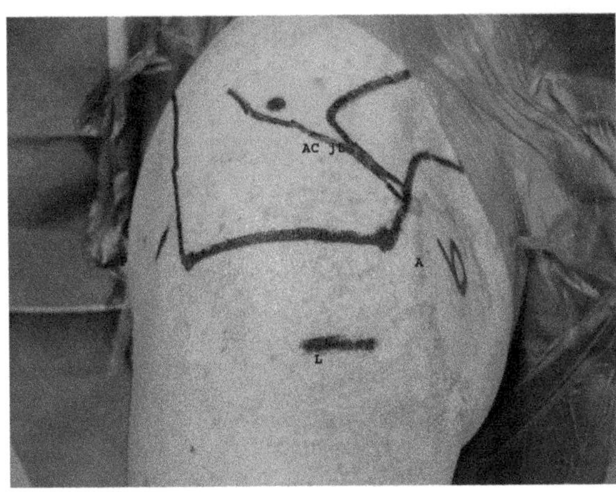

FIGURE 3 Arthroscopic portals. The boney anatomy, including the acromioclavicular (AC) joint, has been outlined. *Abbreviations*: A, anterior portal, 1.5 cm inferior to the anterior aspect of the AC joint at the lateral edge of the coracoid; L, lateral portal, two fingerbreadths lateral to the acromion centered over the posterior aspect of the AC joint; P, posterior portal, located in the posterior soft spot of the shoulder.

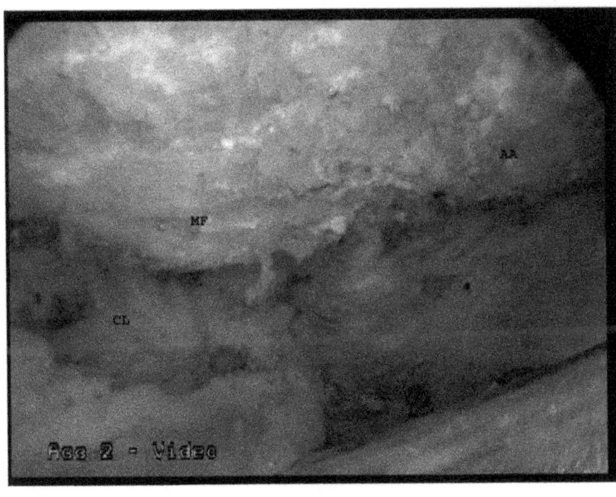

FIGURE 4 Subacromial landmarks. With the arthroscope in the posterior portal, acromial borders are outlined with cautery working from lateral to medial. *Abbreviations*: AA, anterior acromion; CL, clavicle; MF, medial facet of acromion.

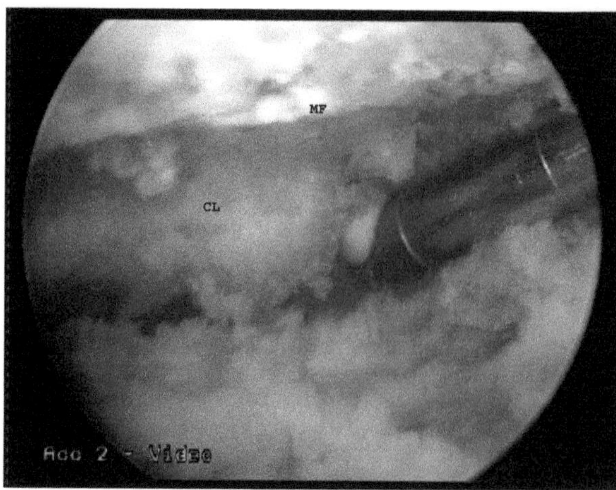

FIGURE 5 Acromioplasty of medial facet. If needed, access to the distal clavicle is facilitated by removing bone from the inferior aspect of the medial facet of the acromion. *Abbreviations*: CL, clavicle; MF, medial fact.

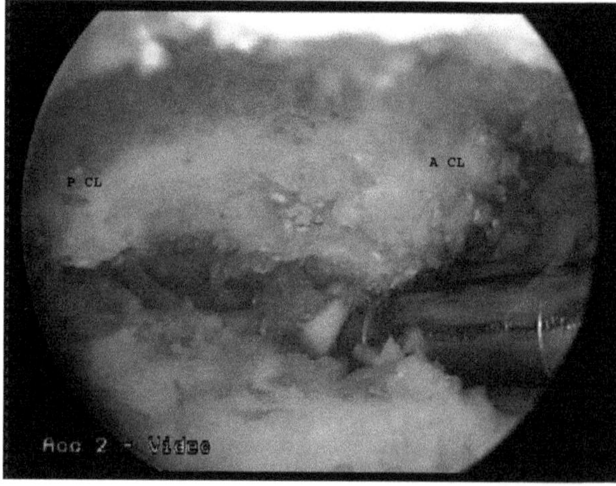

FIGURE 6 The clavicle is skeletonized. With the arthroscope in the posterior portal, the soft tissues are removed from the clavicle circumferentially. The cautery wand is in the lateral portal. *Abbreviations*: A CL, anterior clavicle; P CL, posterior clavicle.

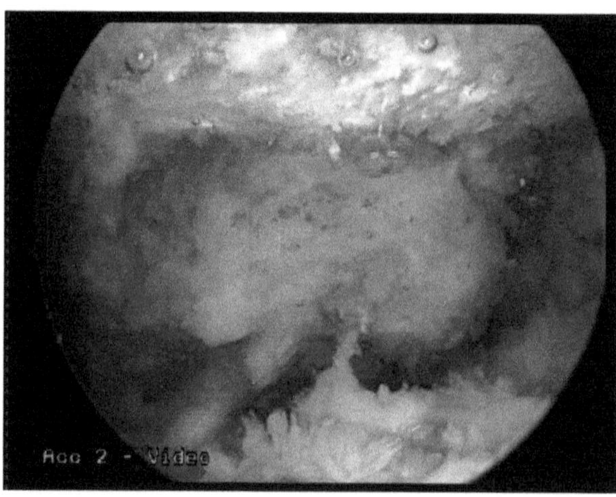

FIGURE 7 Circumferential exposure of the clavicle. The clavicle is completely exposed. The soft tissue at the posterior aspect of the clavicle must be carefully removed because of the vascularity of the tissue.

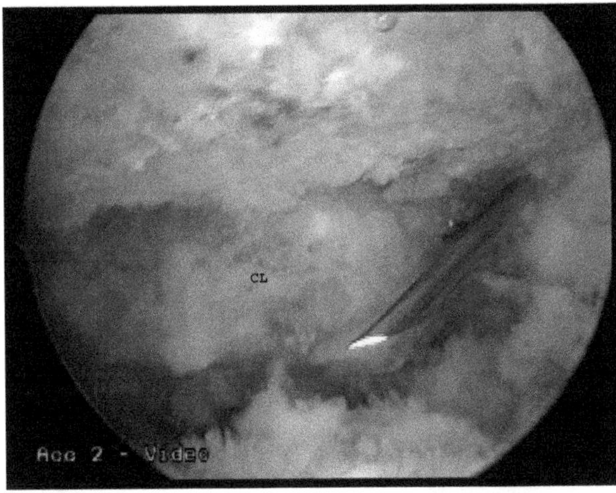

FIGURE 8 Localization of the acromioclavicular (AC) joint. A spinal needle is introduced through the anterior portal at the anterior aspect of the AC joint. The arthroscope has been transferred to the lateral portal. Entry should allow parallel access to the distal clavicle to facilitate bone removal. *Abbreviation*: CL, clavicle.

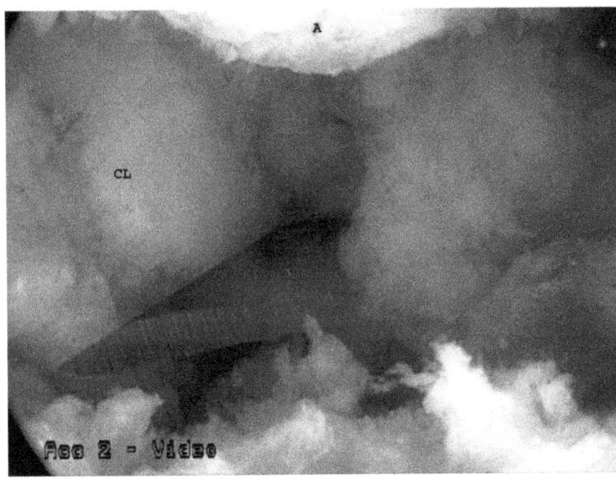

FIGURE 9 Release of the anterior acromioclavicular (AC) joint capsule. The anterior portal is enlarged by releasing the anterior aspect of the AC joint capsule. Care is taken to protect the deltoid muscle. *Abbreviations*: A, acromion; CL, clavicle.

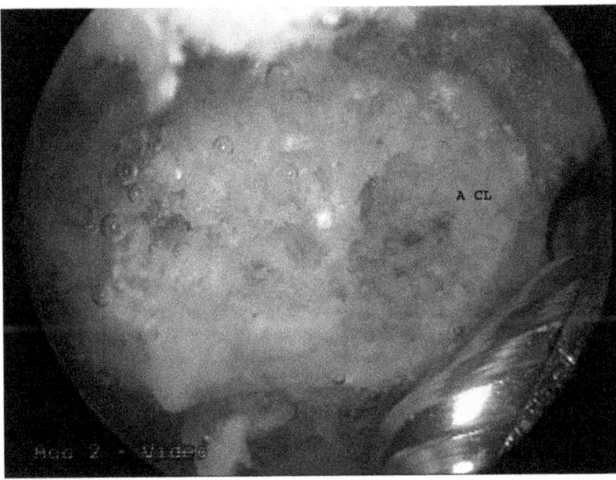

FIGURE 10 Resection of the anterior clavicle. Using a 5.5 mm burr through the anterior portal. A 5 to 6 mm of bone is removed from the anterior clavicle. Bone removal proceeds from an anterior to posterior and inferior to superior direction. Manual pressure can be applied to the clavicle to facilitate access to the clavicle. *Abbreviation*: A CL, anterior clavicle.

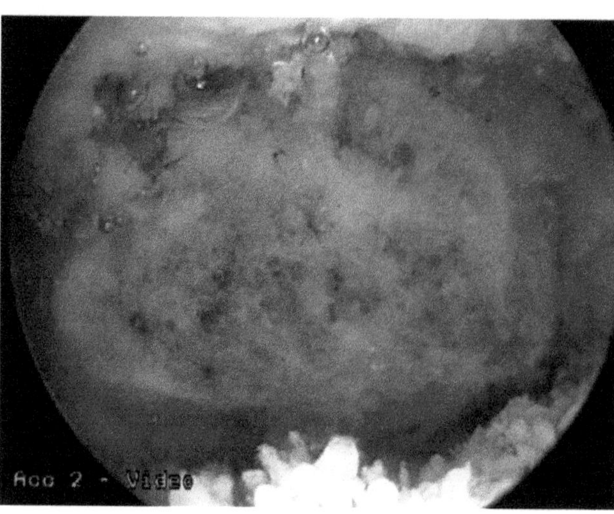

FIGURE 11 Full clavicle resection. A smooth, even line of bone resection has been performed. Care is taken to remove the posterior and superior aspect of the clavicle to prevent residual boney impingement.

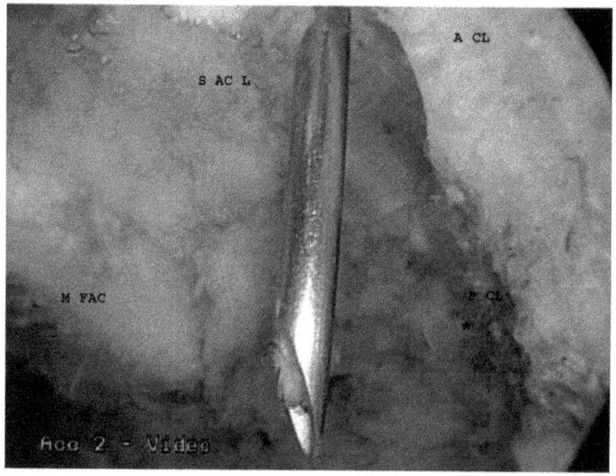

FIGURE 12 Anterior view. The arthroscope is placed in the anterior portal to confirm an adequate and even resection of bone. A spinal needle can be used to feel for residual ridges of bone. *Note*: "*" denotes small retained ridge of posterior clavicle cortex. *Abbreviations*: A CL, anterior clavicle; M FAC, medial acromial facet; P CL, posterior clavicle; S AC L, superior acromioclavicular joint ligament.

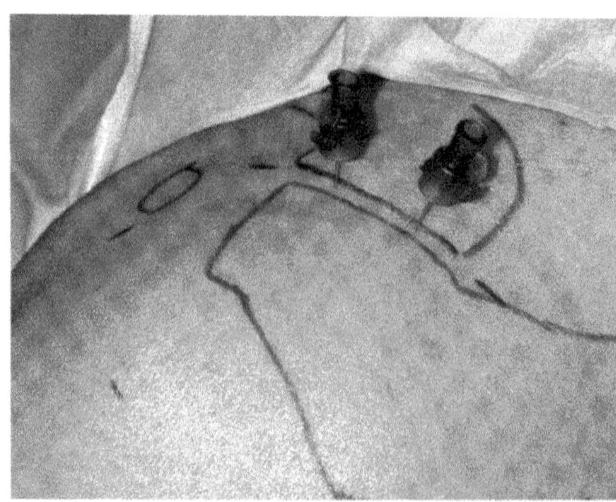

FIGURE 13 Needle localization of the acromioclavicular (AC) joint. Two small caliber needles are inserted at the anterior and posterior margins of the left AC joint. These serve as reference points for marking the anterosuperior and posterosuperior AC joint portals. *Source*: From Ref. 53.

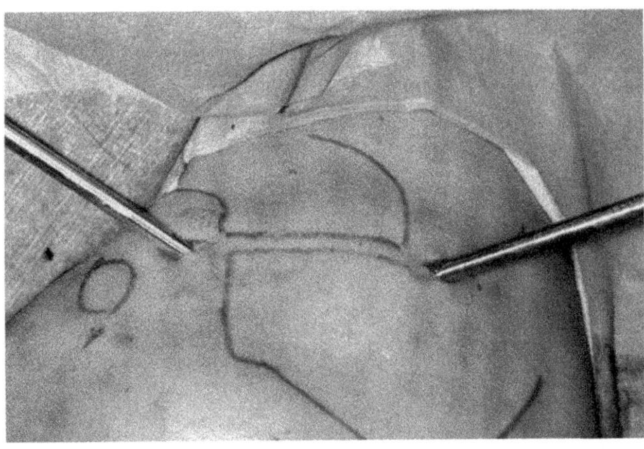

FIGURE 14 Distal clavicle resection from the direct approach. The arthroscope is located in the posterosuperior portal and the burr is in the anterosuperior portal. *Source*: From Ref. 53.

REFERENCES

1. Gurd FB. The treatment of complete dislocation of the outer end of the clavicle. Ann Surg 1941; 113:1094–1098.
2. Mumford EB. Acromioclavicular dislocation—a new treatment. J Bone Joint Surg 1941; 23:799–802.
3. Tyurina TV. Age-related characteristics of the human acromioclavicular joint. Arkh Anat Gistol Embriol 1985; 89:75–81.
4. Depalma AF. The role of the disks of the sternoclavicular and acromioclavicular joints. Clin Orthop 1959; 13:7–12.
5. Depalma AF. Surgery of the Shoulder. 2nd ed. Philadelphia: JB Lippincott, 1973.
6. Urist MR. Complete dislocation of the acromioclavicular joint: the nature of the traumatic lesion and effective methods of treatment with an analysis of 41 cases. J Bone Joint Surg 1946; 28:813–837.
7. Shaffer BS. Painful conditions of the acromioclavicular joint. J Am Ac Orthop Surg 1999; 7:176–188.
8. Fukuda K, Craig EV, An KN, Cofield RH, Chao EY. Biomechanical study of the ligamentous system of the acromioclavicular joint. J Bone Joint Surg Am 1986; 68(3):434–440.
9. Klimkiewicz JJ, Williams GR, Sher JS, Karduna A, Des Jardins J, Iannotti JP. The acromioclavicular capsule as a restraint to posterior translation of the clavicle: a biomechanical analysis. J Shoulder Elbow Surg 1999; 8(2):119–124.
10. Lee KW, Debski RE, Chen CH, Woo SL, Fu FH. Functional evaluation of the ligaments at the acromioclavicular joint during anteroposterior and superoinferior translation. Am J Sports Med 1997; 25(6):858–862.
11. Cadenat FM. The treatment of dislocations and fractures of the outer end of the clavicle. Int Clin 1917; 1:145–169.
12. Inman VT, Saunders JB, Abbott LC. Observations on the function of the shoulder joint. J Bone Joint Surg 1944; 26:1–30.
13. Rockwood CA, Williams GR, Young DC. Disorders of the acromioclavicular joint. In: Rockwood CA, Matsen FA, eds. The Shoulder. Philadelphia: W.B. Saunders Company, 1998:483–553.
14. Bergfeld JA, Andrish JT, Clancy WG. Evaluation of the acromioclavicular joint following first- and second-degree sprains. Am J Sports Med 1978; 6(4):153–159.
15. Taft TN, Wilson FC, Oglesby JW. Dislocation of the acromioclavicular joint. An end-result study. J Bone Joint Surg Am 1987; 69(7):1045–1051.
16. Petersson CJ, Redlund-Johnell I. Radiographic joint space in normal acromioclavicular joints. Acta Orthop Scand 1983; 54(3):431–433.
17. Cahill BR. Osteolysis of the distal part of the clavicle in male athletes. J Bone Joint Surg Am 1982; 64(7):1053–1058.
18. Slawski DP, Cahill BR. Atraumatic osteolysis of the distal clavicle. Results of open surgical excision. Am J Sports Med 1994; 22(2):267–271.
19. Auge WK II, Fischer RA. Arthroscopic distal clavicle resection for isolated atraumatic osteolysis in weight lifters. Am J Sports Med 1998; 26(2):189–192.
20. Murphy OB, Bellamy R, Wheeler W, Brower TD. Post-traumatic osteolysis of the distal clavicle. Clin Orthop Relat Res 1975; (109):108–114.
21. Gerber C, Galantay RV, Hersche O. The pattern of pain produced by irritation of the acromioclavicular joint and the subacromial space. J Shoulder Elbow Surg 1998; 7(4):352–355.
22. Chronopoulos E, Kim TK, Park HB, Ashenbrenner D, McFarland EG. Diagnostic value of physical tests for isolated chronic acromioclavicular lesions. Am J Sports Med 2004; 32(3):655–661.
23. Neer CS II. Shoulder Reconstruction. Philadelphia: WB Saunders, 1990.
24. Sher JS, Uribe JW, Posada A, Murphy BJ, Zlatkin MB. Abnormal findings on magnetic resonance images of asymptomatic shoulders. J Bone Joint Surg Am 1995; 77(1):10–15.
25. Bonsell S, Pearsall AWt, Heitman RJ, Helms CA, Major NM, Speer KP. The relationship of age, gender, and degenerative changes observed on radiographs of the shoulder in asymptomatic individuals. J Bone Joint Surg Br 2000; 82(8):1135–1139.
26. Horvath F, Kery L. Degenerative deformations of the acromioclavicular joint in the elderly. Arch Gerontol Geriatr 1984; 3(3):259–265.
27. Depalma AF, Callery GE, Bennett GA. Varaitional anatomy and degenerative lesions of the shoulder joint. Instr Course Lect 1949; 6:255–281.
28. Neer CS II. Impingement lesions. Clin Orthop 1983; 173:70–77.
29. Brown JN, Roberts SN, Hayes MG, Sales AD. Shoulder pathology associated with symptomatic acromioclavicular joint degeneration. J Shoulder Elbow Surg 2000; 9(3):173–176.
30. Zanca P. Shoulder pain: involvement of the acromioclavicular joint (analysis of 1000 cases). Am J Roentgenol Radium Ther Nucl Med 1971; 112(3):493–506.
31. Strobel K, Pfirrmann CW, Zanetti M, Nagy L, Hodler J. MRI features of the acromioclavicular joint that predict pain relief from intraarticular injection. Am J Roentgenol 2003; 181(3):755–760.
32. Fiorella D, Helms CA, Speer KP. Increased T2 signal intensity in the distal clavicle: incidence and clinical implications. Skeletal Radiol 2000; 29(12):697–702.

33. Stein BE, Wiater JM, Pfaff HC, Bigliani LU, Levine WN. Detection of acromioclavicular joint pathology in asymptomatic shoulders with magnetic resonance imaging. J Shoulder Elbow Surg 2001; 10(3):204–208.
34. Shubin-Stein BE, Ahmad CS, Pfaff CH, Bigliani LU, Levine WN. A comparison of magnetic resonance imaging findings of the acromioclavicular joint is symptomatic versus asymptomatic patients. J Shoulder Elbow Surg 2006; 15(1):56–59.
35. Snyder SJ, Banas MP, Karzel RP. The arthroscopic Mumford procedure: an analysis of results. Arthroscopy 1995; 11(2):157–164.
36. Gartsman GM. Arthroscopic resection of the acromioclavicular joint. Am J Sports Med 1993; 21(1): 71–77.
37. Zawadsky M, Marra G, Wiater JM, et al. Osteolysis of the distal clavicle: long-term results of arthroscopic resection. Arthroscopy 2000; 16(6):600–605.
38. Kay SP, Dragoo JL, Lee R. Long-term results of arthroscopic resection of the distal clavicle with concomitant subacromial decompression. Arthroscopy 2003; 19(8):805–809.
39. Martin SD, Baumgarten TE, Andrews JR. Arthroscopic resection of the distal aspect of the clavicle with concomitant subacromial decompression. J Bone Joint Surg Am 2001; 83-A(3):328–335.
40. Levine WN, Barron OA, Yamaguchi K, Pollock RG, Flatow EL, Bigliani LU. Arthroscopic distal clavicle resection from a bursal approach. Arthroscopy 1998; 14(1):52–56.
41. Flatow EL, Duralde XA, Nicholson GP, Pollock RG, Bigliani LU. Arthroscopic resection of the distal clavicle with a superior approach. J Shoulder Elbow Surg 1995; 4(1 Pt 1):41–50.
42. Levine WN, Soong M, Ahmad CS, Blaine TA, Bigliani LU. Arthroscopic distal clavicle resection: a comparison of bursal and direct approaches. Arthroscopy 2006; 22(5):516–520.
43. Basmania CJ, Wirth MA, Rockwood CA, Moya D. Failed distal clavicle excisions. Orthop Trans 1995; 19:355.
44. Tolin BS, Snyder SJ. Our technique for the arthroscopic Mumford procedure. Orthop Clin North Am 1993; 24(1):143–151.
45. Cook FF, Tibone JE. The Mumford procedure in athletes. An objective analysis of function. Am J Sports Med 1988; 16(2):97–100.
46. Blazar PE, Iannotti JP, Williams GR. Anteroposterior instability of the distal clavicle after distal clavicle resection. Clin Orthop Relat Res 1998; (348):114–120.
47. Miller CA, Ong BC, Jazrawi LM, et al. Assessment of clavicular translation after arthroscopic Mumford procedure: direct versus indirect resection—a cadaveric study. Arthroscopy 2005; 21: 64–68.
48. Berg EE, Ciullo JV. The SLAP lesion: a cause of failure after distal clavicle resection. Arthroscopy 1997; 13(1):85–89.
49. Bigliani LU, Nicholson GP, Flatow EL. Arthroscopic resection of the distal clavicle. Orthop Clin North Am 1993; 24(1):133–141.
50. Matthews LS, Parks BG, Pavlovich LJ Jr, Giudice MA. Arthroscopic versus open distal clavicle resection: a biomechanical analysis on a cadaveric model. Arthroscopy 1999; 15(3):237–240.
51. Branch TP, Burdette HL, Shahriairi AS, Carter FM, Hutton WC. The role of the acromioclavicular ligaments and the effect of distal clavicle resection. Am J Sports Med 1996; 24:293–297.
52. Berg EE, Ciullo JV. Heterotopic ossification after acromioplasty and distal clavicle resection. J Shoulder Elbow Surg 1995; 4(3):188–193.
53. Sellards R, Nicholson GP. Arthroscopic distal clavicle resection. Oper Tech Sports Med 2004; 12(1): 18–26.

7 Calcific Tendinitis of the Shoulder

Walter J. Song and Augustus D. Mazzocca
Department of Orthopedic Surgery, University of Connecticut Health Center, Farmington, Connecticut, U.S.A.

INTRODUCTION

Calcific tendinitis is a clinical entity of unknown cause. Calcific deposits can occur in any tendon in the body, but most commonly it involves the shoulder. Clinically, calcific tendinitis presents as an acute or chronically painful condition that is caused by inflammation around calcific deposits located in or around the rotator cuff tendons. The process involves multifocal, cell-mediated calcification of a living tendon that is usually followed by spontaneous, phagocytic resorption (1). During the deposition of calcium, the patient may have only mild or moderate pain or may be completely asymptomatic. It is believed that the condition only becomes acutely painful once the calcific deposits start to undergo resorption. After resorption or surgical removal of deposits, the tendon reconstitutes itself (2). The diagnosis is made by careful history and physical examination, with careful analysis of radiographic evidence of calcification. Initial treatment is always conservative. Nonoperative interventions include rest, immobilization, heat and cold therapy, range of motion and pendulum exercises, oral nonsteroidal anti-inflammatory medications, and subacromial steroid injections. Localized disruption of the calcifications using a "needling" technique or an extracorporeal shock wave therapy has had some success. Failure of conservative measures may lead to the need for surgical excision of the lesion, which may be performed open or arthroscopically.

HISTORY

Painter (3) in 1907 was the first to describe the radiographic findings associated with calcific tendinitis. Originally, the subacromial bursa was suspected to be the origin of calcific deposits in the shoulder. Later, Codman and others showed that the place of origin of the calcifications was the rotator cuff. Codman (4) proposed that degeneration of cuff fibers preceded calcific deposition. Bosworth (5) in 1941 prospectively reviewed radiographs, and examined 6061 employees of an insurance company and found an incidence of 2.7% of calcific deposits in the shoulder. Of these patients, 51.5% of the deposits were in the supraspinatus tendon, and 35% were previously symptomatic. Bateman made the observation in 1978 that the deposits were often near the insertion of the tendon on the greater tuberosity at the "zone of stress," an area of relative hypovascularity analogous to the current concept of the "critical zone" (6).

Over the years, many treatment options designed to reduce pain have been described. Many authors agree that calcific tendinitis is most likely self-limiting and will spontaneously resolve (7). Most authors also agree that operative treatment should only be performed when nonoperative measures are unsuccessful over 6 to 12 months. In 1902, Codman performed the first reported operative open excision of a calcific deposit (4). More recent reports of arthroscopic treatment for these deposits have shown successful results (8,9). This method continues to be the trend in current surgical management and will be the focus of this chapter.

PATHOGENESIS

The etiology of calcific tendinitis is a matter of controversy. The most common site of occurrence is the supraspinatus tendon, followed in order by the infraspinatus, teres minor,

---

Please refer to pages 83–89 for the figures in this chapter.

and subscapularis. In most reports, females are more commonly affected than males. There is up to a 10% incidence of bilaterality. Most patients with calcific deposits are asymptomatic, and patients with diabetes are more likely to be asymptomatic. According to Hurt (10), more than 30% of patients with insulin-dependent diabetes have tendon calcification. A rotator cuff tear may be seen in up to 25% of patients presenting with calcific tendinitis (11). Smaller amounts of calcification were more likely to be associated with a cuff tear.

Degenerative Calcification

Localized tissue hypoxia and compression have often been suggested as causative factors. Codman (4) and others believe that reduced tissue perfusion with subsequent degeneration and necrosis of the tendon is the starting point for the calcific deposits. McLaughlin believed that the earliest lesion is focal hyalinization of the tendon fibers, which eventually become fibrillated and locally detached. Continued motion of the tendon grinds the detached ends forming necrotic debris, which becomes calcified (12).

Opponents of the theory of degenerative calcification point out the disconnect in the age distribution of affected patients, as well as the course of the disease. Calcific tendinitis occurs most frequently in the fourth or fifth decades of life, whereas a calcification secondary to a degenerative process would increase with age. Uhthoff also believes that a degenerative process would never exhibit a potential for self-healing, whereas calcific tendinosis is ultimately self-limited. He also believes that the histologic and ultrastructural features of degenerative calcification and calcific tendinitis are different (2).

Reactive Calcification

Uhthoff has proposed the theory of reactive calcification, based on the idea that the process of calcification is actively mediated by cells in an ideal environment and the concept that formation of the calcium deposit must precede its resorption. He has divided the evolution of the disease state into three distinct stages: precalcific, calcific, and postcalcific (2).

Precalcific Stage

In the precalcific stage, there is initial fibrocartilaginous transformation of the normal tendon at the site of predilection. Histologically, there is metaplasia of tenocytes to chondrocytes, accompanied by elaboration of proteoglycans. What exactly triggers this fibrocartilaginous transformation is unknown, but tissue hypoxia remains an attractive hypothesis. There also may be an increased frequency of HLA-A1 antigen in patients with calcific tendinitis, indicating a genetic predisposition to the disease (11).

Calcific Stage

This stage is subdivided into the formative phase, the resting phase, and the resorptive phase. During the formative phase, calcium crystals are deposited in tendon matrix vesicles, which coalesce to form large deposits. Initially, there are fibrocartilaginous septa between the foci of deposits, which are generally avascular. These fibrocartilaginous septa are gradually eroded by the enlarging deposits. Grossly, the deposits during this stage have a chalky consistency.

The resting phase is heralded by the presence of fibrocollagenous tissue bordering the calcific deposits. The presence of fibrocollagen indicates that deposition of calcium at that site has terminated.

The resorptive phase begins after a variable period of inactivity of the disease process. Thin-walled vascular channels appear at the borders of the deposits, signaling the beginning of spontaneous resorption. This is followed by the appearance of macrophages and multinucleated giant cells at the periphery of the deposits. These cells phagocytose and remove the calcium. Grossly, the deposits during the resorptive phase take on the characteristic thick, toothpaste-like consistency, and the deposits are often under pressure.

Postcalcific Stage

The postcalcific stage is characterized by tendon healing. As the calcium is phagocytosed, granulation tissue containing fibroblasts and new vascular channels begin to remodel the void left by the deposits. Initially type III collagen is layed down, followed by replacement of type I collagen. Eventually, the fibroblasts and collagen fibers mature, aligning with the longitudinal axis of the tendon. Factors that precipitate the resorptive process are also unknown.

RADIOGRAPHIC EVALUATION

Calcium deposits can, for the most part, be fully evaluated on plain radiographs. A full shoulder series including an anteroposterior (AP), internal and external rotation AP, outlet view, and axillary lateral is recommended. These views can help localize the deposits to a specific tendon and show signs of possible impingement (Figs. 1–3).

DePalma and Kruper (13) classified two types of calcific deposits on plain radiographs. Type I deposits have a fluffy, cloudy appearance with a poorly defined periphery and are usually seen in patients with acute pain. Type II deposits have a well-defined periphery, with uniform density in a discrete lesion. Type II lesions are associated with subacute or chronic cases. The work of Uhthoff confirmed the observations of DePalma and Kruper. During the formative phase, pain is chronic or absent, and the deposit is dense, well defined, and homogeneous on X-ray. During the resorptive phase, the lesions are less well-defined and cloud-like, and the patient typically experiences acute pain. Rupture of the deposit can also occur during the resorptive phase, when the deposit is under pressure and has a creamy consistency. In these cases X-rays show a crescent of increased density in the subacromial space. In long-term studies, the conversion of a type II lesion to a type I is seen, but not the reverse (2).

Patte and Goutallier (14) classified lesions according to their radiographic appearance, with four types. Type I is characterized by a sharp/dense lesion, type II by blunt/dense, type III by sharp translucent, and type IV by blunt/translucent.

Magnetic resonance imaging (MRI) evaluation for isolated calcific tendinitis is not routinely indicated. Calcific deposits typically have heterogeneous low signal on both T1- and T2-weighted sequences, and generally are best seen on gradient echo sequences where the low signal "blooms" or is accentuated. T2-weighted images may show an artifactual increased signal intensity surrounding the deposit similar to edema, which can be mistaken for a full thickness rotator cuff tear. MRI is also helpful in delineating any concomitant shoulder pathology, for example, rotator cuff tear, biceps tendinopathy, and so on (Figs. 4 and 5).

NONOPERATIVE MANAGEMENT

A myriad of nonsurgical modalities have been employed to treat painful, calcific tendinitis. The goal of therapy is to control pain and maintain function. Nonsteroidal anti-inflammatory medications and a brief period of immobilization remain first line treatment options. Cold therapy is also instituted for acute pain flare-ups. The symptoms usually decrease after one week, at which time physical therapy can be instituted. Pendulum and gentle range of motion exercises may be employed to help maintain range of motion, and the patient is advised to do home exercises three to four times per day. Application of moist heat may be beneficial when the symptoms are subacute.

There is a paucity of data in regards to intrabursal steroid injection. If the patient presents with an impingement syndrome during the formative phase, an injection of steroid may be beneficial. There is some concern, however, that corticosteroid injections should not be used in a patient presenting in acute pain. If the patient is in the resorptive phase, steroids may impede spontaneous resolution (15).

During the resorptive phase, when symptoms are acute and radiographs indicate ongoing resorption, some groups advocate needling and lavage of the deposit (2). This may be useful in the resorptive phase because the deposit may be under pressure, and the consistency is more liquid than in the formative phase. The site of lavage is determined radiographically and clinically, and two large bore needles are used as inflow and outflow. Two percent lidocaine is then lavaged through the deposit, and calcium particles can be seen as they elute through the outflow needle. Ultrasound guidance at some centers has shown increased precision and promising results. Using ultrasound guided needle puncture, Farin (16) found favorable results in more than 70% of patients.

Extracorporeal shockwave therapy has been recently used to treat calcific deposits. In a series of 40 patients, Rompe (17) showed that 25 had a partial or complete disappearance of the calcific deposit after a single therapy session.

In a prospective randomized trial, Daecke et al. (18) analyzed the outcome after treatment with shock wave therapy of 115 patients with symptomatic calcific tendinitis. About 60% of patients benefited from either one or two sessions. Patients with radiographic disappearance of the lesions had higher outcome scores. At this time the procedure is still considered experimental in the United States. Longer follow-up studies, a larger patient population, and further reports from other centers are needed before recommending its routine usage.

SURGICAL MANAGEMENT

Approximately 10% of patients who do not respond to nonoperative measures require surgery. Uhthoff (2) has proposed that during the resorptive phase surgery is rarely indicated, as the process of spontaneous resolution has begun. De Seze and Welfling (19) have also stated that during the acute phase, the disease usually heals itself with only supportive measures.

Surgery is indicated for patients who have progression of their symptoms, constant pain that interferes with activities of daily living, and failure of nonoperative therapies (20). Open procedures have been performed since Codman first performed his open excision in 1902. Rochwerger (21) had favorable results in 22 patients who underwent open excision and acromioplasty. They concluded that the most favorable results were seen in those patients with more than one year between onset of disease and surgery and in those with a progressive course.

Arthroscopic excision has been shown to have outcomes equivalent to those of open procedures with shorter rehabilitation times, the possibility of better functional results, and better cosmesis (8). Ark et al. described the results of 22 patients at an average follow-up of 26 months. All patients had a minimum of one year of symptoms. Subacromial bursectomy was performed in all, 13 patients had partial removal of calcium deposits and nine had complete removal. Intraoperative fluoroscopy was not used. Results were good in 50% of patients, with full motion and complete pain relief. Forty-one percent of patients had satisfactory results with occasional pain, and 9% had unsatisfactory results with persistent pain. The two patients with persistent pain had only partial excision, however, all remaining patients with partial excision had significant pain relief. The 91% of patients who achieved good or satisfactory results is comparable to the results of open excision.

Jerosch (9) described the results of 48 patients treated with deposit removal and acromioplasty and CA ligament resection, if there was a type III acromion or mechanical changes at the bursal surface of the cuff. Intraoperative fluoroscopy was not used. Results showed that patients who had reduction or elimination of calcific deposits by postoperative radiographs had significantly better outcomes than patients without radiographic change. The addition of an acromioplasty did not significantly improve results. The authors concluded that removal of as much of the calcific deposit as possible is the ideal situation for excision.

PREFERRED METHOD

Instrumentation

Basic arthroscopic shoulder instrumentation including a standard 30° arthroscope is needed for this procedure (Fig. 6). We use disposable arthroscopic cannulas when possible to avoid fluid extravasation into the soft tissues. Our preference are The translucent Twist-In Cannulas (Arthrex, Inc., Naples, Florida, U.S.A.) for their versatility and ease of insertion. An 18-gauge spinal needle is used for localization of the calcific deposit, and a standard arthroscopic scalpel may be used for incision of the tendon. Any combination of arthroscopic curettes, rasps, and motorized shaver may be used to debride the calcific deposit. Use of a commercially available radiofrequency ablation device is useful for debridement as well.

Positioning/Setup

Debridement of calcific deposits in the rotator cuff tendon can be performed in either the beach chair or lateral decubitus position. Preference at this institution is to perform the procedure with an interscalene regional block, with the patient in the beach chair position. The block is typically administered in the preoperative holding area by the anesthesia team. The patient is then transferred to the operating room and placed supine on the operating table. A preoperative dose of prophylactic antibiotic is given before induction of anesthesia, usually a 2nd generation cephalosporin unless contraindicated. The patient is then placed in the upright beach chair position. Any positioning device that allows unobstructed mini C-arm fluoroscopy of the shoulder may be used. Disposable Velcro chinstraps and forehead restraints are used to stabilize the head and neck within the headrest, during the procedure. The bed should be slightly flexed with several pillows behind the knees to prevent the patient from sliding down the table. All bony prominences are carefully padded, and nonsterile, adhesive U-drapes are applied to the affected shoulder, taking care to allow exposure to the entire surgical field. The main video monitor is placed at the patient's feet, such that the operating surgeon behind the shoulder has an unobstructed view. A second monitor is then placed across the patient, opposite the nonoperative shoulder. This allows the assistant an unhindered view of the surgery.

An important aspect of our surgical protocol is the use of intraoperative fluoroscopy to localize the calcific deposits. Once the patient is appropriately positioned, the mini C-arm fluoroscopy unit is brought in to verify access for unobstructed internal and external rotation AP views (Fig. 7). A lead apron is placed across the patient's reproductive organs prior to any X-rays being taken. It has been our experience that an axillary lateral view is not necessary for localization of the deposits. If needed, the C-arm can be tilted to obtain 45° obliques in either direction in the transverse plane, and in combination with internal and external rotation of the arm, near orthogonal views can be obtained. Preliminary fluoroscopy images are obtained to visualize the deposits within the rotator cuff, and then the C-arm unit is withdrawn. A full examination under anesthesia is performed before the usual sterile preparation and draping. Specifically, any limitation in range of motion must be documented preoperatively. After prepping and draping, we prefer the use of a commercially available pneumatic arm positioner that obviates the need of an assistant to hold the extremity. The forearm is secured into the sterile portion of the positioning device using elastic bandages, which is then secured to the nonsterile portion of the positioning device that is attached to the operating table. A foot pedal allows the hands-free modulation of the pneumatic pump, allowing positioning of the extremity anywhere in space (Fig. 8).

Surgical Technique

The major bony anatomical landmarks are first outlined with a surgical marker. These include the borders of the acromion, the clavicle, the scapular spine, the acromioclavicular joint, and the coracoid process. The posterior soft spot of the shoulder is then palpated and marked. Typically, this is about 2 cm inferior and 1 cm medial to the posterior lateral corner of the acromion. A standard posterior viewing portal is then created. A stab incision in skin is made using an 11 blade, and the blunt obturator and trocar is used to access the joint. We typically do not insufflate the joint prior to camera insertion, nor do we turn on the inflow until the joint is visualized. This "dry" view can give some idea of any intra-articular synovitis before the joint is bathed in fluid (Fig. 9).

The inflow is then turned on, aided by an arthroscopic pump. A complete diagnostic arthroscopy is then performed, including visualization of the cartilage, labrum, biceps anchor and tendon, and the articular surface of the rotator cuff. Any intra-articular pathology can be addressed as appropriate at this point. A careful evaluation of the rotator cuff can be performed by abducting the arm to 30° with downward traction (Fig. 10). Any thickened areas or areas of hyperemia or tearing can be marked with an absorbable monofilament suture, such as a #1 PDS (Ethicon, Inc., Somerville, New Jersey, U.S.A.), to facilitate locating the corresponding cuff area on the bursal side. This is accomplished by introducing an 18-gauge spinal needle from laterally inferior to the lateral edge of the acromion directly into the area of question until the needle passes intra-articular. Again, the area of involvement is most commonly at the leading edge of the supraspinatus tendon, about 1 cm proximal to the insertion on the greater tuberosity. Once the needle passes through the tendon, there is often a small amount of calcium debris lodged in the needle tip. The suture is then threaded through the needle and brought out through a standard anterior portal in the region of the rotator interval. We like to establish our anterior portal using an outside-in technique, localizing with an 18-gauge spinal needle, making a stab incision, and then inserting a Twist-In disposable cannula. Once the suture end is brought out the anterior cannula, the lateral spinal needle is removed taking care not to pull out the PDS suture. Care must be taken to place the suture in a position away from the site of the lateral portal that will be created during the subacromial portion of this procedure.

At this point, the glenohumeral portion of the procedure is complete, and the arm is positioned to view the subacromial bursa. The arthroscopic sheath and the blunt trocar are redirected superiorly into the subacromial space. A gentle sweeping motion can help to release any bursal adhesions. A partial bursectomy allows complete visualization of the rotator cuff, and this is best accomplished using a 4.85 mm arthroscopic shaver and the radiofrequency ablation device through a lateral portal. The lateral portal is established at the level of the posterior border of the acromioclavicular joint, approximately 2 to 3 cm inferior to the lateral border of the acromion. An 18-gauge spinal needle is first introduced and visualized, followed by a stab incision and visualization of a blunt trocar. A Twist-In plastic cannula may be inserted at this point, and accessory lateral portals may be created as needed. Once an adequate bursectomy is performed, the cuff may be evaluated. If a PDS suture was passed previously, the corresponding cuff on the bursal side can be located and evaluated. Often there will be fraying or partial thickness tearing at the site of involvement (Fig. 11).

After the subacromial examination is complete, the precise localization of the calcific deposits using mini C-arm fluoroscopy is performed. The C-arm unit is dressed with a sterile plastic cover and is brought back into position for AP X-rays. An 18-gauge spinal needle is inserted from a lateral position, near to the established lateral portal. It is placed into the cuff in the area of the suspicion as seen from the bursal side or into the corresponding area marked with our PDS suture. Fluoroscopic images are then taken in internal and external rotation, with 45° oblique views if needed. Images should demonstrate the needle entering the deposit on all views, and the A-P and medial-lateral dimensions can be approximated (Figs. 12A–C). The needle is then left in the center of the deposit, and the C-arm unit is withdrawn (Fig. 13). A second 18-gauge spinal needle may be used to "needle" the area marked by the localization needle. After each puncture, the tip of the needle should be observed for any evidence of calcium captured in the central bore. If the deposit is of especially liquid consistency or under pressure, calcium may extravasate directly from the needle holes, creating the so-called "snow-storm" effect. After the deposit is confirmed, a knife is introduced through the lateral cannula to incise the involved area in line with the fibers of the cuff (Fig. 14). At this point the deposit is unroofed, and a probe can be introduced to agitate and loosen up the deposit. A curette or motorized shaver can now be introduced into the deposit to debride out the calcium, and the contents should be clearly visible (Figs. 15 and 16). Switching the viewing portal to lateral and working from the anterior, posterior, or accessory lateral portal is often necessary to adequately debride the deposit. The goal should be complete removal of the calcific deposit. Once the deposit is completely removed, the subacromial space is thoroughly irrigated to remove any remaining debris.

After complete debridement, the defect in the rotator cuff should be inspected, and the surgeon must decide if any repair of the cuff is necessary. We feel that if the residual defect is small, the depth of involvement is less than 50%, and the tendon edges are smooth and well opposed, then allowing the cuff to heal primarily can be considered. Our preference is to try and completely excise the calcific deposit, and rarely is this possible through such a limited tenotomy. Sometimes a side-to-side cuff repair with #2 FiberWire suture (Arthrex, Inc., Naples, Florida, U.S.A.) is adequate for repair if the tendon ends are well opposed and tension free at the longitudinal split. If the defect is large, greater than 50% in depth, or if the insertion of the tendon has been debrided off of bone at its base, then we prefer to perform a suture anchor repair.

With the arthroscope in the lateral viewing portal, a 5.0 mm Corkscrew anchor preloaded with two #2 FiberWire sutures is inserted just off the edge of the articular surface of the humerus, at the site of tendon debridement. The anchor is usually inserted through an accessory anterolateral portal. Care is taken to maintain an approximately 45° angle of entry relative to the greater tuberosity. The suture limbs are pulled out of the anterior cannula with a crochet hook and a 3 cm, crescent shaped Spectrum suture needle (Linvatec, Inc., Largo, Florida, U.S.A.) loaded with a strand of #1 PDS suture is placed through the posterior cannula. The needle and suture are passed from deep to superficial, at either the anterior or posterior aspect of the cuff defect. The PDS suture is retrieved out the anterolateral portal. Now the single limb of FiberWire in the anterolateral cannula to the PDS is tied using a simple knot, with a dilator knot placed in the PDS as far away from the FiberWire as possible. The FiberWire is now passed through the cuff by pulling the PDS through the posterior cannula and retrieve the FiberWire (Fig. 17). After isolating the corresponding opposite limb of the suture in the anterior cannula, it is transferred to the anterolateral cannula using a crochet hook making sure not to unload the anchor. The first limb of the suture is then brought out through the anterolateral cannula in a similar manner. A simple knot is tied using a Duncan Loop or other sliding knot. The process is then repeated for the second suture, spacing the sutures to achieve a tight, tension-free repair (Figs. 18 and 19).

After cuff repair, an acromioplasty is performed if indicated. We typically perform an acromioplasty if there is a large spur on preoperative outlet view radiographs, and the patient clinically has signs of an impingement syndrome. We use a cutting block technique using an acromial burr from the posterior portal, finishing with a handheld rasp, which provides tactile feedback as to the adequacy of resection.

Postoperative Care

We support the arm in an Ultra Sling (dj Orthopedics, Inc., Carlsbad, California, U.S.A.) postoperatively. If no rotator cuff repair has been performed, then full passive- and active-assisted range of motion exercises are started immediately. Patients with calcific tendonitis are prone to postoperative stiffness, and home exercises should be encouraged at least three to four times daily. Once full range of motion has been restored, active range of motion exercises are started with progressive shoulder strengthening. If a rotator cuff repair has been performed, then active motion is not allowed for six weeks. Active-assisted range of motion is instituted from 6 to 12 weeks, and strengthening is instituted from 12 to 24 weeks. The goal of rehabilitation is to achieve full motion and strength by six months postoperatively.

Complications

Intraoperative complications are rare and usually associated with the technical aspects of the procedure. Complications associated with surgical treatment of calcific tendinitis include failure to provide pain relief, insufficient calcium deposit debridement, rotator cuff damage, and postoperative stiffness. These complications can be avoided with meticulous surgical technique and appropriate rehabilitation.

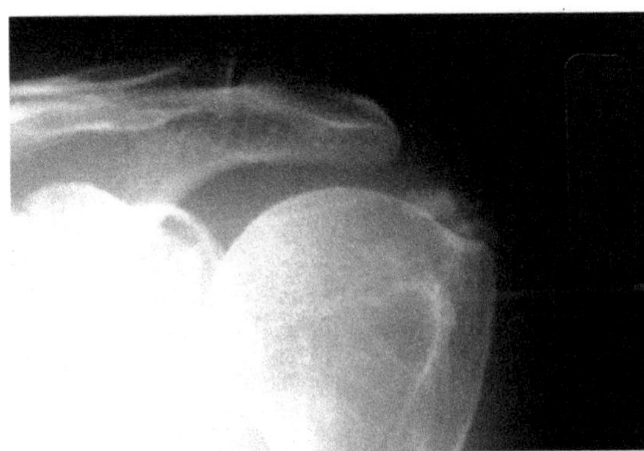

FIGURE 1 External rotation AP radiograph demonstrates the presence of a large calcific deposit within the supraspinatus tendon, just proximal to its insertion at the greater tuberosity.

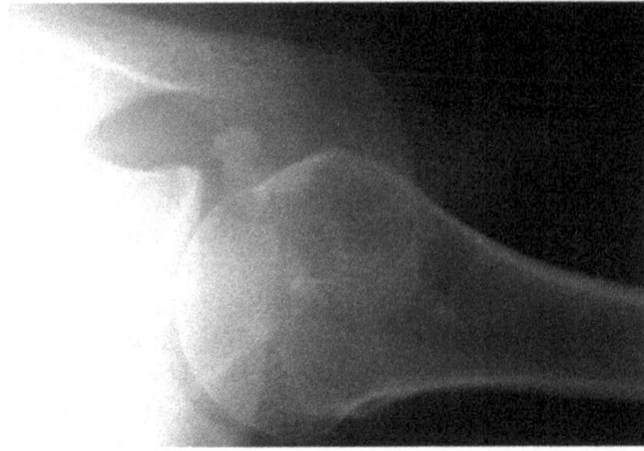

FIGURE 2 Axillary lateral radiograph demonstrating the calcific deposit at the leading edge of the supraspinatus tendon. This view is useful in localizing the deposit in the AP plane.

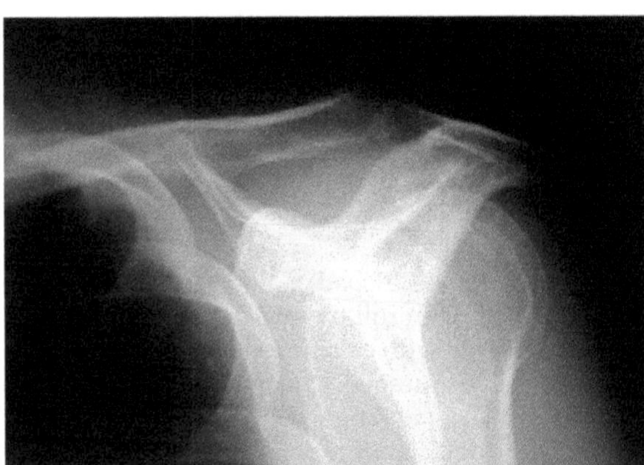

FIGURE 3 Outlet view radiograph demonstrating calcific deposit in the supraspinatus tendon. Acromion morphology may be viewed on this view.

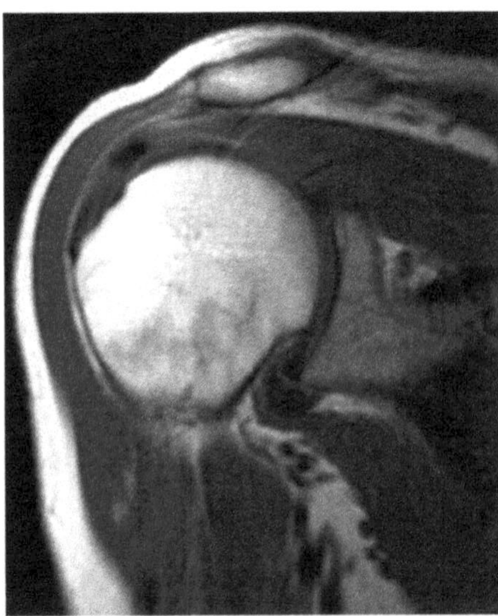

FIGURE 4 T1-weighted coronal-oblique magnetic resonance imaging shows the area of calcification as a discrete focus of low signal.

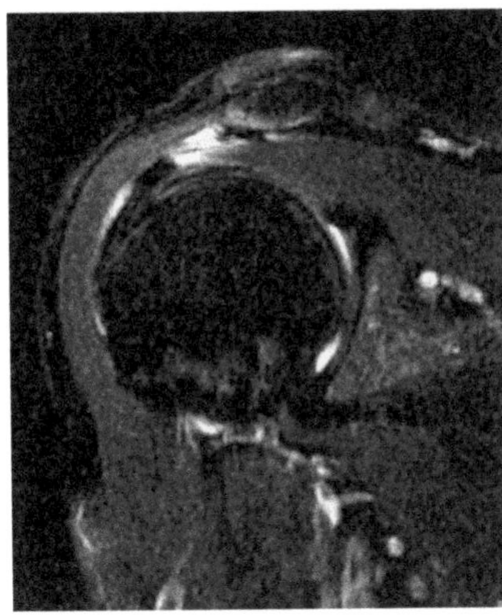

FIGURE 5 T2-weighted coronal oblique images show area of low signal corresponding to the calcification seen on T1-weighted images. Surrounding increased signal may be artifactual and could be misinterpreted as a rotator cuff tear.

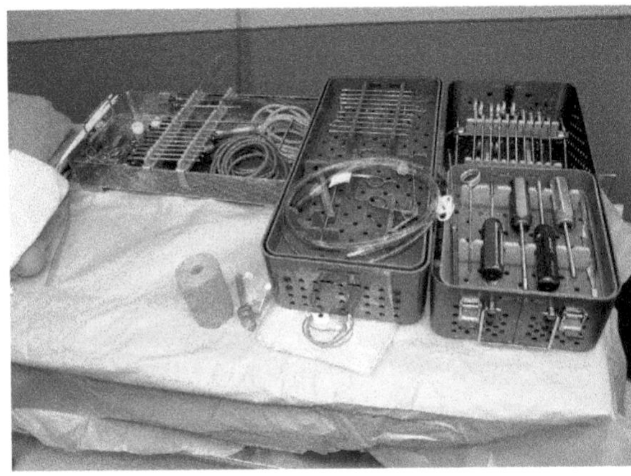

FIGURE 6 Basic arthroscopic shoulder instrumentation set, with disposable cannulas.

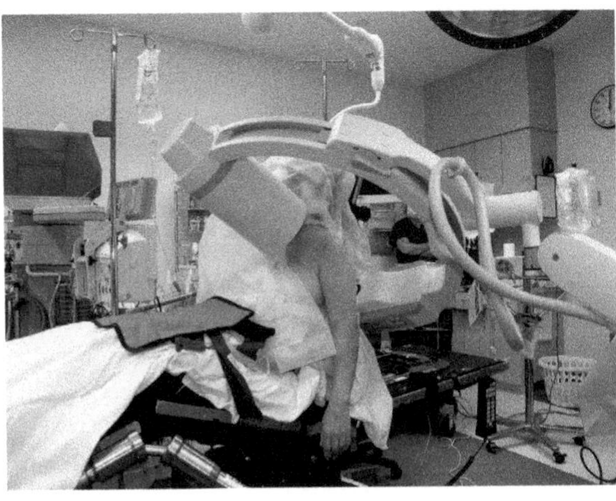

FIGURE 7 Patient setup in beach chair positioner with mini C-arm fluoroscopy unit in appropriate position.

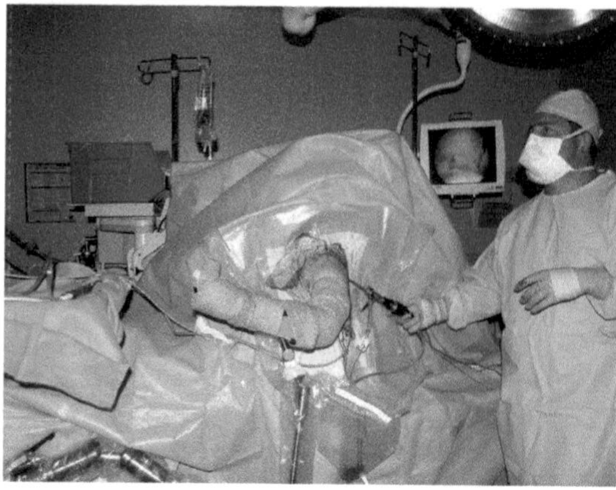

FIGURE 8 Patient prepped and draped in beach chair positioner. Note the pneumatic arm holding device, positioning the arm in space. The main monitor is at the patient's feet, and the secondary monitor is behind the patient's right shoulder.

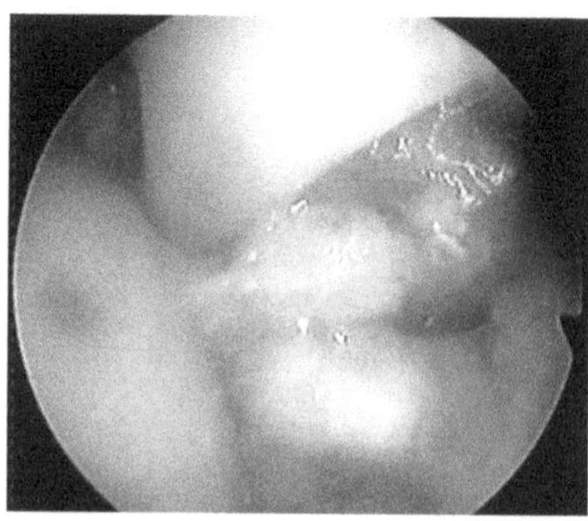

FIGURE 9 "Dry" intra-articular view from posterior portal to access synovitis. After pump aided inflow is turned on, any evidence of synovitis may be masked by a tamponade effect secondary to increased intra-articular pressure.

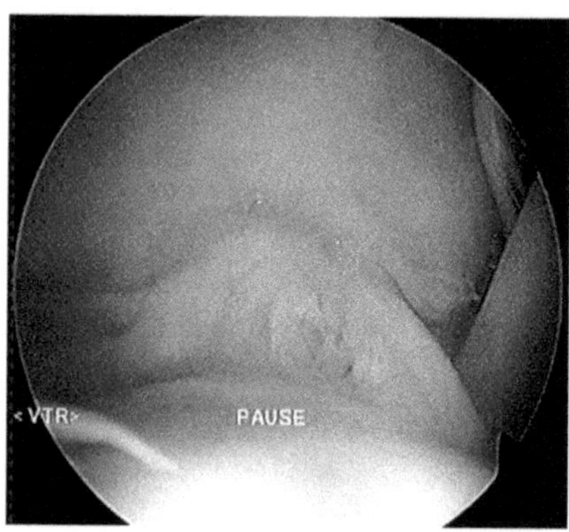

FIGURE 10 Arthroscopic photograph of the articular surface of the rotator cuff viewed from the posterior portal. Any areas that are thickened, hyperemic, or damaged can be examined and marked with a PDS suture. Note the bulging and fraying at the leading edge of the tendon.

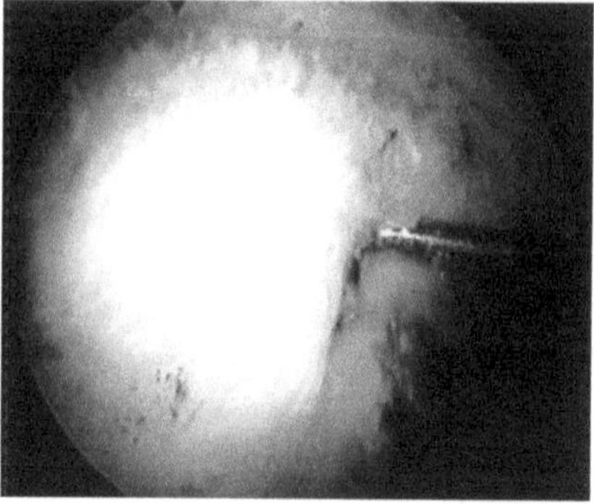

FIGURE 11 Arthroscopic photograph of the bursal surface of the rotator cuff. Note the bulging and fraying. The area of calcific deposit is firm to palpation with the probe.

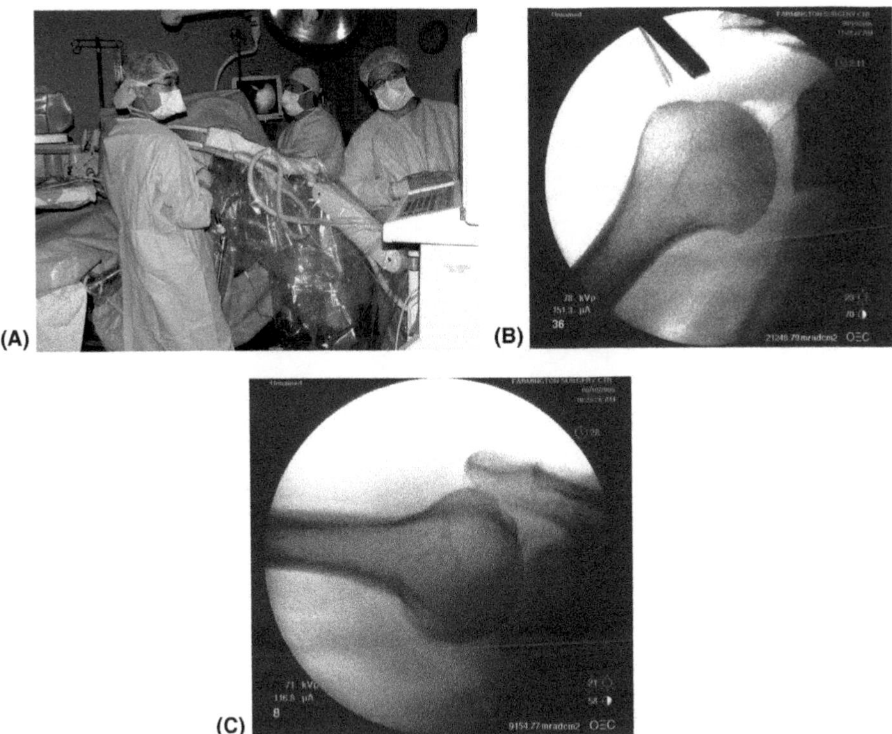

FIGURE 12 (**A**) Mini C-arm fluoroscopy used intraoperatively to precisely localize the calcific deposit. (**B**) Internal rotation AP fluoroscopic image shows spinal needle penetrating the calcific deposit. (**C**) External rotation AP fluoroscopic image shows spinal needle in the deposit. The orthogonal views of the deposit can be provided by 45° oblique views with internal and external rotation of the arm.

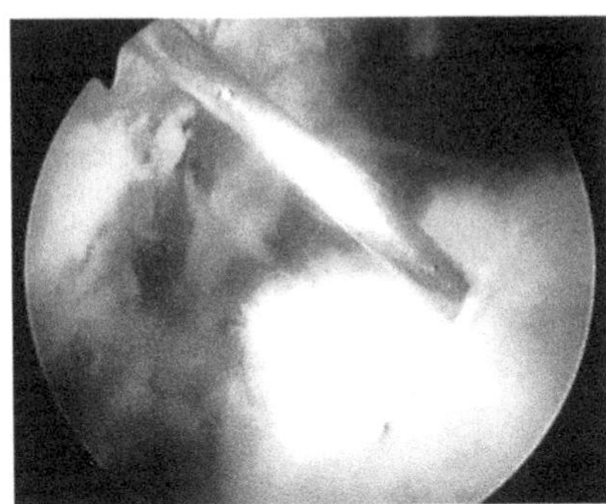

FIGURE 13 Arthroscopic photograph demonstrating the spinal needle inserted into the calcific deposit, as viewed from the posterior portal into the subacromial space of left shoulder.

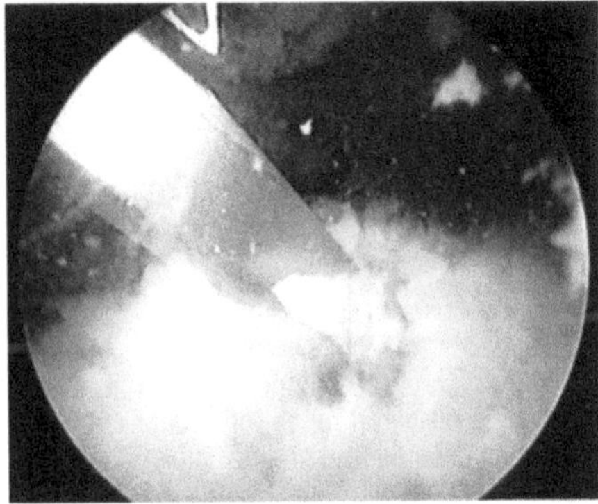

FIGURE 14 A #11 blade is used to incise the tendon directly overlying the deposit, in line with the tendon fibers. Note the localizing needle has been withdrawn just off tendon.

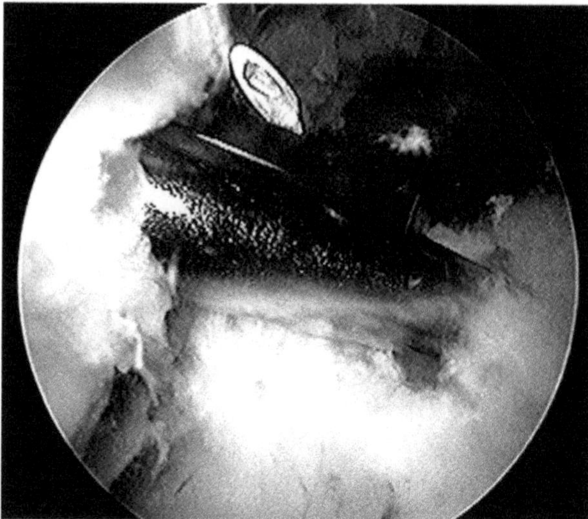

FIGURE 15 Motorized arthroscopic shaver is used to debride the calcific deposit.

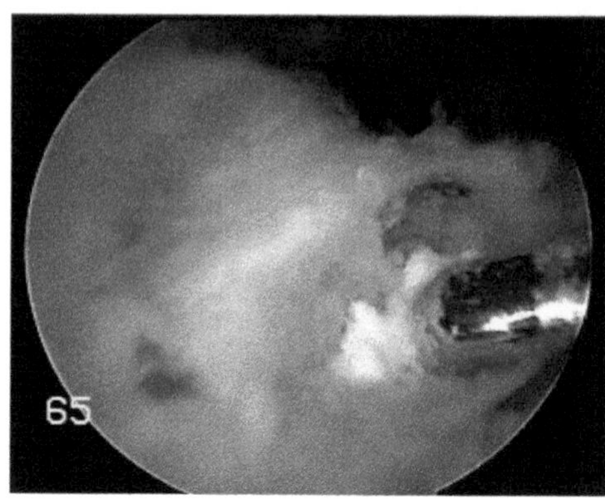

FIGURE 16 Arthroscopic photograph of a calcific deposit being debrided with a motorized shaver. The calcium is often characterized by a cheesy or toothpaste-like consistency and is often under pressure. Note the localizing PDS suture that was placed previously during the intra-articular portion of the procedure.

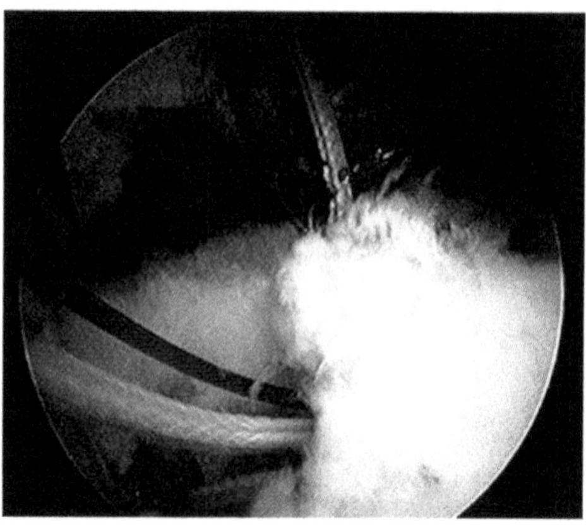

FIGURE 17 Photograph of the second limb of a horizontal mattress suture being relayed through the rotator cuff. The first limb has already been passed and is visible in the anterior cannula.

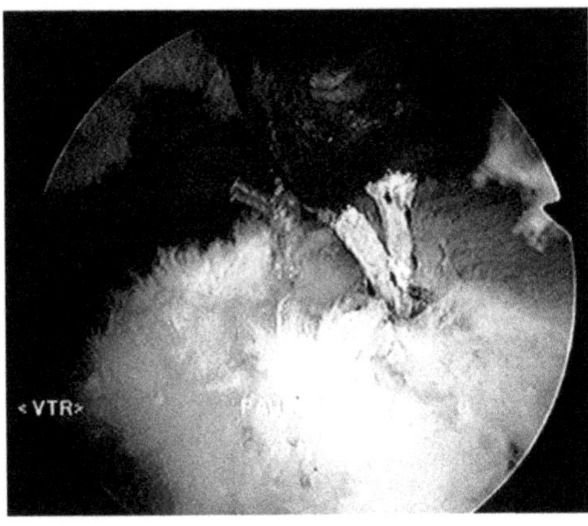

FIGURE 18 Completed rotator cuff repair with two horizontal mattress sutures tied over a single metal suture anchor. The repair is anatomic and tension free.

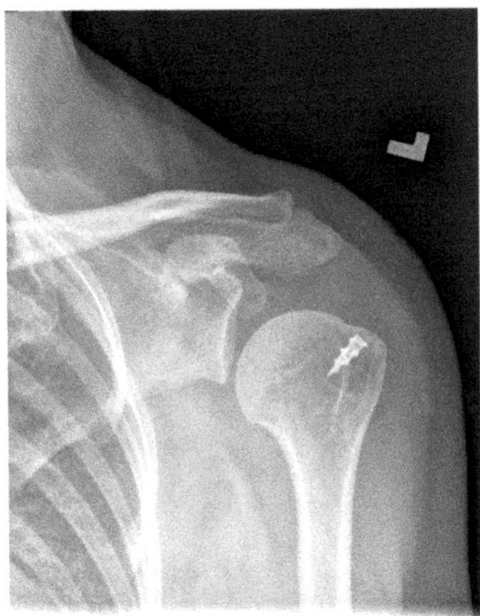

FIGURE 19 Postoperative external rotation AP radiograph demonstrating complete excision of the calcific deposit. The metal suture anchor is in good position.

REFERENCES

1. Uhthoff HK, Sarkar K. Calcifying tendonitis. In: Rockwood Jr CA, Matsen III FA, eds. The Shoulder. Vol. 2. Philadelphia: W.B. Saunders, 1990:774–790.
2. Uhthoff HK, Loehr JW. Calcific tendinopathy of the rotator cuff: pathogenesis, diagnosis, and management. J Am Acad Orthop Surg 1997; 5(4):183–191.
3. Painter C. Subdeltoid bursitis. Boston Med Surg J 1907; 156:345–349.
4. Codman EA. The Shoulder: Rupture of the Supraspinatus Tendon and Other Lesions in or About the Subacromial Bursa. Boston: Thomas Todd Co., 1934:178–215.
5. Bosworth BM. Calcium deposits in the shoulder and subacromial bursitis, a survey of 12,122 shoulders. JAMA 1941; 116(22):2477–2482.
6. Bateman JE. The Neck and Shoulder. Philadelphia: W.B. Saunders, 1978:211–218.
7. Wainner RS, Hasz M. Management of acute calcific tendinitis of the shoulder. JOSPT 1998; 27(3): 231–237.
8. Ark JW, Flock TJ, Flatow EL, et al. Arthroscopic treatment of calcific tendinitis of the shoulder. Arthroscopy 1992; 8(2):183–188.
9. Jerosch J, Strauss JM, Schmiel S. Arthroscopic treatment of calcific tendinitis of the shoulder. J Shoulder Elbow Surg 1998; 7(1):30–37.
10. Hurt G, Baker CL. Calcific tendinitis of the shoulder. Orthop Clin North Am 2003; 34:567–575.
11. Sengar DPS, McKendryl RJ, Uhthoff HK. Increased frequency of HLA-A1 in calcifying tendinitis. Tissue Antigens 1987; 29:173–174.
12. McLaughlin HL. Lesions of the musculotendinous cuff of the shoulder. Ann Surg 1946; 124:354–362.
13. DePalma AF, Kruper JS. Long term study of shoulder joints affected with and treated for calcific tendinitis. Clin Orthop 1961; 20:61–72.
14. Patte CF, Goutallier D. Calcifications. Rev Chir Orthop 1988; 74:277–278.
15. Dalton SE. The Shoulder. In: Klippel JH, Dieppe PA, eds. Rheumatology. 2nd ed. Vol. 1. London: Mosby, 1998:4.7.1–4.7.14.
16. Farin PU, Rasanen H, Jaroma H, et al. Rotator cuff calcifications: treatment with modified US-guided fine-needle technique. Radiology 2001; 221(2):45–61.
17. Rompe JD, Rumler F, Hopf C, et al. Extracorporoeal shock wave therapy for calcifying tendinitis of the shoulder. Clin Orthop 1995; 321:196–201.
18. Daecke W, Kusnierczak D, Loew M. Extracorporeal shockwave therapy (ESWT) in tendinosis calcarea of the rotator cuff: long-term results and efficacy. Orthopade 2002; 31:645–651.
19. De Seze S, Welfling J. Tendinites calcifiantes. Rhumatologie 1970; 22:45–50.
20. Gschwend N, Scherer M, Lohr J. Die tendinitis calcarea des schultergelenks (T.c.). Orthopade 1981; 10:196–205.
21. Rochwerger A, Franceschi JP, Viton JM, et al. Surgical management of calcific tendinitis of the shoulder: an analysis of 26 cases. Clin Rheumatol 1999; 18(4):313–316.

8 Arthroscopic Anterior Instability Repair

Jeffrey S. Abrams
Princeton Orthopaedic & Rehabilitation Associates, Princeton, New Jersey, U.S.A.

INTRODUCTION

Arthroscopic techniques to treat shoulder instability are fast becoming the gold standard of treatment (1). Reasons for this increased popularity extend beyond the morbidity of an arthrotomy and incision. Many surgeons have recognized improved visualization of the articular damage, access to multiple quadrants of the shoulder, the ability to create an anatomical repair, and the avoidance of some of the complications associated with the open surgical approach. Patient satisfaction is no longer limited to whether or not a shoulder dislocation will recur, but rather whether they can return to overhead activities that often require external rotation of the shoulder. As recurrence rates of open and arthroscopic techniques become comparable, and improved life-style with return to sports has been accomplished, arthroscopic instability repairs have been embraced by patients who wish to continue with athletics.

Anterior shoulder instability was once regarded in terms of the presence or absence of dislocation. Orthopedic and sports medicine physicians have identified athletes who have been disabled as a result of abnormal symptomatic shoulder translations that have resulted in pain and loss of function. Although many athletes may be able to demonstrate a "loose" shoulder, this is not unstable unless symptoms of instability are reproduced with excessive glenohumeral translation. We now know there are loose shoulders that acquire a minor traumatic event to create symptomatic shoulder instability, as well as severe trauma that can create shoulder instability in a normal or tight shoulder.

When trying to decide on proper treatment for a patient following a shoulder dislocation or subluxation, we have to recognize the importance of instability recurrences. A common theme in identifying failure in arthroscopic stabilization has been bone loss involving the anterior glenoid rim (bony bankart) or the posterior humeral head (Hill-Sachs). Shoulders that have experienced multiple dislocations are more likely to have greater degrees of bone loss than those with infrequent or rare recurrence (Fig. 1). As we identify individuals at greater risk for recurrence due to young age or patients who participate in activities that place the shoulder at risk, surgeons may argue that early intervention may be necessary to prevent the development of bone loss. Patients can be evaluated preoperatively with X-rays, computed tomography (CT) scans, or magnetic resonance imaging (MRI), and intraoperatively with arthroscopy to determine whether the remaining articular surface is adequate for an arthroscopic repair or whether a bone graft should be considered.

Results of open stabilization judged as the ability to prevent future dislocations have been excellent and have been considered the gold standard of treatment. Patients who had experienced pain, continued to have apprehension, or who avoided sports and activities may still be considered successful results, if dislocation recurrence was avoided. Persistent shoulder dysfunction was equally apparent after nonoperative treatment in some of the patients with first-time dislocations. It was demonstrated that life-style parameters according to the patients were reduced when surgical repair was delayed (2). However, patient expectations include additional variables other than the future risk of shoulder dislocation; patients expect to return to overhead sports, expect near normal range of motion, the ability to participate in pain-free activities, as well as the avoidance of instability recurrence.

Technological advances have allowed the arthroscopic approach to create an anatomical repair. This begins with articular evaluation and identification of tissue damage that has resulted

---

Please refer to pages 100–103 for the figures in this chapter.

from instability events. Anterior shoulder instability can have multiple lesions, including labral avulsion, labral tears, incompetent or torn middle and inferior glenohumeral ligaments, lateral capsule detachments, superior labral and rotator interval tears, rotator cuff tears, glenoid rim fractures, and impression defects on the humeral head. The arthroscope has its greatest success at anatomically repairing the soft tissue deficiencies. Although bone loss is recognized as a risk factor for postsurgical recurrence, the amount of bone loss placing shoulders at risk continues to be evaluated. Arthroscopic solutions to bone loss are being developed and will likely be an option in the future.

The anatomic repair has become the gold standard of shoulder instability reconstruction. Extra-articular repairs that created an excessive loss of external rotation have been replaced with capsular repairs (3). Techniques of tissue fixation to the glenoid articular margin using suture anchors have demonstrated improved arthroscopic stabilization rates. Capsular plication techniques to reinforce deficient ligaments and to create a balanced surgical repair have continued to demonstrate improved outcomes. Instrumentation and technology continue to evolve and become more familiar to surgeons who have become proficient with shoulder arthroscopic repairs.

In order for new technology to replace the old, surgical complications need to be avoided. Articular cartilage injury from displaced suture anchors can be minimized with proper anchor placement. The replacement of metallic anchors with other biologic materials may reduce this risk. Techniques that alter the viability of the capsular ligaments, that is, thermal, have had reduced enthusiasm due to complications, including capsular ablation and axillary nerve injury (4). Recent reported complications of chondrolysis have been associated with thermal techniques, reduced articular outflow resulting in temperature and pressure elevations, suture materials, and catheter pain pump utilization (5,6). Although the etiology of this catastrophic complication is unknown, current recommendations of implants and techniques attempt to minimize this risk. Degenerative arthritis of the shoulder due to overconstraint has improved with anatomical repairs that do not attempt to over-constrain the shoulder. Future developments will include direct tissue stabilization to prepared glenoid margins, management of bone deficits, and techniques to accelerate the biologic soft tissue reattachment to bone, allowing for an accelerated rehabilitation program.

INDICATIONS

The indications for arthroscopic instability repair have expanded due to technological advances, improved surgical results, patients' interests in returning to preinjury levels of activity. Patients with symptomatic anterior instability can be considered for arthroscopic instability repair. There are several subcategories that have been identified, including first-time dislocators, recurrent shoulder dislocators or subluxators, and patients undergoing revision surgery after prior surgical repair.

Patients with an initial shoulder dislocation may have experienced a single isolated event or may experience subluxation, following the index dislocation. Age and activity level are the greatest risk factors associated with recurrence. Patients under the age of 19, contact and collision sport athletes, and those with overhead positioning as in basketball are at high risk. The surgical success rates of initial dislocators are over 95% (2,7,8).

Patients with lower risk of recurrence are often placed in a nonoperative program. This includes immobilization, followed by selective strengthening of the cuff and scapular stabilizers. Immobilization of the shoulder in external rotation has recently been introduced and may reduce recurrence rates in moderate-risk individuals (9).

The most common indication for arthroscopic stabilization is multiple episodes of recurrent shoulder instability. Patients and physicians have to weigh the degree of disability associated with the dislocation event and the potential interruption of athletic season versus the rehabilitation time required for arthroscopic repair. Earlier surgical intervention may offer improved outcomes (10). Pathologic injuries (i.e., bony bankart, Hill-Sachs, and labral tears) associated with multiple dislocations may be additive, and may lead to more extensive surgery if the decision for surgical repair is delayed or prolonged (11,12).

Patients may be considered for revision of failed prior stabilization. Early nonanatomic open procedures that did not address the Bankart lesion emphasized tensioning of extra-articular structures or bony block procedures. Patients with recurrent instability following these procedures may consider arthroscopic evaluation and repair without disruption of the prior surgery. In patients who have had prior anatomic reconstruction, including arthroscopic or open bankart, with capsular shift procedures, failures have occurred due to a new traumatic event, failure to reduce prior capsule and labral detachment, anterior rim fracture, and soft tissue and bone deficiencies. These patients can be considered for arthroscopic revision surgery if there is sufficient bone stock remaining. Although recurrence rates are not as good as index surgery, many patients can be returned to full activities (13). Currently, the contraindications to arthroscopic anterior stabilization surgery include habitual dislocators, uncooperative or noncompliant patients, and shoulders that have developed extensive bone or cartilage deficiency.

Patients with significant bone loss must be corrected with open surgical augmentation. In some cases, structural changes may be compensated for with soft tissue interposition and tensioning. However, this may have a limited role in an athlete that requires maximum abduction and external rotation. In other cases, extra-articular and intra-articular glenoid bone grafts may be used to the glenoid or to the humeral head defect. Since minor bone losses are common even with the first dislocation, the acceptable range of glenoid deficiency has been reported 20% to 30%. An engaging Hill-Sachs lesion places the shoulder at risk for dislocation recurrence (12). Others have looked at the geometry of the rim defect as the most important feature (14). In the author's experience, patients with defects greater than 30% are candidates for bone grafting procedures. Patients with bone loss of 25% to 30% and those wishing to resume contact or collision athletics, or overhead athletes that allow minor reductions of external rotation are candidates for open repair.

PREOPERATIVE EVALUATION

The preoperative history should include the nature (subluxation or dislocation), number and temporal assessment of dislocations. After the initial traumatic event, the treatment and length of time interval prior to a recurrence should be noted. If a previous operation was performed, it is helpful to have a copy of the operative report to identify initial pathology, use of implants, and treatment provided. Additional traumatic events that recreated symptoms are important. The position of the arm and shoulder, degree of force needed to recreate the symptoms, and whether there was symptomatic relief with avoidance of provocative positions should also be assessed.

The examination begins with asking the patient to position the arm to reproduce symptoms. Standard testing includes range of motion and strength testing. Atrophy is uncommon, but may be seen if axillary nerve or brachial plexus injury has occurred. If so, additional neurologic testing, including electromyogram (EMG) and nerve conduction velocity, should be performed, including deltoid, biceps, and brachial plexus. A load-and-shift maneuver is helpful to identify increased translation, reproduce symptoms, and identify an asymmetry from the uninvolved extremity (15). This is easily done with the arm at the side and with arm abduction of 25° in anterior, inferior, and posterior directions. If increased translation is noted, abduction and external rotation can be increased to further qualify the inferior glenohumeral ligament superior third (Fig. 2). Patients may express or demonstrate apprehension during this test if anterior dislocation is anticipated.

The sulcus sign is not uncommon after a significant Bankart lesion (16). This should be further tested with the arm in external rotation to see if the rotator interval is competent. Sulcus signs that are similar in spite of rotation suggest a widened rotator interval. Careful discussion on degree of external rotation following stabilization is important prior to surgery.

Imaging begins with a trauma radiographic series of anteroposterior to the glenoid, outlet view, and an axillary view. Additional views may be helpful to identify fractures, bone loss, or identify hardware placement. Other radiographic studies may be helpful in measuring the glenoid and humeral articular surface. Transverse cuts using CT scan and three-dimensional reconstructions can be used to quantitate glenoid width. An MRI can be used to measure glenoid articular margin and identify soft tissue deficits, including anterior capsule and labrum, and rotator cuff insertion.

ARTHROSCOPIC TECHNIQUES

Surgery begins with an examination under anesthesia. Range of motion and translation testing is important. Performing a load-and-shift maneuver in neutral and in 45° abduction and 45° external rotation can identify a dislocating shoulder, engaging Hill-Sachs lesion, and increased inferior translation. An appreciation of degree of excessive translation and bone loss can determine the amount of capsular re-tensioning that is required to repair the unstable shoulder.

The patient is positioned in either lateral decubitus or beach chair. Both of these positions can be easily converted to open surgery. The lateral decubitus makes combined anterior and posterior approaches easy to accomplish with unimpeded access to anterior, superior, and posterior aspects of the glenoid. The torso is rolled 20° posteriorly, and the shoulder is abducted 30°. The arm is placed in gentle longitudinal traction, and a second lateral traction sling allows for humeral head distraction and easy access to the axillary pouch. Additional padding is placed under the dependent axillae, along the torso and between the legs.

Diagnostic arthroscopy begins with the development of a posterior portal 2 cm inferior to the junction of the acromion and spine of the scapula. The arthroscope is introduced and two anterior portals are established (Fig. 3). An anterior superior portal is placed below the acromioclavicular joint and enters below the biceps. An anterior inferior portal is placed lateral to the coracoid process entering the joint above the subscapularis tendon. The inferior cannula is the larger working cannula allowing for instrumentation and improved access to the inferior glenoid.

Diagnostic arthroscopy begins with visualizing the joint from the posterior portal. The biceps and superior labrum are evaluated and probed. The rotator interval is visualized, including the superior labrum, superior and middle glenohumeral ligaments. The anterior glenoid, labrum, and capsular ligaments are probed, as the humeral head is gently distracted. The inferior pouch and posterior labrum are probed, as the scope is rotated and withdrawn. Rotator cuff evaluation includes the undersurface of supraspinatus, superior border of subscapularis, and posterior inferior teres minor. The relative position of the humeral head without traction and the Hill-Sachs defect relative to the glenoid articular surface are visualized. Rotating the humeral head in provocative positions can demonstrate potential engagement of this lesion.

The arthroscope is moved to the anterior superior portal. The anterior labrum is probed, and the lateral capsular attachments are visualized with the head in internal rotation. Glenoid articular width is quantitated to confirm adequate inferior bone width. In most cases, 1 cm of glenoid anterior to the "bare spot" can result in satisfactory stabilization. As the scope is advanced posterior to the head, the Hill-Sachs lesion can be visualized and degree of anterior translation relative to the glenoid appreciated.

A number of arthroscopic procedures have been used to repair anterior instability. Procedures include (*i*) suture anchor repair of Bankart lesions, (*ii*) capsular plication, (*iii*) rotator interval closure, (*iv*) humeral capsular avulsion repair, and (*v*) posterior soft tissue transfer into Hill-Sachs defect.

Suture Anchor Technique

The most commonly used technique to reattach the labrum and re-establish proper capsular tension utilizes suture anchors. The goal is to reposition and secure the labrum above the glenoid rim, advance the inferior glenohumeral ligament superiorly, and to eliminate any pouches that would permit additional humeral head subluxation. The steps include (*i*) soft tissue mobilization, (*ii*) glenoid preparation, (*iii*) inferior capsule plications, (*iv*) suture anchor placement, (*v*) suture passage, and (*vi*) capsular tensioning. This procedure can be performed in both the lateral decubitus and the beach chair positions.

Intraoperative confirmation of a detached labrum or scarred capsular ligaments along the medial glenoid neck termed an ALPSA (anterior labral periosteal sleeve avulsion) are confirmed. The repair begins with careful mobilization of the labrum and capsular ligaments. An elevator-type instrument is used to free the scar between the glenoid neck and the soft tissues (Fig. 4). The more superior labrum is thinner and needs a gentler approach to avoid tearing the ring. The elevator-type instrument works superiorly to inferiorly until it reaches the normal labral structures. As the structures are elevated off of the glenoid, one can view the subscapularis muscle medially. With release of these adhesions and attachments, the capsule labrum will often reduce to a resting position adjacent to the glenoid rim. A grasping instrument can confirm capsular mobility.

An assessment of capsular laxity in the inferior pouch is made. In most cases, there is a pouch anterior inferiorly permitting the excessive head translation. A curved spectrum suture hook (ConMed Linvatec, Largo, Florida, U.S.A.) is used to introduce a monofilament suture to plicate the pouch (Fig. 5). A pleat technique will avoid potential injury to the axillary nerve. The hook is passed in the anteroinferior cannula. A right curved hook (45° or 60°) is used on a right shoulder. Full-thickness capsule is grasped as the hook enters the capsule and reappears using a supination movement with the hook. The hook is drawn superiorly and is reintroduced through the labrum. As the suture is delivered, the size of the capsule transfer can be appreciated. The most frequent location of this anchoring stitch is at 6 o'clock, which is often coexistent with the most inferior aspect of the capsular derangement. In cases where the damage has extended to more posterior aspects of the inferior glenohumeral ligament, switching the scope to the anterior portal and using the posterior portal with the opposite curved hook allows for anchoring the posterior band of the inferior glenohumeral ligament (IGHL). The additional plication sutures can be used in shoulders with multidirectional laxity.

The glenoid rim and neck need to be prepared for soft tissue reattachment. A shaver and nonaggressive burr can be used to remove loose tissue from the anterior and inferior glenoid. Loose pieces of articular cartilage along the rim can be smoothed. The shape of the glenoid can best be visualized from the anterior superior portals. It is common to have fractures of the glenoid rim creating the remaining glenoid surface as flat, convex, or concave. Using a burr, gently abrade the surface to maximize surface contact with the soft tissues. Loose pieces of bone can be removed, but bone embedded in the detached labrum can be left in place for reattachment.

A drill is passed in the anterior inferior working portal and directed along the inferior edge of the glenoid. The first hole is drilled on the articular surface at the most inferior aspect of the labrum detachment. Drill guides are helpful to elevate the humeral head and depress the subscapularis tendon to make a favorable angle of entry into the glenoid. The drill hole needs to be placed on the articular margin to allow access to the glenoid between 5 and 7 o'clock (Fig. 6A). The soft tissue transfer will cover the articular defect. Additional glenoid holes are prepared at 8 to 10 mm intervals along the glenoid rim from inferior to superior. Spacing of the anchors is important, particularly if absorbable anchors are selected. The holes are drilled, sounded and, occasionally, a tap is used if a screw-in anchor is used in hard glenoid bone.

The first inferior suture anchor is placed. It is critical to make sure the anchor is below the articular cartilage. There are markings on the instruments that indicate when the anchor is deep enough. Remember, there is an acute angle of entry and this often needs additional depth to completely bury the anchor. The anchor should be evaluated from the posterior and anterior viewing portals to confirm proper placement. The sutures and anchor should be tested by pulling and sliding the suture. A reinforced #2 braided suture allows for additional strength of the anchor complex. These suture materials are resistant to fraying along the eyelet of the anchor and edge of the drill hole. Suture materials are nonabsorbable, strong, and malleable, allowing for secure knot tying.

A suture hook is introduced in the inferior cannula to retrieve the anchor stitch. The hook is passed through the inferior glenohumeral ligament. It is critical to grasp the ligament inferior to the anchor to create a capsular shift. A right curved hook is placed in a right shoulder. The tip of the needle enters the capsule 1 cm inferior and medial to the anchor placement. Supination allows for the tip of the needle to reappear. Drawing the hook superiorly, a second pass can be made under the detached labrum. Once the tip of the instrument becomes visible, a suture shuttle (ConMed Linvatec, Largo, Florida, U.S.A.) is introduced (Fig. 6B). The shuttle is retrieved through the superior cannula. The suture arm closest to the labrum is retrieved in the superior cannula to prepare for shuttling. Grasp the suture arm close to the shuttle to avoid twists or entanglements. The shuttle can be used to draw the braided suture under the labrum and through the capsular ligament as the shuttle is drawn out of the inferior working cannula. The suture sliding through this complex is tested. A sliding knot is created on the part of the suture that passed through the capsular ligament. As the knot is tied, the inferior ligament is shifted superiorly, and the labrum is pushed on top of the glenoid rim covering the anchor hole.

Additional anchors are placed and sutures secured in a similar fashion. It is most common to use three or four anchors to secure the anterior labrum, depending on the length of detachment (Fig. 6C). As the sutures are tied, the inferior pouch is further reduced. The superior band of the inferior glenohumeral ligament is re-established, and the middle glenohumeral ligament is repaired. An additional anchor may be necessary to repair the superior labrum if traumatic detachment has occurred. Nontraumatic foveas in the superior quadrant should not be closed with suture anchors, but rather tensioned with capsular plication.

Typical repairs require additional capsular tensioning. This is often coexistent with the patient's history and physical findings. A prolonged history of repetitive subluxation or increased inherited laxity associated with a traumatic labral detachment may benefit from the additional capsular plication. An initial dislocator may require an anatomical labral repair as opposed to an individual with three to five episodes, which may require additional capsular tensioning. Suture hooks are used to grasp the capsule and pleat it to adjacent labrum or capsule.

The interval between the middle and superior glenohumeral ligaments may be closed in selected cases (17). This has been termed the rotator interval, since it is deep to the tendinous interval between the supraspinatus and the subscapularis. The capsular plication sutures are most often monofilament absorbable sutures. A right hook can grasp the superior edge of the middle ligament and draw it superiorly before it is secure to the capsule adjacent to the biceps. The reverse suture hook is used to grasp the capsule behind the biceps and reattach this to the middle ligament (Fig. 7A). This stitch will not only incorporate the superior and middle capsular ligaments, but also the coracohumeral ligament, which is adherent to this capsule (Fig. 7B).

Once the repair is complete, or during the process, remove the traction and rotate the humerus in provocative positions. The humerus should remain seated over the center of the glenoid. The Hill-Sachs defect should remain posterior to the glenoid margin in the externally rotated posture. Anterior translation should be tested, and additional plication sutures are added if needed. The portals are closed and a sling is applied.

Capsular Plication

Creating pleats in the capsule can be used to retension and thicken the ligaments surrounding the shoulder. This technique can be used to augment suture anchor labral repairs, balance repairs with tensioning opposite the site of injury, or be an independent operation when ligaments have been stretched, but not torn or detached.

The most common ligament to be stretched and deformed is the inferior glenohumeral ligament (18,19). This allows the humeral head to translate anteroinferiorly into a pouch. The inferior ligament extends anterior and posterior to the humeral head. After arthroscopic confirmation that the ligament remains firmly attached to the humeral head and glenoid, a capsular plication repair can be performed in the symptomatic unstable shoulder.

A large, working cannula is placed in the anterior portal, below the acromion and entering in the rotator interval. A soft tissue shaver or rasp is used to roughen the capsule. A curved suture hook is placed in the inferior pouch, and a full-thickness bite is created using a supination technique. The capsule is grasped, drawn anteriorly and superiorly, and the hook is passed under the labrum (Fig. 8A). The monofilament suture is introduced and retrieved through the same cannula. The suture choice can be monofilament or braided. If a braided selection is desired, a shuttle is introduced through the spectrum hook. The braided suture is shuttled into position and the suture is tied (Fig. 8B). The steps are repeated as additional sutures are added. The sutures are generally spaced 1 cm apart, which appears to resemble a clock, that is, 6 o'clock, 5 o'clock, and so on.

In patients with pre-existing multidirectional laxity, several surgeons have preferred balancing sutures posteriorly. The purpose is to avoid pushing the humeral head into a posterior resting position on the face of the glenoid. The additional sutures create additional tension in the posterior third of the inferior glenohumeral ligament. When posterior stitches are added, the scope is placed in the anterior portal and the working cannula is transferred to the posterior portal. The opposite curved suture hook is used to create the pleats after the ligament is roughened.

Capsular plication is a subtle operation that can treat multiple symptoms from painful translation, internal impingement syndrome in throwers, to recurrent subluxators with multidirectional instability, to frank dislocators. The size of the tissue transfer should be appropriate to the amount of shortening of the ligament that is desirable. Postoperative motion restrictions should be consistent with desired outcome, and close monitoring is important.

Rotator Interval Closure

The rotator interval is the anatomic region between the supraspinatus and the subscapularis. The tendon gap is necessary for normal shoulder motion since the coracoid process separates these two tendons. There is a capsular interval that is visible to the arthroscopist between the superior and middle anterior glenohumeral ligaments. This interval can be torn or stretched as the result of anterior inferior subluxation. There is controversy on whether or not an interval closure should be routinely performed when repairing anterior stability. The interval closure would appear to resist anterior translation and reduce inferior translation in the adducted shoulder. This may be due to intimate contact of the coracohumeral ligament to these capsular structures. Shoulders that have an excessive sulcus sign that does not reduce with shoulder external rotation are candidates for capsular interval plication. As the interval is reduced with sutures, these ligaments are retensioned (Fig. 7).

There are a number of shoulders that have capsular tears that extend through the superior labrum and rotator interval, continuous with the Bankart lesion. The labral tears and interval tears should be repaired as part of the stabilization surgery. Structural damage to the labrum and interval is repaired with permanent sutures (Fig. 9). Retensioning the interval is commonly performed with absorbable monofilament sutures.

The technique uses a series of suture hooks. The first hook is the same used to repair the inferior quadrant. A single working cannula is used in the anterior portal. The initial hook is introduced, and a full-thickness bite of the middle ligament is made and transferred superiorly. The tip of the hook grasps the superior labrum, advances the suture, and is tied. The opposite-shaped hook is now placed above the biceps to grasp the full-thickness capsule (Fig. 7A). As this hook is advanced across the interval, the tip re-enters the middle ligament and the suture is advanced. As the knot is tied, the interval is reduced. A third suture can be placed as the cannula is withdrawn, to further reduce the size of the interval. Both anterior capsular ligament structures, including the coracohumeral ligament, are incorporated into this plication.

Humeral Capsular Ligament Avulsion

A HAGL injury refers to humeral avulsion of the anterior glenohumeral ligament. This injury can be an isolated finding or may be associated with the Bankart avulsion. This avulsion is most common in the inferior quadrant and best visualized with the arthroscope in the anterior portal (Fig. 10A). Gentle rotation of the humeral head will demonstrate capsular integrity or deficit. Lesions can be seen as avulsions or combined splits in the inferior pouch.

The HAGL repair has to be carefully performed to minimize risk to the nearby axillary nerve. The choices of repair include a side-to-side plication, suture anchor repair of the humeral head, or conversion to an open repair through a deltopectoral approach. The initial step is to correctly diagnose and quantify the size of the capsular tear. It is best to use both anterior and posterior portals. A new posterior and inferior portal can be created to allow visualization within the pouch. With rotation of the arthroscope, the capsular attachments can be visualized with minimal adjustment to shoulder rotation. Using the anterior portal, suture hooks can introduce monofilament sutures that can cross the tear in a sideways fashion (Fig. 10B). If an anchor is preferred, a spinal needle is used to identify the best angle of insertion, superior and lateral to the axillary nerve pathway. A suture shuttle can be used to retrieve the braided sutures through the capsular tear to reinforce the repair.

Humeral Head Defect

The Hill-Sachs lesion is a defect created in the humeral head as the shoulder dislocates anteriorly created by the glenoid rim. With greater frequency of recurrence, the duration that the head is dislocated prior to reduction, and violent pectoralis muscle contraction, this defect can become larger and deeper. Anterior repairs often limit anterior translation and external rotation, preventing this lesion from engaging with the anterior glenoid rim. As the defect enlarges, the loss of rotation can be problematic for return to certain activities.

Treatment of this lesion can include bone grafting or soft tissue transfer into the defect. Bone grafting is considered when the defect is larger than 25% and is currently an open reconstructive procedure from either an anterior or posterior arthrotomy. The soft tissue transfer is being performed arthroscopically by Wolf, and results are short term. The open procedure of transferring the infraspinatus tendon into the posterior humeral head defect was described by Connolly (20).

Two posterior portals and one anterior portal are necessary for soft tissue transfer into the Hill-Sachs defect performed through the arthroscope. Using the scope in the superior posterior portal, 2 cm inferior to the angle of the spine of the scapula, the lesion can be well defined. A second portal is created 2 cm inferiorly using a spinal needle to identify the best angle of entry. A burr is introduced to abrade the surface. Through a puncture between the two cannulas, a suture anchor can be introduced. Using a spinal needle, a shuttle can be introduced parallel to the anchor passing through the infraspinatus tendon and posterior capsule. Another alternative is to use a pointed piercing instrument to retrieve sutures into the subdeltoid space. The scope is reintroduced into a lateral or posterior portal into the subacromial space. The sutures are retrieved into the cannula and tied. This procedure is considered in revision surgical cases. It is combined with anterior repair to limit humeral head anterior translation and prevention of bone defect engagement that may occur with chronic recurrent instability.

POSTOPERATIVE MANAGEMENT

Surgical repair of the anterior Bankart lesion requires protection of the repaired structures. Most commonly, this is done with limits to external rotation and the use of a sling. External rotation is limited to 20° or less for the first two to four weeks. External rotation with the elbow at the side can be increased to 30° after four weeks. Shoulder shrugs, elbow flexion, extension, and grip strength can be started early. Overhead shoulder flexion can be started at four weeks and should approach normal elevation by 8 to 10 weeks.

Return to sports is based on biological healing of the repaired structures. Contact sports are usually delayed four to six months to maximize the strength of the repair. Other criteria for return to sport are appropriate pain-free range of motion for the desired activities and protective strength and endurance of the supporting scapular and rotator cuff structures. Aggressive strengthening and ballistic techniques for power are usually started 10 weeks following repair. Premature return to sports is a well-known cause for treatment failure.

RESULTS

The results or arthroscopic shoulder stabilization continue to improve. Failure rates that were greater than traditional open procedures conflicted with the potential benefits from minimally invasive surgery. As the goals of success were expanded to return to overhead activity and sport, the anatomic repair became desirable. Three major features distinguish the arthroscopic repair from the open approach (21): (*i*) the ability of directly operating on multiple quadrants of the shoulder without the need for additional incisions; (*ii*) previously unrecognized pathology, that is, superior labral anterior to posterior (SLAP) and interval lesions, can be recognized and repaired arthroscopically; and (*iii*) the subscapularis tendon does not need to be disturbed in an arthroscopic approach. Complications, including subscapularis dehiscence and persistent dysfunction, can be avoided when the tendon is left undisturbed.

The most common determinant in patient selection involves the issue of bone loss. It is common for shoulders to experience glenoid rim fractures, impaction defects, and humeral head Hill-Sachs lesions after shoulder dislocations. Moderate bone loss less than 25% can be compensated for with a stable soft tissue reconstruction. As the bone loss increases, shoulders are at risk for dislocation recurrence, particularly in collision and contact sports (10,12–14). Bone grafting procedures are most commonly being performed as an open procedure, although new innovation may offer an arthroscopic alternative.

Compliance in the postoperative period remains an important aspect of soft tissue healing. The soft tissue reattachment is made with simple and mattress sutures placed along the articular margin. Healing does not occur to the articular cartilage, but rather the soft tissue to the abraded glenoid neck between the anchor supports. Patients who do not allow adequate time to permit biological healing may jeopardize the repair. There have been technological advances in suture anchor choices and suture material that may allow earlier activities. Absorbable and nonmetallic anchors may create less friction on the suture material, reducing a stress riser in the suture loop. The suture material is reinforced creating greater strength of the repair prior to the healing. Although instability recurrence is often multifactorial, a common finding at the time of revision surgery is broken sutures and soft tissue detachment.

Using the modern techniques of arthroscopic shoulder stabilization, recurrence rates are comparable to open Bankart repairs. Recent comparative studies have shown high levels of success when bone integrity and patient cooperation are taken into account (22–27). These results have ranged from 0% to 11% recurrence for treatment of repetitive instability. Arthroscopic treatment following a single initial dislocation may be desirable in selected cases due to earlier recognition of pathology, less soft tissue and bone deformity, and improved patient grading when compared to delayed treatment (2,7,8).

The author reports a personal series of 415 patients repaired with arthroscopic anterior stabilization: 300 patients had suture anchor repairs, and 115 patients had capsular plication and HAGL repairs (1993–2006). Follow-up of 15 first-time dislocators have had 100% remaining stable, and all returned to their desired sport. Overall, risk of recurrence of chronic instability was 5.05% after suture anchor repair. If compliance or delay in return to sport and recognition of bone loss exceeding 25% are considered, recurrence was reduced to 3%.

Physicians who manage failed surgical procedures may consider arthroscopy to diagnose and treat failed prior surgeries. Although success rates of open and arthroscopic revision surgery are not as good as primary procedures (77–78%), reasons for recurrence need further evaluation (13,28). Combining patient selection with arthroscopic evaluation prior to committing to the surgical approach has improved results.

The athlete has great expectations of "stable mobility" of the shoulder without apprehension or pain. Anatomic restoration of the shoulder is the best way to achieve this result. As repetitive instability events occur, further deterioration of the articular structures make reconstruction more challenging. Although controversy remains in whether an athlete with an initial dislocation should undergo an arthroscopic repair, the potential for further bony deformity with recurrent dislocations makes early stabilization an attractive option for most patients.

AVOIDING FAILURE AND COMPLICATIONS

The keys to a successful arthroscopic anterior stabilization include careful patient selection, proper technical skill, and proper rehabilitation to provide the best environment for biological healing.

Patient selection begins with an understanding of the history, exam, and imaging. A determination should be made on bone quality and structural restraints to the shoulder. Loss of the articular surface cannot be totally compensated for with soft tissue repair. Significant bony deformity may necessitate an open stabilization procedure. Prior thermal treatment with capsular ablation may need soft tissue grafting to replace the missing structures.

Technical issues include proper suture anchor placement. This includes anchor spacing and depth. Regardless of anchor material, the depth of the anchor needs to be below the articular surface to avoid chondral damage to the humeral head. Spacing of anchors 8 to 10 mm may avoid creating a stress riser in the glenoid rim. Creating proper capsule tension is a combination of location and spacing of sutures. Using suture hooks to create, pleats may be incorporated into the anchor repair or used independently in the mid-substance of the capsular ligaments. A balanced repair with the humeral head remaining centered is the goal of surgical treatment.

Proper rehabilitation requires adequate time for the repaired tissue to become adherent to the prepared surface on the glenoid. A period of restricted activity is important to allow the reattachment process to occur. Noncompliant patients are at great risk for disruptions of their repair prior to adequate soft tissue healing. Although minimally invasive surgery may create less postoperative discomfort, athletes may mistakenly believe that postoperative rehabilitation may be accelerated, following arthroscopic procedures. It is important that the patient, coaches, and family understand the postoperative restrictions on activity required to ensure a successful result.

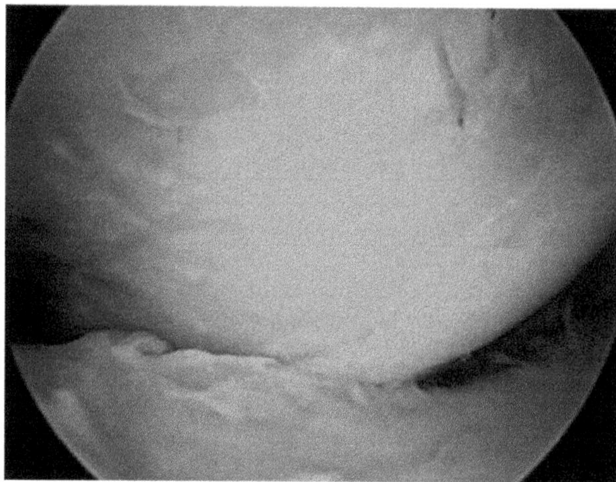

FIGURE 1 Engaging Hill-Sachs lesion: humeral head defect engaged with glenoid rim defect.

(A) 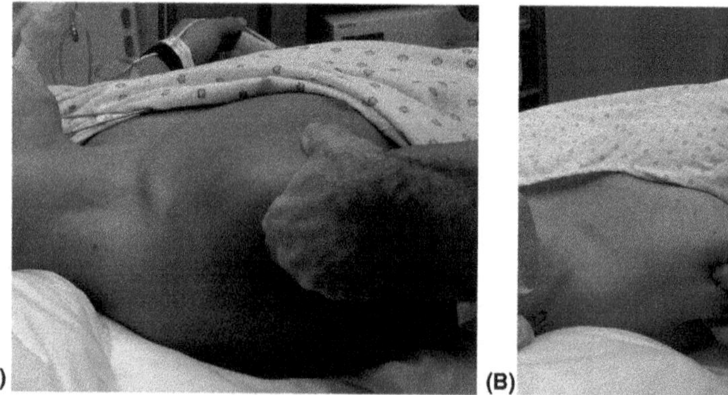

(B) 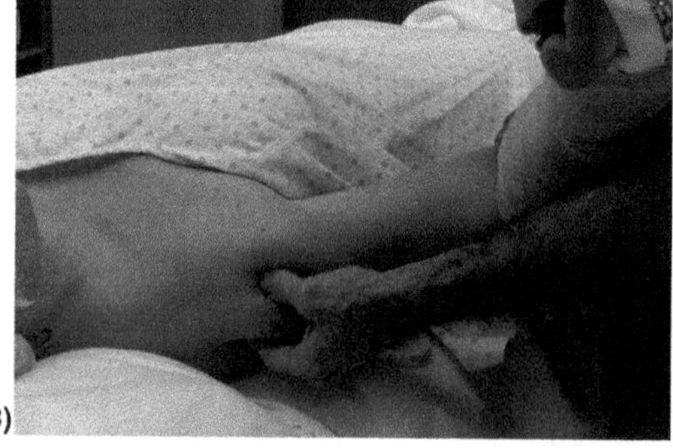

FIGURE 2 Load-and-shift examination. (**A**) Exam performed in neutral orientation. (**B**) Shoulder abducted 45° and externally rotated to test inferior glenohumeral ligament (IGHL) superior third.

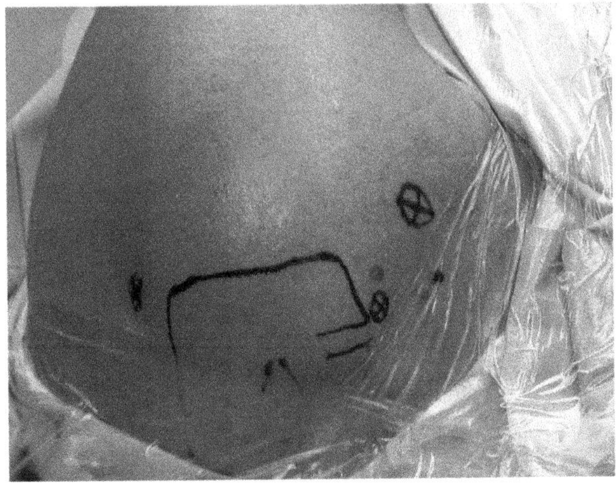

FIGURE 3 Portals for anterior stabilization. Two anterior portals entering rotator interval. The anchors and hooks are placed through the inferior portal, lateral to the coracoid (left shoulder).

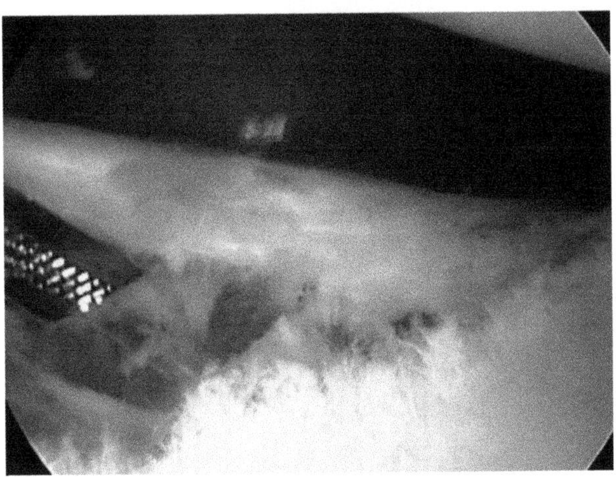

FIGURE 4 A liberator assists labral elevation, capsular mobilization, and glenoid neck abrasion. *Source*: Instrument from ConMed Linvatec, Largo, Florida, U.S.A.

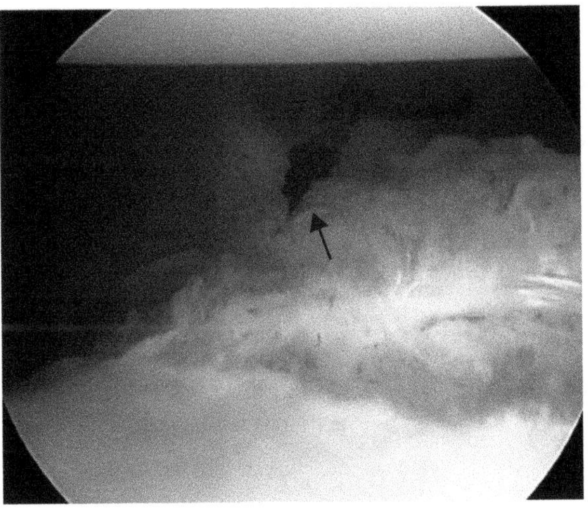

FIGURE 5 A suture hook can place a plication stitch in the inferior capsular pouch.

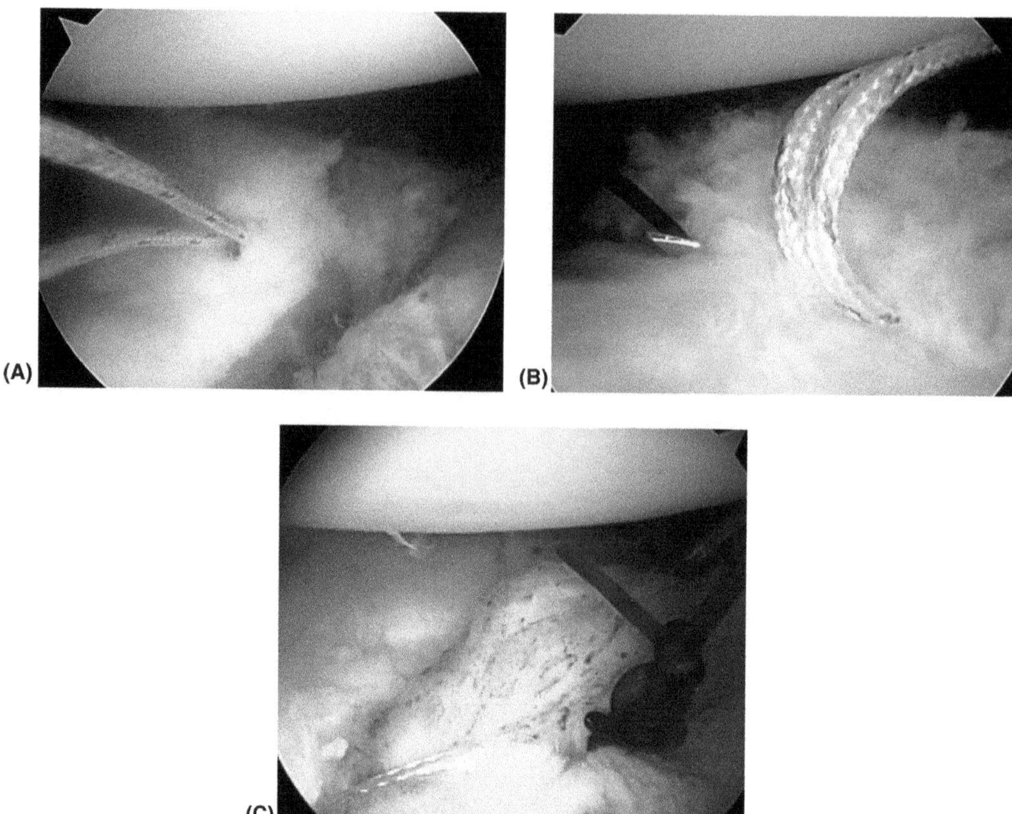

FIGURE 6 Arthroscopic suture anchor repair. (**A**) An anchor is placed along the anterior glenoid margin adjacent to the defect. (**B**) A suture hook can introduce a shuttle to retrieve a suture arm incorporating the labrum and inferior glenohumeral ligament. (**C**) Anterior view of a completed capsule labral repair.

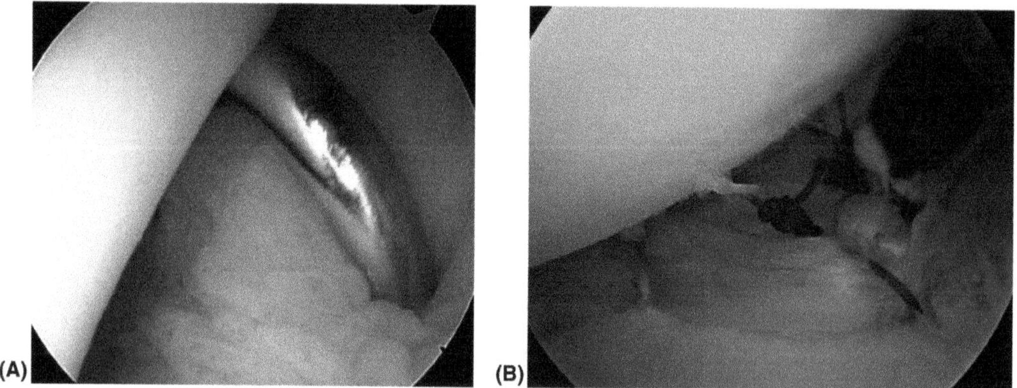

FIGURE 7 Rotator interval closure. (**A**) A suture hook is placed behind the biceps and full-thickness pass is made through the superior glenohumeral ligament. (**B**) Interval closure incorporates superior, middle, and coracohumeral ligament.

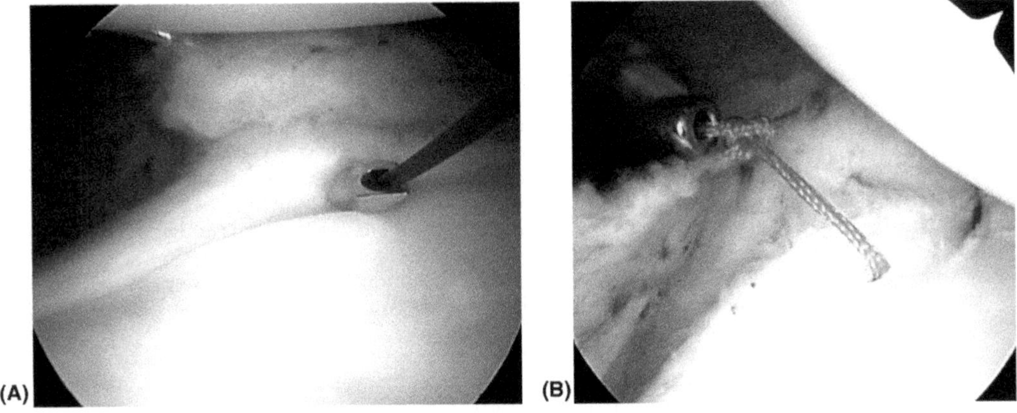

FIGURE 8 Capsular plication. (**A**) After the pouch is abraded, a suture hook takes full-thickness capsule bite and is advanced under the labrum. (**B**) Braided plication sutures can be shuttled and tied.

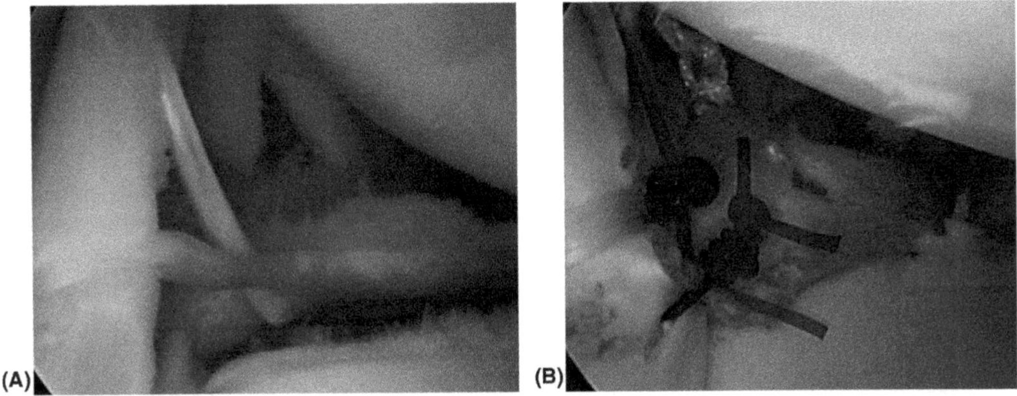

FIGURE 9 Rotator interval tear. (**A**) A Bankart tear can extend through the anterior capsular interval and labrum. (**B**) A Bankart repair should include the torn capsule and superior labrum.

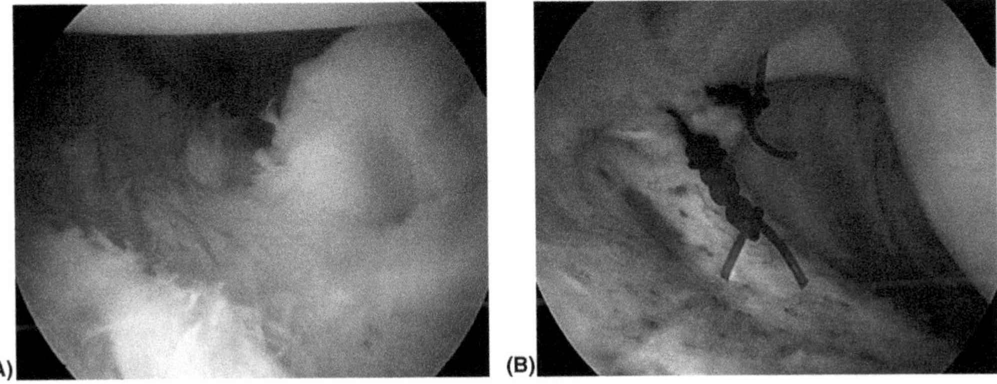

FIGURE 10 Humeral avulsion glenohumeral ligament. (**A**) Capsular tear adjacent to the humeral head. (**B**) The viewing arthroscope is in the posteroinferior portal. Monofilament sutures are placed to repair the defect.

REFERENCES

1. Abrams JS, Savoie FH III, moderators. Symposium, arthroscopic shoulder surgery: Is this the new gold standard? American Academy of Orthopaedic Surgeons 2005 Annual Meeting, Washington, DC.
2. Kirkley A, Griffen S, Richards C, et al. Prospective randomized clinical trial comparing the effectiveness of immediate arthroscopic stabilization versus immobilization and rehabilitation in first traumatic anterior dislocations of the shoulder. Arthroscopy 1999; 15:507–514.
3. Thomas SC, Matsen FA. An approach to the repair of avulsion of the glenohumeral ligaments in the management of traumatic anterior glenohumeral instability. J Bone Joint Surg (Am) 1989; 71:506–513.
4. Abrams JS. Thermal capsulorrhaphy for instability of the shoulder: concerns and applications of the heat probe. Instructional Course Lectures, Am Acad of Ortho Surg 2001; 50:29–36.
5. Andrews JR, Petty DH, Jazrawi L, et al. Glenohumeral chondrolysis after shoulder arthroscopy: case reports. American Shoulder and Elbow Surgeons 20th Annual Meeting, Dana Point, California, October 8–10, 2003. Abstract p. 29.
6. Watson KC. Devastating complication following arthroscopic capsulorrhaphy. American Shoulder and Elbow Surgeons 20th Annual Meeting, Dana Point, California, October 8–10, 2003. Abstract p. 30.
7. Larrain MV, Botto GJ, Montenegro HJ, et al. Arthroscopic repair of acute traumatic anterior shoulder dislocations in young athletes. Arthroscopy 2001; 17(4):373–377.
8. Abrams JS, Savoie FH III, Tauro JT, Bradley JP. Recent advances in the evaluation and treatment of shoulder instability: anterior, posterior, and multidirectional. Arthroscopy 2002; 18(9):1–13.
9. Itoi E, Hatakayama Y, Kido T, et al. A new method of immobilization after traumatic anterior dislocation of the shoulder: a preliminary study. J Shoulder Elbow Surg 2003; 12:413–415.
10. Bacilla P, Field LD, Savoie FH III. Arthroscopic Bankart repair in a high-demand patient population. Arthroscopy 1997; 13(1):51–60.
11. Habermeyer P, Bleyze P, Rickert M, et al. Evolution of lesions of the labrum-ligament complex in post-traumatic anterior shoulder instability: a prospective study. J Shoulder Elbow Surg 1999; 8(1):66–74.
12. Burkhart SS, DeBeer JF. Traumatic glenohumeral bone defects and their relationship to failure of arthroscopic Bankart repairs: significance of the inverted-pear glenoid and humeral engaging Hill-Sachs lesion. Arthroscopy 2000; 16:677–694.
13. Kim SH, Ha KI, Kim YM. Arthroscopic revision Bankart repair: a prospective outcome study. Arthroscopy 2002; 18:469–482.
14. Sugaya H, Moriishi J, Dohi M, et al. Glenoid rim morphology in recurrent anterior glenohumeral instability. J Bone Joint Surg 2003; 85A:878–884.
15. Hawkins RJ, Abrams JS, Schutte JP. Multidirectional instability of the shoulder: an approach to diagnosis. Ortho Trans 1987; 11:246.
16. Hawkins RJ, Schutte JP, Huckel JH, Abrams JS. The assessment of glenohumeral translation using manual and fluoroscopic techniques. Orthop Trans 1988; 12:727.
17. Harryman DT II, Sidles JA, Harris SL, Matsen FA. The role of the rotator interval capsule in passive motion and stability of the shoulder. J Bone Joint Surg 1992; 74:53–66.
18. Speer KP, Deng X, Borrero S, Torzilli PA, Altchek DW, Warren RC. Biomechanical evaluation of the Bankart lesion. J Bone Joint Surgery 1994; 76:1819–1826.
19. Bigliani LJ, Pollock RG, Soslowsky LJ, Flatow EL, Pawluk RJ, Mow VC. The tensile properties of the inferior glenohumeral ligament. J Orthop Res 1992; 10:187–197.
20. Connolly JF. Humeral head defects associated with shoulder dislocation: their diagnostic and surgical significance. Instructional Course Lectures, Am Acad of Ortho Surg 1972; 21:42–54.
21. Abrams JS. Shoulder stabilization and evolving trends in arthroscopic repair. Sports Med and Arthro Rev 1999; 7(2):104–116.
22. Fabbriciani C, Milano G, Demontis A, et al. Arthroscopic versus open treatment of Bankart lesion of the shoulder: a prospective randomized study. Arthroscopy 2004; 20(5):456–462.
23. Mazzocca AD, Brown FM, Carreira DJ, et al. Arthroscopic anterior shoulder stabilization of collision and contact athletes. Am J Sports Med 2005; 33(1):52–60.
24. Bottoni CR, Smith EL, Berkowitz MJ, et al. Arthroscopic versus open stabilization for recurrent instability: a prospective, randomized clinical trial. Am J Sports Med 2006; 34(11):1730–1737.
25. Kim SH, Ha KI, Cho YB, et al. Arthroscopic anterior stabilization of the shoulder: two-to-six-year follow-up. J Bone Joint Surg 2003; 85(8):1511–1528.
26. Gartsman GM, Roddey TS, Hammerman SM. Arthroscopic treatment of anterior inferior glenohumeral instability: two-to-five-year follow-up. J Bone Joint Surg 2006; 82:991–1003.
27. Cole BJ, L'Insalata J, Irrigary J, Warner JJP. Comparison of arthroscopic and open anterior shoulder stabilization: a two- to six-year follow-up study. J Bone Joint Surg 2000; 82:1108–1114.
28. Levine WN, Arroyo JS, Pollock RG, et al. Open revision stabilization surgery for recurrent anterior glenohumeral instability. Am J Sports Med 2000; 28:156–160.

9 Arthroscopic Posterior Instability Repair

Kent Jackson and Beth E. Shubin Stein
Hospital for Special Surgery, New York, New York, U.S.A.

INTRODUCTION

Compared to anterior instability, posterior shoulder instability is a relatively rare condition, comprising only about 5% of all shoulder instability patients (1). In a study performed on college football players at the NFL combine, posterior shoulder instability made up 4% of all shoulder injuries (2). Posterior shoulder instability can range in presentation from frank dislocation requiring emergent reduction, to symptomatic subluxation, to subclinical microinstability that presents with pain and functional deficits. Historically, this condition has been difficult with regard to both diagnosis and treatment. With increased understanding of this pathologic entity and improved diagnostic modalities this diagnosis is being made more frequently. A focused rehabilitation program remains the mainstay of initial management. However, patients who fail an appropriate course of conservative management may benefit from surgical intervention. A number of open and arthroscopic procedures have been described with satisfactory medium-term outcomes (3,4,5,6,7,8–11). In this chapter, we will describe the arthroscopic treatment of recurrent posterior shoulder instability that can provide a predictable result with a high rate of success for the appropriately selected patient.

HISTORICAL

Posterior shoulder instability was first described by Cooper in 1839 in patients with seizure disorders (12). In the last 50 years, the surgical treatment of recurrent posterior shoulder instability has evolved considerably.

Several nonanatomic procedures have been described. In the treatment of recurrent posterior shoulder instability and locked posterior dislocations, McLaughlin described a subscapularis tenodesis in which the subscapularis tendon was transferred into the anterior humeral head defect (13). This procedure has been successful for the treatment of reverse Hill-Sachs lesions with posterior instability, although results have been mixed (14).

The reverse Putti-Platt procedure or infraspinatus tenodesis has also been used to treat recurrent posterior instability, however, a high rate of recurrent instability has been reported with this procedure (3,4).

Subdeltoid transfer of the biceps tendon, lateral to the humeral head to the posterior glenoid, was described by Boyd and Sisk for the treatment of recurrent posterior shoulder instability, with mixed results reported (15,16).

Osteotomies of both the humerus and the glenoid have been described to address the osseous etiologies in recurrent posterior shoulder instability. An external rotation osteotomy of the humerus was described by Surin et al. (5). Ten of 12 patients had good or excellent results with one nonunion and one recurrence of instability. Scott initially described glenoplasty with successful results in two of three patients in his initial report (6). However, Hawkins et al. (3) found both a high rate of complication and recurrence with glenoid osteotomy.

With continued improvements in technology and arthroscopic techniques in addition to the promising results in the treatment of anterior instability, there has been expanded interest in the arthroscopic treatment of posterior shoulder instability. Arthroscopic approaches provide a number of advantages over open techniques. Most importantly, arthroscopy allows accurate identification of the specific posterior pathology in addition to any

---

Please refer to pages 111–112 for the figures in this chapter.

concomitant pathology in the gleno–humeral joint and subacromial space. This allows any unsuspected pathology to be addressed at the same time. Arthroscopy produces less morbidity, less soft-tissue dissection, improved cosmesis, less pain, and improved functional recovery.

INDICATIONS AND CONTRAINDICATIONS

A detailed patient history is critical to the establishment of the correct diagnosis in the setting of recurrent posterior shoulder instability. Patients may present with a wide range of complaints from frank dislocation to more vague complaints of pain and dysfunction of the shoulder. The history should focus on any antecedent traumatic events to the shoulder and the arm position at the time of the injury and during symptoms. This can provide clues regarding the exact pathologic process that may be encountered at the time of arthroscopy and the direction of the instability. The duration, quality, and severity of symptoms as well as any associated functional limitations should be explored. Most patients will report some degree of pain or discomfort with excessive shoulder activity in addition to provocation of symptoms in the flexed, adducted, and internally rotated position. Patients will often describe the sensation of instability or that the shoulder will "slip" or "pop out." When dealing with athletes, the specific sport played and more importantly the exact position can be useful information. Athletes in sports such as football (particularly interior lineman) and lacrosse are at an increased risk due to a repetitive posteriorly directed force in combination with a shearing force to the posterior labrum (7).

Patients who can voluntarily sublux or dislocate their shoulders should be probed regarding their psychiatric history. Patients with certain psychiatric disorders who can voluntarily dislocate their shoulders for "secondary gains" have an increased risk of failure with both operative and nonoperative treatment (17).

The past medical history of the patient should be explored for other systemic illnesses, connective tissue disorders, or comorbidities. Questions about the type, quality, duration, and compliance with physical therapy can provide insight into the patient's motivation. The prior surgical history is important and any available operative notes or pictures from the previous procedures can provide clues as to the pathologic anatomy in addition to the type of procedure and quality of tissue encountered.

PHYSICAL EXAMINATION

A thorough physical examination should be performed to determine the degree and direction of instability. All examinations performed should be compared to the contralateral side. The patient's shoulder girdle should be inspected at rest looking for any obvious atrophy or static abnormalities. In addition, the patient should be inspected during active range of motion looking for evidence of scapulothoracic dyskinesis. A standard shoulder examination including an assessment of active and passive range of motion, strength of the rotator cuff, and evaluation of the acromio-clavicular joint, biceps, and posterior shoulder for tenderness to palpation should be performed. A neurovascular examination should be performed looking for any evidence of focal neurologic deficit or alteration in circulation. A complete examination of the cervical spine should also be included to rule out any radicular pathology.

The load and shift test should be performed and laxity assessed both anteriorly and posteriorly. During this examination laxity should be graded as humeral head translation to the glenoid rim (1+), translation over the glenoid rim (2+), and locked dislocation over the glenoid rim (3+). Provocative testing such as the jerk test can be virtually diagnostic of posterior instability (18). The jerk test is performed by stabilizing the scapula while applying an axial load to the humerus in 90° of abduction and internal rotation. The arm is then brought horizontally across the body into adduction. A positive test includes a clunk indicative of humeral head dislocation with or without pain. A second clunk can be appreciated upon relocation, as the shoulder is then brought into abduction in the horizontal plane. Special tests including the posterior load and shift test can be performed looking for subclinical instability.

The posterior load and shift test is performed with the patient in either the standing or supine position. A posteriorly directed force is applied with the arm in 90° of forward flexion and internal rotation. A positive test is characterized by the reproduction of pain, a mechanical grind, or both. Evidence of inferior laxity should be assessed by placing downward traction on both arms simultaneously with the patient relaxed looking for a sulcus sign. The degree of laxity is based on the distance between the humeral head and lateral acromion. Performing this examination again with the arms externally rotated can be helpful in assessing the integrity of the rotator interval. If the sulcus sign persists with external rotation, this is suggestive of rotator interval laxity and should be addressed with rotator interval closure at the time of surgery (8). The patient should also be examined for signs of generalized ligamentous laxity that may contribute to their instability. A number of useful examinations can be performed including abduction of the thumb to the forearm, or hyperextension of the elbow, or metacarpophalangeal joints.

RADIOLOGY

Standard radiographs of the shoulder including an anterior–posterior (AP) view, Grashey true AP view, scapular Y view, and axillary view should be obtained on all patients with posterior shoulder instability. These studies should be examined for evidence of osseous abnormalities including fractures of the posterior glenoid or reverse Hill Sachs lesions. The axillary view should be part of any standard shoulder series and is critical in assuring that the shoulder is located with the humerus seated in the glenoid. It is also very useful in evaluating the posterior glenoid for bony erosions or fractures and getting a sense of the glenoid version.

Magnetic resonance imaging (MRI) should be obtained on patients to document any capsulolabral pathology. MRI performed with the appropriate sequences has been shown to be useful in detecting tears of the posterior labrum and lesions of the posterior capsule (Fig. 1). MRI arthrography has been shown to be highly sensitive and specific for detecting capsulolabral lesions (19,20).

Computed tomography (CT), although not required on all patients, is useful when evaluating the osseous anatomy of the shoulder. CT is very useful in detecting subtle fractures, reverse Hill Sachs lesions, and in evaluating the version of the glenoid.

NONOPERATIVE TREATMENT

All patients with a diagnosis of posterior shoulder instability should initially be treated with a course of nonoperative treatment. Activity modification should be undertaken to eliminate any provocative movements or activities during rehabilitation. A course of nonsteroidal anti-inflammatory medications should be prescribed to control inflammation and to aid in compliance with the therapy program. Most importantly, all patients should be enrolled in a directed physical therapy program with a knowledgeable therapist. The therapy program should focus on pain control, maintenance of motion, and strengthening of the rotator cuff, deltoid, and periscapular musculature. Other studies have reported good results with nonsurgical treatment of posterior instability, particularly in those patients without a history of trauma (9).

Surgical intervention is indicated in patients with persistent symptoms after an appropriate course of physical therapy. Indications for arthroscopic treatment of recurrent unidirectional posterior instability include isolated labral tears or capsular pathology. In those patients with both posterior instability and a positive sulcus sign indicating inferior instability, arthroscopic treatment of the capsulolabral pathology in combination with a rotator interval closure is appropriate.

Although this chapter deals primarily with arthroscopic treatment of posterior instability, it is important to discuss the indications for open treatment as well. Patients with bony abnormalities are often best treated with open reconstruction. These abnormalities include alterations in glenoid or humeral version and deficiencies of the humeral head or glenoid. In addition to bony abnormalities, a history of failed arthroscopic stabilizations is often an indication for open reconstruction as well. A relative indication for open surgery would be in a patient with excessive generalized ligamentous laxity.

SURGICAL TECHNIQUE

Although surgery may be performed in the lateral decubitus position, we prefer regional interscalene anesthesia in the modified beach chair position. Care is taken during positioning to ensure access to the entire shoulder girdle. Preoperative antibiotics are administered intravenously. The examination under anesthesia is then performed, checking passive range of motion and documenting instability in the anterior, posterior, and inferior directions. The affected extremity and shoulder are then prepped and draped in the usual sterile fashion. The bony landmarks of the shoulder are outlined with a marker as the intended portal sites. The standard posterior portal is used and is located 2 cm inferior and 2 cm medial to the posterolateral border of the acromion. The portal site is first injected subcutaneously with 3 cc of local anesthetic and epinephrine. A vertical incision is made with a #11 blade through the skin and subcutaneous tissue. The blunt trochar and camera cannula are introduced into the glenohumeral joint with a palpable "pop" as they advance through the posterior capsule. The arthroscope is then exchanged for the trochar and the joint is insufflated with saline containing epinephrine to a pressure of 40 mmHg using an arthroscopic pump. An anterior portal is needed for viewing the posterior capsulolabral complex, and rather than a standard anterior portal, we prefer using an anterolateral portal for improved visualization of the posterior structures. This portal is located roughly one to two centimeters distal to the anterolateral edge of the acromion. While viewing arthroscopically, the portal is marked first with a spinal needle, followed by placement of the cannula in the rotator interval anterior to the supraspinatus tendon, and above the biceps tendon. A systematic diagnostic arthroscopy is undertaken at this time evaluating the biceps tendon, biceps anchor, articular surfaces, anterior capsule, anterior, posterior, and inferior labrum, axillary pouch, rotator cuff and glenoid, and humeral head cartilage. To obtain a better view of the posterior structures, the arthroscope is exchanged over a wissinger rod to the anterolateral portal and a 5.0 mm cannula is placed in the posterior portal. The posterior and inferior glenoid, capsule, and labrum can further be assessed visually from this portal while probing from the posterior portal for labral tears (Fig. 2).

CAPSULOLABRAL REPAIR

After identification of a posterior labral tear an accessory posterolateral portal will be necessary for instrumentation. The location of this portal is 2 cm inferior to the posterolateral aspect of the acromion at the same level as the posterior portal. While viewing from an intra-articular location this portal is marked with a spinal needle. The correct placement of this portal is critical to have access to all portions of the glenoid including the six O'clock position for capsular advancement and labral reattachment. This portal traverses the infraspinatus tendon, and as a result the size of the cannula should be minimized when possible (preferably no larger than a 6 mm canula).

After establishment of the portals the glenoid and labrum are prepared for repair. From the posterolateral portal the torn labrum is debrided with a 4.5 mm shaver back to stable tissue. Next, an arthroscopic elevator is used to release the scarred labrum and adhesions from the glenoid neck. The release is adequate once muscle fibers can be visualized medially and the labrum is adequately mobilized for anatomic repair. After the release is complete the 4.5 mm shaver is used to abrade the glenoid rim and neck and stimulate bleeding to aid the healing process (Fig. 3).

Bioabsorbable anchors single loaded with #2 Fiberwire® suture (Arthrex, Naples, Florida, U.S.A.) are used for the capsulolabral repair. The drill guide and trochar are placed on the glenoid rim in the appropriate position (Fig. 4). The guide should be placed so that the anchor could be placed at the junction of the articular margin and glenoid neck with the appropriate angle, to avoid sliding posteriorly out of the bone or anteriorly onto the articular surface. We have found that erring with the anchor slightly on the articular side produces the most predictable result. This step is critical for the recreation of the capsulolabral complex and the "bumper." After using the trochar to make a small pilot hole, the drill is introduced and drilled to the appropriate depth. The drill is then removed and while continuing to hold the guide in position the anchor is introduced and malleted into position. The guide is then removed and the security of the anchor is tested by pulling on the sutures. The sutures are then retrieved out of the posterior portal with an arthroscopic claw. Next, a Suture Lasso (Arthrex, Naples, Florida, U.S.A.) is introduced through the posterolateral portal and used to penetrate both the capsule and labrum approximately 1 cm inferior to the anchor. The looped wire of the Suture Lasso is then fed into the joint and retrieved out of the posterior portal with an arthroscopic grasper (Fig. 5A and 5B). The suture that is situated more peripherally in regards to the glenoid is placed through the Lasso (approximately 5 cm) and then it is shuttled with the suture through the labrum and capsule and out of the posterolateral portal. Both the suture limbs are retrieved out of the posterolateral portal, and a knot is tied in standard arthroscopic fashion using the limb passing through the capsule and labrum as the post. We use a sliding knot of two half hitches thrown in the same direction, followed by three alternating half hitches (changing the post with each throw). The suture tails are then cut using arthroscopic scissors. This technique achieves not only an anatomic restoration of the labrum, but also superior and medial advancement of the capsule as well. Additional anchors can be placed depending on the size of the tear. The repair should proceed from inferior to superior, tying the knots in the process (Fig. 6).

SUTURE PLICATION

In cases of posterior instability, where the patient has no recognizable labral tear, an arthroscopic capsular plication is an excellent option. Using the same portals as described earlier, a 4.5 mm shaver, is introduced through the posterolateral portal and used to abrade the posterior capsule to stimulate bleeding for the reparative process. To provide improved access to the posterior capsule an assistant can provide anterior and lateral pressure on the humerus. Next, the Arthrex Suture Lasso is introduced through the posterolateral portal and is used to pierce the inferior capsule at roughly the six o'clock position. Care must be taken not to penetrate the capsule greater than 1 cm from the inferior glenoid or too deeply to avoid injury of the axillary nerve. The Lasso is then passed through the labrum at the seven o'clock position, with the device entering the joint at the articular surface labrum margin. The wire loop is then advanced into the joint and retrieved through the posterior portal using an arthroscopic grasper. A #2 Arthrex Fiberwire suture is placed in the end of the wire loop and shuttled through the capsule and labrum. A standard arthroscopic knot is tied using the limb through the capsule as the post. Suture ends are cut with arthroscopic scissors. Additional capsular plications can be performed at 1 cm intervals proceeding from inferior to superior. This technique not only achieves the intended capsular plication but superior advancement of the capsule as well.

ROTATOR INTERVAL CLOSURE

In patients with both posterior and inferior instability, rotator interval closure in combination with posterior stabilization should be performed. Arthroscopic interval closure is performed while viewing intra-articularly from the posterior portal. From the anterior portal, a tissue penetrator loaded with #2 Fiberwire is advanced through the superior edge of the subscapularis tendon and left in the glenohumeral joint. The anterior cannula is withdrawn slightly and placed just anterior to the rotator interval. The same tissue penetrator is then passed through the leading edge of the supraspinatus tendon into the glenohumeral joint where the free suture is grasped and retrieved through the supraspinatus into the subacromial space. We then introduce the arthroscope into the subacromial space. After performance of a subacromial bursectomy with a 4.5 mm shaver and identification of the sutures, an arthroscopic knot is tied in the subacromial space in a standard fashion with the arm in 45° of external rotation and neutral adduction to minimize the risk of loss of motion. Suture tails are cut with arthroscopic scissors. A single well-placed knot is sufficient for secure rotator interval closure in most cases.

PEARLS AND PITFALLS

The key to making the procedure go smoothly is portal placement. Time should be spent making sure the portals are positioned appropriately so that they allow adequate visualization of the repair and access to the needed structures. An assistant can also be helpful by placing anterolateral traction on the humerus if visualization is difficult. In addition, the Suture Lasso comes is a variety of curves that can be of help, especially with the difficult angles encountered in posterior repairs.

Care should be taken not to injure the glenoid cartilage when passing the sharp tip of this device through the labrum. Advancing the Lasso slowly and with adequate visualization to avoid this risk is suggested.

REHABILITATION

Patients are placed in an abduction sling postoperatively. The sling is worn round the clock for the first four weeks. Patients will work on hand, wrist, and elbow range of motion, as well as shoulder and scapular isometric exercises during this time. At four weeks gentle passive and active assisted range of motion exercises are started and advanced to full active range of motion usually by eight to 10 weeks. Functional or sports specific training can be started at three to four months and should be continued until full range of motion and normal strength are achieved. We do not recommend return to contact sports prior to six months.

RESULTS

Although several studies have been performed looking at the results of treatment of posterior shoulder instability, objective comparison can be difficult due to a number of confounding variables including surgical technique, sample size, outcome assessments, and inclusion criteria. Most studies evaluate instability as the chief outcome measure, defining failure as a recurrence of instability. In addition, most studies use some type of functional measure to assess outcome. In patients with unidirectional posterior shoulder instability, the recurrence rate reported in the literature is 5%. In patients with posteroinferior instability the recurrence rates are generally thought to be higher, however, there have been no studies that bear this out, due to the heterogeneity of the population.

Williams et al. (10) reported 26 patients treated arthroscopically with Suretac fixation of a discrete traumatic capsulolabral detachment from the glenoid rim. At follow up averaging 5.1 years, no patients had greater than 1+ instability in any direction with mean L'Insalata shoulder scores of 90. They felt arthroscopic repair of the posterior capsulolabral complex was an effective means of eliminating symptoms of pain and instability associated with posterior instability.

Using more current techniques, Provenchar et al. (11) treated 33 patients with posterior instability using arthroscopic shoulder stabilization with suture anchors, or suture capsulolabral plication, or both. At a mean follow up of 39.1 months there were seven failures (four recurrent instability and three symptoms of pain) with American Shoulder and Elbow Surgeons Ratings Scale of 94.6. They noted that patients with voluntary instability were the only patients that demonstrated recurrent instability at follow up. They also noted that patients with prior surgery and those with an intact capsulolabral complex, treated with suture plication alone, generally did worse with regards to outcome scores.

CONCLUSION

With appropriate patient selection based on an indepth history, physical examination, and radiographic findings, arthroscopic treatment of posterior instability is an excellent option for patients who have failed an appropriate course of nonoperative management.

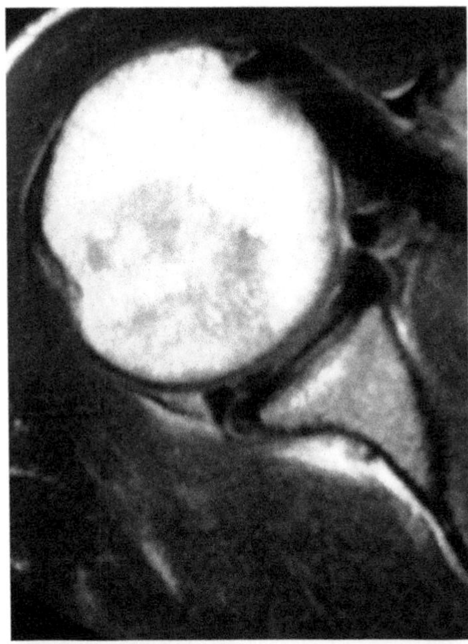

FIGURE 1 Axial T1 weighted MRI of posterior labral tear.

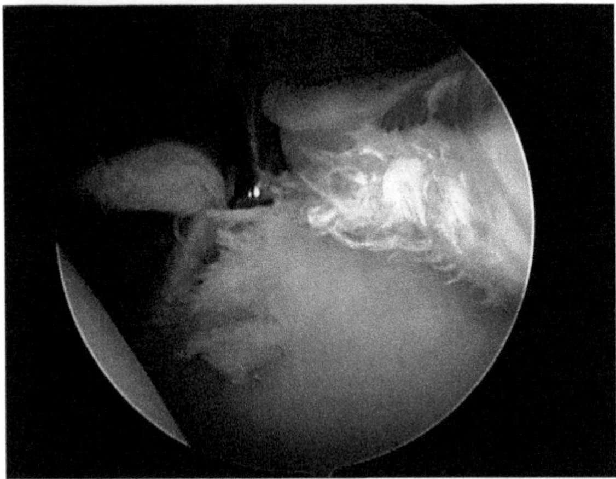

FIGURE 2 Arthroscopic picture of posterior labral tear.

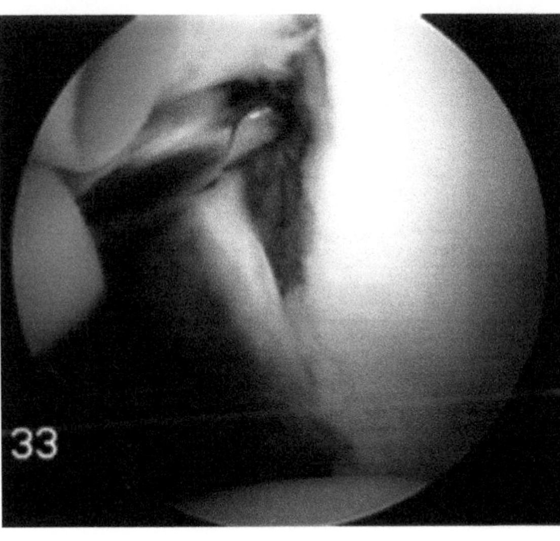

FIGURE 3 Debridement of tear and glenoid bone preparation.

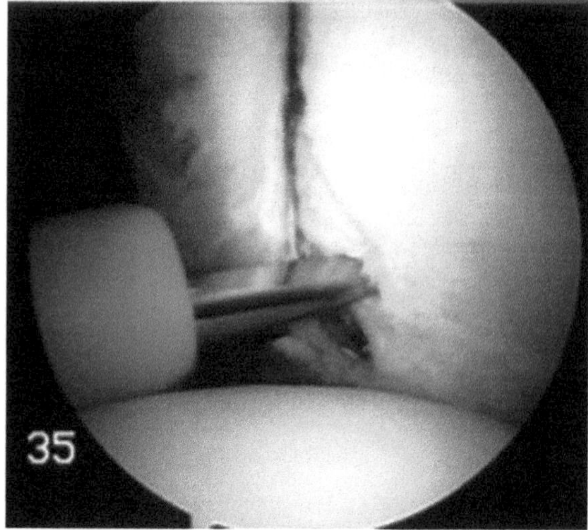

FIGURE 4 Placement of drill guide onto glenoid.

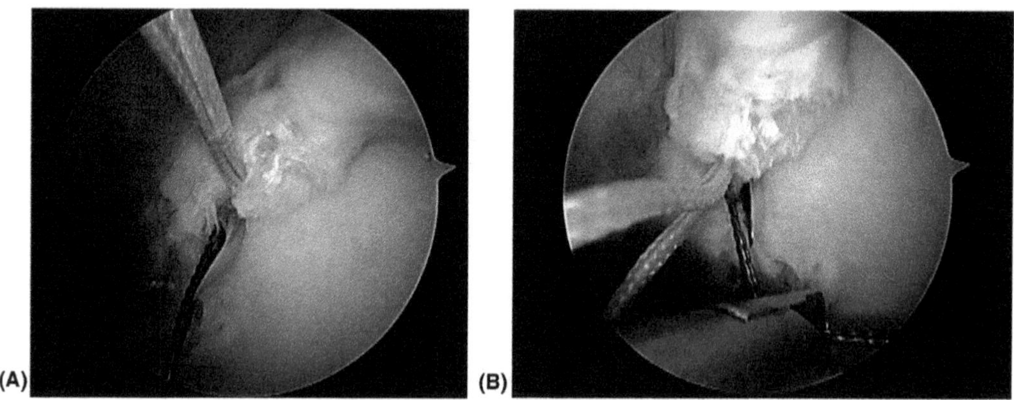

FIGURE 5 (**A**) Suture lasso thru labrum; (**B**) retreive suture lasso shuttle suture.

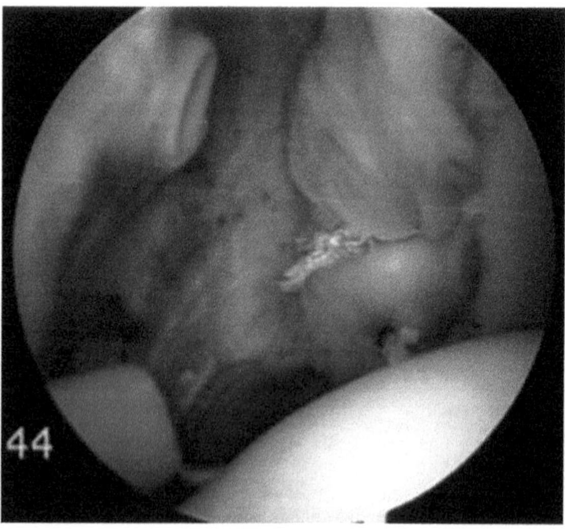

FIGURE 6 Finished repair.

REFERENCES

1. Wolf EM, Eaking CL. Arthroscopic capsular plication for posterior shoulder instability. Arthroscopy 1998; 14:153–63.
2. Kaplan LD, Flanigan DC, Norwig J, et al. Prevalence and variance of shoulder injuries in elite collegiate football players. Am J Sports Med 2005; 33:1142–1146.
3. Hawkins RJ, Koppert G, Johnston G.'Recurrent posterior instability (subluxation) of the shoulder. J'Bone Joint Surg Am 1984; 66:169–174.
4. Hurley JA, Anderson TE, Dear W, et al. Posterior shoulder instability. Surgical versus conservative results with evaluation of glenoid version. Am J Sports Med 1992; 20:396–400.
5. Surin V, Blader S, Markhede G, et al. Rotational osteotomy of the humerus for posterior instability of the shoulder. J Bone Joint Surg Am 1990; 72:181–186.
6. Scott DJ, Jr. Treatment of recurrent posterior dislocations of the shoulder by glenoplasty. Report of three cases. J Bone Joint Surg Am 1967; 49:471–476.
7. Mair SD, Zarzour RH, Speer KP. Posterior labral injury in contact athletes. Am J Sports Med 1998; 26:753–758.
8. Millet PJ, Clavert P, Warner JP. Arthrscopic management of anterior, posterior, and multidirectional shoulder instability: pearls and pitfalls. Arthroscopy 2003; 19(suppl 1):86–93.
9. Tibone JE, Bradley JP. The treatment of posterior subluxation in athletes. Clin Orthop Relat Res 1993; 291:124–137.
10. Williams RJ, Strickland S, Cohen M, et al. Arthroscopic repair for traumatic posterior shoulder instability. Am J Sports Med 2003; 31:203–209.
11. Provenchar MT, Bell J, Menzel KA, et al. Arthroscopic treatment of posterior shoulder instability. Am J Sports Med 2005; 33:1463–1471.
12. Cooper A.'On the dislocations of the os humeri upon the dorsum scapulae and upon fractures near the shoulder joint. Guys Hosp Rep 1839; 4:265–284.
13. McLaughlin HL. Posterior dislocation of the shoulder. J Bone Joint Surg Am 1952; 24-A-3:584–590.
14. McLaughlin HL. Posterior dislocation of the shoulder. J Bone Joint Surg Am 1962; 44A:1477.
15. Boyd HB, Sisk TD. Recurrent posterior dislocation of the shoulder. J Bone Joint Surg Am 1972; 54: 779–786.
16. Hawkins RJ, Janda DH. Posterior instability of the gleno-humeral joint. A technique of repair. Am J Sports Med 1996; 24:275–278.
17. Rowe CR, Pierce DS, Clark JG. Voluntary dislocation of the shoulder. A preliminary report on a clinical, electromyographic, and psychiatric study of twenty-six patients. J Bone Joint Surg Am 1973; 55:445–460.
18. Speer KP, Hannafin JA, Altchek DW, et al. Am J Sports Med 1994; 22:177–183.
19. Green M, Christensen K.'Magnetic resonance imaging of the glenoid labrum: MR imaging of 88 arthroscopically confirmed cases. Am J Sports Med 1994; 22:493–498.
20. Iannotti J, Zlatkin M, Esterhai J.'Magnetic resonance imaging of the shoulder. Sensitivity, specificity, and predictive value. J Bone Joint Surg Am 1991; 73:17–29.

10 Arthroscopic Multidirectional Instability Repair

Cordelia Carter and William N. Levine
Center for Shoulder, Elbow, and Sports Medicine, Department of Orthopedic Surgery, Columbia Presbyterian Medical Center, New York, New York, U.S.A.

INTRODUCTION

Neer and Foster (1) described a open inferior capsular shift for patients with symptomatic multidirectional instability (MDI), which quickly became a mainstay of treatment after documented failure of nonoperative management. Since that time, other surgeons have replicated this technique, or variations upon it, with equally satisfactory results, and the inferior capsular shift has remained the gold standard of MDI treatment for years. However, with the advent of minimally invasive surgery and its associated emphasis on maximizing surgical outcomes while minimizing surgery-related morbidities, numerous arthroscopic techniques to address glenohumeral pathology traditionally treated by open methods have evolved, and the arthroscopic capsular shift is not an exception.

This chapter will describe the indications, contraindications, surgical technique, pearls and pitfalls, and rehabilitation program for arthroscopic capsular plication in the treatment of patients with MDI.

INDICATIONS

Patients with MDI should always be treated nonoperatively for a minimum of six months since many will be successfully treated with this approach. The goals of nonoperative management are to improve the dynamic stabilizers for improving stability in the face of suboptimal ligamentous support.

"Classic" MDI patients will demonstrate generalized ligamentous laxity and hypermobile joints. Patients who have symptomatic instability in two or more directions (anterior, posterior, and inferior) and have failed nonoperative management for six months are considered appropriate candidates for surgical intervention. Examination will typically show anterior load and shift of 2+ (translation of the humeral head beyond the glenoid but reduces with removal of the force), 2+ posterior load and shift (translation of the humeral head beyond the glenoid posteriorly, but reduces with removal of the force), and 2+ sulcus sign (inferior translation of 1 to 2 cm measured as the sulcus between the lateral acromion and the greater tuberosity). Rotator interval incompetence is commonly found in these patients as well. An incompetent rotator interval is demonstrated on physical examination as a positive sulcus sign that does not diminish with arm adduction and external rotation (Fig. 1).

CONTRAINDICATIONS

Patients who have voluntary instability are poor candidates for surgical intervention. Also, patients with connective tissue disorders and hyperlaxity are also often poor candidates for surgery, due to the high recurrence of the instability from their underlying collagen deficiency (Figs. 2A–C).

Please refer to pages 118–122 for the figures in this chapter.

TECHNIQUES

Exam Under Anesthesia

Exam under anesthesia (EUA) of the glenohumeral joint should always be performed and allows the examiner to assess the degree and direction of glenohumeral laxity in each shoulder, as well as to make side-to-side comparisons. Importantly, the EUA should confirm the preoperative diagnosis established through careful history taking, physical examination, and radiographic evaluation prior to surgical intervention.

Patient Positioning and Anesthesia

We perform the majority of these procedures with regional interscalene anesthesia. We have a regional anesthesia department and work closely with our anesthesia colleagues to assure appropriate pain relief, sedation, and blood pressure maintenance. After appropriate anesthesia is obtained, we place the patient in the lateral decubitus position (Fig. 3). Although the procedure can be performed in the beach chair position (depending on surgeon's preference, of course), we prefer the lateral decubitus position for this procedure, as the entire capsule can more easily be addressed.

Arthroscopic Capsular Plication

Standard diagnostic arthroscopy is carried out from a posterior portal (Fig. 4). Typical intra-articular findings of shoulders with MDI include the following:

1. Widened rotator interval (capsule between anterior supraspinatus and top of subscapularis)
2. Patulous capsule (typically not just anterior, but posterior as well)
3. Positive "drive-through" sign: the arthroscope can be "driven" from posterior to anterior below the glenoid equator without any resistance
4. Normal labrum (entire labrum superiorly, anteriorly, and posteriorly)
5. Normal biceps tendon
6. Normal articular cartilage
7. Normal rotator cuff

Next, anterior working portals are made dependent on the pathology found. Typically, two rotator interval portals are made—one high in the rotator interval and the other low just proximal to the subscapularis. These working portals need to be separated as much as possible, externally, to avoid crowding in the intra-articular joint space (Fig. 5).

Background

In general, the goal is to shift the redundant capsular tissue and gather it onto the glenoid rim to enhance the existing labrum and deepen the effective glenoid concavity.

Ability of this type of capsular plication procedure using a "pinch-tuck" technique, in which a pleat is formed by suturing the capsule to itself, has been shown to significantly decrease humeral translation without excessive loss of rotational motion (2–8). The capsule can either be advanced to an intact labrum or repaired with suture anchors into the glenoid, incorporating the labrum as well. In either case, we first abrade the capsule to enhance healing of the plicated capsule.

General Principles

In general, we begin posteriorly and place one to three posterior capsular plication sutures from six to eight o'clock (right shoulder) as necessary. This is best performed with the arthroscope in the anterosuperior viewing portal, and then the posterior and anteroinferior portal can be used for suture passage and tying. We typically use a disposable suture shuttling device (Suture lasso, Arthex; Naples, Florida, U.S.A.) for this part of the procedure (Fig. 6). In some cases, an additional posterolateral portal may be necessary for better orientation of suture passing devices and/or suture anchor placement if necessary.

The arthroscope is then placed back in the posterior viewing portal and the rest of the anteroinferior capsular plication can be performed from the six to three o'clock position. Typically, two to four anterior capsular plication sutures will be placed, thereby eliminating the redundant anteroinferior and posteroinferior capsule.

Next, the rotator interval is assessed for pathologic laxity (as described earlier). There are three options for rotator interval closure: intra-articular repair, extracapsular repair in a single cannula, and subacromial repair. All have distinct advantages and disadvantages, and more extensive description can be found in chapter 12.

When performing the capsular plication procedure, the capsule can be advanced to an intact labrum or directly to the glenoid with the use of suture anchors (with or without incorporation of the labrum if present). We will detail both of these procedures subsequently.

Intact Labrum

In shoulders with an intact labrum, the capsule can be repaired directly to the labrum without the need for suture anchor placement (Fig. 7). The advantages of this procedure are that a suture anchor is not necessary, thereby allowing as inferior placement as desirable. In the example shown in Figure 6, this is a right shoulder viewed from the posterior viewing portal, and the suture is seen in the capsule and through the intact posteroinferior labrum at seven o'clock prior to tying. Care should be taken, however, when this technique is used to observe the labrum when the suture is being tied—on some occasions, the labrum can be seen to pull away from the glenoid when the suture is tied. If this is identified, stop before the suture is secured and place a suture anchor in the glenoid at the desired location. Then the suture from the anchor can be shuttled through the capsule with the previously placed capsular plication suture.

Final evaluation should demonstrate obliteration of the capsular redundancy and elimination of the drive-through sign (Figs. 8A and B).

Labral Tear or Incompetent Labrum

In shoulders where the labrum is deficient, torn, or seen to pull away from the glenoid, suture anchors should be used (Fig. 9). The glenoid should be abraded to enhance healing, as is the capsule. Suture anchors are placed in routine fashion, beginning as inferiorly as possible. Care is taken to perform a south–north shift with the capsular sutures in each case (avoid east–west shift that will cause additional loss of external rotation and possible over-tightening).

Specific Pearls and Pitfalls of Capsular Plication

1. Begin as inferiorly as possible to avoid being shut out of the working space.
2. View from anterosuperior portal to work on the posteroinferior capsule.
3. Abrade capsule to enhance healing.
4. If labrum is intact and competent, perform capsular plication to the intact labrum. Pass suture through posteroinferior cannula and retrieve other limb from anteroinferior cannula. Then take both limbs out of the posteroinferior cannula and tie the first posterior capsular plication suture. Repeat as many times as necessary for posterior plication.
5. Switch to posterior viewing portal and perform anteroinferior plication using the anterosuperior and anteroinferior working portals. In general, always have one viewing and two working portals to facilitate suture passage, tying, and management.
6. If the labrum is not intact or deficient, then simply perform identical procedure using suture anchors and follow the steps 3 to 5 mentioned earlier.
7. Goal is to achieve "balanced" plication—view from anterosuperior portal is helpful to determine that humeral head is well centered and that there is not over-tightening on either anterior or posterior side.

Finally, the rotator interval needs to be assessed. In the majority of patients with MDI and posterior instability, the rotator interval does require closure. More specific details on rotator interval closure can be found in chapter 12. We generally place one rotator interval closure suture laterally taking care to not place it to medially, which will lead to contracture of the middle glenohumeral ligament (MGHL) and superior glenohumeral ligament (SGHL) and limit external rotation (Fig. 10).

Techniques for rotator interval closure:

1. A penetrating suture passer loaded with permanent suture is used to perforate the upper edge of the MGHL, and the suture is retrieved into the anterosuperior (AS) cannula.
2. The AS cannula is withdrawn until it sits just external to the capsule and the end of the suture is reloaded into the straight penetrator, which is used to repierce the superior capsule and advance the suture into the joint.
3. A sliding arthroscopic knot is tied extracapsularly in the cannula and cut.

POSTOP REHABILITATION

Immobilization in a sling in slight external rotation (Fig. 11) or gunslinger brace is used for six weeks. Range of motion exercises are deferred for four weeks in most patients with gross laxity and no labral tearing or traumatic instability. Gentle range of motion exercises at home, in addition to supervised physical therapy, are then begun at the fourth postoperative week. The goals are to achieve full passive range of motion by six to eight weeks and to start progressive strengthening exercises from 8 to 12 weeks. Although rare, stiffness can occur, so we generally evaluate the patients every two weeks in the beginning to assure that the patient is not getting early stiffness. If stiffness if felt to be developing early, then the patient will be referred to physical therapy earlier. Typically, resistance exercises and sports-specific rehabilitation start in 12 to 16 weeks and return to sports is possible at six months.

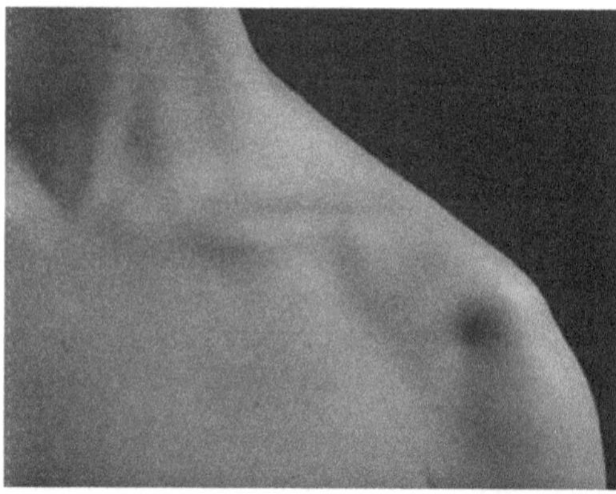

FIGURE 1 Pathologic rotator interval—the sulcus sign does not reduce with external rotation of the arm at the side.

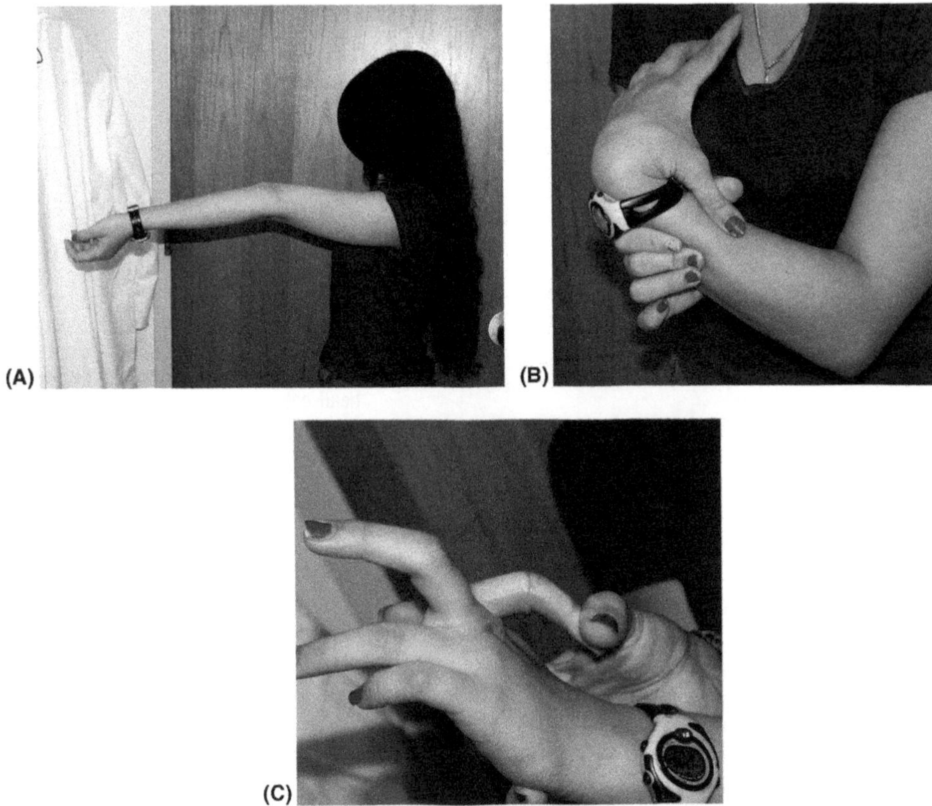

FIGURE 2 A sixteen-year-old RHD female with multidirectional instability and profound ligamentous laxity: (**A**) elbow recurvatum, (**B**) thumb to forearm, and (**C**) metacarpophalangeal hyperextension.

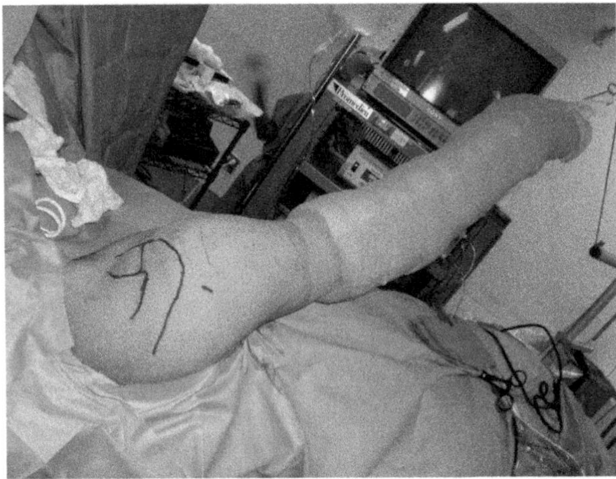

FIGURE 3 Patient is in the lateral decubitus position—the right upper extremity is being suspended in a traction device (Arthrex; Naples, Florida, U.S.A.) applying 10 pounds of traction.

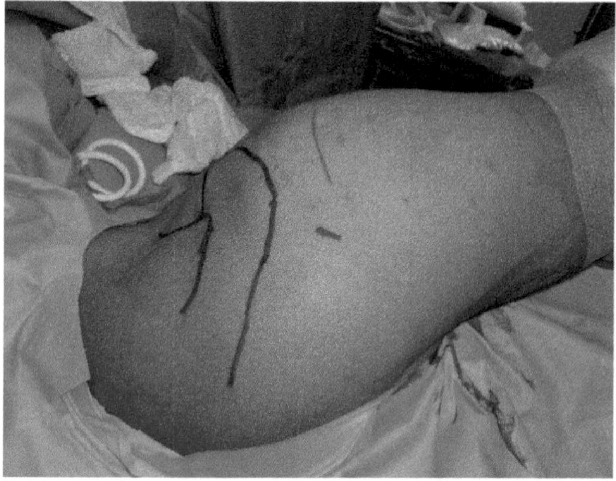

FIGURE 4 In the same patient seen in Figure 3, the routine posterior portal is made in the soft spot felt by shucking the humeral head between the thumb and index finger—typically, 2 cm inferior and 1 cm medial to the posterolateral edge of the acromion.

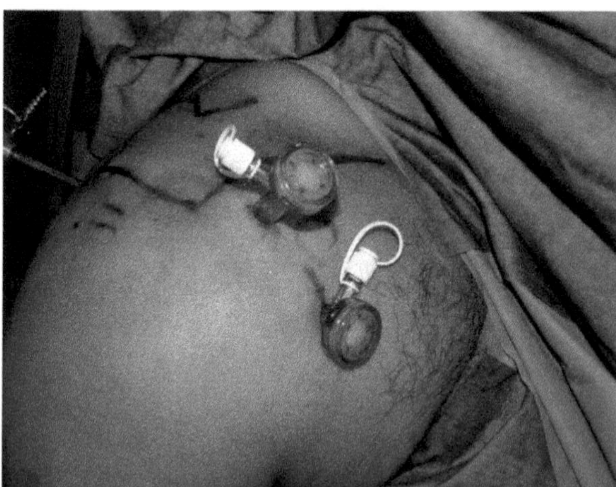

FIGURE 5 External view of two rotator interval portals—one cannula is seen high in the rotator interval and the other is just proximal to the subscapularis tendon.

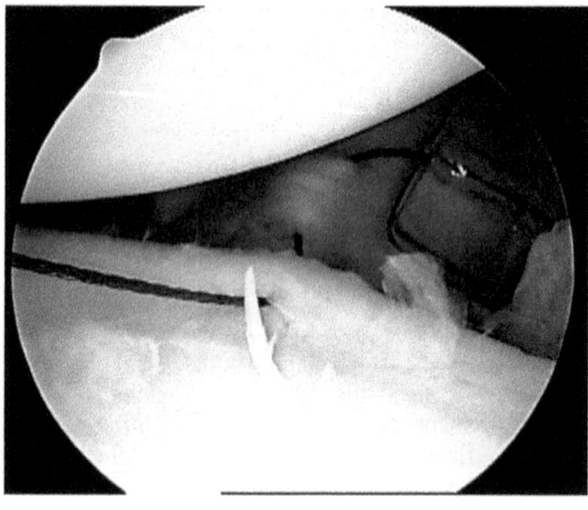

FIGURE 6 Right shoulder—lateral decubitus position, anterosuperior viewing portal. Nitenol wire loop from a disposable suture lasso (Arthrex; Naples, Florida, U.S.A.) is seen through the posteroinferior capsule and the intact posteroinferior labrum.

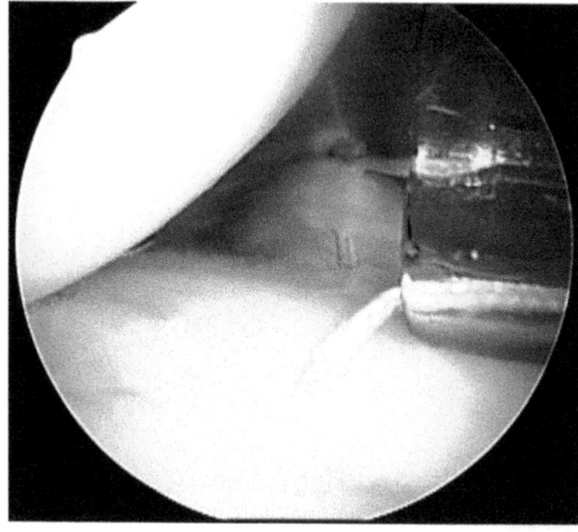

FIGURE 7 Right shoulder—lateral decubitus position, anterosuperior viewing portal. Permanent suture in postero-inferior capsule and the corresponding posteroinferior labrum prior to tying.

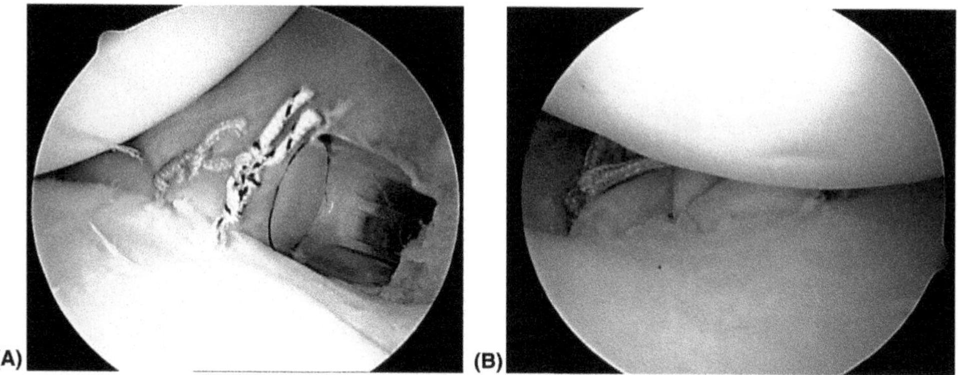

FIGURE 8 Right shoulder—lateral decubitus position. Final view of (**A**) posterior plication and (**B**) anterior plication in an 18-year-old RHD female with generalized ligamentous laxity, multidirectional instability, and no labral pathology.

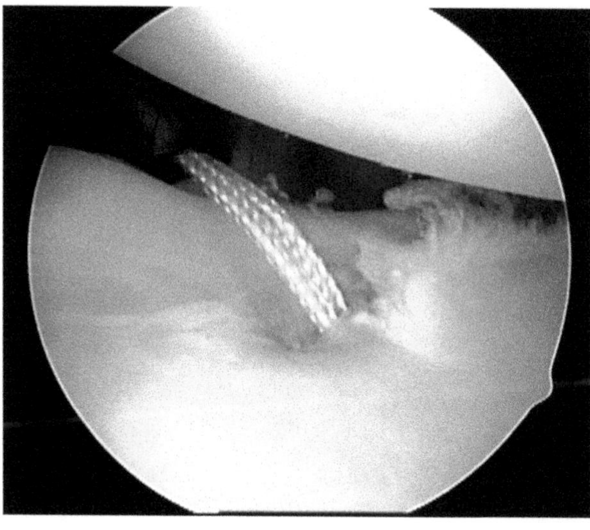

FIGURE 9 Right shoulder—lateral decubitus position posterior viewing portal. Suture anchor placed at the four o'clock position in this patient with an anteroinferior labral tear in association with multidirectional instability.

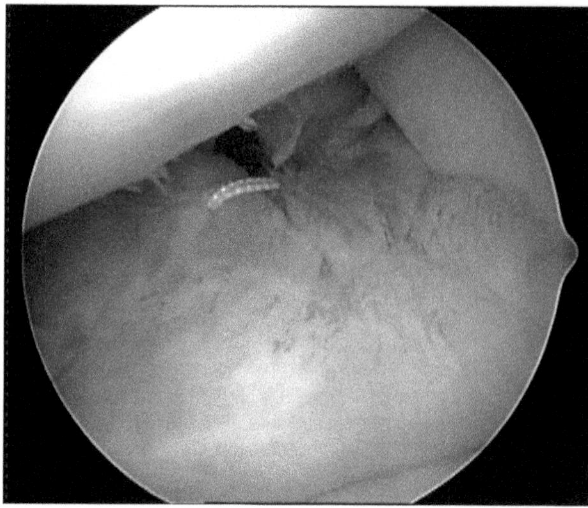

FIGURE 10 Left shoulder—lateral decubitus position. One rotator interval closure suture placed and tied in the cannula on the extra-articular side of the capsule.

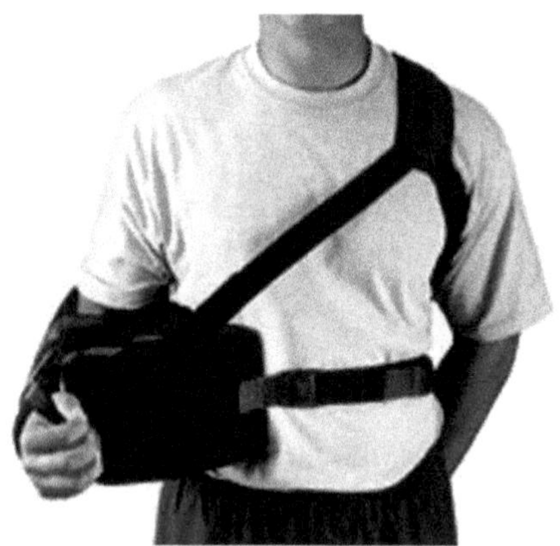

FIGURE 11 Patient following arthroscopic capsular plication with external rotation sling.

REFERENCES

1. Neer CS, II, Foster CR. Inferior capsular shift for involuntary inferior and multidirectional instability of the shoulder. A preliminary report. J Bone Joint Surg Am 1980; 62(6):897–908.
2. Flanigan DC, Forsythe T, Orwin J, Kaplan L. Volume analysis of arthroscopic capsular shift. Arthroscopy 2006; 22(5):528–533.
3. Karas SG, Creighton RA, DeMorat GJ. Glenohumeral volume reduction in arthroscopic shoulder reconstruction: a cadaveric analysis of suture plication and thermal capsulorrhaphy. Arthroscopy 2004; 20(2):179–184.
4. Werner CM, Nyffeler RW, Jacob HA, Gerber C. The effect of capsular tightening on humeral head translations. J Orthop Res 2004; 22(1):194–201.
5. Westerheide KJ, Dopirak RM, Snyder SJ. Arthroscopic anterior stabilization and posterior capsular plication for anterior glenohumeral instability: a report of 71 cases. Arthroscopy 2006; 22(5):539–547.
6. Wiley WB, Goradia VK, Pearson SE. Arthroscopic capsular plication-shift. Arthroscopy 2005; 21(1): 119–121.
7. Alberta FG, ElAttrache NS, Mihata T, McGarry MH, Tibone JE, Lee TQ. Arthroscopic anteroinferior suture plication resulting in decreased glenohumeral translation and external rotation. Study of a cadaver model. J Bone Joint Surg Am 2006; 88(1):179–187.
8. Cohen SB et al. Anterior capsulorrhaphy: an in vitro comparison of volume reduction–arthroscopic plication versus open capsular shift. Arthroscopy 2005; 21(6):659–664.

11 Arthroscopic Superior Labrum Anterior Posterior Repair

Christopher S. Ahmad
Center for Shoulder, Elbow, and Sports Medicine, Department of Orthopedic Surgery, Columbia Presbyterian Medical Center, New York, New York, U.S.A.

INDICATIONS

Superior labral anterior to posterior (SLAP) lesions describe injuries to the superior labrum (1) and are classified into four basic types. Type I lesions consist of fraying and degeneration (Fig. 1), type II consists of detachment of the biceps anchor (Fig. 2), type III lesions consist of a bucket-handle tear (Fig. 3), and type IV lesions are similar to a type III lesion with extension of the tear into the biceps tendon (Fig. 4). Combinations of these lesions may also be observed.

Indications for surgery include those patients with a suspected SLAP lesion who have failed nonoperative treatment. Symptoms include anterior–superior or posterior–superior shoulder pain exacerbated by activity with the arm overhead. Popping, locking, and snapping may occur with unstable labral tears. Symptoms of shoulder instability may be present especially if the tear extends anterior and inferior or posterior and inferior.

Examination tests suggestive of SLAP tears include the active compression test, compression–rotation test, Speed's biceps tension test, Yergason test, Jobe relocation test, and tenderness of the bicipital groove. Magnetic resonance imaging (MRI)-enhanced arthrography is superior to plain MRI for diagnosing SLAP lesions (Fig. 5) (2). It is emphasized, however, that the ultimate diagnosis is made and confirmed during arthroscopy.

CONTRAINDICATIONS

Contraindications for SLAP repair include patients who are unwillingly to comply with necessary postop rehabilitation. Relative contraindications to SLAP repair include older patients with degenerative glenohumeral joint arthritis in which a biceps tenodesis may be preferred. Patients who are minimally symptomatic should also avoid surgery.

TECHNIQUE

Type I SLAP lesions are treated with debridement of the frayed labrum and typically is in addition to the treatment of other associated shoulder pathology. Type II SLAP lesions are repaired using a suture anchor technique for fixation. Type III SLAP lesions are treated by resection of the unstable bucket-handle labral fragment. For larger tears, repair may be preferred. Type IV SLAP lesions are treated similarly to type III lesions unless the biceps tendon split is severe, which requires either repair as with a type II SLAP or biceps tenodesis. Age and activity level of the patient as well as the condition of the remainder of the biceps tendon should factor in to the decision making for biceps tenodesis. If the tendon contains greater than 50% degeneration, a tenodesis is performed in the younger active patient, and a tenotomy is performed in the older less-active patient.

Positioning

General or regional anesthesia is induced and an exam under anesthesia is performed with the patient in the supine position. SLAP repairs may be performed in either the beach chair or

---

Please refer to pages 127–131 for the figures in this chapter.

lateral decubitus position. We prefer the lateral decubitus position with traction to improve superior visualization as well as ability to repair combined anterior and posterior labral tears if they exist. The patient is tilted 20° posteriorly and 20° reverse trendelenburg to position the glenoid parallel to the floor. Typically, 10 lbs of traction is applied and excess should be limited to avoid brachial plexus injury.

Diagnostic Arthroscopy

A standard posterior portal is created and an examination is performed to assess all pathology prior to committing to the anterior and other portal placement (Fig. 6). Common associated pathology includes partial thickness rotator cuff tears, anterior labral tears, and posterior labral tears. A spinal needle introduced anteriorly may be used to probe the superior labrum before committing to the location of the anterior portal. Proper placement of the suture anchors requires exact placement of the anterosuperior portal in the superior aspect of the rotator interval and slightly inferior to the biceps tendon. A probe is used then to test the stability of the biceps/superior labrum attachments to the glenoid (Fig. 2). To perform the peel-back test, the arm is positioned to 90° abduction and 90° external rotation. Existence of a posterior SLAP lesion will cause the biceps/superior labrum complex to drop medially over the edge of the glenoid.

After confirming the presence of a reparable lesion, a motorized shaver from the anterior working portal is used to prepare the superior neck of the glenoid beneath the detached labrum (Fig. 7). The soft tissues are removed and the bone is abraded to enhance healing. A Wilmington portal is then established with a clear cannula to allow suture anchor placement and suture management. This portal is established at the lateral edge of the acromion at its posterior one-third (Fig. 8). A suture anchor is placed through this cannulae adjacent to the biceps tendon at the glenoid articular surface margin (Fig. 6). The suture anchor must be visualized and confirmed to be seated in bone, and tested with tension to confirm security (Fig. 9). Suture passage through the labrum is performed next with many devices available. Nonshuttling devices penetrate the labrum from superior to inferior, followed by grasping the suture. The device is then withdrawn to pull the suture out the anterosuperior cannula. Other devices that require suture shuttling are often smaller in diameter and less traumatic to the injured labrum. The limb of suture facing the labrum is retrieved out the anterior portal. The suture passing device is passed through the labrum, and the suture shuttle is retrieved out the anterior portal (Fig. 10). Outside the cannulae, the suture is then passed through the shuttle loop, and the suture passer with shuttle is withdrawn through the labrum and to the posterior and cannula. Arthroscopic knot tying is then performed. Sliding knots that are locking or nonlocking are typically used (Fig. 11). A probe is used to assess the repair. The process of anchor placement, suture passing, and knot tying is repeated anteriorly and posteriorly, as needed with anchors spaced 3 to 4 mm apart until the labrum is secured. For meniscoid type labrums, suture may be placed in a horizontal fashion to achieve a more anatomic repair.

If minimizing morbidity to the rotator cuff from creation of the Wilmington Portal is desired, a percutaneous and transtendinous technique may be employed. A small stab incision is made at the location of the Wilmington portal. The guide for anchor placement is then introduced percutaneously and transtendinously (Fig. 12). The anchor is placed and the sutures are visualized from the entrance of the capsule (Fig. 13). The suture to be passed through the labrum is retrieved out the anterior cannulae. Suture passing is then performed by introducing the suture passer percutaneously and transtendinously (Fig. 14), and then used to penetrate the labrum (Fig. 15). Next, the suture is shuttled creating a simple suture through the labrum (Fig. 16). The anterior cannulae is then placed over the anchor and the sutures are retrieved (Fig. 17). Subsequently, knot tying is performed and the steps are repeated for additional anchors. Figure 18 depicts the completion of the first anchor.

PEARLS AND PITFALLS

An important aspect of SLAP repair is differentiating a true SLAP lesion from a meniscoid type labrum. Exact portal placement enhances ease of tissue preparation and anchor placement. Anchors should be visually confirmed to be in bone and tested with tension for fixation security. The glenoid has a high curvature and suture anchors may be errantly placed in soft tissue adjacent to bone. An errantly placed anchor could result in migration and joint damage. Optimal loop security and knot security favors biologic healing. Small knots may reduce glenohumeral irritation.

REHABILITATION

Postoperatively, the shoulder is protected in a sling for six weeks. The patient begins elbow, wrist, and hand exercises immediately postoperatively, and gentle pendulum exercises in one week. The shoulder is protected to avoid stress on the biceps tendon for six weeks. Strengthening of the rotator cuff, scapular stabilizers, and deltoid in addition to exercises to restore terminal range of motion are initiated at six weeks. Biceps strengthening is begun eight weeks postoperatively. Vigorous or strenuous lifting activities are allowed after three months. At four months, throwing athletes begin an interval throwing program on a level surface. They continue a stretching and strengthening program, with particular emphasis on posterior–inferior capsular stretching. At six months, pitchers may begin throwing full-speed, and at seven months pitchers are allowed maximal effort throwing from the mound.

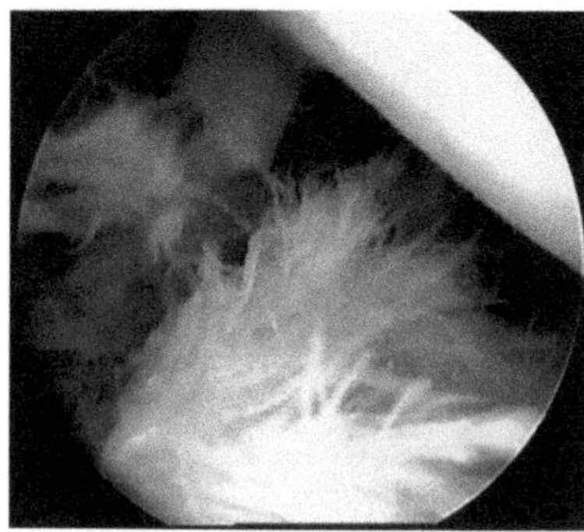

FIGURE 1 Type I superior labral anterior to posterior (SLAP) tear demonstrating fraying of the labrum.

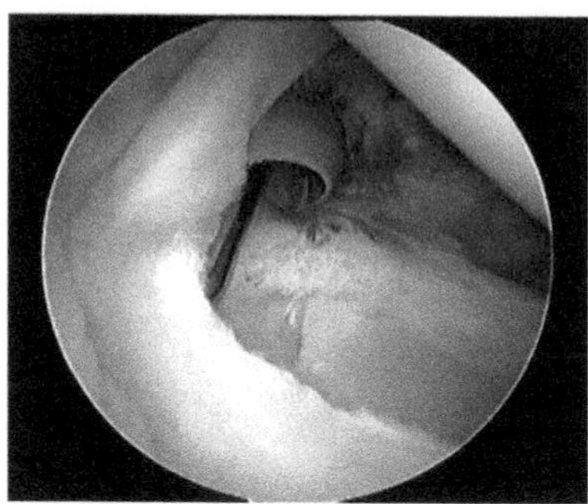

FIGURE 2 Type II superior labral anterior to posterior (SLAP) tear with probe demonstrating instability of labrum and biceps anchor.

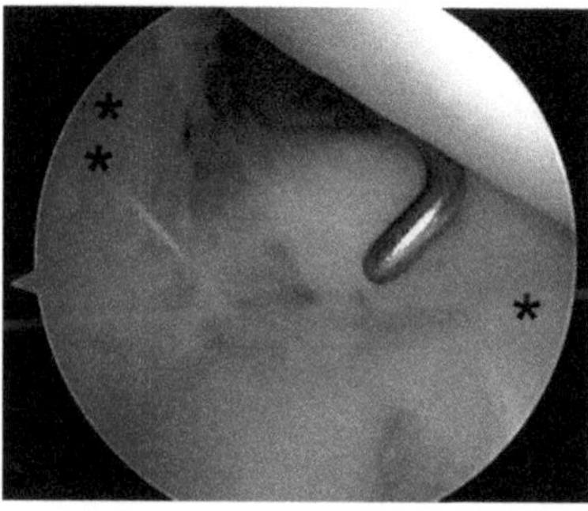

FIGURE 3 Type III superior labral anterior to posterior (SLAP) tear demonstrating bucket handle type tear with "*" indicating the labral tear displaced and "**" indicating the biceps tendon.

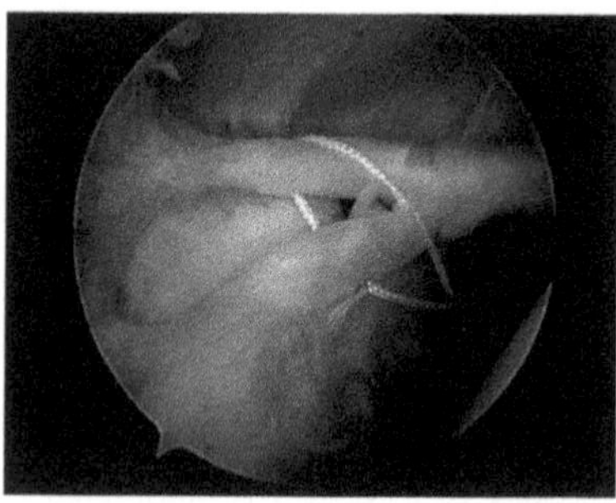

FIGURE 4 Type IV superior labral anterior to posterior (SLAP) tear demonstrating a split in the biceps tendon.

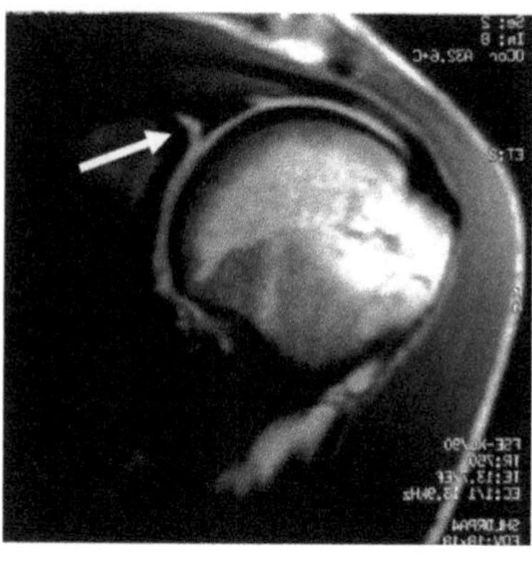

FIGURE 5 Gadolinium enhanced magnetic resonance imaging coronal oblique with dye under biceps anchor indicating type II superior labral anterior to posterior (SLAP) tear.

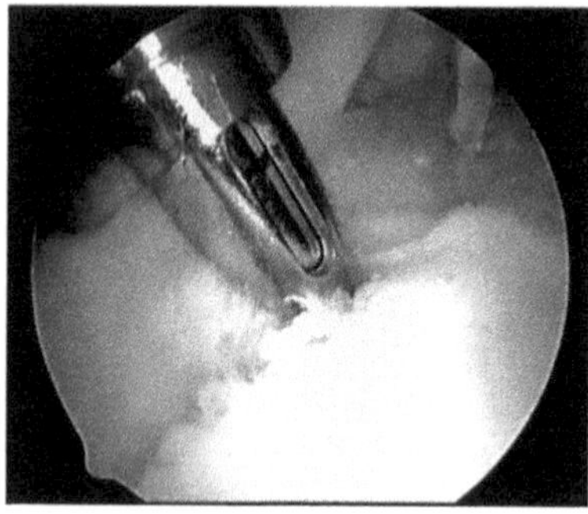

FIGURE 6 Drill guide for suture anchor placement introduced through Wilmington portal.

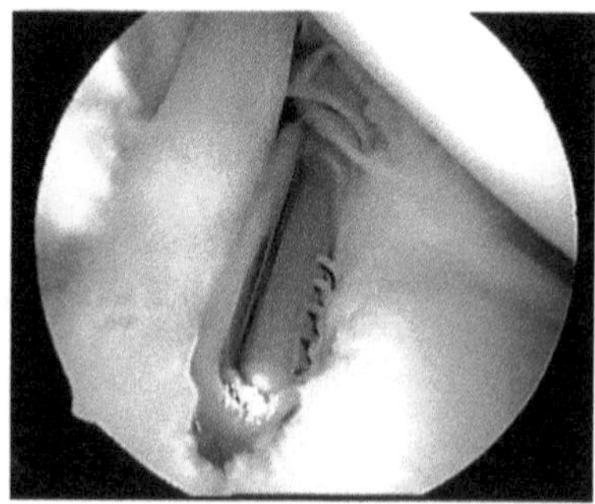

FIGURE 7 Debridement of superior glenoid.

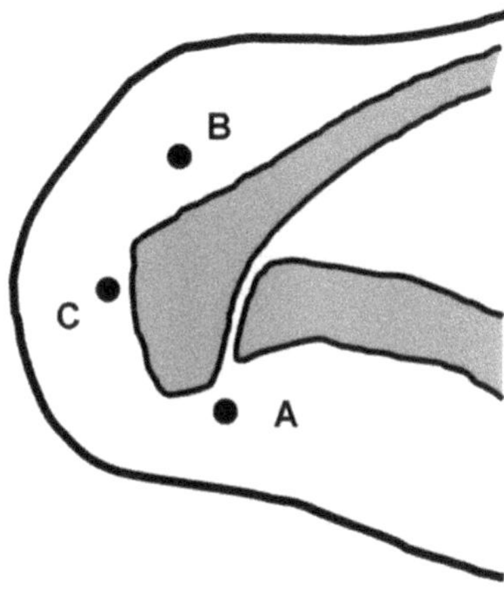

FIGURE 8 (**A**) Anterior working portal, (**B**) standard viewing portal, and (**C**) Wilmington portal located adjacent to acromion in posterior one-third.

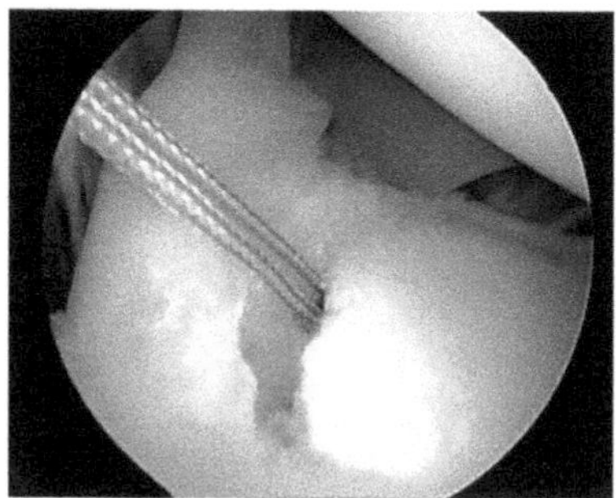

FIGURE 9 Suture anchor placement adjacent to articular cartilage.

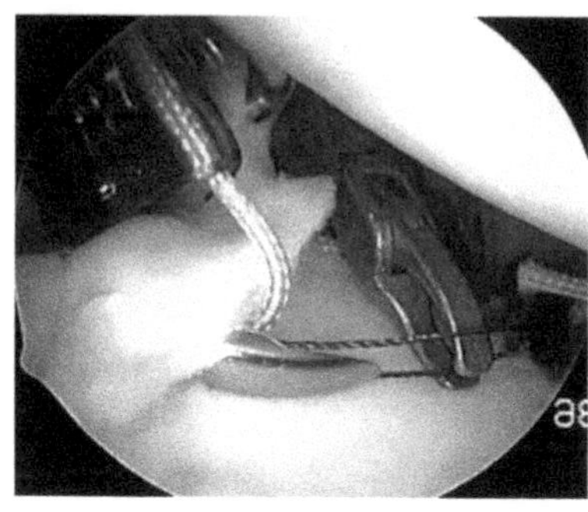

FIGURE 10 Suture passer placed through the labrum and wire shuttle advanced into joint.

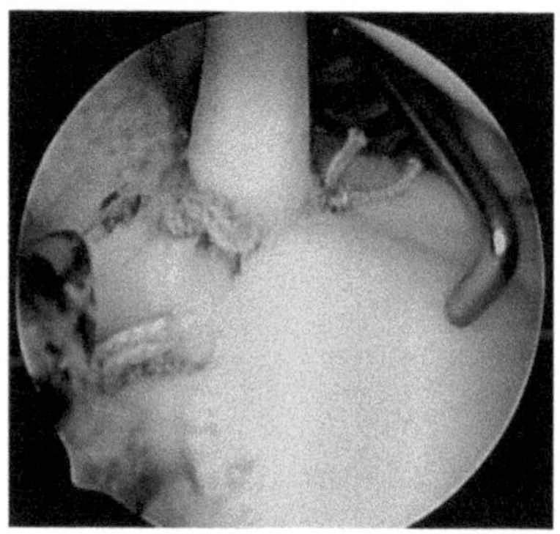

FIGURE 11 Completed repair with several anchors placed and knots tied.

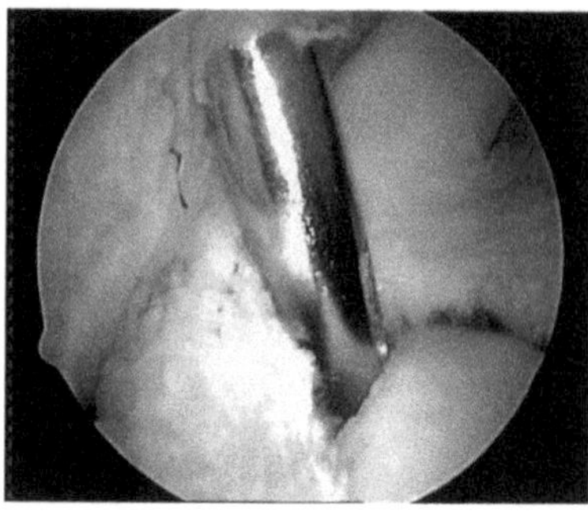

FIGURE 12 Percutaneous and transtendi-nous drill guide placement.

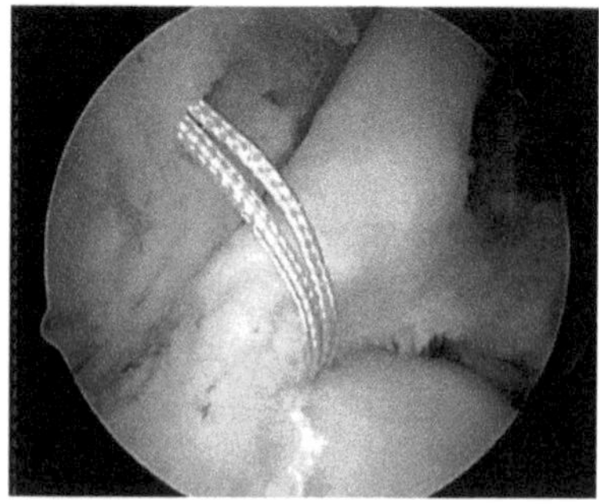

FIGURE 13 Anchor placed with sutures penetrating capsule.

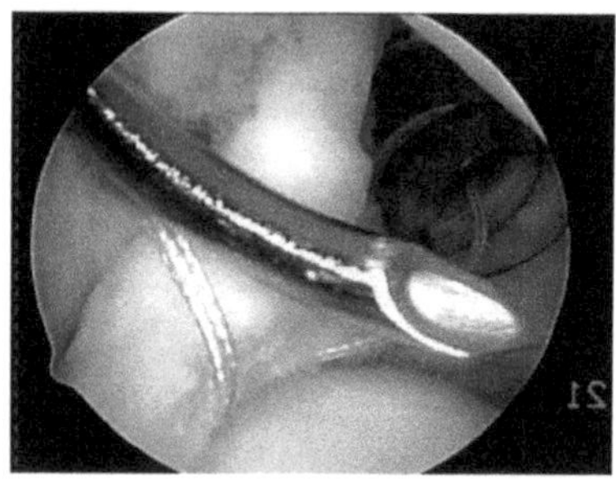

FIGURE 14 Percutaneous and transtendinous introduction of suture passer.

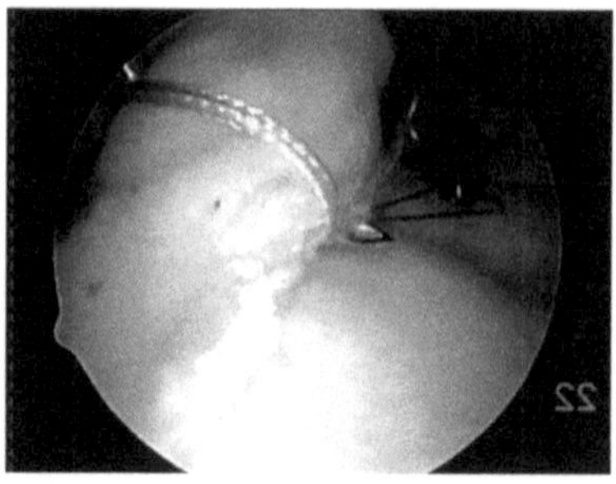

FIGURE 15 Suture passer placed through labrum and shuttle wire advanced into glenohumeral joint.

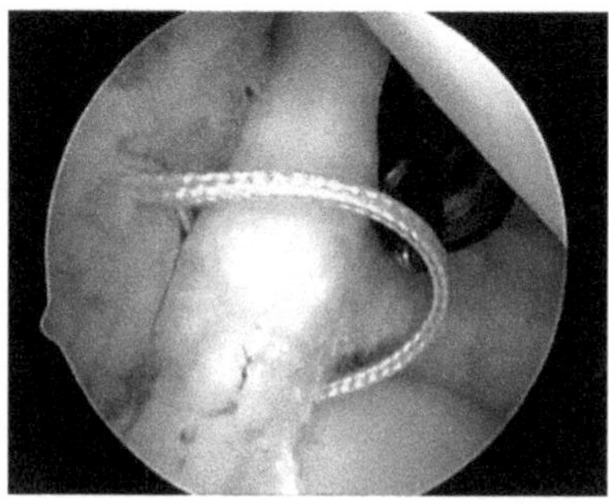

FIGURE 16 Suture shuttled through labrum for simple suture passing configuration.

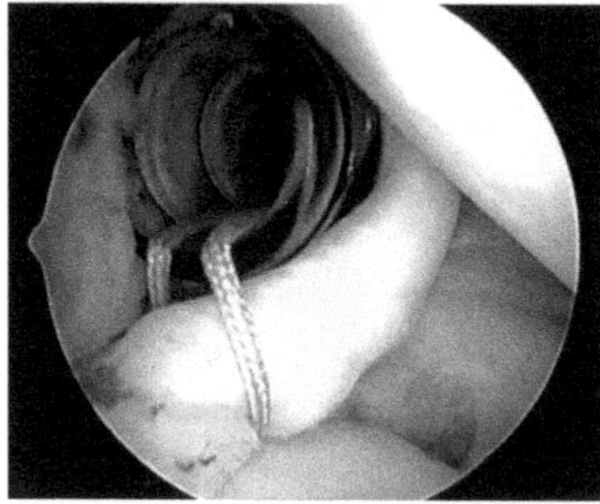

FIGURE 17 Anterior cannulae positioned posterior to biceps with sutures retrieved.

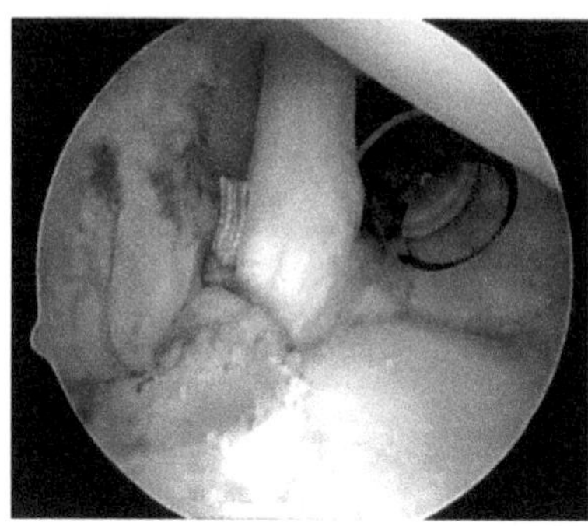

FIGURE 18 Placement, passing, and tying of first anchor completed.

REFERENCES

1. Snyder SJ, Karzel RP, Del Pizzo W, Ferkel RD, Friedman MJ. SLAP lesions of the shoulder. Arthroscopy 1990; 6(4):274–279.
2. Bencardino JT, Beltran J, Rosenberg ZS, et al. Superior labrum anterior-posterior lesions: diagnosis with MR arthrography of the shoulder. Radiology 2000; 214(1):267–271.

12 Arthroscopic Rotator Interval Closure

Andreas H. Gomoll
Department of Orthopedic Surgery, Brigham and Women's Hospital, Harvard Medical School, Boston, Massachusetts, U.S.A.

Brian J. Cole
Departments of Orthopedics and Anatomy and Cell Biology, and Division of Shoulder and Elbow Surgery, Department of Orthopedic Surgery, Rush University Medical Center, Rush Medical College, Chicago, Illinois, U.S.A.

INTRODUCTION

The rotator interval has been identified as an important anatomic structure contributing to shoulder stability. It is defined as the articular capsule bordered by the superior margin of the subscapularis inferiorly, the leading edge of the supraspinatus superiorly, the base of the coracoid medially, and the long head of the biceps tendon laterally (Fig. 1). It varies in size (1), and its incompetency results in increased glenohumeral translation in all planes (2). Glenohumeral instability is rarely the result of an isolated deficiency of the rotator interval and, therefore, its closure is usually only an adjunct to standard arthroscopic instability repair. While indications remain for rotator interval closure, there is emerging conservatism amongst surgeons specializing in shoulder instability. As such, it should be performed at the end of the procedure, when inferior or posteroinferior instability persists in spite of adequate labral repair and capsular plication (3). Overtightening of the rotator interval is associated with significant loss of external rotation. Various techniques for arthroscopic rotator interval closure have been reported (4–6), which will be presented in this chapter.

INDICATIONS FOR SURGERY

The main indication for rotator interval closure is as an adjunct in patients who present with symptomatic shoulder instability (chronic traumatic anteroinferior, bi-directional, posterior, or multi-directional instability) with pain and functional impairment refractory to nonoperative treatment and, thus, who are candidates for surgical management.

Patients frequently report a traumatic shoulder dislocation as the initial event, followed by persistent subluxation or frank dislocation. However, instability can also present with vague symptoms, such as pain, fatigue, or popping with repetitive physical activity. Typically, patients with bi-directional or multi-directional instability may complain of pain in various positions of glenohumeral rotation and, possibly, "dead-arm" type symptoms during provocative activities. Physical examination findings depend upon the instability pattern being addressed. Traumatic anteroinferior instability reveals glenohumeral instability with varying degrees of humeral translation on the load-shift test, positive apprehension, and sulcus signs. Patients with bi-directional or multi-directional instability may have pain with provocative testing, but typically lack signs of apprehension. They too will often have a sulcus sign. A sulcus sign that does not decrease with external rotation at the side in association with any instability pattern signifies a rotator interval lesion with functional incompetence and should be surgically addressed in conjunction with labral repair and capsular plication as necessary.

Unfortunately, there are currently no imaging modalities that have good sensitivity and specificity to detect rotator interval lesions.

Please refer to pages 135–137 for the figures in this chapter.

CONTRAINDICATIONS

Contraindications include inability to tolerate surgery, active infection, or restricted motion. A relative contraindication is concurrent rotator cuff repair, due to concerns of a higher incidence of postoperative stiffness.

TECHNIQUE

Anesthesia and Positioning

The procedure can be performed under general or regional anesthesia, or a combination thereof. After appropriate antibiotic prophylaxis and induction of anesthesia, the patient is placed in the beach-chair position or lateral decubitus depending on surgeon preference and instability pattern.

Examination Under Anesthesia

After positioning, and before the extremity is prepped and draped, the surgeon should examine shoulder motion and stability in all planes. The major direction of instability should be determined, and the amount of inferior translation (sulcus sign) should be assessed both in neutral and external rotation. A persistent sulcus sign with the shoulder adducted and externally rotated suggests rotator interval incompetency that may contribute to pathologic glenohumeral translation and to symptomatic instability.

Portal Placement and Arthroscopic Examination

A diagnostic arthroscopy of the glenohumeral joint is performed through standard anterior and posterior portals. Findings such as redundancy of the capsule in the rotator interval and tearing or fraying of the superior glenohumeral ligament, biceps tendon, or superior border of the subscapularis tendon are common in rotator interval incompetency (3). Associated pathology such as a superior labrum anterior to posterior (SLAP) tear should be repaired first; subsequently, glenohumeral instability should be addressed by labral repair and capsular plication as needed. If repeat examination demonstrates persistent inferior or posteroinferior instability, rotator interval closure can provide additional stability.

Rotator Interval Closure

The capsule within the rotator interval is gently abraded with an arthroscopic rasp or a synovial shaver (without suction) to encourage healing. A spinal needle is then placed percutaneously, or through an existing anteroinferior portal, penetrating the middle glenohumeral ligament and capsule just superior to the subscapularis tendon, and a monofilament suture is threaded into the glenohumeral joint (Fig. 2). If this tissue is inadequate for repair, the superior edge of the subscapularis can be incorporated in this repair, although we have rarely found this necessary. Subsequently, a tissue penetrator is placed through the anterosuperior portal to pierce the superior glenohumeral ligament and capsule just anterior to the leading edge of the supraspinatus tendon (Fig. 3). It is important to direct the penetrator anterior to the long head of the biceps to avoid incorporating the tendon into the repair. The monofilament suture is retrieved with the tissue penetrator, withdrawn though the anterosuperior portal, and used to shuttle a braided nonabsorbable suture through the capsular tissue (Fig. 4).

A knot pusher is threaded over the inferior limb of the suture and passed through the anteroinferior portal to deliver the suture out the anterosuperior portal (Fig. 5). If the inferior limb was placed percutaneously, without establishment of a formal anteroinferior portal, a small stab incision facilitates passage of the knot pusher. It is important to ensure that the knot pusher is passed in the subacromial space just anterior to the capsule and underneath the deltoid muscle. This is accomplished by a combination of external palpation of the deltoid muscle and intra-articular visualization of the knot pusher tenting the anterior capsule. Both suture limbs are now protruding through the anterosuperior portal (Fig. 6) and can be tied by an appropriate sliding knot. Under direct arthroscopic visualization, tension is applied to the suture to draw the superior glenohumeral ligament and the inferior rotator interval tissue together, thus demonstrating the degree of rotator interval closure (Fig. 7). To avoid loss of external rotation, the shoulder is placed in adduction and 30° to 40° of external rotation, before knot tying. If needed, additional sutures can be placed, progressing from lateral to medial. Most commonly, no more than two sutures are placed in the lateral aspect of the interval.

Alternatively, the knot can be tied under direct visualization in the subacromial space. In this technique, the arthroscope and anterosuperior cannula are placed in the subacromial space after initial suture passage. The inferior limb of the suture is then retrieved through the anterosuperior portal and tied under direct visualization.

After suture placement, the shoulder should be gently ranged to ensure that rotator interval closure did not result in excessive limitation of external rotation. Finally, the portals are closed with simple sutures, a sterile dressing is applied, and the arm is placed in a shoulder immobilizer.

PEARLS AND PITFALLS

If the inferior limb of the suture is placed percutaneously, without the use of a formal anteroinferior portal, a small stab incision facilitates subsequent passage of a knot pusher to deliver the suture out the anterosuperior portal. This stab incision should be made before the spinal needle is withdrawn, to avoid cutting the suture in the process.

Care must be taken to ensure that the knot is placed deep to the deltoid and does not capture any muscle tissue in the process.

If the knot is tied under direct visualization in the subacromial space, selective bursectomy should be performed prior to suture passage to avoid cutting the suture with the shaver.

The knot should be tied with the shoulder in 30° to 40° of external rotation to avoid significant loss of motion.

REHABILITATION

Postoperatively, the patient is placed in a shoulder immobilizer at all times except during therapy. Rehabilitation consists of active-assisted, range-of-motion exercises with external rotation to 30°, forward flexion to 140°, and free internal rotation. Closed-chain scapular protraction and retraction exercises are begun immediately, postoperatively. After four weeks, the shoulder immobilizer is discontinued, rehabilitation is advanced to free range-of-motion as tolerated in all planes, and gentle strengthening is initiated with therabands at first, progressing to light weights at six weeks. Return to contact-sports is determined on a case-by-case basis, but is usually permitted at the six-month mark.

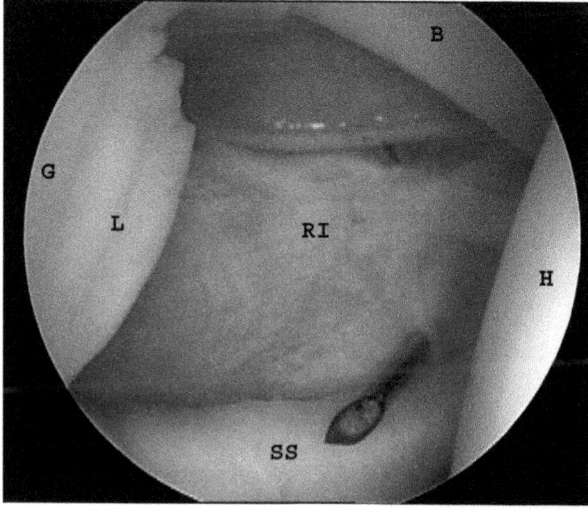

FIGURE 1 Arthroscopic view of the rotator interval. *Abbreviations*: B, biceps tendon; G, glenoid; H, humeral head; L, labrum; RI, rotator interval; SS, subscapularis.

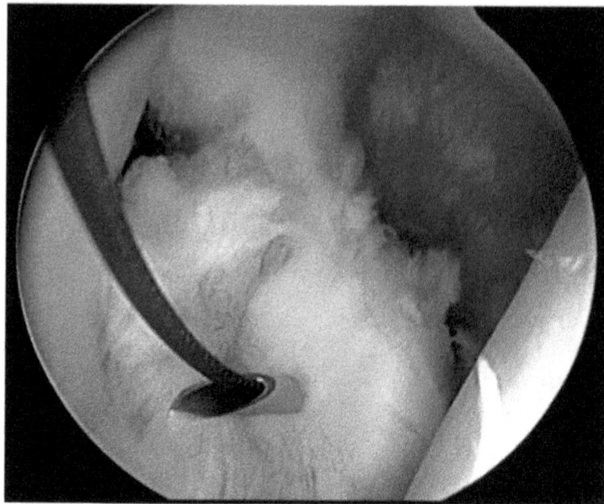

FIGURE 2 Placement of a spinal needle through the middle glenohumeral ligament and capsule.

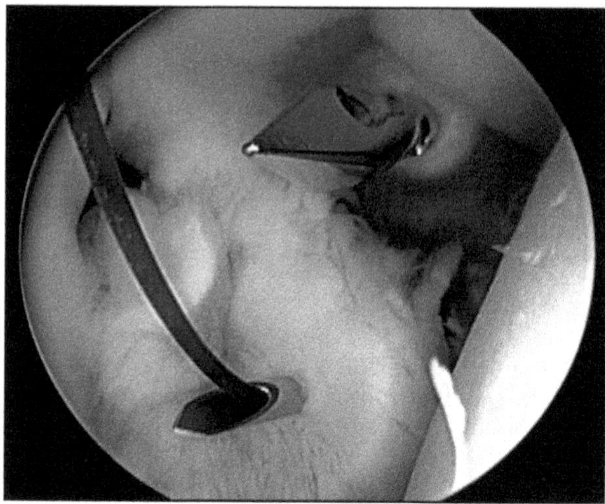

FIGURE 3 Tissue penetrator placed through the superior glenohumeral ligament and anterior capsule.

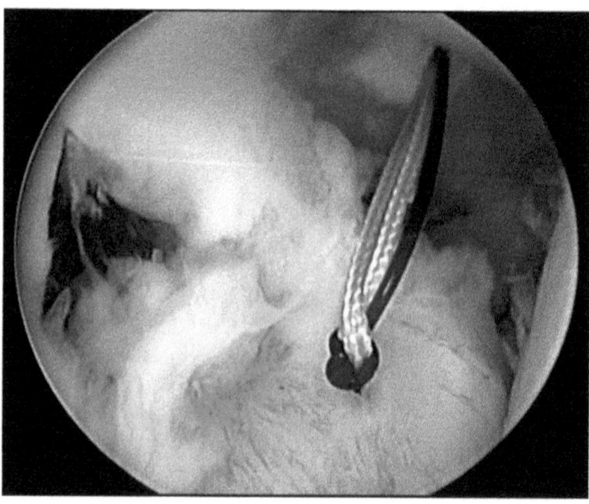

FIGURE 4 Suture shuttled through the tissue.

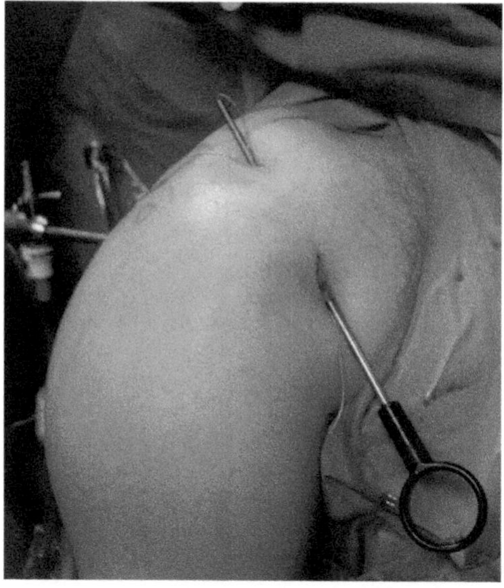

FIGURE 5 Knot pusher delivering the inferior suture limb through the anterosuperior portal.

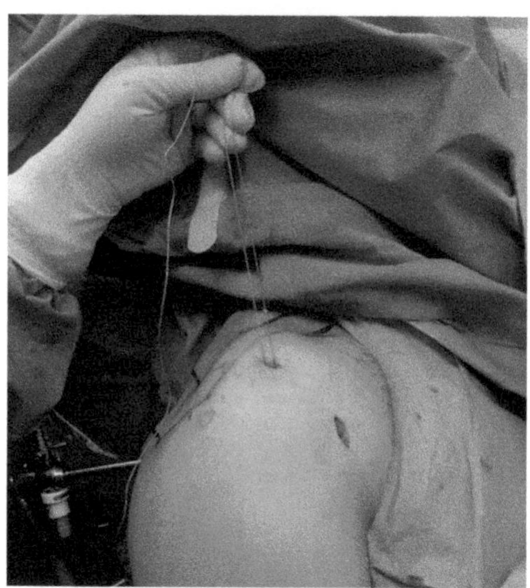

FIGURE 6 Both suture limbs delivered through the anterosuperior portal.

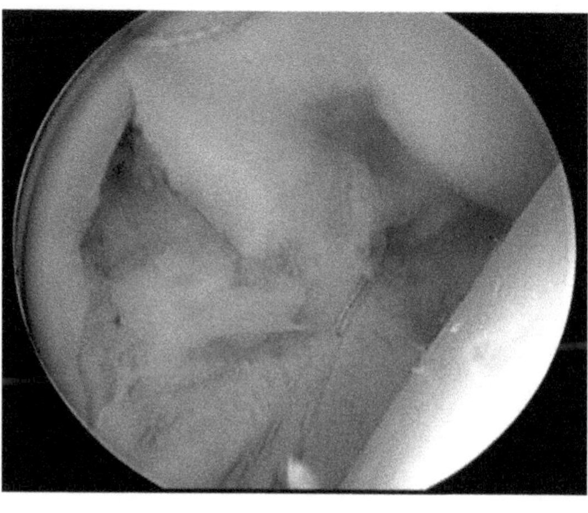

FIGURE 7 Rotator interval closed by tensioning of the suture.

REFERENCES

1. Cole BJ, Rodeo SA, O'Brien SJ, et al. The anatomy and histology of the rotator interval capsule of the shoulder. Clin Orthop Relat Res 2001; (390):129–137.
2. Harryman DT II, Sidles JA, Harris SL, et al. The role of the rotator interval capsule in passive motion and stability of the shoulder. J Bone Joint Surg Am 1992; 74(1):53–66.
3. Gartsman GM, Roddey TS, Hammerman SM. Arthroscopic treatment of anterior-inferior glenohumeral instability. Two to five-year follow-up. J Bone Joint Surg Am 2000; 82-A(7):991–1003.
4. Treacy SH, Field LD, Savoie FH. Rotator interval capsule closure: an arthroscopic technique. Arthroscopy 1997; 13(1):103–106.
5. Gartsman GM, Taverna E, Hammerman SM. Arthroscopic rotator interval repair in glenohumeral instability: description of an operative technique. Arthroscopy 1999; 15(3):330–332.
6. Cole BJ, Mazzocca AD, Meneghini RM. Indirect arthroscopic rotator interval repair. Arthroscopy 2003; 19(6):E28–E31.

13 Arthroscopic Glenoid Debridement for Arthritis

Scott P. Steinmann
Department of Orthopedic Surgery, Mayo Clinic, Rochester, Minnesota, U.S.A.

INDICATIONS AND CONTRAINDICATIONS

Prior attempts at open out debridement of the shoulder with removal of osteophytes and loose bodies were not found to be a very successful procedure and were not recommended as a treatment option (1). Arthroscopic techniques, however, have evolved over the past several years and have made it possible to debride osteophytes, resect capsule, and remove loose bodies. In the patient with primary degenerative arthritis of the shoulder, arthroscopic debridement can potentially be used at any stage of the disease, although best results seem to be achieved when intervention occurs early on in the disease process (2–4). Simple debridement of the glenohumeral joint includes removal of loose bodies, resection of labral tears, and shaving of articular cartilage defects. This has been shown to offer pain relief and results in a high level of patient satisfaction (2,3,5,6).

A more extensive operative approach is to perform a capsular release in addition to glenohumeral joint debridement. This might be done in a patient with limited range of motion in the setting of arthritic changes in the glenohumeral joint. When performing a capsular release, the surgeon has the option of selective capsular release of only the tight area or complete capsular resection, depending on the experience and skill of the operating surgeon. Capsular resection has the added risk of potential damage to neurovascular structures during an overly aggressive debridement.

Additionally, when performing arthroscopic debridement in the patient with glenohumeral arthrosis it is helpful to examine the subacromial space. A thickened subacromial bursa may be encountered in patients with glenohumeral arthritis. When debrided, joint motion is increased and pain is reduced (3). Likewise, viewing of the subacromial space will allow for adequate evaluation of the rotator cuff and determine the possible existence of associated rotator cuff tears. An acromioplasty is not typically performed in the setting of shoulder arthritis, but if a bony spur is encountered, it can be removed.

The most ambitious arthroscopic technique is to attempt to reconstruct a more normal bony architecture of the glenohumeral joint. This involves aggressive resection of osteophytes and recontouring of the glenoid if significant posterior or anterior wear has occurred (Fig. 1A and 1B). This technique also typically involves release of a significant portion of the joint capsule. When the glenoid is recontoured with arthroscopic instruments, this is termed a glenoidplasty (7). If there is significant posterior subluxation, with posterior wear of the glenoid, the anterior glenoid is leveled and the typical biconcavity is removed in an attempt to restore the normal curve of the native glenoid surface. This extensive procedure requires a high level of familiarity with arthroscopy of the shoulder. There is no long-term data on the overall ability of recontouring to change the natural history of glenohumeral arthritis. While better results might be expected in patients with less arthritic changes, presently, there are not enough studies to help orthopedic surgeons to determine which patients should not be candidates for arthroscopic treatment.

In treating patients who might be candidates for arthroscopic techniques, standard nonoperative modalities should be explored first such as nonsteroidal anti-inflammatory medication, steroid injections, and physical therapy. In the geriatric patient, total shoulder arthroplasty remains the standard treatment against which arthroscopy should be measured.

Please refer to pages 143–144 for the figures in this chapter.

There are however some patients for whom total shoulder arthroplasty might not be a suitable option. They might be young or very active. Hemiarthroplasty has often been offered to the younger patient with glenohumeral arthritis, but in the patient with significant posterior wear and subluxation, this is not a good option.

The quality of the patient's pain is also given a consideration. Pain of shoulder arthrosis can be divided into three types. Pain at the extremes of motion is usually due to osteophytes and stretching of inflamed capsule and synovium. Pain at rest is thought to be due to synovitis. Pain at night is not the same as rest pain. Night pain may be due to synovitis but can also represent positional pain due to awkward positions or increased pressure on the joint. Thirdly, pain in the mid arc of motion is usually accompanied by crepitus and typically represents articular surface damage. Some patients have crepitus, which is almost painless, but not a major focus of pain.

The first two types of pain are potentially helped by an arthroscopic procedure (pain at end range of motion or rest pain) but pain during the mid arc of motion is a poor prognostic indication and requires closer examination of the patient. The patient's glenohumeral joint should be compressed while moving through a mid arc of motion. If this causes significant discomfort, the articular surfaces might be damaged to the extent that arthroscopy might not offer significant pain relief.

Limitation of motion can also be related to pain and has several causes. Impinging osteophytes can abut, limit movement and result in pain. Congruous incongruity, with a biconcavity of the glenoid can also result in loss of motion. Capsular contracture from prior injury or surgery might increase joint contact forces and result in pain. A pseudocontracture can also occur if there is significant posterior subluxation or large loose bodies.

On the whole, replacement arthroplasty remains the gold standard of treatment for severe arthritic changes of the glenohumeral joint. There are currently few reports in the literature of arthroscopic treatment of degenerative arthritis of the shoulder (2,3). The ultimate results of these newer nonreplacement, arthroscopic techniques will require longer follow up and more reports in the literature.

SURGICAL TECHNIQUE

Patients may be positioned in either the lateral decubitus position or in the beachchair position for arthroscopic treatment of glenohumeral arthritis. A potential disadvantage of the lateral decubitus position is the need to periodically take the arm out of traction to check the range of motion after capsular resection. Additionally, if working in the area of the axillary nerve, the semi-abducted position used in the lateral decubitus position tends to bring the axillary nerve closer to the capsule (Fig. 2).

The arthroscopic anatomy of the axillary nerve is an important consideration when performing extensive debridement of the glenohumeral joint. The nerve is most at risk at the anteroinferior portion of the joint capsule. Neer (8) initially reported on the dangers of open capsular work in the anteroinferior portion of the shoulder capsule. External rotation of the shoulder tends to relax the nerve (9). The average distance of the nerve to the anteroinferior shoulder capsule has ranged in studies from 3 to 12 mm (10,11).

After the patient is anesthetized, an examination under anesthesia is helpful for two reasons. It can give the surgeon an idea if loss of motion affects the entire shoulder capsule such as in adhesive capsulitis or if there is a more local block to motion such as one that might occur after an open anterior capsular plication. After checking the patients glenohumeral motion, the surgeon has the option to consider manipulation under anesthesia. This is not a necessary step, but gentle pressure might release light adhesions.

When placing portals for debridement of the glenohumeral joint, standard portals are usually adequate. A viewing portal from posterior is initially placed and then a working portal established anteriorly. Instruments needed include a large shaver (4.8 to 5.5 mm) and a cautery or radiofrequency probe for ablation of hypertrophic synovium. It is helpful to place both the posterior and anterior portals a bit more inferior than usual to allow for easier access to the inferior aspect of the joint. As mentioned previously, there are four treatment options possible depending on the needs of the patient and the experience and skill of the operating surgeon. This ranges from the simplest option of synovectomy and loose body removal to a more extensive option of capsular resection and recontouring of the glenoid and humerus. Two portals, one anterior and one posterior are usually enough for simple synovectomy and loose body removal. A switching stick can then be used to view from the front of the joint, and the working portal can be switched to the back.

Debridement of the joint includes initial removal of all hypertrophic synovium. Once a complete synovectomy has been performed, the remainder of the joint can be visualized. Next, resection of labral tears can be performed. In the arthritic patient, it is not usually beneficial to perform labral repairs. Removal of loose bodies is usually done as they are visualized. A long needle driver is sometimes useful at removing large loose bodies that might otherwise damage delicate arthroscopic instruments. Large loose bodies can also be removed by pinning the body between the arthrosopic camera sleeve and the outflow cannula and then pushing the loose body out of the joint.

Osteophyte removal is usually best done before resection of the capsule, and primarily involves working in the inferior aspect of the glenohumeral joint. It is usual for osteophytes to form along the inferior portion of the humeral neck. To gain a working view of this area, it is possible to use two posterior portals. However, the arthroscope and the shaver portals are often too close and the surgeon is soon in a "swordfight" between the closely adjacent instruments. A more efficient way to visualize and remove inferior osteophytes is by viewing from the anterior portal using a standard 30-degree arthroscope and then establishing a posterior inferior working portal. The shaver or burr can then be brought in posteriorly to remove capsule or osteophytes.

The need to release or remove capsule depends on the pathology. If a prior anterior procedure was performed on the patient, then only direct anterior capsule release is often needed. This can be done by viewing from a posterior portal and using an anterior portal to direct a cautery/radiofrequency device or a shaver to release the anterior capsule from the anterior glenoid surface. If the patient has extensive osteoarthritis, with capsular contraction and osteophyte formation, then capsular resection may be required in addition to osteophyte removal to improve range of motion.

The capsule can be removed in two parts. The anterior capsule can be removed as described for anterior capsular release, using an anterior working portal, while visualizing from posterior (Fig. 3). After the anterior capsule is released down to the anteroinferior recess, visualization is switched to the anterior portal and the shaver or resector brought into the joint from posterior to remove the inferior capsule.

The axillary nerve may be encountered, as the resection is carried further anteroinferiorly. The nerve is usually about a centimeter from the capsule and can be located with a nerve hook or Howarth retractor. If the axillary nerve is identified, a total resection of the capsule can then be completed with a combination of shavers and punch resectors. The direct posterior capsule is not generally removed, just as it is not typically resected during a total shoulder replacement. The posterior capsule is often lax from the posterior subluxation and posterior-glenoid wear seen in osteoarthritis. This posterior shift can cause a compensatory pseudocontracture of the anterior capsule.

Once impinging osteophytes have been removed, labral tears debrided, and any capsular contracture addressed, the condition of the glenoid surface can be inspected. If a biconcave glenoid from posterior wear exists, a recontouring of the surface may be performed. This is termed as glenoidplasty. The procedure involves converting the biconcave glenoid into a single concavity (Figs. 4A–D). This might potentially restore the position of the humeral head, reducing the posterior subluxation. Restoration of a single concavity might also increase the surface area of the glenohumeral articulation, decreasing joint pressure. A reversal of the posterior subluxation might also help in relaxing contracted anterior soft tissues. At present, there are no long-term studies of the effect of this technique.

The procedure is performed with an anterior and a posterior portal. Viewing alternatively from the front and the back, the remaining cartilage is first removed from the anterior glenoid facet, and then the central vertical bony ridge is resected. A round 4 mm burr is usually sufficient to accomplish this task. Once a single concave surface is established, a large rasp can be used to smooth the surface. This is similar to the technique of reaming the anterior portion of the glenoid during total shoulder arthroplasty to restore the native version of the glenoid. Since a portion of subchondral bone is removed by this technique, long term follow up will be needed to ascertain if any medial migration of the humeral head occurs as a consequence of the procedure.

The final option in treating arthritis of the shoulder is to inspect and debride the subacromial space. Using standard portals to explore the subacromial space, a shaver or cautery/radiofrequency probe can be placed above the rotator cuff, and removal of any thickened bursa can be performed. Any bursa sided fraying or tearing of the rotator cuff can also be addressed, simultaneously. There is usually no need to perform an acromioplasty, but if a minor spur of the acromion is encountered it can be resected. The coracoacromial ligament should be preserved.

POSTOPERATIVE MANAGEMENT

After completion of the procedure, a drain is usually not needed, and simple suture closure of the portals and placement of a sterile dressing is all that is required. It is an option to place an anesthetic infusion pump into the glenohumeral joint if this is the surgeon's preference. The arm is placed into a simple sling before the patient leaves the operating room.

The patient typically will leave the hospital the day of the surgery. The patient should begin progressive range of motion exercises as soon as possible, beginning on the first postoperative day. Adequate oral pain control should be maintained with narcotic and nonnarcotic medications to enable the patient to perform a therapy regiment. Essentially, there are no limitations to the use of the arm and full active motion should be encouraged. Patients should be allowed to go back to work as soon as they are comfortable. Most patients will benefit from a structured therapy program under the guise of a trained therapist, who can encourage the patient to maintain the range of motion achieved in the operating room. There are no limits and full passive and active motions are allowed. The sling should be removed a few days after surgery to encourage a greater arc of motion.

RESULTS

There are currently few studies examining the benefit of arthroscopic debridement of the shoulder for degenerative arthritis. Ellman (5) demonstrated the benefit of debridement of the glenohumeral joint in patients undergoing surgery for impingement syndrome. His study showed the advantage of arthroscopy over open surgery in detecting coexisting pathology in patients with impingement syndrome. Cofield (4) and others have demonstrated a relief of symptoms in patients with arthroscopic lavage of the glenohumeral joint (12,13).

In two series of patients undergoing debridement for glenohumeral degeneration, a high percentage of patients in both studies reported initial pain relief (100% and 88%) (2,3). The mechanism of pain relief is unclear but may have resulted from removal of painful synovium or by dilution of degenerative debris.

The results of glenoidplasty, the most extensive form of debridement of the glenohumeral joint have been reported in only one article (7). At an early follow up of three years, active motion had increased in the majority and 86% felt they were either significantly improved or improved by the procedure. There were no complications and no evidence of medial migration of the humerus on the axillary view. Importantly, whether simple debridement of the glenohumeral joint is performed, or a more advanced glenoidplasty is done, future potential surgery including total shoulder arthroplasty is not compromised.

Arthroscopic debridement of the glenohumeral joint appears to be useful for short-term pain relief, with a large majority of patients feeling the procedure being worthwhile. Age does not appear to be a factor, but range of motion may not improve significantly after the procedure. Patients with minimal to severe arthritis may benefit from the procedure. In patients with severe arthritis, significant improvements are unlikely unless an extensive debridement such as a glenoidplasty is performed. Although total shoulder replacement is the gold standard against which results are measured, in active patients in whom a replacement is either unsuitable or undesirable, arthroscopic treatment may be of benefit.

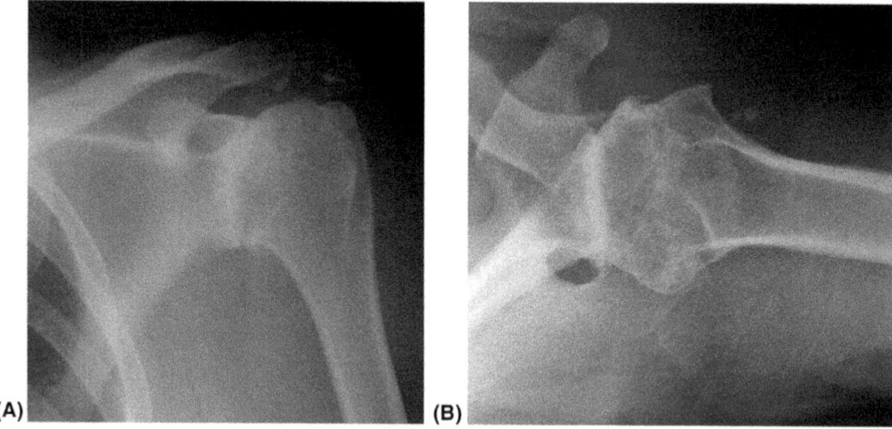

FIGURE 1 (**A**) and (**B**) Anteroposterior and axillary views of an arthritic shoulder with posterior subluxation and wear.

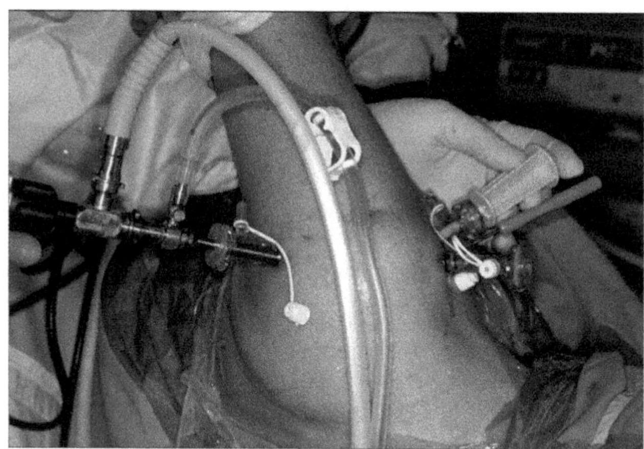

FIGURE 2 Intraoperative view of patient in the lateral decubitus position during glenohumeral debridement and glenoidplasty.

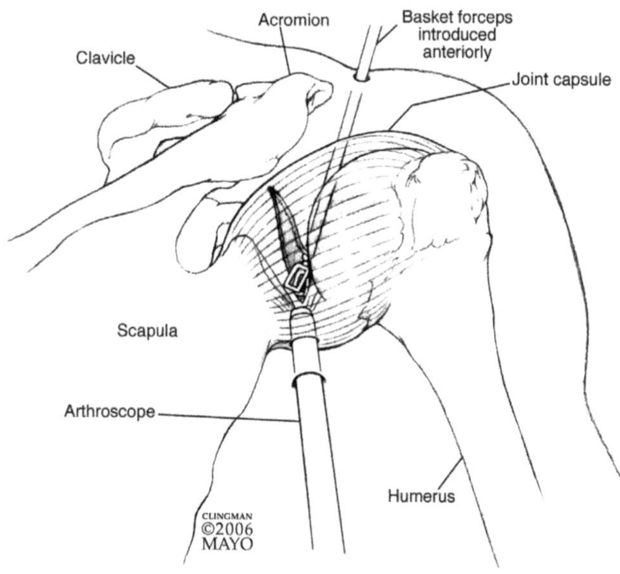

FIGURE 3 Drawing demonstrating release of anterior capsule while viewing from a posterior portal with the arthroscope.

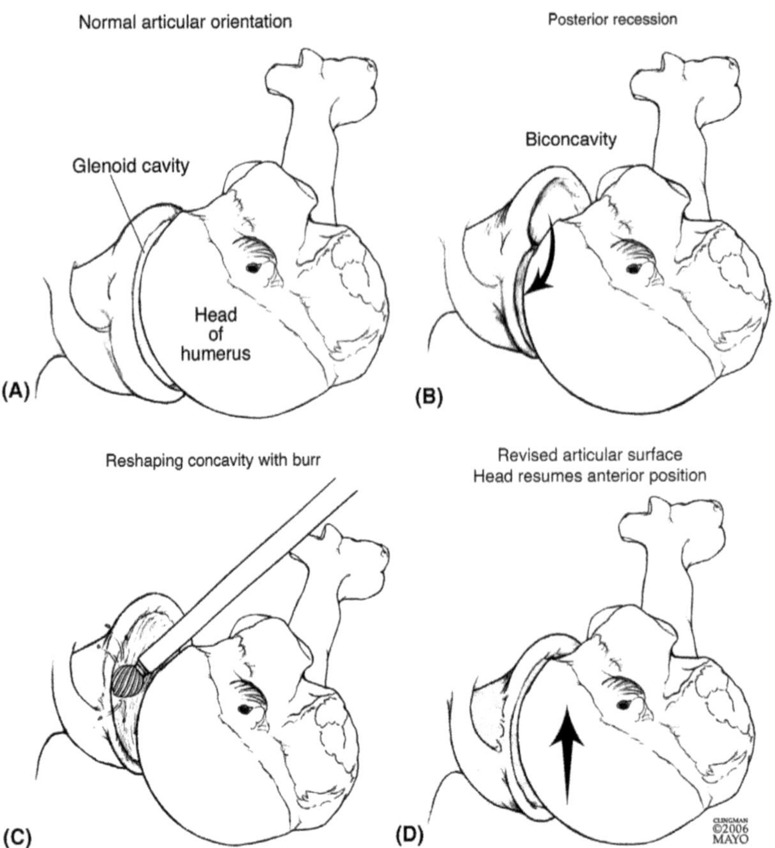

FIGURE 4 (**A**) Drawing demonstrating normal alignment of the glenohumeral joint viewed from a superior perspective, (**B**) posterior recession and biconcavity associated with glenohumeral arthritis, (**C**) reshaping the glenoid to a single concavity, and (**D**) after glenoidplasty, the humeral head resumes a more anatomical position.

REFERENCES

1. Neer CS. Shoulder Reconstruction. Vol. 1. 1st ed. Philadelphia: Saunders, 1990.
2. Cameron BD, Galatz LM, Ramsey ML, Williams GR, Iannotti JP. Non-prosthetic management of grade IV osteochondral lesions of the glenohumeral joint. J Shoulder Elbow Surg 2002; 11:25–32.
3. Weinstein DM, Bucchieri JS, Pollock RG, Flatow EL, Bigliani LU. Arthroscopic debridement of the shoulder for osteoarthritis. Arthroscopy 2000; 16:471–476.
4. Cofield RH. Arthroscopy of the shoulder. Mayo Clin Proc 1983; 58:501–508.
5. Ellman H, Harris E, Kay SP. Early degenerative joint disease simulating impingement syndrome: arthroscopic findings. Arthroscopy 1992; 8:482–487.
6. Midorikawa K, Hara M, Emoto G, Shibata Y, Naito N. Arthroscopic debridement for dialysis shoulders. Arthroscopy 2001; 17:685–693.
7. Kelly E, O'Driscoll S, Steinmann S. Arthroscopic glenoidplasty and osteocapsular arthroplasty for advanced glenohumeral arthritis. Annual Open Meeting of the American Shoulder and Elbow Surgeons 2001, San Francisco, California.
8. Neer CS. Inferior capsular shift for involuntary inferior and multidirectional instability of the shoulder. A preliminary report. J Bone Joint Surg 1980; 62B:897–908.
9. Loomer. Anatomy of the axillary nerve and its relationship to inferior capsular shift. Clin Orthop 1989; 243:100–105.
10. Bryan WJ SK, Tullos HS. The axillary nerve and its relationship to common sports medicine shoulder procedures. Am J Sports Med 1986; 14:113–116.
11. Eakin CL, Dvirnak P, Miller CM, Hawkins RJ. The relationship of the axillary nerve to arthroscopically placed capsulolabral sutures. An anatomic study. Am J Sports Med 1998; 26:505–509.
12. Johnson LL. The shoulder joint: an arthroscopic perspective of anatomy and pathology. Clin Orthop 1987; 223:113–125.
13. Ogilvie-Harris DJ, Wiley AM. Arthroscopic surgery of the shoulder. J Bone Joint Surg 1986; 60:201–207.

14 Arthroscopic Capsular Release

John-Erik Bell and William N. Levine
Center for Shoulder, Elbow, and Sports Medicine, Department of Orthopedic Surgery, Columbia Presbyterian Medical Center, New York, New York, U.S.A.

INDICATIONS FOR SURGERY

Arthroscopic capsular release is an effective technique in the management of shoulder stiffness that is refractory to nonoperative regimens. It is useful for many types of "frozen shoulder,"(1) including primary adhesive capsulitis, post-traumatic, or postsurgical stiffness. Neviaser originally described the pathology as vascular and fibrotic, with a chronic inflammatory appearance, while more recent pathological descriptions have included comparisons with the histology of Dupuytren's disease (2,3). Early reports on adhesive capsulitis described it as a self-limited process, with near complete recovery of motion (1,4–6), and others have shown the importance of physical therapy as well (7). Other studies have drawn different conclusions, reporting that the condition may take much longer to resolve and motion may never fully recover (8,9). Shaffer, for example, reported that 50% of patients had mild pain and stiffness at seven year follow-up, including permanent external rotation deficit and 60% decrease in overall range of motion (9). Nonoperative treatment typically consists of physical therapy, anti-inflammatory agents, intra-articular corticosteroid injections, and manipulation under anesthesia. While recent work at our institution supports the conclusion that most patients with adhesive capsulitis will experience resolution with nonoperative measures in a relatively short time period, a minority of patients will require operative treatment for a successful outcome, and our treatment of choice in this situation is arthroscopic capsular release (10).

Since first described for shoulder stiffness in 1991, arthroscopy has become a widely used technique, with multiple reports documenting its efficacy (11–19). Advantages include the requirement of decreased force and torque on the humerus during manual manipulation, the ability to diagnose and treat concomitant intra-articular and subacromial disease, the ability to perform a synovectomy when inflammation is active, avoidance of disruption of the rotator cuff tendons through the use of selective and precise divisions of the pathologic capsule, and the ability to confirm a complete capsular release including the posterior capsule for increased internal rotation. Operative indications include failure of at least six months of nonoperative treatment, severe pain, significant functional restrictions, and time constraints, precluding prolonged nonoperative treatment.

CONTRAINDICATIONS FOR SURGERY

Arthroscopic release is contraindicated when the source of stiffness is felt to be primarily extra-articular, as in older stabilization procedures such as the Putti-Platt or Magnuson-Stack. Relative contraindications to arthroscopic capsular release include cases in which the bony anatomy of the shoulder is altered and limits motion or may be better treated with arthroplasty, such as severe glenohumeral osteoarthritis, avascular necrosis, and certain post-traumatic situations. Another contraindication to arthroscopic capsular release is lack of experience with shoulder arthroscopy and arthroscopic anatomy, as it is a technically demanding procedure.

Please refer to pages 150–152 for the figures in this chapter.

AUTHORS' PREFERRED TECHNIQUE

Arthroscopic capsular release is performed in either the lateral decubitus or beach-chair position. Interscalene regional anesthesia is used, and frequently this is done via an indwelling catheter to allow continuous postoperative regional anesthesia during early physical therapy sessions. Standard portals are utilized, including a posterior and anterior rotator interval portal. When subacromial adhesions are felt to be contributing to the stiffness, a midlateral portal is also used (Fig. 1). Evaluation under anesthesia is performed in every case to accurately document preoperative passive range of motion. We document forward elevation, abduction, external and internal rotation at the side, and external and internal rotation in 90° of abduction. We do not manipulate the shoulder prior to arthroscopy.

Pertinent anatomic considerations for this procedure include recognition of three portions of the capsule, which require different release techniques; the rotator interval and anterior capsule, the inferior capsule, and the posterior capsule. The rotator interval is always involved and is likely a significant contributor to pain and loss of motion. The coracoacromial ligament is typically not involved and the subacromial space is usually not involved unless the stiffness is postsurgical or post-traumatic. The capsule itself has a greatly reduced volume, with loss of the infraglenoid recess as a result of the capsule scarring to itself where it is redundant.

Rotator Interval and Anterior Capsular Release

The procedure begins with the arthroscope in the posterior portal. Entry into the joint can be more difficult than for a typical shoulder arthroscopy due to thickened capsule and decreased joint space. An 18-gauge spinal needle is carefully inserted into the rotator interval (Fig. 2). Although a cannula can be placed, in some cases the interval is so tight that an electrocautery device is placed directly into the joint (Fig. 3). The cautery is then used to completely release the rotator interval capsule. The release begins superiorly with the coracohumeral and superior glenohumeral ligaments (Figs. 3A and B). This release is considered complete when the coracoid, the conjoint tendon, and the coracoacromial ligament are visualized. Visualization of the coracoacromial (CA) ligament ensures that both the superficial and deep bands of the coracohumeral ligament have been divided (Fig. 3C).

Before releasing the anterior capsule, the subscapularis must be liberated from the anterior capsule. Once this plane is developed, the anterior capsule is released with cautery inferior to approximately the five o'clock position, taking care not to injure the subscapularis (Figs. 3D and E). This release includes the middle glenohumeral ligament and the anterior band of the inferior glenohumeral ligament.

Manipulation Under Anesthesia

At this point, the scope is withdrawn and a gentle manipulation is performed in forward elevation to tear the remainder of the inferior capsule, and in external rotation to tear any remaining anterior adhesions (Fig. 4). Allowing the inferior capsular fibers to tear under manipulation is safer than surgical incision of the inferior capsule since the axillary nerve is intimately related to the capsule between the five o'clock and seven o'clock positions before it dives into the quadrilateral space (20,21). If it is necessary to divide the inferior capsule, we choose a basket punch rather than cautery in between the five o'clock and seven o'clock positions and place the arm in adduction and external rotation to increase the distance between the capsule and the nerve (21,22).

Documentation of range of motion at this juncture should demonstrate full forward elevation, abduction, external rotation at the side, and external rotation in abduction. However, since the posterior capsule has not been addressed, internal rotation in abduction will still be greatly limited.

Posterior Capsular Release

Using switching sticks, the arthroscope is then placed in the anterosuperior portal and a cannula is placed posteriorly. Often, the posterior capsule is inflamed and contracted as well, which can make visualization difficult (Fig. 5A). The posterior capsular release begins at the anterosuperior rotator interval, continues posteriorly behind the biceps tendon and labrum, and is completed when the muscle fibers of the infraspinatus are clearly visible inferiorly (Figs. 5B–D). Once the posterior release to about seven o'clock is completed, manipulation in internal rotation is performed to tear any remaining posterior-inferior capsular fibers below the seven o'clock safe zone. It is important to achieve hemostasis to prevent excessive postoperative bleeding, which can limit motion and increase fibrosis.

Subacromial Release

If a 360° release has been performed and confirmed arthroscopically to be complete, and motion is still not full, there may be adhesions in the subacromial space. This is especially likely in the setting of postsurgical or post-traumatic stiffness. In these situations, we will enter the subacromial space from the posterior portal and create a standard mid-lateral working portal. We use a combination of an electric shaver and cautery to perform a bursectomy and lysis of adhesions to the acromion. Care must be taken in these situations to avoid damage to the rotator cuff tissue.

PEARLS AND PITFALLS

In cases with severe preoperative restriction of motion, the posterior portal should be placed slightly more superiorly than normal. This is helpful because there is often more room for joint entry above the equator of the humerus. The standard, more inferiorly positioned posterior portal allows a better vantage point for most cases of shoulder arthroscopy, but it relies on the ability to laterally displace the humeral head for visualization of the anterior–inferior capsule, however in severe adhesive capsulitis, the humeral head cannot always be laterally displaced.

It is critical to obtain a postoperative X-ray of the shoulder and the entire humerus to document that the shoulder has not been dislocated and that the humerus has not been fractured.

REHABILITATION

Many insurance carriers will no longer allow inpatient hospitalization following arthroscopic capsular release but if they do we will typically admit the patient for one night for postoperative pain management and intensive physical therapy. While we used to routinely utilize indwelling catheters to administer analgesics, we no longer do so due to recent concern raised about possible association with chondrolysis. The patient's shoulder is then passively moved through a full range of motion three times daily.

If outpatient arthroscopic capsular release is performed, however, the postoperative rehabilitation program must be planned preoperatively. Typically, the patient is given their postoperative narcotic prescription prior to surgery so that their narcotic medication is home and waiting for them. A long-acting interscalene anesthetic block is provided (18–24 hours) so that the patient has significant reduction in the early postoperative pain. We have the patient coordinate their postoperative physical therapy visits preoperatively and have the patient see the therapist on postoperative day one and a minimum of three times weekly. In addition, all patients have a family member instructed to perform passive range of motion twice daily in all planes (forward elevation, external rotation, and internal rotation). Finally, the patient is instructed in performing home stretching exercises twice daily as well. Patients are seen for postoperative evaluation at five days, two weeks, four weeks, six weeks, and three months postoperatively. If a patient begins to regress during their early postoperative recovery, an intra-articular glenohumeral corticosteroid injection is usually performed. Most patients achieve their final range of motion by three to four months postoperatively (Figs. 6A and B).

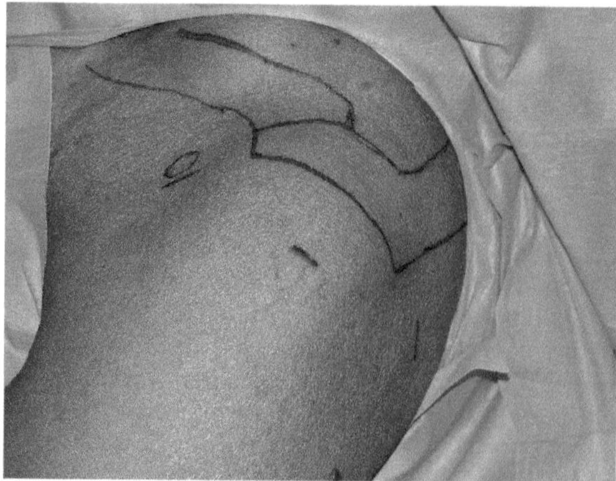

FIGURE 1 Portal placement—posterior and anterior (routine) and optional mid-lateral portal.

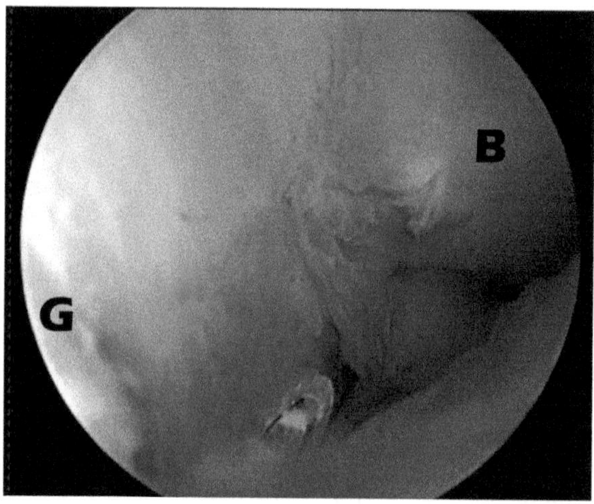

FIGURE 2 52 y.o. Right hand dominant (RHD) female with recalcitrant adhesive capsulitis. Posterior viewing portal demonstrating intense synovitis and contraction along the rotator interval. B = long head of biceps tendon, G = glenoid insertion.

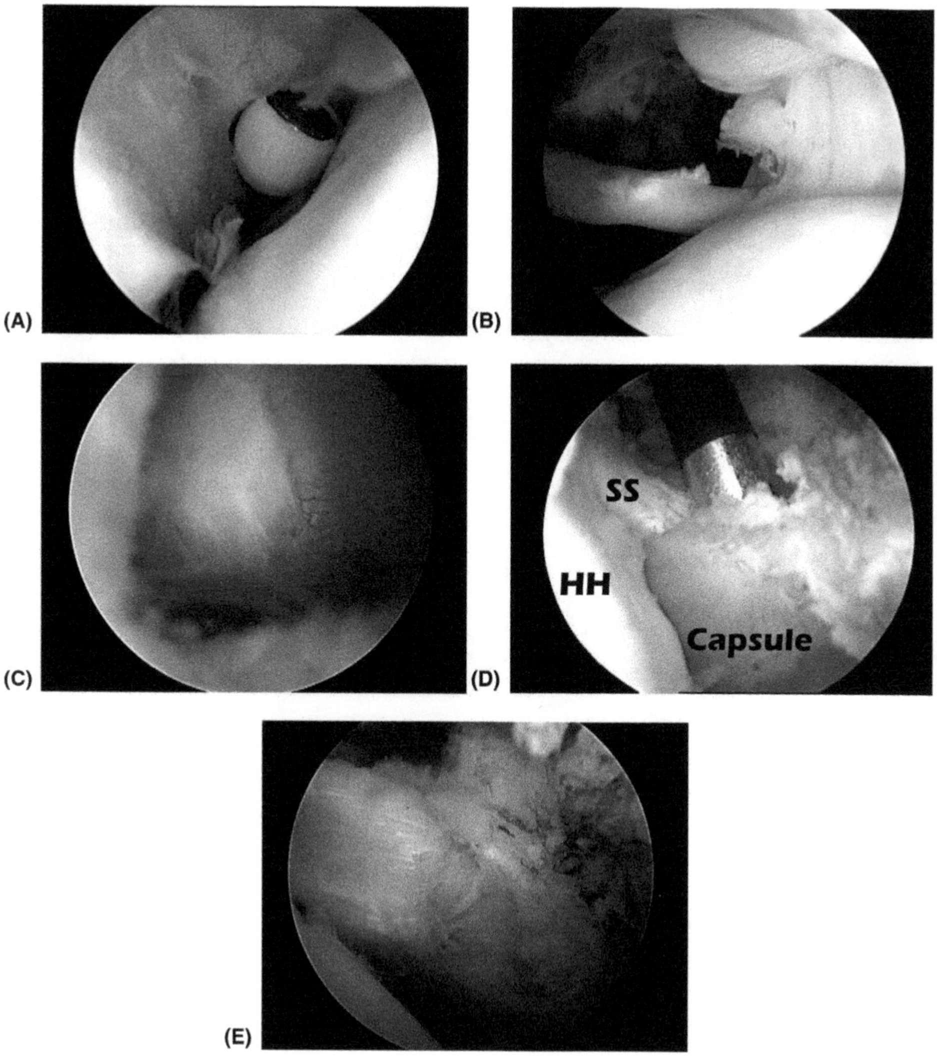

FIGURE 3 (**A**) Same patient—posterior viewing portal showing cautery in the rotator interval; (**B**) complete release of the superior aspect of the rotator interval; (**C**) complete release of the anterior capsule, sparing the subscapularis; (**D**) cautery underneath autoinferior capsule prior to release; (**E**) complete anterior capsular release, sparing the subscapularis. *Abbreviations*: HH, humeral head; SS, subscapularis tendon.

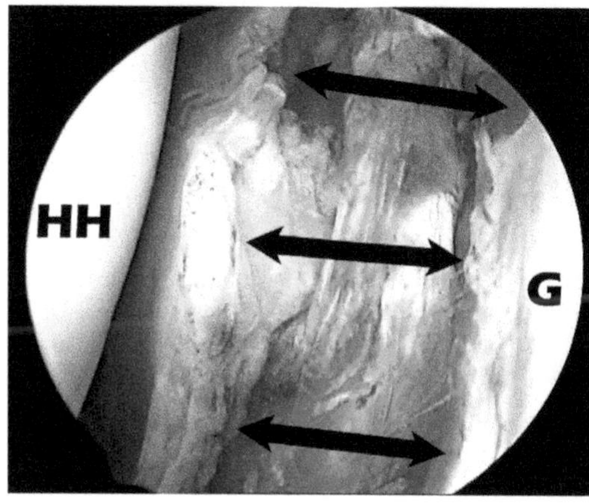

FIGURE 4 Same patient—posterior viewing portal showing tearing of the remaining inferior capsular fibers after manipulation. HH = humeral head, G = glenoid, arrows indicated torn capsule.

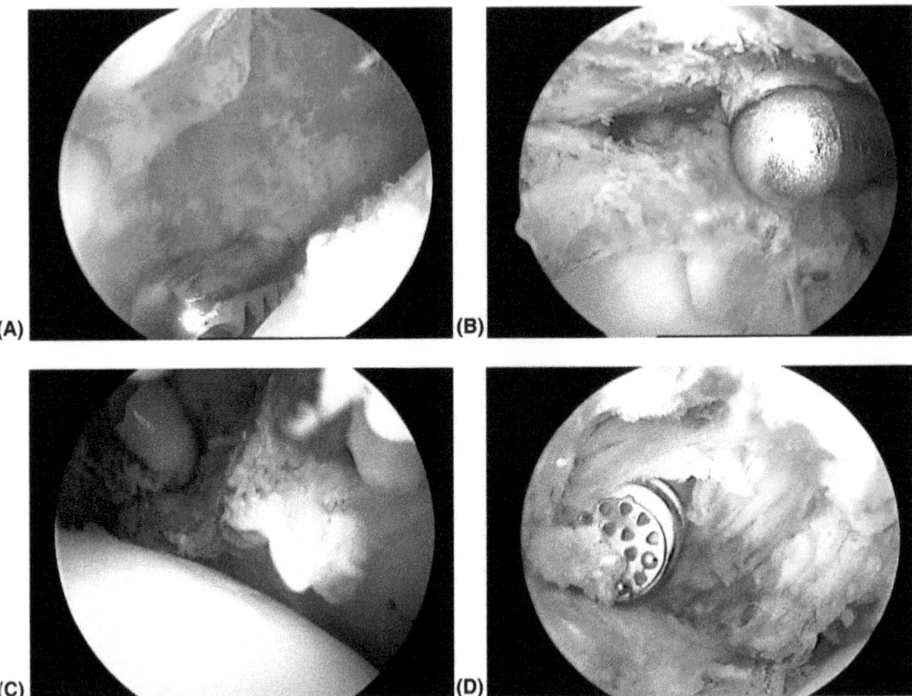

FIGURE 5 Same patient—viewing from anterosuperior portal. Synovitis and contracture of the posterior capsule (**A**); release of the posterior superior capsule with cautery, between superior labrum and rotator cuff (**B**); release of posterior capsule (**C**); and complete posterior release indicated by visualization of infraspinatus muscle fibers (**D**).

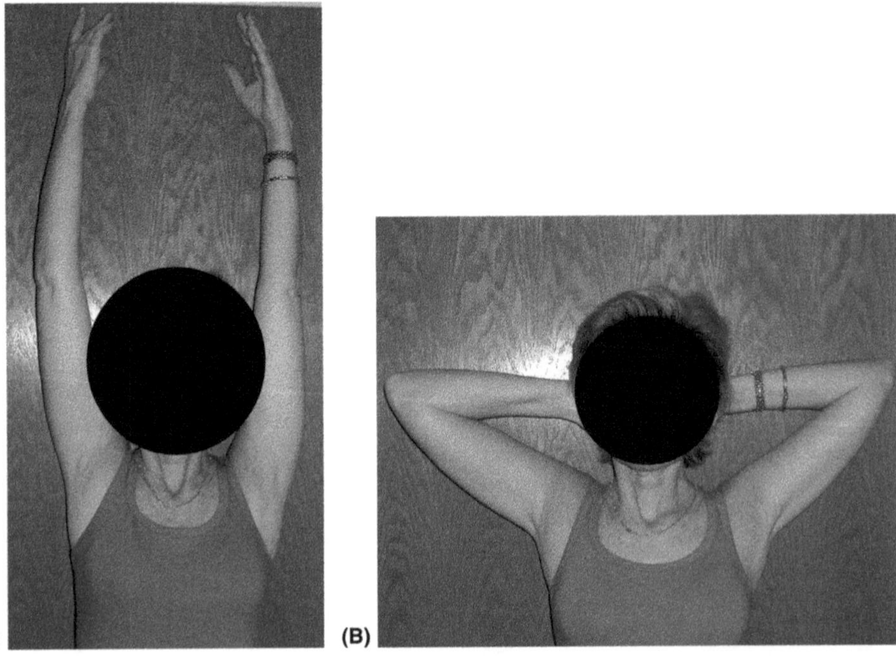

FIGURE 6 Same patient seen at her 3 month postoperative visit demonstrating full, symmetric forward elevation (**A**); and full, symmetric forward elevation, abduction, and external rotation (**B**).

REFERENCES

1. Codman E. The Shoulder: Rupture of the Supraspinatus Tendon and Other Lesions in or About the Subacromial Bursa. Boston: Thomas Todd, 1934.
2. Neviaser J. Adhesive capsulitis of the shoulder. A Study of the Pathologic Findings in Periarthritis of the Shoulder. J Bone Joint Surg Am 1945; 27A:211–222.
3. Bunker TD, Anthony PP. The pathology of frozen shoulder. A Dupuytren-like disease. J Bone Joint Surg Br 1995; 77-B(5):677–683.
4. Grey R. The natural history of "idiopathic" frozen shoulder. J Bone Joint Surg 1978; 60-A:564.
5. Simmonds F. With particular reference to the "frozen" shoulder. J Bone Joint Surg 1949; 31:426–432.
6. Miller M, Wirth M, Rockwood C. Thawing the frozen shoulder: the "patient" patient. Orthopedics 1996; 19(10):849–853.
7. Griggs SM, Ahn A, Green A. Idiopathic adhesive capsulitis: a prospective functional outcome study of nonoperative treatment. J Bone Joint Surg Am 2000; 82(10):1398–1407.
8. Reeves B. The natural history of frozen shoulder syndrome. Scand J Rheumatol 1975; 4:193–196.
9. Shaffer B. Frozen Shoulder: A long-term follow-up. J Bone Joint Surg 1992; 74-A:738–746.
10. Bak S, Kashyap C, Bigliani L, Levine W. Natural History of Conservatively Treated Adhesive Capsulitis. In: ASES Closed Meeting. Miami, Florida, U.S.A., 2005.
11. Warner JJP, Allen A, Marks PH, Wong P. Arthroscopic release for chronic, refractory adhesive capsulitis of the shoulder. J Bone Joint Surg Am 1996; 78(12):1808–1816.
12. Wiley A. Arthroscopic appearance of frozen shoulder. Arthroscopy 1991; 7:138–143.
13. Bradley J. Arthroscopic treatment for frozen capsulitis. Operative Techniques in Orthopaedics 1991; 1:248–252.
14. Pollock R, Duralde X, Flatow E, Bigliani L. The use of arthroscopy in treatment of resistant frozen shoulder. Clin Orthoped 1994; 304:30–36.
15. Segmuller H, Taylor D, Hogan C, Sales A, Hayes M. Arthroscopic treatment of adhesive capsulitis. J Shoulder Elb Surg 1995; 4:403–404.
16. Ogilvie-Harris D, Biggs D, Fitsialos J, MacKay M. The resistant frozen shoulder: manipulation versus arthroscopic release. Clin Orthoped 1995; 319:238–248.
17. Berghs BM, Sole-Molins X, Bunker TD. Arthroscopic release of adhesive capsulitis. J Shoulder Elb Surg 2004; 13(2):180–185.
18. Holloway GB, Schenk T, Williams GR, Ramsey ML, Iannotti JP. Arthroscopic capsular release for the treatment of refractory postoperative or post-fracture shoulder stiffness. J Bone Joint Surg Am 2001; 83(11):1682–1687.
19. Beaufils P, Prevot N, Boyer T, et al. Arthroscopic release of the glenohumeral joint in shoulder stiffness: a review of 26 cases. Arthroscopy: J Arthroscopic & Related Surg 1999; 15(1):49–55.
20. Price MR, Tillett ED, Acland RD, Nettleton GS. Determining the relationship of the axillary nerve to the shoulder joint capsule from an arthroscopic perspective. J Bone Joint Surg Am 2004; 86(10):2135–2142.
21. Uno A, Bain GI, Mehta JA. Arthroscopic relationship of the axillary nerve to the shoulder joint capsule: An anatomic study. J Shoulder Elb Surg 1999; 8(3):226–230.
22. Jerosch, Filler, Peuker. Which joint position puts the axillary nerve at lowest risk when performing arthroscopic capsular release in patients with adhesive capsulitis of the shoulder? Knee Surg, Sports Traumatology, Arthroscopy 2002; 10(2):126–129.

15 Arthroscopic Biceps Tenodesis

Mark W. Rodosky
Department of Orthopedic Surgery, Division of Shoulder Surgery, University of Pittsburgh Sports Medicine, Pittsburgh, Pennsylvania, U.S.A.

Emilio Lopez-Vidriero and Jon K. Sekiya
Center for Sports Medicine, Department of Orthopedic Surgery, University of Pittsburgh Medical Center, Pittsburgh, Pennsylvania, U.S.A.

INDICATIONS

Since Neer defined the so called impingement syndrome, the long head of biceps has been recognized as one of the causes of shoulder pain (1,2) and has been determined to be a significant potential "pain generator" (3). The biceps tendon and its role in shoulder pathology have ranged from describing it as a vestigial structure (3), to a secondary stabilizer of the glenohumeral joint (4). With the increased role and use of minimally invasive diagnostic and therapeutic options, including the widespread use of arthroscopy, the ability to diagnose and treat biceps tendon pathology has increased and great interest in this area has recently arisen.

The value and function of the long head of the biceps brachii becomes compromised in the scenario of shoulder pathology, due to the fact that it may cause discomfort and dysfunction when tendon instability, chronic degeneration, and/or tearing are present. In these situations, biceps tenodesis has been shown to decrease shoulder pain while preserving elbow function (5–7). Several different open techniques have proven successful, but all require the added morbidity of open surgical approaches (5,8–11). In the past several years, arthroscopic techniques have been developed and allow the surgery to be performed with less morbidity and pain (6,12–19).

Long head of the biceps tendon disorders can be categorized into three groups: inflammatory, traumatic, and instability (20). Usually, biceps tendon pathology involves the inflammatory subtype and is most often related to impingement. Those patients who complain of impingement symptoms are often found to have tenderness at the intertubercular groove (2). In most cases in which the inflammation has not progressed to degeneration (Fig. 1A), successful treatment of the rotator cuff disease will eradicate the problem. However, when tendon degeneration has become significant, the swollen or partially torn tendon will continue to abrade the walls of the intertubercular groove (21) (Fig. 1B). The only way to effectively manage this significant pain and dysfunction brought on by the chronically diseased biceps tendon may be biceps tenodesis. Most shoulder specialists consider this technique when the long head of the biceps tendon becomes more than 25% to 50% involved (20). Moreover, normal appearing tendons with recalcitrant symptoms can also be treated successfully with biceps tenodesis. A lidocaine injection test should be performed before any surgical intervention is entertained in order to prove that the biceps is the true cause of pain.

The biceps tendon travels from the supraglenoid tubercle and turns an angle of approximately 35° anteriorly to enter the intertubercular groove. It is held in the groove by a pulley system whose floor consists of the superior glenohumeral ligament, which is reinforced by the subscapularis tendon insertion to the lesser tuberosity (Fig. 2).

Long head of the biceps tendon instability is a less frequent problem than tendinitis, but is usually very symptomatic and can result in unwanted damage to the rotator cuff when left untreated (Fig. 3). The most common form of biceps tendon instability results in the biceps subluxating (Fig. 3A) or dislocating inferiorly into or under the subscapularis tendon

Please refer to pages 161–164 for the figures in this chapter.

(Fig. 3B and C) (22). If left untreated, the unstable tendon can continue to weaken or cause further tearing of the subscapularis tendon.

In rare instances, the biceps tendon can subluxate or dislocate into or under the supraspinatus tendon, which is reinforced by the transverse humeral ligament forming the roof of the pulley system (5). When this happens, further tearing of the supraspinatus tendon can occur. In both types of instability, patients complain of painful popping or clicking as the tendon jumps in and out of the groove. The most important indication for long head of the biceps tenodesis in these instances is when the rotator cuff may be damaged by the unstable tendon. It should also be considered when symptoms persist as a result from the biceps tendon instability.

High-energy force is required to cause acute traumatic rupture of a normal long head of the biceps tendon. However, a chronically diseased tendon may rupture with a lesser force (20). The acute disruption may actually lead to relief of shoulder pain, but can be associated with an unwanted deformity and mild weakness of elbow supination or flexion. In some individuals, painful biceps muscle belly cramping may develop; usually, for the short term. Biceps tenodesis prior to an impending rupture can prevent these undesirable side effects.

CONTRAINDICATIONS

As in other surgical procedures, there are a few contraindications to biceps tenodesis. The patient's pathology must not be so severe that there is insufficient tendon to fix either to soft tissue or to bone. Complete ruptures that have retracted below the intertubercular groove are best left alone or treated with open surgery. While arthoscopic biceps tenodesis can be performed very expeditiously, it will nonetheless always take longer than a biceps tenotomy. In more debilitated patients in which it is important to decrease surgical time, a biceps tenotomy may be a better option.

ALTERNATIVE TREATMENTS

The main purpose of arthroscopic biceps tenodesis is to alleviate pain and dysfunction brought on by a chronically inflamed or diseased long head of the biceps tendon. However, nonoperative treatment should always be tried first for at least three months with rehabilitation and anti-inflammatory medications, either by mouth or injection. Physical therapy is directed at the underlying impingement, which is most often the cause of the biceps tendonitis. Surgery is necessary in cases that fail nonoperative treatment, either from recalcitrant inflammation or significant chronic degeneration of the tendon. Open biceps tenodesis is an option and can be performed through a deltoid split, deltopectoral approach, or via a sub-pectoral approach. All have the added morbidity of open surgery.

Another viable treatment option is biceps tenotomy. The biceps tendon is simply cut at its origin from the supraglenoid tubercle and left to retract into the arm past the intertubercular groove (23). Patients who undergo tenotomy should be forewarned, especially in thin patients, whether male or female, that an unwanted deformity might develop (24). In addition, they may suffer painful cramping of the muscle belly, which is most often temporary. Furthermore, mild weakness in supination and flexion at the elbow can be noted, mainly in overhead exercises, otherwise no other clinical strength deficits usually develop. The cramping and weakness are usually temporary, but the deformity is permanent (23).

In some instances, surgery is necessary to protect the cuff tendons in patients in which the biceps tendon is unstable and continues to inflict damage to the rotator cuff tendons. The groove may be deepened and the damaged soft tissues repaired around the biceps tendon. However, the tendon may stick in the groove, or alternatively, it may continue to subluxate out of the groove and result in failure of the rotator cuff repair. Since the rotator cuff is much more important to the long term outcome of any shoulder and should not be put in jeopardy, arthroscopic biceps tenodesis may be a better choice. As described earlier, tenotomy is another option in this situation.

RESULTS

Biceps tenodesis is an effective procedure with satisfactory results in the literature as can be seen in Table 1. Pain relief is experienced by the vast majority of patients in published series

TABLE 1 Results of Arthroscopic Biceps Tenodesis

Authors (Year)	Number of shoulders	Procedure	Mean patient age (range)	Mean follow-up (range)	Results
Boileau, Krishnan, Coste, and Walch 2002	43	Bioabsorbable interference screw (bone technique)	63 yrs (25–78)	17 mo (12–34)	Mean constant score 79 (43 Pre-op); 90% strength return; Two post-op deformities
Elkousy, Fluhme, O'Connor, and Rodosky 2002	12	PITT technique (soft tissue technique)	55 yrs	25 mo (12–48)	All without deformity or cramping and thought benefited; One still with pain

Abbreviation: PITT, percutaneous intra-articular trans-tendon technique.

(6,7). Most patients in our experience, both male or female, prefer not to have a biceps deformity. In many patients, that is their primary concern. Fortunately, arthroscopic biceps tenodesis is a reliable way to prevent the deformity. In addition, arthroscopic biceps tenodesis permits maintenance of the length–tension relationship of the biceps muscle by establishing a new origin of biceps attachment at the appropriate length to prevent muscle atrophy. Moreover, biceps tenodesis is an effective procedure that relieves pain, prevents deformity, with the added benefit of strength preservation at the elbow.

TECHNIQUES

Soft Tissue Techniques

First, descriptions of biceps tenodesis were related to the open "keyhole" technique (8), a type of procedure in which the long head of the biceps tendon was tied into a knot and stuffed into a keyhole created at the proximal humerus. Many surgeons abandoned this technique, as it was associated with a small number of postoperative proximal humeral fractures stemming from the keyhole serving as a stress-riser.

Other techniques became widely used, attaching the long head of the biceps tendon to proximal soft tissue structures such as the pectoralis major muscle and conjoin tendon insertion; or, to bone via drill holes or anchors, when they became available in the mid 1980s (25). These techniques are based on the premise of scarring in the biceps groove as a result of an immobile tendon, such as occurs in cases of trauma. Many of these techniques require expensive implants or involve creating drill holes in bone.

Due to the increasing knowledge and skills of different shoulder surgeons in arthroscopy, there have been a number of arthroscopic techniques for tenodesis described that differ in the type of fixation and hardware needed. The different types of fixation varies from bony (6,18,26) to soft tissue (13) attachment of the long head of biceps stump including some mixed fixation methods, including anchor fixation (12,19) or the use of the biceps as a graft to be included in rotator cuff repairs (27).

In the late 1990s, Rodosky introduced a simple all-arthroscopic soft tissue technique for long head of the biceps tenodesis. The technique was coined the "PITT" technique (13) or "percutaneous intra-articular trans-tendon technique."

Percutaneous Intra-Articular Trans-Tendon Technique

With standard shoulder arthroscopic knowledge, this technique is simple. Moreover, the technique requires no special hardware and can be performed with two spinal needles, suture material, and standard arthroscopic equipment. As with any of the arthroscopic biceps tenodesis procedures described subsequently, the procedure can be performed in either the beach chair or lateral positions, or any other modified arthroscopic set-up position the surgeon chooses. As we standardly utilize an arthroscopic pump system, we find that is extremely helpful for visualization, but other surgeons who are not used to this may not need it. A standard posterior arthroscopic portal is utilized. An anterior portal is established in the rotator interval, just above or below the superior glenohumeral ligament. In order to identify any associated glenohumeral pathology, a diagnostic arthroscopy is performed prior to evaluating the intra-articular portion of the long head of the biceps tendon (Fig. 4A). By placing the arm in adduction and forward flexion and the elbow in flexion and supination, the biceps tendon is fully evaluated. With a soft-tissue grabber or probe, the inter-tubercular portion of the biceps tendon is pulled into glenohumeral joint (Fig. 4B). This allows evaluation of the biceps tendon where pathology is most commonly encountered.

After confirmation of the biceps tendon pathology, the arm is placed in approximately 20° of external rotation. After that, 1.5 to 2 cm of the proximal biceps tendon is pulled into the joint using a soft-tissue grabber, via the anterior cannula. This provides the optimal tension needed to prevent deformity. The elbow can also be hyperflexed at this point as well if the beach chair position is used. Then, a spinal needle is placed in a percutaneous fashion across skin, deltoid, transverse humeral ligament or lateral rotator cuff interval tissue and biceps tendon, starting approximately 2 cm inferior to the antero-lateral corner of the acromion (Fig. 5A). Under direct visualization, the tip of the needle is seen to traverse the bicipital groove and pierce the biceps tendon to enter the intra-articular space. A second needle is placed in the same fashion. The needles should exit the biceps tendon approximately 5 to 10 mm apart with one more anterior and inferior and one more posterior and superior.

Once both spinal needles are in place, O poly-diaxone monofilament sutures (PDS, Ethicon; Cornelia, Georgia, U.S.A.) are threaded through each needle and into the intra-articular space (Fig. 5B). Both sutures are pulled out through the anterior cannula. Under direct visualization, after exiting the anterior cannula, one of the sutures is tied to one end of a blue no. 2 braided nonabsorbable polyester suture (Tycron; United States Surgical, Norwalk, Connecticut, U.S.A.). The other monofilament suture is tied to the opposite end of the braided nonabsorbable suture (Fig. 6A). Note that two PDS strands shuttle a single definitive braided suture. The surgeon then grabs hold of the two monofilament sutures at the site of their percutaneous insertion and pulls on them. This in turn in shuttles both ends of the braided nonabsorbable suture through the joint, piercing the biceps tendon and traversing the subacromial space to exit the skin at the site of insertion of the needles (Fig. 6B). The biceps tendon is captured with a mattress-type suture whose loop end is on the inside of the joint against the biceps tendon.

In order to perform a criss-cross suture, the whole process is repeated with a second braided nonabsorbable suture, a green no. 2 braided nonabsorbable polyester suture (Surgidac; United States Surgical, Norwalk, Connecticut, U.S.A.) (Figs. 7 and 8). This time, the placement of the needles for the second suture should be done with one needle posterior-inferior and the other anterior-superior (Fig. 7A), allowing the mattress loop to cross the other suture in a locking pattern (Fig. 8B). This provides secure fixation of the biceps tendon in the groove for soft tissue tenodesis. In order to simplify suture management, using two different colored sutures is advisable.

Once the soft tissue fixation is performed and the sutures are placed, a narrow cutting tool is used to cut the biceps tendon laterally (Fig. 9), on the medial side of the sutures (Fig. 9B). In order to prevent cutting through the sutures, they are placed under tension to draw them laterally, away from the cutting device (Fig. 9A). After severing the tendon, the remaining stump is debrided with a large shaver to a smooth margin at the superior labrum (Fig. 9C).

After the intra-articular part of the procedure is completed, the arthroscope is placed in the subacromial space, and bursectomy is performed and sutures are identified (Fig. 10). Using standard arthroscopic knot-tying technique, each suture is tied over the transverse humeral ligament or lateral interval tissue, securing the biceps tendon in the groove for tenodesis (Fig. 11). A spinal needle is used to stab the tendon in the groove several times in order to incite a scarring response and expedite the healing process.

Direct Suture Technique

An alternative soft tissue technique is the direct suture technique. In this technique, the biceps tendon is pulled into the joint in the same fashion as above. One or two percutaneous needles are placed, and O poly-diaxone monofilament sutures are threaded through each needle and into the intra-articular space. The sutures are pulled out of the anterior cannula and used to hold the tendon in position. The intra-articular portion of the tendon is resected in the same fashion as above. The sutures are kept in position for temporary fixation and subacromial arthroscopy is performed, including a bursectomy. The transverse humeral ligament tissue spanning from lesser to greater tuberosity over the biceps groove is identified distal to the needles. Using a curved needle suture passing device (Spectrum, CONMED Linvatec; Largo, Florida, U.S.A.), a single strand of O polydiaxone monofilament suture is passed across the transverse humeral ligament, through the biceps tendon and back through the transverse humeral ligament tissue. The suture is then exchanged for a blue no. 2 braided nonabsorbable polyester suture. It is tied using standard arthroscopic knot-tying techniques. The process is repeated at least one more time for adequate fixation. The temporary fixation sutures are removed after the biceps tendon is secured in the groove with the braided non-absorbable sutures.

Bony Repair Techniques

Soft tissue techniques are dependent upon having intact or adequate transverse humeral ligamentous tissue or rotator cuff/interval tissue. When these tissues are inadequate, the surgeon must perform bony repair of the biceps tendon for tenodesis. Some surgeons prefer to use bony techniques rather than soft tissue techniques, as they feel more confident with a repair to bone. However, biomechanical studies have not shown any significant advantage for the bony techniques, when the soft tissue structures are adequate. The quality of the biceps tendon is the most important aspect in determining the success or failure of the tenodesis, whichever technique is utilized.

Suture Anchor Technique

This technique has been described by Gartsman (12). Standard anterior, lateral, and posterior portals are established and the arm is placed in neutral to slight external rotation. When the cuff is intact, a spinal needle is introduced percutaneously as describe above, piercing the biceps tendon. However, it is advanced until lodged into bone at the biceps groove. Subacromial arthroscopy, including bursectomy, is performed until the needle is identified. Immediately distal to the needle, the transverse humeral ligament tissue is resected until the biceps is seen within the groove. In the case of a rotator cuff tear, the biceps is identified directly as it enters the groove. In either situation, single-loaded suture anchors are placed either next to or in the groove. Both suture limbs of both anchors are shuttled through the tendon and tied in a mattress fashion. Following secure fixation, the intra-articular portion of the biceps tendon is excised. When the cuff is intact, intra-articular resection can be made easier by transecting the tendon at its insertion into the superior labrum prior to exiting the glenohumeral joint.

Bioabsorbable Interference Screw Fixation

The arthroscopic bioabsorbable interference screw fixation technique was first described by Boileau (6). The procedure is performed with the shoulder in approximately 30° of flexion, 30° of internal rotation, and 30° of abduction. The procedure is done with three portals: standard posterior portal and two anterior portals. The anterior portals are 1.5 cm on each side of the groove (anteromedial and anterolateral). The posterior and anterolateral portals are used for viewing, and the anteromedial portal is used as the working portal.

As described in the aforementioned techniques, glenohumeral arthroscopy is performed with the arthroscope in the posterior portal and a probe in the anterior cannula. Biceps pathology is confirmed and the tendon is held in position with a percutaneously placed spinal needle at the mouth of the groove. The tendon is transected at its junction with the superior labrum.

Subacromial arthroscopy, including bursectomy, is performed with the arthroscope in the anterolateral portal. The transverse humeral ligament spanning from lesser to greater tuberosity over the biceps groove is incised with an electrocautery device and the biceps tendon is exposed. The biceps tendon is pulled out of the glenohumeral joint to the exterior via the anteromedial portal.

Techniques for placement of the tendon into the hole vary depending on the type of interference screw. Usually, a humeral socket large enough to allow placement of the biceps tendon into, usually 7 to 8 mm, is drilled to a depth of 25 to 30 mm in the center of the groove and at least 10 mm from the top of the groove.

In the Boileau technique, a standard cannulated screw system is used. The end of the biceps tendon is doubled over for 2 cm and sewn together using a running baseball stitch with a heavy nonabsorbable suture. A guide (Shoulder-Guide, Future Medical System; Glen Burnie, Maryland, U.S.A.) is used to pass a guide wire through and out the posterior aspect of the humerus exiting the skin. It is directed away from the axillary nerve with the guide. The humeral socket is drilled over the guide wire. A Beath pin is placed through the socket and exits the posterior shoulder, penetrating the skin in the same location as the guide pin, away from the axillary nerve. A heavy nonabsorbable suture is placed through the end of the biceps tendon. The heavy suture is then threaded through the Beath pin, which is pulled through the humeral socket and used to pull the tendon back into the subacromial space and into the humeral socket. A guide wire is placed into the socket next to the tendon and used for placement of the cannulated interference screw. The screw is then finally placed to fix the tendon into the socket.

In other interference screw techniques, a heavy nonabsorbable suture is placed through the end of the biceps tendon and then one limb of the suture is drawn through the canulated hole of the interference screw. The other limb of the suture remains outside the interference screw. This allows the end of the tendon to be pulled and held into the socket with the cannulation device, avoiding the need for drilling across the humerus (10) (Bio-Tenodesis driver, Arthrex, Inc.; Naples, Florida, U.S.A.) (Fig. 12). This is a safer and easier technique for most surgeons, as it avoids the possibility of injuring the axillary nerve.

Rehabilitation

Postoperative rehabilitation after isolated arthroscopic biceps tenodesis is initiated within the first week of surgery. Pendulum exercises and gentle active and passive shoulder and elbow motion can begin immediately. A sling is worn for three to four weeks. The patient is instructed to avoid any significant pushing, pulling, or lifting with the involved arm for eight weeks. This especially includes avoiding any significant elbow supination activities. At that point, gentle progressive strengthening can begin. Heavy lifting and sports are avoided for a full six months. When concomitant surgery, such as rotator cuff repair, is performed, the rehabilitation protocol is altered so as not to conflict with the postoperative protection of the rotator cuff and/or other concomitant repairs.

PITFALLS AND COMPLICATIONS

Arthroscopic biceps tenodesis is a relatively safe technique with few potential pitfalls. Biomechanical studies have shown little difference in fixation strength between the various techniques. Wolf et al. (28) reported the superiority of the bioabsorbable interference screw over tenotomy in terms of load failure and migration. Moreover, Jayamoorthy (29) showed that there were no differences with the classic open keyhole technique and the bioabsorbable screw, and Mazzoca (30) compared three different open techniques using interferential screw with the anchor technique and found no differences between them for load to failure and displacement.

The major determinant appears to be the quality of the biceps tendon itself. This issue should be considered for the postoperative rehabilitation. In term of forces, the biceps tendon ranges from 75 N to support the weight of the forearm against gravity up to 300 N if a 20 N weight is held in the hand, depending on the activities and how it is tested (29,31).

In Rodosky's studies (32), there are no significant differences between the PITT technique and the double anchor technique showing ultimate load failures around 150 N, and due to this observation, absolute immobilization might not be needed and passive and light active movements could be permitted in the early postoperative period.

In cases where the portion of the tendon that is being fixed is of poor quality, the surgeon may need to go more distal to find better quality tendon. In some instances, this may require an open technique. An alternative to this approach would be to simply perform the arthroscopic technique of choice, realizing that failure of the poor quality tendon would be the equivalent of a biceps tenotomy. If this is not acceptable, the surgeon should proceed with an alternative approach for fixation.

Neurovascular complications are extremely rare. When placing an interference screw using the transhumeral technique, it is important to direct the transhumeral pin away from the axillary nerve. This is facilitated by the use of a standard drill guide.

Stiffness is a rare complication after arthroscopic biceps tenodesis. It is important to resect the intra-articular portion of the biceps tendon in order to prevent tethering of the glenohumeral joint. This could lead to loss of motion, especially external rotation in adducted positions. Active and passive motion of the glenohumeral joint can begin immediately after surgery.

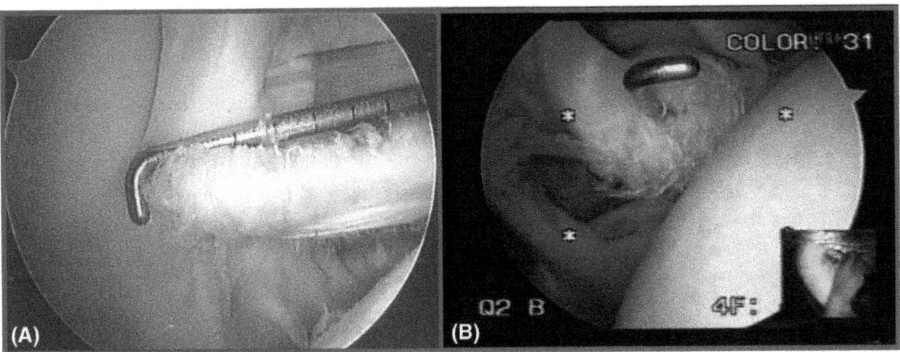

FIGURE 1 Intra-articular view of two different stages of biceps tendinitis. (**A**) Chronic inflammation; (**B**) significant fibrotic degeneration.

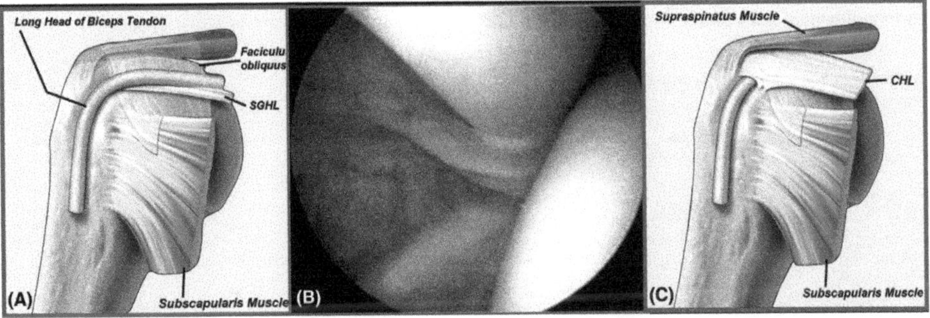

FIGURE 2 Anatomy of biceps tendon held in the groove by the pulley system. (**A**) The floor of the bicipital groove consists of the superior glenohumeral ligament, which is reinforced by the subscapularis tendon insertion to the lesser tuberosity. (**B**) Athroscopic view showing the floor of the pulley system. (**C**) The roof is formed by the supraspinatus tendon reinforced by the coracohumeral and the transverse humeral ligaments. *Abbreviations*: CHL, coracohumeral ligament; SGHL, superior glenohumeral ligament.

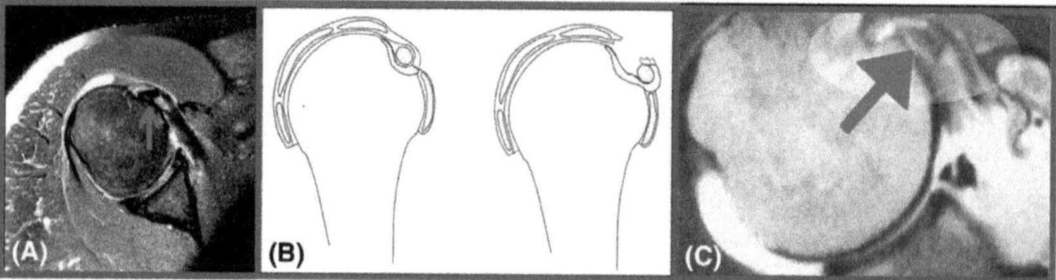

FIGURE 3 Biceps instability. (**A**) The most common form of biceps tendon instability results in the biceps subluxating inferiorly into or under the subscapularis tendon. (**B**) If left untreated, the unstable tendon can continue to weaken or cause further tearing of the subscapularis tendon. (**C**) Complete dislocation of the biceps tendon under the subscapularis tendon.

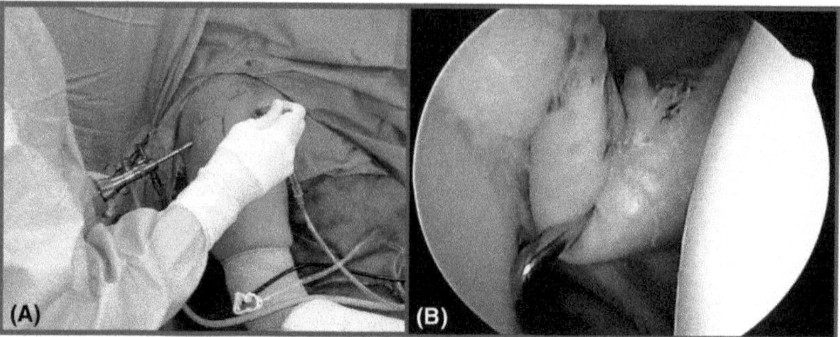

FIGURE 4 (**A**) Beach chair position and use of the probe through the anterior portal. (**B**) Intra-articular diagnosis of long head of biceps by pulling the intertubercular portion into glenohumeral joint with the probe.

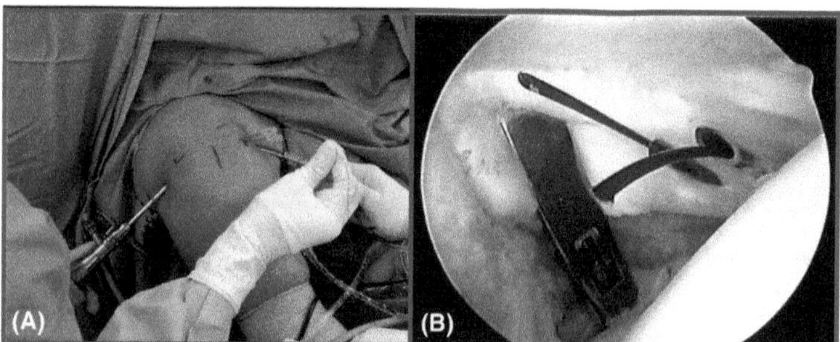

FIGURE 5 (**A**) Spinal needles are placed in a percutaneous fashion across skin, deltoid, transverse humeral ligament or lateral rotator cuff interval tissue and biceps tendon. (**B**) Under direct arthroscopic control, 0 poly-diaxone monofilament sutures are threaded through each needle and into the intra-articular space.

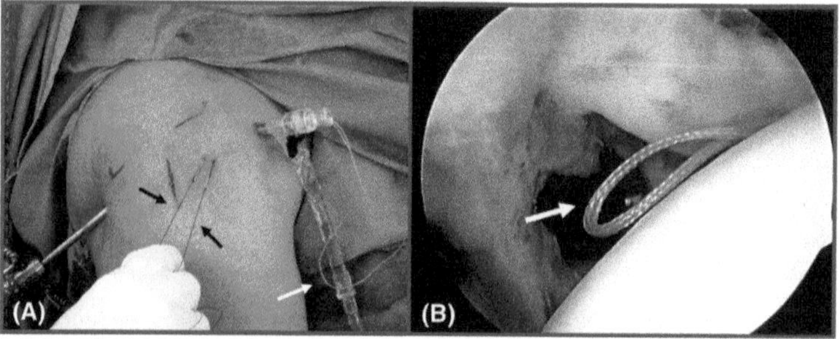

FIGURE 6 (**A**) Both threads of 0 poly-diaxone monofilament sutures (*black arrows*) are tied to both ends of a single braided nonabsorbable suture (*white arrow*). (**B**) Intra-articular view showing the biceps tendon captured with a mattress-type suture with the loop (white arrow) end on the inside of the joint against the biceps tendon.

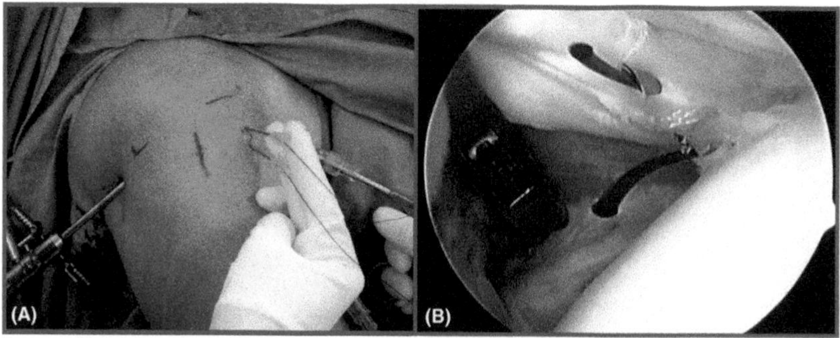

FIGURE 7 (**A**) The process is repeated again, placing the spinal needles first posterior-inferior and the other anterior-superior. (**B**) The 0 poly-diaxone monofilament sutures strands are passed again through the respective spinal needle, while the biceps tendon is held with a grasper placed through the anterior portal.

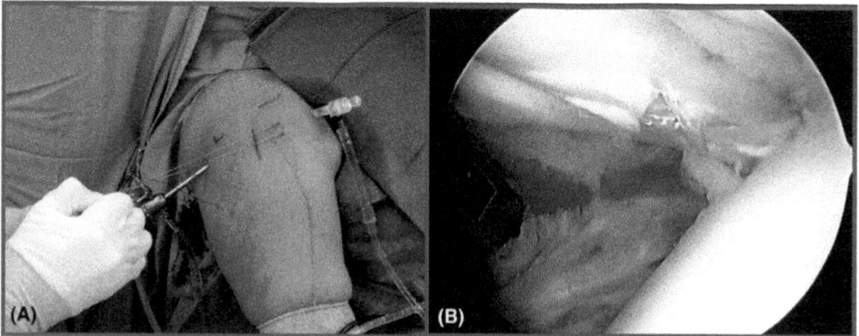

FIGURE 8 (**A**) The criss-cross stitch is completed by pulling the other colored polyester mattress stitch using the 0 poly-diaxone monofilament sutures as a shuttle as previously described. (**B**) The criss-cross suture is seen in this intra-articular view holding the biceps tendon in a secure fashion.

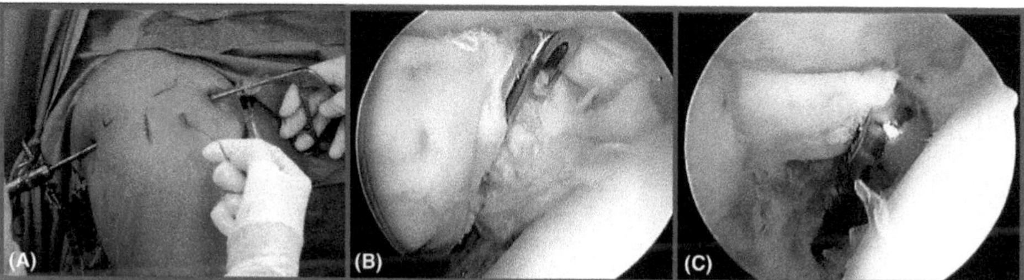

FIGURE 9 (**A**) Sutures are then placed under tension to draw them laterally in order to prevent inadvertent injury during transaction of the biceps tendon. (**B**) A narrow cutting tool is used to cut the biceps tendon just lateral to its insertion on the superior labrum, on the medial side of the sutures. (**C**) After severing the tendon, the remaining stump is debrided with a large shaver to a smooth margin at the superior labrum.

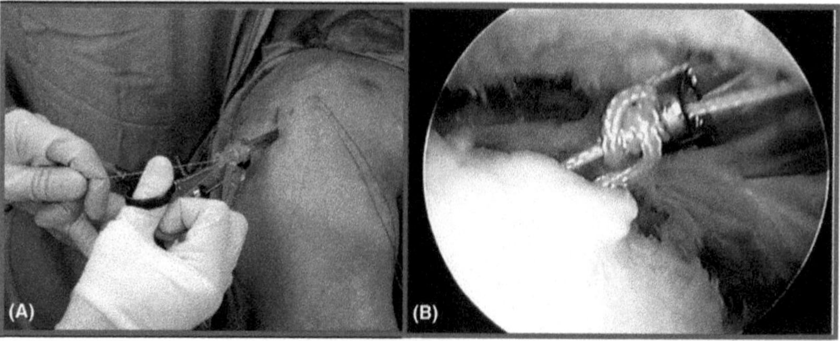

FIGURE 10 Arthroscopic knot tying is performed in the subacromial space to secure the biceps tendon. (**A**) Exterior view of the arthroscopic knot tying through a standard cannula. (**B**) Arthroscopic view of Nicky's sliding knot being secured using a knot pusher in the subacromial space.

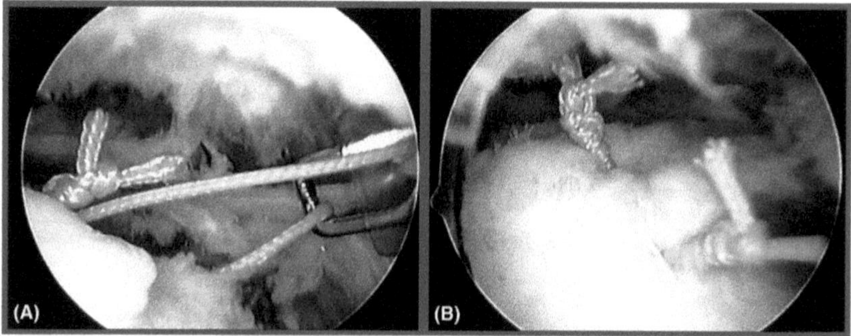

FIGURE 11 (**A**) The second set of sutures are identified and then tied in a similar fashion. (**B**) Final appearance of the biceps tenodesis with both knots tied as viewed in the subacromial space.

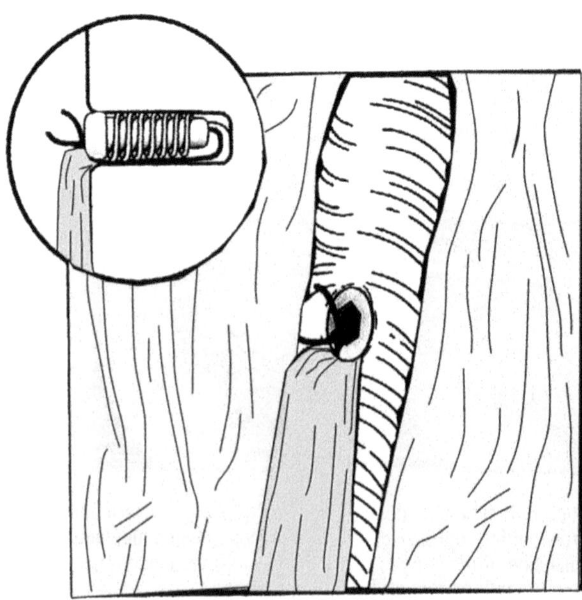

FIGURE 12 One of the several interference screws used to perform biceps tenodesis. The biotenodesis screw with a knot tied over the top of the screw securing the tendon.

REFERENCES

1. Dinnes J, Loveman E, McIntyre L, Waugh N. The effectiveness of diagnostic tests for the assessment of shoulder pain due to soft tissue disorders: a systematic review. Health Technol Assess 2003; 7(29):iii, 1–166.
2. Neer CS II. Impingement lesions. Clin Orthop Relat Res 1983; 173:70–77.
3. Lippmann R. Bicipital tenosynovitis. N Y State J Med 1944; 44:2235–2240.
4. Rodosky MW, Harner CS, Fu FH. The role of the long head of the biceps muscle and superior glenoid labrum in anterior stability of the shoulder. Am J Sports Med 1994; 22(1):121–130.
5. Michele AA, Krueger FJ. Tenodesis of biceps tendons; a preliminary report. Surgery 1951; 29(4):555–559.
6. Boileau P, Krishan SG, Coste JS, Walch G. Arthroscopic biceps tenodesis: a new technique using bioabsorbable interference screw fixation. Arthroscopy 2002; 18(9):1002–1012.
7. Elkousy HA, Fluhme DJ, O'Connor DP, Rodosky MW. Arthroscopic biceps tenodesis using the percutaneous, intra-articular trans-tendon technique: preliminary results. Orthopedics 2005; 28(11):1316–1319.
8. Froimson AI, OI. Keyhole tenodesis of biceps origin at the shoulder. Clin Orthop Relat Res 1975; (112):245–249.
9. Pinzur MS, Hopkins GE. Biceps tenodesis for painful inferior subluxation of the shoulder in adult acquired hemiplegia. Clin Orthop Relat Res 1986; 206:100–103.
10. Mazzocca AD NM, Romeo AA. Open and sub pectoral biceps tenodesis. Oper Tech Sports Med 2003; 11:24–31.
11. Mazzocca AD, Rios CG, Romeo AA, Arciero RA. Subpectoral biceps tenodesis with interference screw fixation. Arthroscopy 2005; 21(7):896.
12. Gartsman GM, Hammerman SM. Arthroscopic biceps tenodesis: operative technique. Arthroscopy 2000; 16(5):550–552.
13. Sekiya LC, Elkousy HA, Rodosky MW. Arthroscopic biceps tenodesis using the percutaneous intra-articular transtendon technique. Arthroscopy 2003; 19(10):1137–1141.
14. Ozalay M, Akpinar S, Hersekli MA, Ozkoc G, Tandooan RN. Arthroscopic assisted biceps tenodesis. Acta Orthop Traumatol Turc 2003; 37(2):144–149.
15. Wiley WB, Meyers JF, Weber SC, Pearson SE. Arthroscopic assisted mini-open biceps tenodesis: surgical technique. Arthroscopy 2004; 20(4):444–446.
16. Romeo AA, Mazzocca AD, Tauro JC. Arthroscopic biceps tenodesis. Arthroscopy 2004; 20(2):206–213.
17. Lo IK, Burkhart SS. Arthroscopic biceps tenodesis using a bioabsorbable interference screw. Arthroscopy 2004; 20(1):85–95.
18. Kim SH, Yoo JC. Arthroscopic biceps tenodesis using interference screw: end-tunnel technique. Arthroscopy 2005; 21(11):1405.
19. Castagna A, Conti M, Mouhsine E, Bungaro P, Garofalo R. Arthroscopic biceps tendon tenodesis: the anchorage technical note. Knee Surg Sports Traumatol Arthrosc 2006; 14(6):581–585.
20. Ahmad CS, ElAttrache NS. Arthroscopic biceps tenodesis. Orthop Clin North Am 2003; 34(4):499–506.
21. Neviaser TJ. The role of the biceps tendon in the impingement syndrome. Orthop Clin North Am 1987; 18(3):383–386.
22. Habermeyer P, Magosch P, Pritsch M, Schelbel MT, Lichtenberg S. Anterosuperior impingement of the shoulder as a result of pulley lesions: a prospective arthroscopic study. J Shoulder Elbow Surg 2004; 13(1):5–12.
23. Gill TJ, McIrvin E, Mair SD, Hawkins RJ. Results of biceps tenotomy for treatment of pathology of the long head of the biceps brachii. J Shoulder Elbow Surg 2001; 10(3):247–249.
24. Osbahr DC, Diamond AB, Speer K.P. The cosmetic appearance of the biceps muscle after long-head tenotomy versus tenodesis. Arthroscopy 2002; 18(5):483–487.
25. Dines D Warren RF, Inglis AE. Surgical treatment of lesions of the long head of the biceps. Clin Orthop Relat Res 1982; 164:165–171.
26. Boileau P, Neyton L. Arthroscopic tenodesis for lesions of the long head of the biceps. Oper Orthop Traumatol 2005; 17(6):601–623.
27. Checchia SL, Doneux PS, Mivazaki, Silva LA, Fregoneze M, Ossada A, et al. Biceps tenodesis associated with arthroscopic repair of rotator cuff tears. J Shoulder Elbow Surg 2005; 14(2):138–144.
28. Wolf RS, Zheng N, Weichel D. Long head biceps tenotomy versus tenodesis: a cadaveric biomechanical analysis. Arthroscopy 2005; 21(2):182–185.
29. Jayamoorthy T, Field JR, Costi JJ, Martin DK, Stanley RM, Hearn TC. Biceps tenodesis: a biomechanical study of fixation methods. J Shoulder Elbow Surg 2004; 13(2):160–164.

30. Mazzocca AD, Bicos J, Santangelo S, Romeo AA, Arciero RA. The biomechanical evaluation of four fixation techniques for proximal biceps tenodesis. Arthroscopy 2005; 21(11):1296–1306.
31. Langenderfer J, LaScaiza S, Mell A, Carpenter JE, KuhnJE, Hughes RE. An EMG-driven model of the upper extremity and estimation of long head biceps force. Comput Biol Med 2005; 35(1):25–39.
32. Rodosky MW. Failure strength of arthroscopic biceps tenodesis repairs: suture anchor vs. P.I.T.T. technique. Arthroscopy 2006; 22(6):e14–e15.

16 | Arthroscopic Treatment of Para-Labral Cysts

Mitchell F. Fagelman, Charles L. Getz, and Gerald R. Williams, Jr.
Department of Orthopedic Surgery, University of Pennsylvania School of Medicine, Philadelphia, Pennsylvania, U.S.A.

INTRODUCTION

Shoulder pain is a common ailment for which patients seek medical attention. Common causes of shoulder pain include rotator cuff tears, impingement syndrome, glenohumeral arthrosis, acromioclavicular arthrosis, and instability. Less common causes include cervical radiculopathy, thoracic outlet syndrome, para-labral (ganglion) cysts, and nerve compression. This chapter will focus on the pathogenesis of para-labral cysts, diagnosis of para-labral cysts with and without nerve compression, and treatment options and results of operative and nonoperative intervention of para-labral cysts.

HISTORICAL PERSPECTIVE

Suprascapular nerve entrapment at the suprascapular notch was first documented in the literature in 1959 by Kopell and Thompson (1) and cited by other authors (2,3) as a source of shoulder pain (Table 1). In 1982, Aiello et al. (4) helped to differentiate between suprascapular nerve compression at the spinoglenoid notch and the suprascapular notch. However, recognition of the para-labral cyst as a source of suprascapular nerve palsy and shoulder pain has only, more recently, been described with the arrival of shoulder magnetic resonance imaging (MRI). Initial reports recognizing para-labral cysts were sparse with only 21 cases reported in the Japanese and English literature combined from 1970–1989 (5). Para-labral cysts may be clinically important as they have been associated with shoulder pain, labral tears (6–10), and suprascapular nerve compression (5–8,11–22). Although relatively uncommon, compression neuropathy from cysts (especially spinoglenoid cysts) may be the cause of shoulder disability.

PATHOGENESIS

The exact etiology of para-labral cysts is unknown. Most authors would agree that para-labral cysts are a collection of extra-articular joint fluid. Whether this fluid leak is caused by injury to the capsule or an inherent weakness in the capsulolabral complex is a matter of debate. It is postulated that synovial fluid may leak out of the joint, creating this labral (ganglion) cyst via a one-way-valve mechanism (7,20,21). Furthermore, Neviaser (23) reported a ganglion cyst connected to a subacromial bursa.

An association between cartilaginous tears and intra-articular pathology with periarticular cysts around the knee has been made (24). A similar association between labral tears and para-labral cysts around glenohumeral joint has been reported (6,8,20,25,26). Lichtenberg (21) reported six of eight patients undergoing decompression of a ganglion cyst were found to have a superior labrum anterior posterior (SLAP) lesion at the time of surgery. Similarly, Moore found superior labral tears in 11 of 12 patients who underwent arthroscopy for cyst decompression. Although some authors report a high incidence of associated labral tears and ganglion cysts (10), up to 53% of cysts are not associated with an identifiable labral lesion by MRI (9).

Please refer to pages 175–176 for the figures in this chapter.

TABLE 1 Causes of Suprascapular Neuropathy

Direct trauma to suprascapular nerve
Clavicle fractures
Scapular fractures
Anterior shoulder dislocations
Traction injuries
Injury at Erb's point
Repetitive microtrauma/stretch
Calcification
Transverse scapular ligament
Spinoglenoid ligament
Fracture Callus
Ganglion cyst
Tumor
Iatrogenic injury

ANATOMY

The anatomy of the suprascapular nerve and its surrounding structures is well described in the literature. The suprascapular nerve is a mixed motor and sensory nerve arising from the upper trunk of the brachial plexus formed by the fifth and sixth cervical roots, with variable contribution by the fourth cervical root (27). The nerve courses through the posterior cervical triangle deep to the trapezius and omohyoid muscles to reach the suprascapular notch. The suprascapular nerve passes through the notch below the transverse scapular ligament, and then bifurcates into two main branches (28,29). Upon entering the supraspinatus fossa, the nerve innervates the supraspinatus muscle and receives sensory branches from the glenohumeral and acromioclavicular joints, subacromial bursa, and posterior capsule (7,30–32). The suprascapular nerve then travels around the lateral edge of the scapular spine to enter the infraspinatus fossa via the spinoglenoid notch. A cutaneous branch of the suprascapular nerve has been described and supplies sensation to the lateral part of the deltoid (as supplied by axillary nerve) in up to 15% of the population (30,32,16).

Lesions of the suprascapular nerve generally occur at two regions: the suprascapular notch and the spinoglenoid notch. Therefore, further detail of the anatomy around these two areas is worth mentioning. In a cadaveric study of 211 scapula, Rengachary et al. (33) described six different types of suprascapular notch abnormalities. In a later study, Ticker et al. (34) described a "U"-shaped (77%) and "V"-shaped (23%) suprascapular notch in 79 shoulders, with 89% of cadavers having the same shape bilaterally (34). Although the suprascapular notch may have different morphology, no study has linked a specific notch morphology with a higher incidence of nerve entrapment. However, an ossified or anomalous superior transverse ligament can lead to suprascapular nerve compression (34,35).

The spinoglenoid ligament (inferior transverse scapular ligament) is variable in morphology and prevalence in the population (34,36–39). Kaspi (36) reported the presence of a spinoglenoid ligament in 87% of men and only 50% of women in 25 cadaveric shoulders. Cummins classified the ligament into three categories: (*i*) absent, (*ii*) Type I (insubstantial thin fibrous band), or (*iii*) Type II (distinct ligament) (Table 2). They found no ligament in 20%, type I ligament in 61%, and type II ligament in 20% of the shoulders. Overall, 80% of the shoulders had some type of band, creating a tunnel through which the suprascapular nerve could travel (37). In a more recent study, Plancher et al. (39) found the presence of a spinoglenoid ligament in all 58 cadaveric shoulders and were the first to report the histological characteristics of the ligament. Based on their histological analysis, the ligament consisted of a highly organized collagen and was found to insert onto the scapula via Sharpey's fibers.

TABLE 2 Classification of the Spinoglenoid Ligament (According to Cummins)

Ligament type	Prevalence (%)
Absent/insubstantial	20
Type I	61
Type II	20

The suprascapular nerve is more vulnerable to injury at the spinoglenoid notch due to the tethering effect of the spinoglenoid ligament and the close proximity of the nerve to the posterior glenoid. In a cadaveric study, Warner et al. (29) noted three or more motor branches to the infraspinatus muscle, which passed on an average 2 cm posterior to the glenoid rim in 15 of 31 shoulders (48%). Furthermore, Bigliani et al. (28) showed the average distance between the suprascapular nerve and the posterior glenoid rim was 1.8 cm. Hence, even small para-labral cysts can cause encroachment on the suprascapular nerve, leading to clinical signs of nerve compression.

CLINICAL EVALUATION

Patients with a para-labral cyst can present to the office in a variety of ways. A thorough history and systematic evaluation of the shoulder girdle and cervical spine are essential to determine the underlying pathology that may be very subtle in the case of para-labral cysts. More common causes of shoulder pain and dysfunction such as rotator cuff tears, impingement syndrome, arthritis, and instability should first be sought as a reason for the patient's shoulder complaints. However, if the diagnosis remains uncertain, the presence of a para-labral cyst should be ruled-in or ruled-out. Para-labral cysts fall into three presenting categories: (*i*) associated with suprascapular nerve palsy, (*ii*) pain without neurologic involvement, or (*iii*) incidental.

The clinical findings from para-labral cysts are directly related to the location of the cyst in the shoulder. Patients with suprascapular nerve palsy often present with a deep, dull ache that may be poorly localized over the lateral and posterior aspects of the shoulder (7,16,20,25). Patients may often relate an inability to lie on the affected shoulder and difficulty sleeping. Furthermore, the pain may be exacerbated by overhead or recurrent activities. Patients with suprascapular nerve compression at the suprascapular notch may have more significant pain complaints than those with compression at the spinoglenoid notch (7,16). Often, patients will give a history of trauma to the shoulder, or repetitive use of the shoulder during various activities such as volleyball, basketball, tennis, swimming, throwing, or weightlifting (7,40–46).

Because some patients may have neck symptoms or pain down the affected arm, a cervical spine exam with provocative testing is important. Patients may have limited range of motion of the shoulder mimicking adhesive capsulitis. Palpation over the suprascapular notch, between the posterior clavicle and scapular spine, may produce tenderness if the nerve is compressed in this area. Furthermore, cross-body adduction with the arm extended may cause increased tenderness in the area of the suprascapular notch, but exact localization can be difficult (16). Long-standing nerve compression may cause atrophy of both the supraspinatus and infraspinatus muscles. However, in muscular, athletic individuals, supraspinatus atrophy may be difficult to appreciate due to the large, overlying trapezius. Strength testing of the affected shoulder may reveal weakness in external rotation and abduction.

Complaints from compression of the suprascapular nerve at the spinoglenoid notch can vary from pain-free shoulders to severe, debilitating shoulder pain. Moore et al. (8) reported the results of 22 patients with symptomatic spinoglenoid cysts. Fourteen patients presented with both pain and weakness, whereas only eight presented with pain alone. No patient had discrete areas of tenderness on palpation. Patients may exhibit significant wasting of the infraspinatus, which is easily seen due to the subcutaneous position of the muscle. However, even with significant infraspinatus wasting, severe weakness in external rotation may not be present due to the compensation by the deltoid and teres minor (16,47).

Diagnostic nerve blocks around either the spinoglenoid or suprascapular notches can be used to confirm the diagnosis of nerve compression. However, clinically locating these anatomic structures can be difficult, making injections less reliable (7,48).

DIAGNOSTIC TESTING

Plain radiographs of the shoulder may reveal healed fractures of the clavicle or scapula and/or callus formation around the suprascapular and spinoglenoid notches. An anterior-posterior

(AP) radiograph of the scapula, with the beam directed 15° to 30° caudally, offers a good view of the suprascapular notch to look for calcification or other potential causes of suprascapular nerve entrapment (16,49). However, because para-labral cysts consist of soft tissue, few, if any radiographic findings will be seen on plain X ray.

MRI now serves as the diagnostic tool of choice to evaluate para-labral cysts (7,9,12,16,20,21,50–52). Oftentimes, para-labral cysts will just be an incidental finding on an MRI ordered for evaluation of a possible rotator cuff tear or labral injury. Para-labral cysts will typically appear as a homogenous mass with decreased signal intensity on T1-weighted imaging and increased signal intensity on T2-weighted imaging. Tung et al. (9) found 51 cysts in 46 patients with a mean cyst diameter of 2.2 cm. In addition to cyst evaluation, muscle denervation from nerve compression can be seen on MRI (9,53,54). Characteristics of muscle denervation include increased signal intensity in the muscle on T2-weighted imaging (with or without muscle atrophy). McDonald et al. (55) compared short T1 recovery (STIR) MRI to needle electromyography (EMG) in detecting denervation of skeletal muscle. They found that the increased signal intensity on STIR MRI corresponds closely with spontaneous activity on EMG in denervated muscles. However, STIR MRI was less sensitive overall.

Tirman et al. (6) reported that all 20 patients who underwent surgery for glenoid labral cysts had evidence of a labral tear on a preoperative MRI after retrospective review. Moore et al. (8) used MRI to diagnose cysts in 20 of 22 patients and denervation of the infraspinatus muscle in six patients. They did not find SLAP tears on preoperative MRIs, but found SLAP lesions in 10 of 11 patients who underwent arthroscopic surgery. In contrast, Piatt et al. (10) found superior labral pathology in 89% of patients with a spinoglenoid cyst, with atrophy of the infraspinatus or supraspinatus muscle present in 38% of patients. These MRI discrepancies between studies can be attributed to the fact that MRI is insensitive to some labral tears (9,56,57). MR arthrography can improve the sensitivity for identifying labral pathology, especially SLAP tears (9,58). In a prospective study of 30 patients, Chandnani et al. compared plain MRI, MR arthrography, and computed tomographic (CT) arthrography to determine the sensitivity of each technique in detecting labral tears. Of the 28 labral tears found at surgery, 93% were detected preoperatively by plain MRI, 96% by MR arthrography, and 73% by CT arthrography. They concluded MR arthrography was the most sensitive of the three imaging modalities for detecting labral tears and labral degeneration (59).

EMG and nerve conduction studies (NCS) are essential tools for the evaluation of suprascapular nerve compression from associated para-labral cysts. These tests are indicated when patients exhibit muscle weakness when other, more common, sources of weakness have been ruled out. EMG/NCS can be used to differentiate the site of nerve entrapment and dysfunction between the suprascapular and spinoglenoid notches (60). Electrophysiological evaluation of the suprascapular nerve is usually limited to data acquired from motor distal latency and motor response amplitudes from the supraspinatus and infraspinatus muscles, after stimulation at Erb's point (20,61). With nerve injury, EMG studies will show increased spontaneous activity, polyphasic activity, sharp waves, fibrillation, and reduced evoked potentials (16,60).

Although abnormal EMG/NCS are common in the presence of suprascapular nerve compression, inaccuracies with false-negative examinations are possible (8,16,20). Moore et al. (8) reported difficulty with the use of EMG/NCS in four patients. On initial interpretation, these four studies were reported as normal despite obvious clinical evidence of infraspinatus atrophy. However, upon redirecting the neurologist to specifically evaluate the suprascapular nerve, the appropriate diagnosis was made. Moore et al. (8) attributed these false-negative results to several possible explanations. First, a cyst may only compress one of the three or four motor branches that supply the infraspinatus muscle. Therefore, needle studies and NCS must be placed in multiple areas of the infraspinatus during testing, and the person performing the test should be informed of the specific details wanted by the treating physician. Second, because of the mixed motor and sensory composition of the suprascapular nerve, the cyst may only be compressing the sensory portion of the nerve without any effect on the motor branches. Therefore, the EMG and NCV will be unable to detect this sensory compression and a normal test will be reported.

In addition to the diagnostic value of EMG/NCS for the detection of suprascapular neuropathy, EMG studies have been shown to partly predict functional outcomes after treatment

(60). In a study of 64 consecutive patients, Antoniou et al. (60) found that more severe EMG changes were associated with more significant improvement following treatment. In contrast, 19 patients with spinoglenoid notch cysts and less severe pretreatment EMGs showed the least improvement, following either operative or nonoperative treatment. Although this failure of functional improvement following treatment may seem contrary to conventional thinking, the authors attribute the low preoperative functional scores to the pain and disability caused by secondary pathology (a labral tear causing a cyst) rather than directly to nerve compression. Therefore, isolated treatment of nerve compression without identification or treatment of the other pathology would not expect to improve pain or function postoperatively.

TREATMENT AND RESULTS

Treatment options for patients with para-labral cysts vary from nonoperative management to surgical intervention. The initial treatment for most patients with para-labral cysts should be conservative, especially if patients are minimally symptomatic or the cyst was found incidentally on MRI. Patients should be told to avoid aggravating or repetitive activities, and consideration for nonsteroidal anti-inflammatory drug (NSAID) therapy is given. If used, physical therapy should focus on range-of-motion, scapular stabilization, and rotator cuff strengthening. Furthermore, special attention should focus on scapular retraction exercises and strengthening of the trapezius, rhomboids, and serratus muscles (16). Moore et al. (8) reported the conservative treatment of 6 of 21 patients with spinoglenoid cysts. Two patients had improvement with one having essentially complete resolution of symptoms. At a minimum of one-year follow-up, four of the six patients were unchanged. Piatt (10) reported their results in 19 patients following conservative management consisting of physiotherapy and NSAIDs. Overall, 53% of the patients were satisfied with their outcome, including two patients who showed improvement of their muscle atrophy.

In the face of muscle atrophy or an abnormal EMG, the role of nonoperative treatment is limited. Image-guided aspiration of cysts around the shoulder has been reported in the literature (6,9,10,12,21,52,62,). Tung et al. (9) performed four cyst aspirations under sonographic guidance. Repeat shoulder sonography at four months showed recurrence of the para-labral cyst in three of the four shoulders, including one cyst that was injected with corticosteriods following cyst aspiration. Piatt et al. (10) reported cyst aspiration in 11 patients with recurrence in five patients at final follow-up.

Surgical treatment of para-labral cysts of the shoulder includes either open or arthroscopic techniques. The traditional "gold standard" for surgical treatment of ganglion cysts causing nerve compression is open decompression. Reports in the literature from open cyst decompression or a combined open/arthroscopic cyst decompression are favorable (7,8,10,16). Moore et al. (8) reported their results in 16 patients with spinoglenoid cysts. Six patients underwent a combined arthroscopic and open procedure, five underwent open procedures alone, and five underwent arthroscopic treatment alone. At arthroscopy, 10 of 11 patients were noted to have a concomitant SLAP lesion, but only five of these cases were treated with a repair. Postoperative MRI scans were obtained in 15 of 16 patients treated with surgery. Four patients had only partial resolution of the cyst, three of which were treated with open surgery alone. In the other case, the patient was treated with a combined open/arthroscopic procedure. A SLAP lesion was not identified at the index arthroscopic procedure. Following a period of improvement, the patient's symptoms returned and a repeat arthroscopy was performed. A SLAP lesion was then identified, which was probably missed during the first procedure. Although open surgery does allow for direct visualization of the cyst and the suprascapular nerve, open decompression may increase morbidity from longer incisions and muscle detachment.

Fehrman et al. (7) reported their results using a combined open/arthroscopic approach for treatment of ganglion cysts. All six patients were found to have posterior labral tears that were only debrided. Five of six patients had complete relief at final follow-up, but one patient's pain had not completely resolved. In cases of suprascapular nerve compression affecting both the supraspinatus and infraspinatus muscles, these authors advocated early intervention with arthroscopic evaluation of the glenohumeral joint, followed by open cyst excision to prevent irreversible damage. Furthermore, they stated that treatment of associated intra-articular pathology is "paramount" in eliminating both the pain and root cause (labral pathology) of the ganglion cyst.

Iannotti and Ramsey (14) were the first to report an all-arthroscopic decompression of ganglion cysts in three patients. All cysts were decompressed through the concurrent labral tear and all the three became symptom-free following surgery. Postoperative MRI did not show recurrence of the cyst in any of the cases. Several other authors (10,14,16,19,21,25,60) have since published their results of cyst decompression using arthroscopic techniques alone. Piatt (10) reported arthroscopic cyst decompression and fixation of a posterosuperior labral tear in 10 patients. All were satisfied and none had pain at rest or with activities of daily living, following the procedure. Antoniou (60) reported the results of 10 patients who underwent arthroscopic decompression of a ganglion cyst compared to seven patients who had open decompression and found no difference between the two techniques. Although a posterosuperior or posterior labral tear (fissure) was seen in all 10 arthroscopic cases, no formal repair of the labrum was done. Both interventions resulted in a significant improvement compared to nonoperative treatment.

Chen reported results from three patients treated with arthroscopic cyst excision and type II SLAP repairs associated with suprascapular neuropathy. This was the first report to document both preoperative and postoperative MRI and EMG findings. Postoperatively, patients not only had good clinical results, but also EMG studies showed recovery of the suprascapular nerve. Furthermore, postoperative MRIs confirmed cyst resolution and labral healing (19). More recently, Lichtenberg et al. (21) reported their results following an all arthroscopic technique for treating a ganglion cyst of the spinoglenoid notch in eight patients (21). Six patients had associated SLAP lesions (one type I, one type IV, and four type II) that were repaired. In the two cases without a SLAP lesion, a capsulotomy was performed. After a mean follow-up of 27 months, all patients had significant improvement in their symptoms and normal external rotation strength. EMG studies showed reversal of the neurologic lesion and MRIs revealed no recurrence of the cyst in seven of the eight patients. The one patient with recurrence (or persistence) of the cyst had no clinical evidence of nerve entrapment.

AUTHOR'S PREFERRED APPROACH

As previously mentioned, para-labral cysts fall into three presenting categories: (*i*) associated with suprascapular nerve palsy, (*ii*) painful without neurologic involvement, or (*iii*) incidental (63). Our approach aims to place the patient into one of the three arms of the following treatment algorithm, by eliciting a positive history or exam of weakness of the infraspinatus, and then confirming our clinical suspicions with EMG.

Cyst Associated with Suprascapular Nerve Palsy

In our experience, lesions of the suprascapular nerve usually produce painful atrophy of the affected muscles. However, the presenting complaint may range from difficulty in throwing or volleyball spiking (associated with overhead athletes), pain, or simply weakness. In the face of motor atrophy or an abnormal EMG, the role of nonoperative treatment is limited. Although cysts have been reported to resolve spontaneously, strong consideration for surgery is made once nerve compression has been identified (8).

Posterior Shoulder Pain without Nerve Involvement

Pain can be produced locally by the presence of the cyst without compression of the suprascapular nerve. Typically the pain is located in the posterior aspect of the shoulder and can be painful to palpation. In these cases, EMG studies can be helpful to confirm whether or not there is nerve compression. Once the isolated ganglion cyst is confirmed by MRI, a trial of observation can be undertaken. Currently, the natural history of para-labral cysts is unknown. Furthermore, there is no means of predicting which lesions may progress to compress the suprascapular nerve or which will not. If nerve compression becomes evident or the patient is unwilling to live with his or her current symptoms, surgical treatment can be entertained.

If a patient becomes asymptomatic, a discussion is needed to inform the patient of the types of symptoms that might develop if the cyst were to become problematic. If either pain or weakness develops, the patient must return for re-evaluation. Repeated evaluation of external rotation strength and the presence or absence of atrophy in 6 to 12 months might be helpful to ensure that the cyst has not started compressing the suprascapular nerve.

Incidental Finding

Cysts that are found on MRI scan, but do not correlate with the history or exam, are observed. For example, patients with typical impingement-type symptoms who respond to subacromial injection, likely have rotator cuff pathology. If an MRI of this particular patient revealed a cyst, liberal use of EMG can be helpful to confirm that no concurrent nerve compression exists. In the face of a negative EMG, the cuff-based symptoms would drive the treatment algorithm. If the patient continued to have cuff symptoms after prolonged nonoperative treatment, then athroscopic examination and decompression of the cyst can be combined with techniques to address the cuff pathology. The possibility of the cyst causing problems in the future may not constitute enough of a reason for surgery when found incidentally. However, if surgery is needed for a separate reason, little morbidity is added by addressing the cyst at the same setting.

PREOPERATIVE PLANNING

As previously written, posterior shoulder pain with external rotation weakness are red flags for a possible para-labral cyst. If no imaging studies are brought with the patient at the time of the initial visit, an MRI with intra-articular gadolinium is ordered. This has the best ability to show a labral lesion and to demonstrate the size and location of a para-labral cyst. If the patient presents with a noncontrast MRI that demonstrates a cyst but no labral lesion, the study is not repeated.

Preoperatively, the MRI can be used to determine the center of the cyst, which can help focus dissection during decompression. Another essential preoperative test is the EMG. The degree of denervation already present can be documented, and the results are used as a baseline for future comparative studies following surgery.

TECHNIQUE

The type of anesthesia is at the anesthesiologist's and patient's discretion and may consist of either a general or regional (interscalene block) anesthetic alone or a combination of a general and a regional anesthetic. The patient is positioned in the beach-chair position with their back 10° to 20° from vertical. After sterile prep and drape, the bony anatomy is palpated and drawn onto the skin. A standard posterior portal is made into the glenohumeral joint. The camera is inserted and the joint lavaged. A standard diagnostic arthroscopy is performed with special attention drawn to the following structures: biceps tendon, rotator cuff, articular surfaces, posterior labrum, anterior labrum, and axillary recess.

Next, an anterior portal is established in the rotator interval using needle localization. A probe is inserted and the superior labrum, biceps, and anterior labrum are examined. The camera may be switched to the anterior portal to aid in diagnosing posterior labral pathology or anterior capsular pathology. Once the extent of the concurrent pathology is established, the para-labral cyst is decompressed first. Repair of any concurrent pathology follows the cyst decompression.

Cyst decompression begins with placing the viewing camera through the posterior portal. Next, an electrocautery device is placed through the anterior portal. Starting just posterior to the biceps tendon, the superior and posterior capsules are released as far around the back as possible (Fig. 1). Keys to this release are as follows: (*i*) stay close to the labrum to help prevent injury to the rotator cuff and (*ii*) try to open a rather generous portion of the capsule to facilitate cyst decompression. Even in the presence of a concurrent type II SLAP tear, adequate visualization and decompression of the cyst can be difficult when working between the glenoid edge and the detached labrum.

After the capsular opening is created, the arthroscope is placed in the anterior portal. A posterolateral portal is created using an 18-gage spinal needle to locate the ideal position for an accessory viewing portal. It is essential that the needle easily reach the labrum just posterior to the biceps anchor. Typically, this accessory portal is located lateral to the posterior acromion. A skin incision is made and the arthroscopic canula is placed into the joint with the aid of a switching stick. The camera is then placed into the newly established portal (Fig. 2).

The arthroscope is passed through the posterosuperior glenohumeral capsulotomy previously created to visualize the posterior and posterosuperior portion of the scapula. It is important to remember that the suprascapular nerve lies deep (ventral) to the deep wall of the cyst. The superficial soft-tissues on the posterior surface of the scapula are carefully dissected and cleared, using a combination of instruments through either the previously placed anterior portal or a separate anterolateral portal. First, a blunt instrument, such as the blunt obturator from the arthroscope, can be used for the initial dissection. Next, a combination of an arthroscopic shaver and judiciously used electrocautery can be used. With careful dissection, the cyst will be visualized as a bluish structure protruding from the deep soft-tissues (Fig. 3). In most cases, the scapular spine can also be visualized or palpated. This, along with intraoperative reference to the MRI will help confirm the cyst location. The superficial wall is then punctured using the arthroscopic shaver and intermittent suction. The interior of the cyst cavity is then visualized and can be evacuated using the suction on the arthroscopic shaver (Fig. 4). Care should be taken to avoid penetrating the deep wall of the cyst with the shaver, as the nerve is adjacent to the deep wall of the cyst. After cyst decompression, any concurrent pathology, including SLAP tears, are addressed according to surgeon preference.

POSTOPERATIVE MANAGEMENT

The arthroscopic procedure described earlier is performed on an outpatient basis. The use of regional anesthesia may aid greatly in the postoperative pain management. The patients are placed into a sling immediately following surgery. The sling is removed only for showers, dressing, and pendulum exercises during the first week. Patients return to the office 7 to 10 days later for removal of sutures. At this time, patients are allowed to be out of the sling while at home, but remain in the sling while out of the house. If no labral repair was performed, passive forward flexion and external rotation exercises of the arm are added to the pendulum exercises, and the patients are encouraged to use their arm for all daily activities within their limits of pain. If a labral tear was repaired, passive exercises are maintained for six weeks to prevent stiffness, and active exercises are added at that time.

At six weeks, strengthening of the rotator cuff, deltoid, and scapular muscles may begin, and the sling is removed full-time. By 10 weeks, progress in the patient's external rotation strength should be seen. If progress is sluggish, a new EMG is ordered (hopefully performed by the original doctor). Atrophy of the muscle typically lags behind functional recovery. Therefore, visual inspection of the muscles is not very helpful when evaluating the patient in the early postoperative period.

If there has been no labral repair, soft tossing for throwers begins at four months, with a gradual increase in number and distance of throws over the next month. Hard throwing is allowed at five months and return to competitive pitching at six months. If the labrum was repaired, soft tossing is started at six months, with an anticipated return to full throwing activities at 9 to 12 months.

POSSIBLE CONCERNS AND FUTURE OF THE TECHNIQUE

Although no significant complications have been reported with all-arthroscopic cyst decompression, several potential problems may develop with its use. The first is failure to decompress the cyst. Several small series have shown that the cyst is decompressed on postoperative MRI or ultrasound (19). However, recurrences have been reported (8).

To ensure successful para-labral cyst decompression, certain steps during the procedure must be taken. First, care must be taken to establish both the posterolateral and anterolateral (if needed) portals in the proper locations. If the instruments are not able to reach the location of the cyst, then adequate decompression is impossible.

Second, one must thoroughly evaluate the preoperative MRI to establish the location of the cyst and direct instrument placement. Postoperatively, if any question arises as to success of the cyst decompression during surgery, another ultrasound or MRI can locate a residual fluid collection that may be amenable to drainage. Since the intra-articular pathology should at this point be addressed, percutaneous drainage is probably an acceptable treatment.

Third, one must be keenly aware of iatrogenic injury to the suprascapular nerve during arthroscopic decompression. Four technical points may be helpful to decrease the risk for neurologic injury: (*i*) avoid electrocautery more than 1.5 cm medial to the edge of the glenoid, (*ii*) limit the amount of suction that is used with the shaver more than 1.5 cm medial to the glenoid, (*iii*) using blunt dissection under the rotator cuff will allow for a more limited use of the shaver, and (*iv*) stop any shaving and dissection before penetrating the deep or medial wall of the cyst.

CONCLUSION

Symptomatic para-labral cysts are continually being recognized, as a condition treatable by arthroscopy. This surgical technique is increasingly acknowledged as advantageous to open decompression, due to its ability to address both the intra-articular and extra-articular pathology with minimal tissue disruption. Advances in arthroscopy will only help to improve the surgical treatment of para-labral cysts. The number of arthroscopic cyst decompressions may increase as this clinical diagnosis is on the rise with the increased use of MRI.

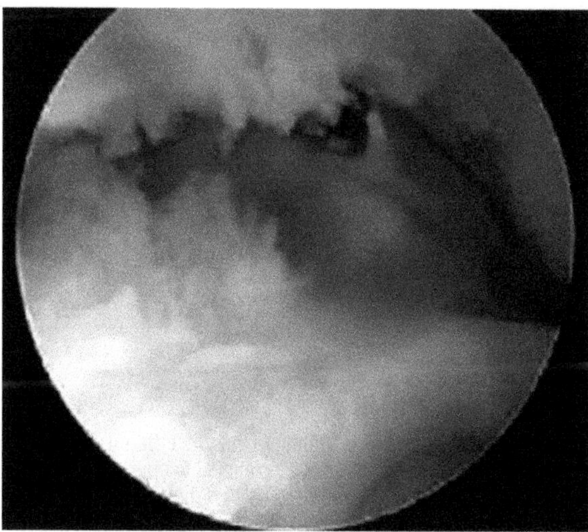

FIGURE 1 The image demonstrates a posterosuperior capsulotomy, as viewed from a standard posterior portal in a right shoulder. Supraspinatus muscle fibers can be visualized through the capsulotomy. *Source*: From Ref. 63.

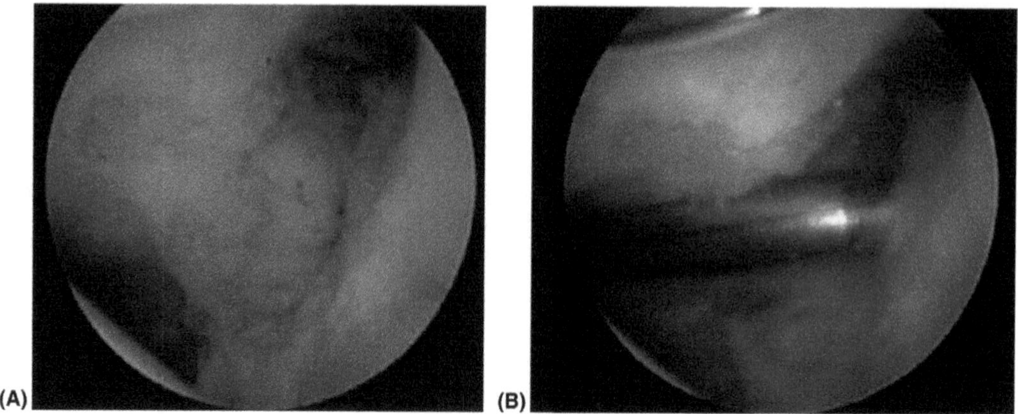

FIGURE 2 (**A**) The arthroscope has been moved to the anterior portal to visualize the posterosuperior capsulotomy. A posterolateral portal is then created, after localization with a spinal needle that passes easily through the capsulotomy. (**B**) A switching stick is placed through the posterolateral portal into the capsulotomy. The arthroscopic canula is then passed over the switching stick. *Source*: From Ref. 63.

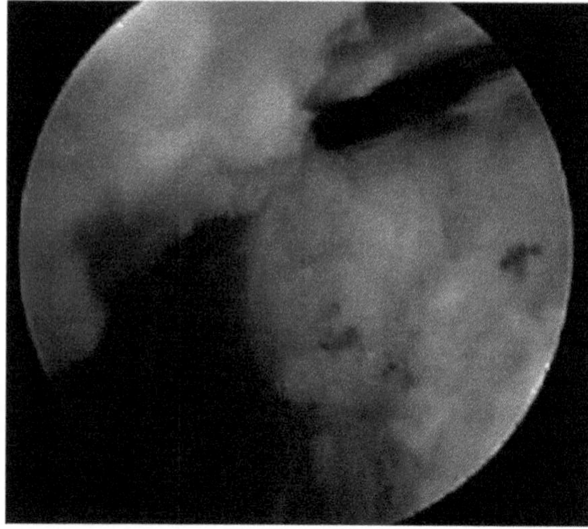

FIGURE 3 After blunt dissection, the cyst can be visualized as a bluish structure within the yellow fat and connective tissue. *Source*: From Ref. 63.

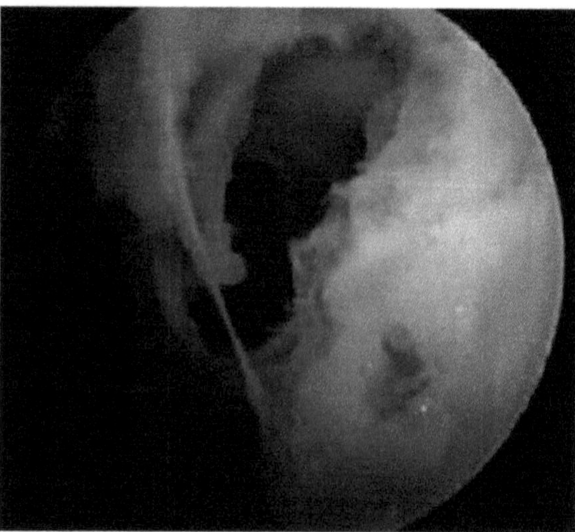

FIGURE 4 The cyst cavity is entered by resecting the superficial cyst wall, usually with a shaver. The contents can then be suctioned out. *Source*: From Ref. 63.

REFERENCES

1. Kopell HP, Thompson W. Pain and the frozen shoulder. Surg Gynecol Obstet 1959; 109:92–96.
2. Clein L. Suprascapular entrapment neuropathy. J Neurosurg 1975; 43(3):337–342.
3. Hirayama T, Takemitsu Y. Compression of the suprascapular nerve by a ganglion at the suprascapular notch. Clin Orthop Relat Res 1981; 155:95–96.
4. Aiello I, Serra G, Traina GC, et al. Entrapment of the suprascapular nerve at the spinoglenoid notch. Ann Neurol 1982; 12(3):314–316.
5. Ogino T, Minami A, Kato H, et al. Entrapment neuropathy of the suprascapular nerve by a ganglion. A report of three cases. J Bone Joint Surg Am 1991; 73(1):141–147.
6. Tirman PF, Feller J, Janzen DL, et al. Association of glenoid labral cysts with labral tears and glenohumeral instability: Radiologic findings and clinical significance. Radiology 1994; 190(3):653–658.
7. Fehrman DA, Orwin JF, Jennings R. Suprascapular nerve entrapment by ganglion cysts: a report of six cases with arthroscopic findings and review of the literature. Arthroscopy 1995; 11(6):727–734.
8. Moore TP, Fritts HM, Quick DC, et al. Suprascapular nerve entrapment caused by supraglenoid cyst compression. J Shoulder Elbow Surg 1997; 6(5):455–462.
9. Tung GA, Entzian D, Stern JB, et al. MR imaging and MR arthrography of paraglenoid labral cysts. AJR 2000; 175:1707–1715.
10. Piatt BE, Hawkins RJ, Fritz RC, et al. Clinical evaluation and treatment of spinoglenoid notch ganglion cysts. J Shoulder Elbow Surg 2002; 11(6):600–604.
11. Steinwachs MR, Haag M, Krug C, et al. A ganglion of the spinoglenoid notch. J Shoulder Elbow Surg 1988; 7(5):550–554.
12. Fritz R, Helms C, Steinbach L, et al. Suprascapular nerve entrapment: evaluation with MR imaging. Radiology 1992; 182:437–444.
13. Skirving AP, Kozak TK, Davis S. Infraspinatus paralysis due to spinoglenoid notch ganglion. J Bone Joint Surg Br 1994; 76(4):588–591.
14. Iannotti JP, Ramsey M. Arthroscopic decompression of a ganglion cyst causing suprascapular nerve compression. Arthroscopy 1996; 12(6):739–745.
15. Sjoden GO, Movin T, Guntner P, et al. Spinoglenoid bone cyst causing suprascapular nerve compression. J Shoulder Elbow Surg 1996; 5(2):147–149.
16. Romeo AA, Rotenberg DD, Bach JB. Suprascapular neuropathy. J Am Acad Orthop Surg 1999; 7(6):358–367.
17. Sheets J, Ford K. Aunt Minnie's Corner. Superior labral tear with associated paralabral cyst in the spinoglenoid notch, and infraspinatus denervation myositis. J Comput Assist Tomogr 1999; 23(1):167.
18. Van Zandijcke M, Casselman J. Suprascapular nerve entrapment at the spinoglenoid notch due to a ganglion cyst. J Neurol Neurosurg Psychiatry 1999; 66(2):245.
19. Chen AL, Ong BC, Rose D. Arthroscopic management of spinoglenoid cysts associated with SLAP lesions and suprascapular neuropathy. Arthroscopy 2003; 19(6):E15–E21.
20. Westerheide KJ, Karzel R. Ganglion cysts of the shoulder: technique of arthroscopic decompression and fixation of associated type II superior labral anterior to posterior lesions. Orthop Clin North Am 2003; 34(4):521–528.
21. Lichtenberg S, Magosch P, Habermeyer P. Compression of the suprascapular nerve by a ganglion cyst of the spinoglenoid notch: the arthroscopic solution. Knee Surg Sports Traumatol Arthrosc 2004; 12(1):72–79.
22. Bouzaidi K, Ravard-Marsot C, Debroucker F, et al. Ganglion cyst at the spinoglenoid notch. A case report and literature review. Rev Med Interne 2005; 26(4):335–338.
23. Neviaser TJ, Ain BR, Neviaser R. Suprascapular nerve denervation secondary to attenuation by a ganglionic cyst. J Bone Joint Surg Am 1986; 68(4):627–629.
24. Lantz B, Singer K. Meniscal cysts. Clin Sports Med 1990; 9(3):707–725.
25. Chochole MH, Senker W, Meznik C, et al. Glenoid-labral cyst entrapping the suprascapular nerve: dissolution after arthroscopic debridement of an extended SLAP lesion. Arthroscopy 1997; 13(3):753–755.
26. Ferrick MR, Marzo J. Ganglion cyst of the shoulder associated with a glenoid labral tear and symptomatic glenohumeral instability. A case report. Am J Sports Med 1997; 25(5):717–719.
27. Lee HY, Chung IH, Sir WS, et al. Variations of the ventral rami of the brachial plexus. J Korean Med Sci 1992; 7(1):19–24.
28. Bigliani LU, Dalsey RM, McCann PD, et al. An anatomical study of the suprascapular nerve. Arthroscopy 1990; 6(4):301–305.
29. Warner JP, Krushell RJ, Masquelet A, et al. Anatomy and relationships of the suprascapular nerve: anatomical constraints to mobilization of the supraspinatus and infraspinatus muscles in the management of massive rotator-cuff tears. J Bone Joint Surg Am 1992; 74(1):36–45.

30. Horiguchi M. The cutaneous branch of some human suprascapular nerves. J Anat 1980; 130(1):191–195.
31. Mestdagh H, Drizenko A, Ghestem P. Anatomical basis of suprascapular nerve syndrome. Anat Clin 1981; 3:67–71.
32. Ajmani M. The cutaneous branch of the human suprascapular nerve. J Anat 1994; 185(2): 439–442.
33. Rengachary SS, Burr D, Lucas S, et al. Suprascapular entrapment neuropathy: a clinical, anatomical, and comparative study. Part 2: anatomical study. Neurosurgery 1979; 5(4):447–451.
34. Ticker JB, Djurasovic M, Strauch RJ, et al. The incidence of ganglion cysts and other variations in anatomy along the course of the suprascapular nerve. J Shoulder Elbow Surg 1998; 7(5):472–478.
35. Alon M, Weiss S, Fishel B, et al. Bilateral suprascapular nerve entrapment syndrome due to an anomalous transverse scapular ligament. Clin Orthop Relat Res 1988; 234:31–33.
36. Kaspi A, Yanai J, Pick CG, et al. Entrapment of the distal suprascapular nerve. An anatomical study. Int Orthop 1988; 12(4):273–275.
37. Cummins CA, Anderson K, Bowen M, et al. Anatomy and histological characteristics of the spinoglenoid ligament. J Bone Joint Surg Am 1998; 80(11):1622–1625.
38. Demirhan M, Imhoff AB, Debski RE, et al. The spinoglenoid ligament and its relationship to the suprascapular nerve. J Shoulder Elbow Surg 1998; 7(3):238–243.
39. Plancher KD, Peterson RK, Johnston JC, et al. The spinoglenoid ligament. Anatomy, morphology, and histological findings. J Bone Joint Surg Am 2005; 87(2):361–365.
40. Zeiss J, Woldenberg LS, Saddemi SR, et al. MRI of suprascapular neuropathy in a weight lifter. J Comput Assist Tomogr 1993; 17(2):303–308.
41. Antoniadis G, Richter HP, Rath S, et al. Suprascapular nerve entrapment: experience with 28 cases. J Neurosurg 1996; 85(6):1020–1025.
42. Martin SD, Warren RF, Martin TL, et al. Suprascapular neuropathy. Results of non-operative treatment. J Bone Joint Surg Am 1997; 79(8):1159–1165.
43. Ferretti A, De Carli A, Fontana M. Injury of the suprascapular nerve at the spinoglenoid notch. The natural history of infraspinatus atrophy in volleyball players. Am J Sports Med 1998; 26(6):759–763.
44. Cummins CA, Bowen M, Anderson K, et al. Suprascapular nerve entrapment at the spinoglenoid notch in a professional baseball pitcher. Am J Sports Med 1999; 27(6):810–812.
45. Dramis A, Pimpalnerkar A. Suprascapular neuropathy in volleyball players. Acta Orthop Belg 2005; 71(3):269–272.
46. Kim DH, Murovic JA, Tiel RL, et al. Management and outcomes of 42 surgical suprascapular nerve injuries and entrapments. Neurosurgery 2005; 57(1):120–127.
47. Ferretti A, Cerullo G, Russo G. Suprascapular neuropathy in volleyball players. J Bone Joint Surg Am 1987; 69(2):260–263.
48. Murray J. A surgical apprach for entrapment neuropathy. Orthop Rev 1974; 3:33–35.
49. Post M, Mayer J. Suprascapular nerve entrapment. Diagnosis and treatment. Clin Orthop Relat Res 1987; 223:126–136.
50. Goss TP, Aronow MS, Coumas J. The use of MRI to diagnose suprascapular nerve entrapment caused by a ganglion. Orthopedics 1994; 17(4):359–362.
51. Inokuchi W, Ogawa K, Horiuchi Y. Magnetic resonance imaging of suprascapular nerve palsy. J Shoulder Elbow Surg 1998; 7(3):223–227.
52. Leitschuh PH, Bone CM, Bouska W. Magnetic resonance imaging diagnosis, sonographically directed percutaneous aspiration, and arthroscopic treatment of a painful shoulder ganglion cyst associated with a SLAP lesion. Arthroscopy 1999; 15(1):85–87.
53. Fleckenstein JL, Watumull D, Conner KE, et al. Denervated human skeletal muscle: MR imaging evaluation. Radiology 1993; 187(1):213–218.
54. Uetani M, Hayashi K, Matsunaga N, et al. Denervated skeletal muscle: MR imaging. Work in progress. Radiology 1993; 189(2):511–515.
55. McDonald CM, Carter GT, Fritz RC, et al. Magnetic resonance imaging of denervated muscle: comparison to electromyography. Muscle Nerve 2000; 23(9):1431–1434.
56. Legan JM, Burkhard TK, Goff WB II, et al. Tears of the glenoid labrum: MR imaging of 88 arthroscopically confirmed cases. Radiology 1991; 179(1):241–246.
57. McCauley TR, Pope CF, Jokl P. Normal and abnormal glenoid labrum: assessment with multiplanar gradient-echo MR imaging. Radiology 1992; 183(1):35–37.
58. Jee WH, McCauley TR, Katz LD, et al. Superior labral anterior posterior (SLAP) lesions of the glenoid labrum: reliability and accuracy of MR arthrography for diagnosis. Radiology 2001; 218(1):127–132.
59. Chandnani VP, Yeager TD, DeBerardino T, et al. Glenoid labral tears: prospective evaluation with MRI imaging, MR arthrography, and CT arthrography. AJR Am J Roentgenol 1993; 161(6):1229–1235.

60. Antoniou J, Tae SK, Williams GR, et al. Suprascapular neuropathy. Variability in the diagnosis, treatment, and outcome. Clin Orthop Relat Res 2001; 386:131–138.
61. McCluskey L, Feinberg D, Dolinskas C. Suprascapular neuropathy related to a glenohumeral joint cyst. Muscle Nerve 1999; 22(6):772–777.
62. Hashimoto BE, Hayes AS, Ager J. Sonographic diagnosis and treatment of ganglion cysts causing suprascapular nerve entrapment. J Ultrasound Med 1994; 13(9):671–674.
63. Getz CL, Ramsey ML, Glaser D, et al. Arthroscopic decompression of spinoglenoid cysts. Tech Shoulder Elbow Surg 2005; 6(1):36–42.

17 Arthroscopic Treatment of Inflammatory Synovitis and Related Tumor Conditions

Adam M. Smith
Kentucky Sports Medicine Clinic, Lexington, Kentucky, U.S.A.

John W. Sperling
Department of Orthopedics, Mayo Clinic, Rochester, Minnesota, U.S.A.

INDICATIONS

In recent times, there is little information in the literature to guide surgical treatment of the shoulder in patients with inflammatory arthritis. The spectrum of pathology is broad ranging from occasional mild synovitis that is well controlled by oral medications to severe shoulder dysfunction with bone deficiency. This wide range of pathology creates difficulty in assessing the effectiveness of surgical intervention. Although many disease processes cause synovitis of the shoulder, the most commonly encountered stem is from rheumatoid arthritis and will be the focus of this chapter.

Only recently has the role of arthroscopic treatment been explored for the treatment of these disorders. Furthermore, although surgical intervention may be indicated in patients with shoulder synovitis, patients are best managed with a team approach with a consulting rheumatologist. Every attempt should be made to maximize medical management, oral medications, and injection therapy in order to avoid operative intervention in this patient population, which may be predisposed to infection and frequently have associated medical comorbidities. With this in mind, arthroscopic treatment of shoulder synovitis offers a minimally invasive approach to a problem that can be debilitating.

The pathophysiology of inflammatory arthritis is thought to be due to a combination of genetic and environmental factors in its etiology (1). Current research in rheumatoid arthritis is centered on interactions of the immune system with antigen presentation to macrophages by T-helper or inducer cells. Complexes of immunoglobins are thought to deposit in blood vessels, leading to vasculitis. In addition to its systemic effects, this vasculitic process leads to cellular infiltration of the synovium causing a reactive effusion. The immune-mediated response leads to destruction of tendon, ligament, and cartilage structures.

Patients with shoulder synovitis usually have a known diagnosis of inflammatory arthritis, rarely presenting with shoulder pain as the initial complaint. Frequently, patients are seen in referral for shoulder pain that has been resistant to nonoperative interventions, including changes in oral medications, and failed trials of therapy. Patients often complain of pain (at rest, at night, and with activities), loss of strength, and motion.

Physical examination demonstrates shoulder swelling with effusion in the subacromial and/or subdeltoid space. There may be a significant crepitance with gentle motion. Limitations in all planes of active and passive motion, including elevation, external, and internal rotations, are common due to underlying arthrofibrosis. Motion may be painful, which may lead to deficits in strength despite structurally intact rotator cuff tendons. Careful examination of the acromioclavicular joint and biceps tendon with provocative maneuvers should be performed to assess for pathology.

Radiographs of the affected shoulder are helpful to assess the underlying arthritic changes of the glenohumeral and acromioclavicular joints (2,3). Advanced imaging with magnetic resonance imaging (MRI) can be helpful for assessment of the underlying soft

---

Please refer to pages 185–186 for the figures in this chapter.

tissue changes such as rotator cuff and biceps tendon abnormalities. Patients with underlying synovitis frequently demonstrate thinning or full-thickness tearing of the rotator cuff tendons and inflammation, fraying, or tearing of the biceps tendon. MRI can also demonstrate the extent of the intra-articular synovitis and subacromial bursitis. Radiographs of the cervical spine, including flexion and extension views, should be obtained to assess for cervical subluxation (4).

SURGICAL TREATMENT

Synovectomy

Synovectomy of the shoulder has been used with limited success in patients with rheumatoid arthritis (5–13). Although most of these studies report good pain relief, concerns exist regarding the efficacy and long-term results of synovectomy in the rheumatoid population, especially when glenohumeral changes are present on radiographs. Furthermore, there is minimal information regarding the efficacy of arthroscopic treatment.

Multiple problems may coexist in the rheumatoid shoulder. Rotator cuff abnormalities have been reported to range from 25% to 80% in patients undergoing other reconstructive procedures (6,14–18), which can make interpreting the success of synovectomy difficult (9). Patients may demonstrate underlying shoulder pathology including limited range of motion (19–21) and radiographic changes including osteopenia, proximal humeral migration, and glenohumeral and acromioclavicular erosions (11,12,18,22,23).

Pahle (9,10) published the largest series of patients (54 shoulders) undergoing open surgical synovectomy, noting good pain relief even in advanced cases of arthritis with increased abduction and external rotation. He did caution, however, that radiographs continued to show advancing disease. Petersson (11) noted similar findings with pain relief and functional gains, with two patients requiring later shoulder arthroplasty. However, both of these studies included patients with rotator cuff tearing limiting the interpretation of outcome in the assessment of isolated shoulder synovectomy.

One study from the Mayo clinic examined 16 shoulders in 13 patients with rheumatoid arthritis, with an intact rotator cuff (24). At average follow-up of 5.5 years, 13 of the 16 shoulders had improved pain. Thirteen of the 16 shoulders had at least satisfactory results (14). Patient satisfaction was high with all but one patient (who required revision surgery with arthroplasty) having a higher level of satisfaction with their shoulder than before surgery. These results were similar to the findings of Pahle (9,10) and Petersson (11,12), in their use of open shoulder synovectomy .

Biceps Tendon

Biceps tendon pathology is common in patients with inflammatory synovitis. MRI may demonstrate inflammation of the biceps tendon sheath. Fraying and frank tearing of the biceps may also be visualized. When biceps tendon pathology is noted, particularly with subluxation, the subscapularis should be closely inspected for tearing from the lesser tuberosity insertion. Treatment of the biceps tendon is controversial. Biceps tendon debridement, tenodesis, and tenotomy are all reasonable options than can be performed arthroscopically with reported excellent results.

Rotator Cuff Pathology

Patients with inflammatory synovitis frequently have inflammation and thickening of the subacromial bursa, which can be tenacious. While excision of the pathologic bursa may be indicated, many authors have cautioned against the sacrifice of the coracoacromial ligament, thus disrupting the coracoacromial arch. Concerns remain about progression of inflammatory disease, increasing rotator cuff deficiency, and the development of severe upward and forward humeral subluxation (8,25). The authors do not routinely divide the coracoacromial ligament or perform acromioplasty in this patient population unless impingement or wear is directly visualized on the rotator cuff tendons.

Rotator cuff tearing is frequently associated with inflammatory arthritis of the shoulder. Although the true incidence of symptomatic tearing is not known in the rheumatoid population, during procedures such as arthroplasty and synovectomy, the rotator cuff has been described as being abnormal in 25% to 80% of shoulders (6,14–18). Decision making in this population can be difficult, as the results of treatment have been less than predictable. Repair of rotator cuff tears in patients with rheumatoid arthritis (RA) can be technically challenging due to the size of tears and adjacent tendon attrition, which makes predicting outcomes of treatment difficult (26).

Although repair of the rotator cuff may be desirable, individual patient factors such as functional demands and poor health status, along with the known risks associated with rheumatoid disease, such as increased risk of infection (27,28), and associated systemic comorbidities may discourage more complex reparative interventions. Although the results of rotator cuff repair have been well documented for the general population, the results of rotator cuff repair in patients with rheumatoid arthritis, until recently, had not been discussed.

In a study from the Mayo clinic, 23 shoulders in 21 patients were identified who underwent open repair of the rotator cuff and were followed at a median of 9.7 years (26). Nine shoulders had partial thickness tears, and 14 had full-thickness tears (nine medium, four large, and one massive) that required repair with an open procedure. Patients with partial and full thickness tears had significantly improved pain and were mostly satisfied with the procedure. Functional gains were less predictable for motion and strength. Of the nine shoulders with partial thickness tears, two had unsatisfactory results. Six of the 14 shoulders with full-thickness tears had unsatisfactory results.

Less complex procedures such as debridement for rotator cuff tears have been investigated in the general population (29–32). However, the success of rotator cuff debridement in patients with inflammatory arthritis has not, until recently, been investigated. In a study from the Mayo clinic, 16 shoulders underwent arthroscopic debridement of a rotator cuff tear, of which six were partial thickness and ten were full thickness tears (33). Five of the six patients with partial tears had improved pain at a median follow-up of 6.8 years. Only five of the 10 patients with full thickness tears had improved pain at a median of 5.2 years. Motion and strength did not improve in either group. The six shoulders with partial thickness tears had two excellent, three satisfactory, and one unsatisfactory result. Of the ten shoulders with full thickness tears none had an excellent, two had satisfactory, and eight had unsatisfactory results. Night pain was not reliably relieved in shoulders with partial or full thickness tears. Patients and surgeons should be aware of these limited, expected outcomes in patients who are deemed to be candidates for rotator cuff debridement.

Acromioclavicular arthritis is routinely encountered in patients with inflammatory arthritis. Radiographic changes and MRI findings can be noted, which are significant. However, surgical intervention is warranted only for patients with symptoms directly referable to the acromioclavicular joint. Patients with a symptomatic acromioclavicular (AC) joint and physical examination findings, consistent with pain to direct palpation or pain with crossed-body adduction, should be considered candidates for resection of the distal clavicle. In the 16 patients treated with arthroscopic synovectomy of the shoulder from Mayo clinic, only one required treatment with distal clavicle excision (24).

SYNOVIAL CHONDROMATOSIS

Synovial chondromatosis is a benign disorder of synovial joints, tendon sheaths, and bursae. The disease process affects large joints, most commonly the knee, hip, elbow, and shoulder. Histologically, synovial cells undergo metaplasia to chondrocytes, which produce cartilage nodules that may also be centrally ossified. Symptoms are similar to inflammatory arthritis and include pain, limited motion, intermittent locking, and crepitation. Radiographs may show impressive loose bodies as shown in Figure 1. MRI is often diagnostic if X rays are negative. The goal of the treatment is removal of loose bodies and synovectomy. Synovectomy may reduce the incidence of recurrence.

OPERATIVE TECHNIQUE

Patients can be positioned in the beach chair or lateral position with the affected shoulder widely prepped. Standard arthroscopic portals should be used to gain access to the shoulder and subacromial space. Debridement of the glenohumeral joint and hypertrophic synovial

(Fig. 2) tissue is usually carried out using an oscillating shaver and a cautery/ablation device. Attempts should be made to perform a complete synovectomy of all pathologic appearing tissues. Intra-articular bleeding can be encountered that makes adequate visualization difficult to achieve. Preoperative discussion with the anesthesiologist is important to emphasize the importance of a hypotensive approach throughout the entirety of the case. Meticulous hemostasis is necessary intraoperatively to facilitate adequate viewing, and hemostasis should be achieved prior to termination of the procedure to avoid a significant hematoma. Caution should be used with the use of cautery or ablation techniques in the inferior capsular recess regions, as injury to the axillary nerve has been reported with other procedures (34).

Arthroscopic treatment of synovial chondromatosis is similar to inflammatory arthritis. Standard portals are created, and loose bodies, as they are encountered, are removed (Figs. 3 and 4). Larger bodies may need to be debrided prior to removal and a large-sized cannula facilitate removal. Thorough evaluation of the glenohumeral joint requires inspection of the subscapularis recess and the biceps tendon sheath. They may require 70° arthroscope and changing the camera to the anterior portal. Figure 5 demonstrates loose bodies removed, and Figure 6 shows the postoperative X ray.

PEARLS AND PITFALLS

Communication with the patient's rheumatologist is necessary to insure that medical treatment has been maximized. Although arthroscopic synovectomy may achieve improvement of symptoms initially, it does not seem to prevent progression of the radiographic changes in the rheumatoid shoulder (35). Kelly (8) recommended that synovectomy must be done before significant damage to articular cartilage occurs. In a study by Wakitani et al. (36), patients with a broad spectrum of radiographic changes were examined, and the authors concluded that patients with severe arthritis had less favorable results with synovectomy compared to those undergoing prosthetic arthroplasty procedures.

Results presented from the Mayo clinic (24) that used an arthroscopic approach are similar to the findings of studies examining an open approach with radiographs, demonstrating progression of arthritis in 88% (7/8) of patients. Although synovectomy would be ideally performed in rheumatoid patients with normal shoulder articular contour, durable pain relief can be achieved despite moderately advanced radiographic changes. All three of the 16 patients with unsatisfactory results had pain that was no better or worse than before surgery and had radiographic arthrosis at last follow-up with advancing periarticular erosions and reduction of glenoid articular space. In patients with rotator cuff tearing, repair of the tear is preferred when possible. Debridement, in our hands, is best reserved for patients with irreparable tears or in patients unable to tolerate the immobilization required for a repair. In the patients with moderate to severe arthritic changes treated at the Mayo clinic, patients were able to be treated successfully with arthroscopic intervention, but the results seemed to be less predictable than in patients with minimal arthritic changes. Although arthroscopic treatment is an excellent option in the appropriately chosen patient, arthroplasty is the most well-understood treatment option with long-term, predictable results in the rheumatoid population (14,16).

REHABILITATION

Postoperative management is dependent upon the additional procedures performed at intervention. Patients undergoing only debridement and synovectomy can be safely managed with a sling for comfort. Rehabilitation can began on the first postoperative day with active-assisted motion and progressed as tolerated. However, postoperative management of patients undergoing reparative procedures such as rotator cuff repair is more controversial. Currently, the authors follow a closely monitored program of therapy with passive motion only until tendon healing can occur.

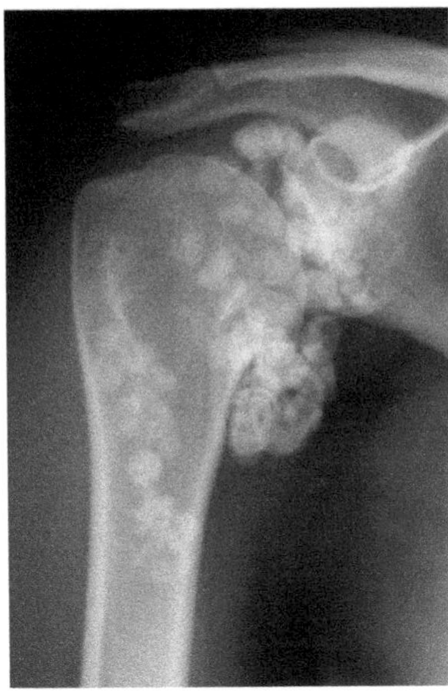

FIGURE 1 Preoperative anterior-posterior (AP) X-ray demonstrating large number of loose bodies typical of synovial chondromatosis.

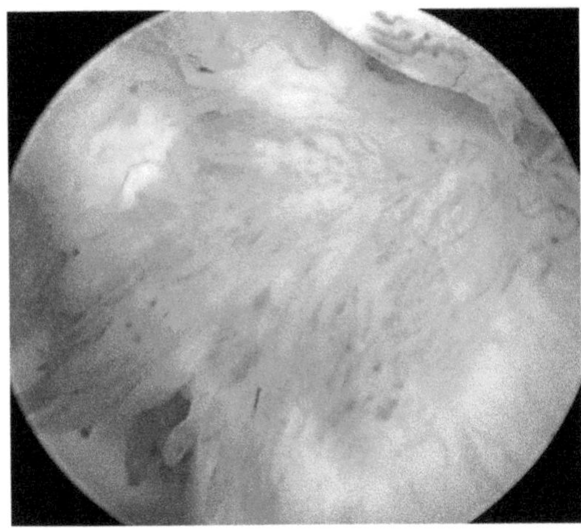

FIGURE 2 This figure demonstrates the typical arthroscopic appearance of inflamed synovium in the shoulder. The frond-like, injected tissue in this figure lies on the subscapularis tendon.

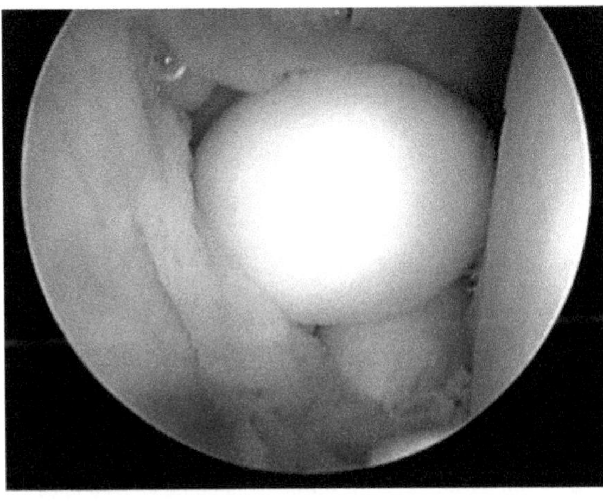

FIGURE 3 Arthroscopic view of loose bodies.

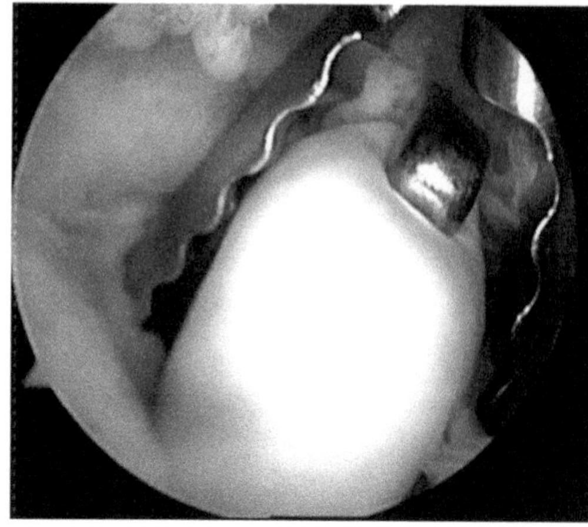

FIGURE 4 Grasper used to remove loose body.

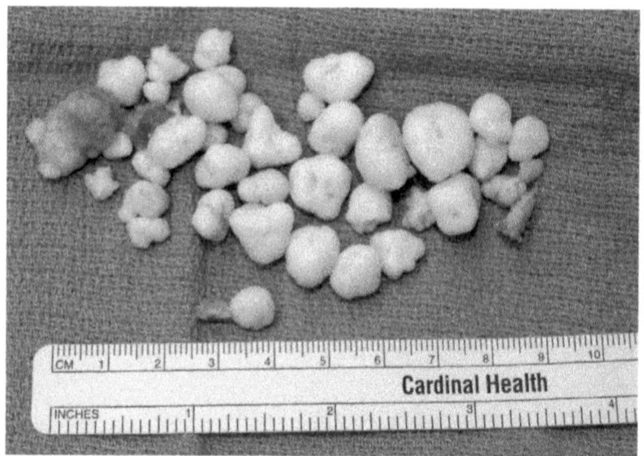

FIGURE 5 Loose bodies obtained arthro-scopically.

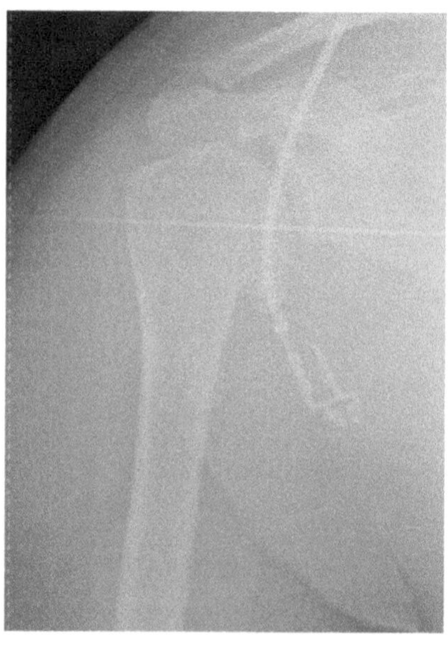

FIGURE 6 Postoperative AP X-ray demonstrating loose bodies removed.

REFERENCES

1. Goronzy JJ, Weyand CM. Rheumatoid arthritis: epidemiology, pathology, and pathogenesis. In: Klippel JH, ed. Primer on the Rheumatic Diseases. 12th ed. Atlanta: Arthritis Foundation, 2001:209–217.
2. Crossan JF, Vallance R. The shoulder joint in rheumatoid arthritis. In: Bayley I, Keddel L, eds. Shoulder Surgery. New York: Springer-Verlag, 1982:131–139.
3. Crossan JF, Vallance R. Clinical and radiological features of the shoulder joint in rheumatoid arthritis. J Bone Joint Surg 1980; 62B:116.
4. Neva MH, Hakkinen A, Makinen H, Hannonen P, Kauppi M, Sokka T. High prevalence of asymptomatic cervical spine subluxations in patients with rheumatoid arthritis waiting for orthopaedic surgery. Ann Rheum Dis 2006; 65:884–888.
5. Bennett WF, Gerber C. Operative treatment of the rheumatoid shoulder. Curr Opin Rheumatol 1994; 6:177–182.
6. Clayton ML, Ferlic DC. Surgery of the shoulder in rheumatoid arthritis: a report of nineteen patients. Clin Orthop 1975; 106:166–174.
7. Cuomo F, Greller MJ, Zuckerman JD. The rheumatoid shoulder. Rheum Dis Clin North Am 1998; 24:67–82.
8. Kelly IG. Surgery of the rheumatoid shoulder. Ann Rheum Dis 1990; 49(suppl 2):824–829.
9. Pahle JA, Kvarnes L. Shoulder synovectomy. Ann Chir Gynaecol Suppl 1985; 198:37–49.
10. Pahle JA. The shoulder joint in rheumatoid arthritis: synovectomy. Reconstr Surg Traumatol 1981; 18:33–47.
11. Petersson CJ. Shoulder surgery in rheumatoid arthritis. Acta Orthop Scand 1986; 57:222–226.
12. Petersson CJ. The acromioclavicular joint in rheumatoid arthritis. Clin Orthop 1987; 223:86–93.
13. Smith-Peterson MN, Aufranc OE, Larson CB. Useful surgical procedures for rheumatoid arthritis involving the upper extremity. Arch Surg 1943; 46:764–770.
14. Cofield RH. Total shoulder arthroplasty with Neer prosthesis. J Bone Joint Surg 1984; 66A:899–906.
15. Ennevarra K. Painful shoulder joint in rheumatoid arthritis: a clinical and radiologic study of 200 cases with special reference to arthrography of the glenohumeral joint. Acta Rheum Scand 1967; (suppl 11):1–108.
16. Kelly IG, Foster RS, Fisher WD. Neer total shoulder replacement in rheumatoid arthritis. J Bone Joint Surg 1987; 69B:723–726.
17. Rozing PM, Brand R. Rotator cuff repair during shoulder arthroplasty in rheumatoid arthritis. J Arthroplasty 1998; 13:311–319.
18. Weiss JJ, Thompson GR, Doust V, Burgener F. Rotator cuff tears in rheumatoid arthritis. Arch Intern Med 1975; 135:521–525.
19. Curran JF, Ellman MH, Brown NL. Rheumatologic aspects of painful conditions affecting the shoulder. Clin Orthop 1983; 173:27.
20. Laine VAI. Shoulder affections in rheumatoid arthritis. Ann Rheum Dis 1954; 13:157–160.
21. Dabrowski W, Fonseka N, Ansell BM, Liyanage IS, Arden GP. Shoulder problems in juvenile chronic polyarthritis. Scand J Rheumatol 1979; 8:49.
22. Hirooka A, Wakitani S, Yoneda M, Ochi T. Shoulder destruction in rheumatoid arthritis: classification and prognostic signs in 83 patients followed 5–23 years. Acta. Acta Orthop Scand 1996; 67(3):258–263.
23. Lehtinen JT, Belt EA, Lyback CO, et al. Subacromial space in the rheumatoid shoulder: A radiographic 15-year follow-up study of 148 shoulders. J Shoulder Elbow Surg 2000; 9:183–187.
24. Smith AM, Sperling JW, O'Driscoll SW, Cofield RH. Arthroscopic shoulder synovectomy in patients with rheumatoid arthritis. Arthroscopy 2006; 22(1):50–56.
25. Chen AL, Joseph TN, Zuckerman JD. Rheumatoid arthritis of the shoulder. J Am Acad Orthop Surg 2003; 11:12–24.
26. Smith AM, Sperling JW, Cofield RH. Rotator cuff repair in patients with rheumatoid arthritis. J Bone Joint Surg Am 2005; 87(8):1782–1787.
27. Doran MF, Crowson CS, Pond GR, O'Fallon WM, Gabriel SE. Predictors of infection in rheumatoid arthritis. Arthritis Rheum 2002; 46:2294–2300.
28. Doran MF, Crowson CS, Pond GR, O'Fallon WM, Gabriel SE. Frequency of infection in patients with rheumatoid arthritis compared with controls: a population-based study. Arthritis Rheum 2002; 46:2287–2293.
29. Ogilvie-Harris DJ, Demaziere A. Arthroscopic debridement versus open repair for rotator cuff tears: a prospective cohort study. J Bone Joint Surg 1993; 75B:416–420.
30. Rockwood CA, Burkhead WZ. Management of patients with massive rotator cuff defects by acromioplasty and rotator cuff debridement. Orthop Trans 1998; 12:190–191.
31. Rockwood CA Jr. Shoulder function following decompression and irreparable cuff lesions. Orthop Trans 1984; 8:92.
32. Weber SC. Arthroscopic debridement and acromioplasty versus mini-open repair in the treatment of significant partial-thickness rotator cuff tears. Arthroscopy 1999; 15:126–131.
33. Smith AM, Sperling, Cofield RH. Arthroscopic rotator cuff debridements in patients with rheumatoid arthritis. J Shoulder Elbow Surg 2006 Oct 18; EPUB ahead of printing.

34. Wong KL, Williams GR. Complications of thermal capsulorrhaphy of the shoulder. J Bone Joint Surg 2001; 3A:S151–S155.
35. Kaarela K, Kautiainen J. Continuous progression of radiologic destruction on seropositive rheumatoid arthritis. J Rheumatol 1997; 24:1285–1287.
36. Wakitani S, Imoto K, Saito M, et al. Evaluation of surgeries for rheumatoid shoulder based on the destruction pattern. J Rheumatol 1999; 26:41–46.

18 Minimally Invasive Management of Proximal Humerus Fractures

Mark Tauber and Herbert Resch
Department of Traumatology and Sports Injuries, University Hospital of Salzburg, Salzburg, Austria

INDICATIONS

The treatment of proximal humerus fractures represents a special challenge for shoulder surgeons. Blood supply to fracture fragments has to be preserved through decreased soft tissue stripping and detachment while simultaneously assuring restoration of normal anatomic relationships and stable internal fixation that permits early range of motion. Primary prosthetic replacement is a treatment option for severe fractures. However, the results are often not satisfactory (1). For treatment to be successful it is crucial to develop an individual concept of therapy, taking into consideration not only fracture pattern and degree of displacement but also bone quality and biological age of the patient. Respecting the limits of minimally invasive osteosynthesis can provide good results in the elderly, with advanced osteoporosis as well.

Brooks (2) reported that the main arterial supply to the humeral head occurs via the ascending branch of the anterior humeral circumflex artery and its intraosseous continuation, the arcuate artery. In four-part fractures the posteromedial arteries play a major role in maintaining the vascularity of the humeral head. At open reduction and internal fixation, the ascending branch of the anterior humeral circumflex artery is at high risk for damage if not already disrupted by the fracture itself. In percutaneous techniques, compromising the arterial supply is unlikely so that the risk of post-traumatic avascular head necrosis is reduced. Preserving soft tissue attachments, especially those containing the posteromedial vessels, may help ensure the vascularity of the humeral head. Hertel et al. (3) reported on a diminished blood supply in cases with 2 mm medialization of the shaft and reduction of 8 mm of the dorsomedial metaphyseal extension. Therefore, initial fracture pattern and amount of interfragmentary displacement are of decisive significance for fracture healing and clinical outcome.

Indications for percutaneous techniques are extraarticular fractures (e.g., fractures of the greater tuberosity) and subcapital fractures. Within intraarticular fractures, good indications are surgical neck fractures with avulsion of the greater tuberosity (three-part fractures according to Neer) and impacted humeral head fractures without severe lateral displacement [valgus impacted four-part fractures (4)].

We consider four-part fractures with severe lateral displacement of the articular segment ("true" four-part fractures, according to Neer) and severely displaced fracture dislocations (type VI, according to Neer) to be poor indications for the percutaneous technique. Head-split-fractures and unreducable fracture dislocations with the necessity of open reduction and internal fixation are considered to be contraindications for minimally invasive fracture management.

SURGICAL TECHNIQUE

Principles of Closed Reduction

According to the injury mechanism, we can basically differentiate between two types of fractures: (*i*) depression fractures in falls on the extended arm with valgus impaction of the head fragment caused by the glenoid and (*ii*) avulsion fractures caused by a combination of rotational, axial, and muscle forces. In this second group the risk of detachment of the

Please refer to pages 194–197 for the figures in this chapter.

periosteum and interruption of the soft tissue bridges is high. The fragments follow the tension of the inserting muscles, so that conclusions about the periosteal connections can indirectly be drawn from the radiographic distance between the fragments.

Before choosing the right implant for osteosynthesis an anatomic reduction of the fracture is necessary. It is of uppermost interest to reconstruct the gliding mechanism in the subacromial space, that is, to anatomically reduce the greater tuberosity and the articular segment to each other. Healing of the greater tuberosity in an anatomical position is also crucial to avoid impingement symptoms and for potential secondary shoulder replacement (5). Preoperative analysis of radiographs in two planes (anterior–posterior and axillary view) is indispensable in order to identify the relationship of the various fragments to each other as well as to identify the soft tissue links between those fragments, which are still intact (Fig. 1). Due to intact interfragmentary soft tissue bridges, anatomical closed reduction is possible (Fig. 2). The relationship between the head fragment and the shaft on the medial side, the greater tuberosity and the shaft, and the lesser tuberosity and the head fragment are especially important in this respect. In case of longitudinal displacement, the periosteum is destroyed. If the head fragment is displaced medially, the periosteum is stripped off from the shaft but, depending on the amount of displacement, is not destroyed, nor are the vessels within the periosteum destroyed. However, in the case of lateral displacement of the head fragment, the periosteum at the medial side is cut by the sharp edge of the shaft fragment. The limits for periosteal disruption are 6 mm of medial displacement and 9 mm of lateral displacement.

The Humerusblock as Minimally Invasive Implant

An implant used in minimally invasive techniques must fulfil certain requirements. The implant size has to be moderate in order to introduce it percutaneously. Sufficient stability must be provided permitting early motion; further, the applicability must be simple, leading to good results. It should also be usable in complex fractures and in porotic bone as most patients with humeral head fractures are of advanced age.

Kirschner wires (K-wires) have shown a high-failure rate in plurifragmentary fractures and in the elderly patients with poor bone quality (6). We developed the so-called "Humerusblock" (Synthes®), a semirigid implant for minimally invasive treatment of proximal humerus fractures consisting of a metallic cylinder and two 2.2 mm K-wires (Fig. 3). In addition to an Arthroscopic and Percutaneous Screw Fixation System (Leibinger®, Freiburg, Germany), three-part and four-part fractures can also be fixed. The Leibinger®-set compromises cannulated, self-tapping screws with a diameter of 2.7 mm and a length of 10 to 40 mm. The use of a cannula set with blunt trocar helps minimize damage to soft tissues.

The Humerusblock is a metallic cylinder with preformed gliding holes inside in an angle of 30°. The holes can be locked by fixation screws inside the metallic cylinder. The metallic button is fixed to the humeral shaft by a cannulated screw and inserted by means of a guiding system (Fig. 4). This guiding device also permits the drilling of the two K-wires through the preformed gliding holes in the cylinder, which are locked at the end of osteosynthesis by the two fixation screws.

The Humerusblock allows for a rotational stable fixation of the head fragment with a three-point locking of the K-wires: first, in the subchondral bone of the articular head fragment, second, in the lateral metaphyseal cortex, and third, in the metallic button of the Humerusblock, itself. This system also provides stability and prevents pin loosening in elderly patients.

Patient Positioning and Operative Steps

The procedure is usually performed under general anaesthesia combined with an interscalene cervical plexus block. The patient is placed in the beachchair position with the respective arm draped to permit mobility. Gross reduction is performed under the image intensifier positioned cranially with the C-arm creating a right angle between the central beam and the humerus shaft.

A 2 to 3 cm long skin incision is performed in the median line on the lateral side of the humerus shaft 5 cm distally to the subcapital fracture line. At the level of the deltoid insertion the muscle is slightly pushed backward and the cylinder, which is inserted by means of a guiding system, is fixed to the bone with a cannulated screw. The screw is not locked until the direction of the two K-wires, drilled through guiding cannules in an angle of 30°, can be varied in the frontal plane. First, the two K-wires are drilled up to the line of the subcapital fracture. Then anatomic reduction in two planes under radiological control with the image intensifier is performed. After successful reduction the two pins are drilled forward into the subchondral bone of the articular fragment. Perforation by pins should be avoided. The tips of the wires should be directed to the area between the superior glenoid pole and the top of the humeral head. In case of secondary impaction, the head fragment glides along the two K-wires distally ("guided sliding" of the head) with perforation of the tips through the articular surface. In this case, if the pins are directed too gently toward the glenoid, damaging of the glenoid cartilage is unavoidable when shoulder motion is started.

The greater and lesser tuberosities are fixed by cannulated titanium screws (Leibinger®), which are inserted over a guide wire. The guide wire is part of a drill guide-wire combination with a thickness of 2.2 mm. This combination is used like a K-wire for temporary fixation of the tuberosities. In case the radiological check shows correct position, the drill is removed, whereas the guide wire remains in place. The screw, usually 40 mm long, is inserted over the wire.

Anatomical Neck Fractures

Reduction in the normally, medially, and slightly posteriorly shifted head fragment is performed with an elevator in this type of fracture. This instrument is inserted through a stab incision and then guided steadily while in contact with the bone anterior to the humeral head to the anatomical neck. While traction is applied to the slightly abducted arm in neutral position the anatomical neck is pushed in a superior direction. Usually, the periosteum on the medial side is stripped off from the shaft but is still intact. In case of additional posterior displacement, the shaft fragment has to be pushed backward at the same time as the head fragment is pushed superiorly. With reduction of the head, the rotator cuff is strained and the greater tuberosity is approximated to its anatomical position.

Surgical Neck Fractures with Avulsion of the Greater Tuberosity

In case of severe displacement of three-part fractures, the head fragment is internally rotated due to the tension of the subscapularis tendon and the absent counteracting force of the infraspinatus tendon by the avulsed greater tuberosity (Fig. 5). Usually, the periosteum between shaft and greater tuberosity is disrupted with consecutive superior migration of the greater tuberosity into the subacromial space. Additionally, the shaft is displaced anteriorly and medially. Depending on the displacement between the humeral head and the shaft, these fractures are characterized by high-graded instability due to the destroyed soft tissue bridges between the fragments. Reduction of head and greater tuberosity has to be performed separately. First, the head has to be raised to allow for reduction of the greater tuberosity. This is performed by means of an elevator, which is inserted through a stab incision into the gap of the intertubercular fracture, located 5 mm lateral to the bicipital groove (Fig. 6). In case of pronounced rotational displacement of the head, the reduction is performed by means of a pointed hook retractor (Fig. 7). This instrument is engaged at the lesser tuberosity, where the subscapularis tendon is attached. Pulling laterally, the rotational displacement of the head fragment can be arrested. The final step consists in drilling the two K-wires into the head fragment, holding the arm in an adducted and internal rotated position. As soon as the head is in good alignment with the shaft and the head shows anatomical profile in the anterior–posterior (AP)-view, the K-wires are drilled into the head. The greater tuberosity is then reduced by means of a hook retractor, which is inserted in the subacromial space through a stab incision. Engaged at the insertion of the supraspinatus tendon, the hook retractor is pulled in an anteroinferior direction until anatomic reduction is achieved (Fig. 8). After temporary fixation with the guiding pin for the cannulated titanium screw, the anatomic position of the greater tuberosity is checked in maximal external and internal rotation and fixation is performed by two to three cannulated titanium screws (Figs. 9 and 10).

Valgus Impacted Fractures

These fractures result from a depression mechanism and are characterized by the impact on the articular segment into the metaphysis. The greater tuberosity is displaced laterally and the lesser tuberosity, anteriorly, in case of a four-part fracture. Caused by the displacement of the head the lesser tuberosity appears to be displaced medially in the axillary view. But both usually remain in a correct longitudinal position indicating an intact periosteal connection although minimally stripped off the shaft. In valgus impacted fractures, the head is not displaced laterally or medially, so that the periosteum remains intact at the medial side. The blood supply is preserved and the intact soft-tissue bridge works as a "hinge" when the humeral head is raised.

The maneuver of raising the head fragment is performed, using an elevator inserted through a separate stab incision. In order to provide orientation for the surgeon to find the correct insert position, the patient's arm is held in adduction by the surgeon's assistant and the incision is made at the border between the anterior and middle-thirds of the head, working under image-intensifier control. The fracture gap between the greater and lesser tuberosity is almost always located 5 mm lateral to the bicipital groove and has to be detected by gently sliding over the bone with the tip of the elevator in an anterior–posterior direction. The elevator is inserted through this fracture gap underneath the head fragment, which can then be raised to its anatomical position. The shape of the humeral head with correct positioning of the greater tuberosity has to be assessed to allow for orientation in order to accomplish anatomical reduction. Then the two 2.2 mm K-wires of the Humerusblock are drilled into the head as far as the subchondral bone of the articular fragment. Due to the ligamentotaxis effect, anatomical alignment of the greater tuberosity can normally be achieved only by raising the impacted head fragment. It is held on the inferior side by the periosteum and on the superior side by the rotator cuff. Fixation of the greater tuberosity in its anatomical position is performed with two cannulated titanium screws inserted through two stab incisions. One screw is located proximally in the greater tuberosity passing through the upper part of the articular segment. The other screw is passed through the inferior part of the greater tuberosity into the fragment of the shaft so that the greater tuberosity has a carrier function between the shaft and the articular segment. For reduction of the lesser tuberosity the arm is held in 70° of abduction with the image intensifier set for an axial view. Then a hook retractor is inserted through a stab incision and engaged at the tip of the lesser tuberosity. The fragment is pulled laterally until the articular step formation has disappeared. Definitive fixation is carried out by insertion of a cannulated screw in an anterior–posterior direction. The length of this screw usually measures 40 mm.

Severely Displaced Humeral Head Fractures

Fortunately this type of fracture ("true" four-part fracture) is rare and seen almost only in the elderly. In young patients such fractures result from high-energy trauma and often occur as fracture dislocations. The extreme variation of this type of fracture is the four-part fracture dislocation. Due to the high degree of displacement, all soft tissue links between the fragments are disrupted and the vascularity is highly impaired. The risk of avascular post-traumatic humeral head necrosis is quite high and in the elderly these fractures represent an indication for primary prosthetic head replacement. Percutaneous treatment as well as open reduction are very difficult and represent a challenge for the surgeon. At least in young patients we recommend reconstructing the head, even if the blood supply seems to be completely interrupted. As patients do well with partial head necrosis, prosthetic replacement remains an option for future treatment, if necessary.

PEARLS AND PITFALLS

Axillary Nerve

The angle for the cannulated screws to fix the greater tuberosity can endanger the axillary nerve, which traverses in a distance of about 6 cm from the acromion under the deltoid muscle. To avoid any harm to the axillary nerve, the surgeon has three options:

1. The stem of the axillary nerve forms terminal branches at the level of the lateral end of the acromion. Where the line of fracture permits, the screws should be set from a slightly anterolateral direction with the arm held in additional internal rotation.

2. If one of the screws has to be inserted in the area of the stem of the axillary nerve, the trocar sheath with the blunt trocar should be used to protect the nerve. After incising the skin, the trocar is advanced in a craniomedial direction until bone contact is made and then slid down the bone caudally.
3. In the area of the axillary nerve no washers should be used to avoid entrapment of the nerve under the washer.

Fracture of the Greater Tuberosity

In comminuted fractures of the greater tuberosity screw fixation alone usually is not sufficient. In these cases additional transosseous sutures or wire cerclage by open surgery is necessary. To control anatomical reduction of the greater tuberosity, the profile of the head has to appear anatomically and the bone density between head and fragment has to be homogenous. A step-off between the tuberosity and the head in maximal internal rotation means persistent posterior displacement of the fragment, and this has to be reduced.

Fracture of the Lesser Tuberosity

The medial displacement of the lesser tuberosity, seen only in the axillary view, is caused by the tension of the subscapularis tendon. The step-off in the articular surface can be taken as measure for the medial displacement. For percutaneous reduction the arm is held by the surgeon's assistant in 70° of abduction with the image intensifier positioned for an axillary view. Then a pointed hook retractor is engaged at the tip of the lesser tuberosity, where the subscapularis tendon is inserted, and pulled laterally under radiographic control until the step-off in the articular surface has disappeared.

Limits of the Humerusblock

As percutaneous technique, the Humerusblock is not the appropriate implant for every type of proximal humerus fracture. As aforementioned, there are some factors, which reduce the indications for our implant. If closed reduction is not possible anatomically, the Humerusblock will fail.

1. In severely displaced fractures and especially fracture dislocations, an anatomical reduction is difficult in most cases and not achievable. In these cases open reduction or even primary humeral head replacement is necessary.
2. In subcapital fractures with extension of the fracture line distally in the proximal humerus shaft involving the lateral cortex, the fixation of the Humerusblock is complicated and stability can not be guaranteed. For these fractures, other implants for osteosynthesis, such as the proximal humerus nail or the humerus plate with locking screws, should be considered.
3. Head-split-fractures should not be treated with the Humerusblock, and represent an absolute contraindication.
4. In the elderly with poor bone quality and four-part humeral head fracture, primary shoulder replacement with the reversed prosthesis is an alternative that should be considered. Early movement and reuptake of functionality is possible and allows the patients to return to their daily activities faster.

If the surgeon is in doubt about whether to opt for minimally invasive or open procedure, an attempt at percutaneous treatment should be made. Switching to the open technique always remains a possibility.

POSTOPERATIVE TREATMENT

The arm is immobilized against the body with light bandaging for three weeks. Depending on the stability achieved, passive exercising in the scapular plane without rotation is begun on the first postoperative day. Active movement and rotation exercises are started after three weeks. At this time, serial radiographs are necessary. Because of the porotic bone of the head fragment, an impaction along the two K-wires can occur with perforation through the articular surface (so called "guided sliding" of the head). To avoid the resulting cartilage damage on the glenoid when rotation is started, a reoperation is carried out, consisting of drawing back the two K-wires under the articular surface again, usually three weeks after the implantation of the Humerusblock. In the elderly, the cannulated screws can show poor purchase in the porotic bone with loosening and loss of reduction. In cases where poor stability is to be expected, post-operative treatment has to be modified and strict immobilization of the shoulder is required. Removal of the Humerusblock is performed after six to eight weeks, if radiological signs of fracture healing are present. The cannulated titanium screws are usually not removed.

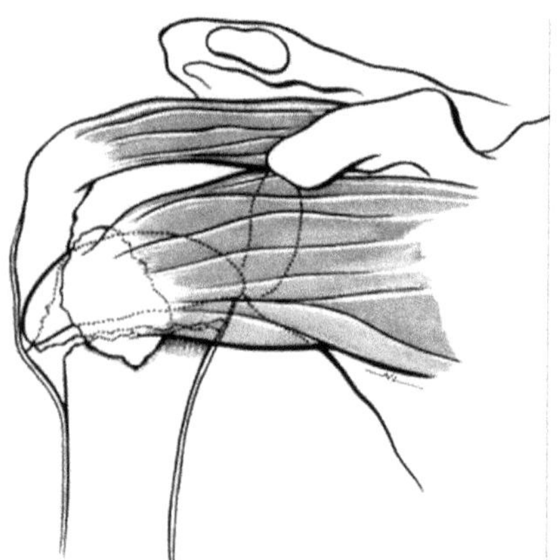

FIGURE 1 Drawing of a four-part valgus impacted humeral head fracture. The head fragment is impacted with intact medial "hinge-periosteum." The greater tuberosity is displaced laterally with stripped off but still intact periosteum.

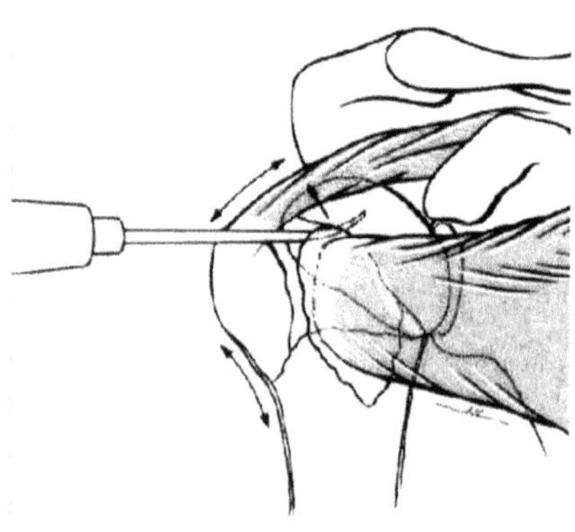

FIGURE 2 Closed reduction by means of an elevator taking full advantage of the ligamentotaxis effect. Due to intact periosteal bridges on the lateral and medial side and tension of the inserting tendons an anatomic reduction is possible by simple raising the head.

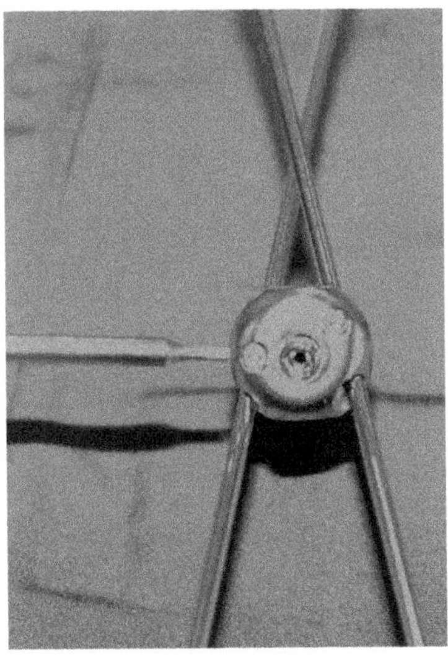

FIGURE 3 The Humerusblock: consisting of a metallic cylinder with two 2.2 mm Kirschner wires (K-wires) passing through in an angle of 30°. The K-wires can be locked by fixation-screws inside the metallic cylinder.

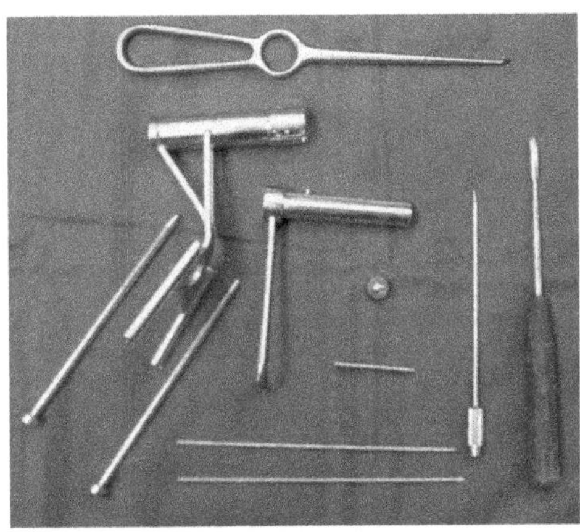

FIGURE 4 Instruments for implantation of the Humerusblock: hook retractor, elevator, guiding system, two 2.2 mm K-wires, screw driver for the locking screws inside the Humerusblock, cannulated screw for fixation of the Humerusblock.

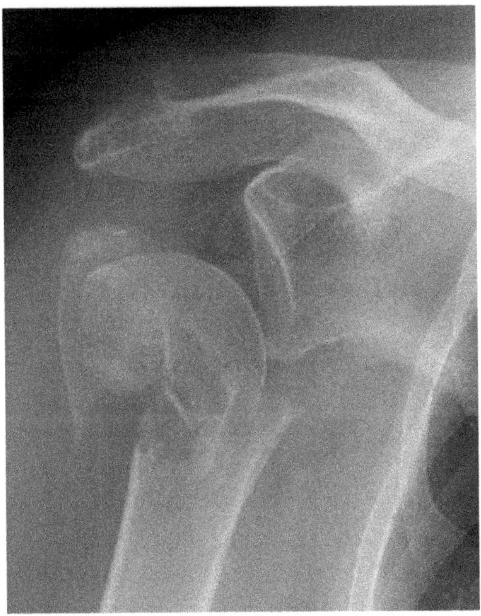

FIGURE 5 Three-part valgus impacted fracture with medialization of the shaft and superior–posterior dislocation of the greater tuberosity. The medialization of the shaft is almost 6 mm and the integrity of the medial periosteum is uncertain. The periosteum at the lateral side is stripped off but still intact.

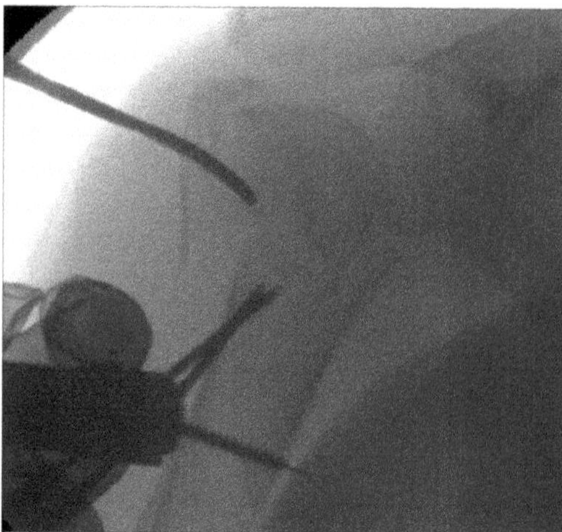

FIGURE 6 Closed reduction of the three-part humerus fracture: after positioning of the K-wires of the Humerusblock at the level of the subcapital fracture, the head is raised by means of an elevator, which is inserted through a stab incision from laterally into the intertubercular fracture gap, which is about 5 mm lateral to the bicipital groove.

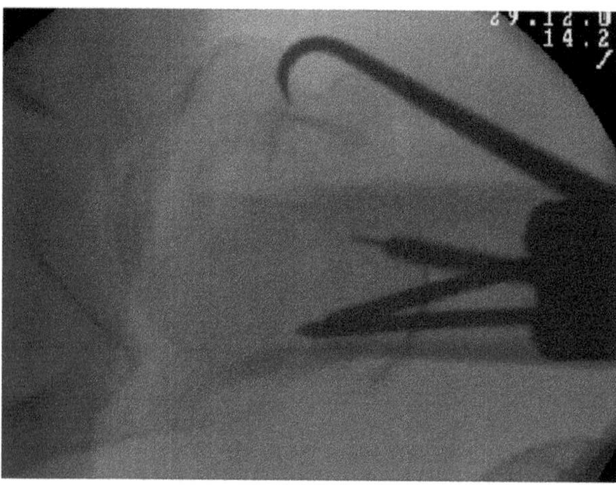

FIGURE 7 Due to the tension forces of the subscapularis tendon the head is rotated internally. This can be verified in an axillary view under the image intensifier and reduced by means of a hook retractor derotating the head fragment. Then the two K-wires of the Humerusblock are drilled into the subchondral cortex of the articular segment.

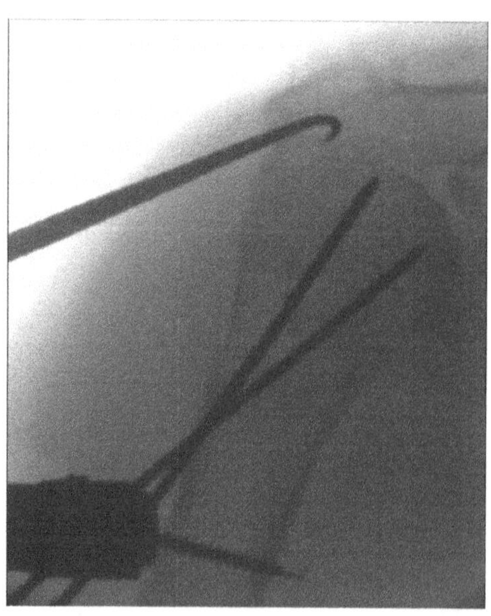

FIGURE 8 The superior–posteriorly displaced greater tuberosity is reduced by means of a hook retractor pulling the fragment in an anterior and inferior direction.

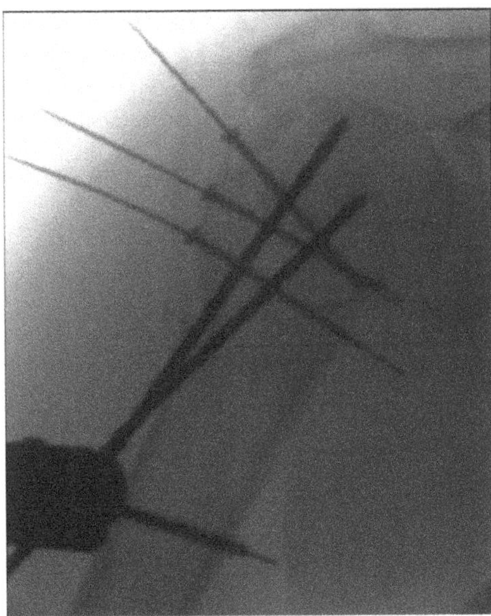

FIGURE 9 Temporary fixation of the fragment is performed by the drill guide-wire combination of the Leibinger®-system and anatomic reduction is controlled rotating the head until maximal internal rotation. If an anatomic shape of the humeral head could be achieved, the cannulated titanium screws are inserted over the guide wires after removal of the drill.

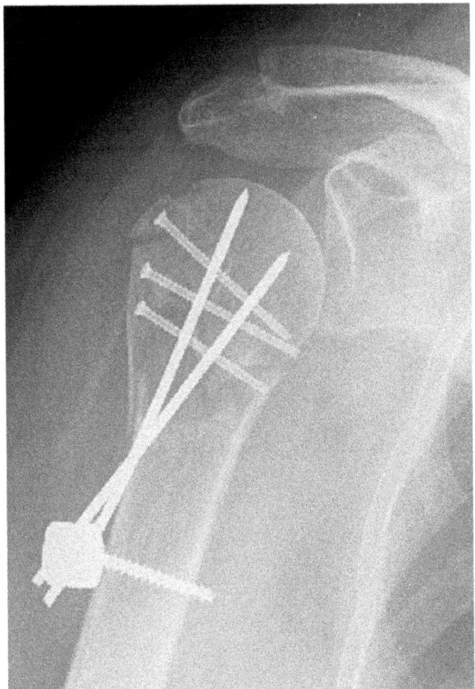

FIGURE 10 The guide wires are removed after definitive anatomic reduction. Removal of the cannulated screw without the guide wire can be difficult.

REFERENCES

1. Zyto K, Wallace WA, Frostick SP, Preston BJ. Outcome after hemiarthroplasty for three- and four-part fractures of the proximal humerus. J Shoulder Elbow Surg 1998; 7(2):85–89.
2. Brooks CH, Revell WJ, Heatley FW. Vascularity of the humeral head after proximal humeral fractures. An anatomical cadaver study. J Bone Joint Surg Br 1993; 75(1):132–136.
3. Hertel R, Hempfing A, Stiehler M, Leunig M. Predictors of humeral head ischemia after intracapsular fracture of the proximal humerus. J Shoulder Elbow Surg 2004; 13(4):427–433.
4. Jakob RP, Miniaci A, Anson PS, Jaberg H, Osterwalder A, Ganz R. Four-part valgus impacted fractures of the proximal humerus. J Bone Joint Surg Br 1991; 73(2):295–298.
5. Frankle MA, Greenwald DP, Markee BA, Ondrovic LE, Lee WE, III. Biomechanical effects of malposition of tuberosity fragments on the humeral prosthetic reconstruction for four-part proximal humerus fractures. J Shoulder Elbow Surg 2001; 10(4):321–326.
6. Herscovici D Jr, Saunders DT, Johnson MP, Sanders R, DiPasquale T. Percutaneous fixation of proximal humeral fractures. Clin Orthop Relat Res 2000; (375):97–104.

19 Evaluation and Tear Recognition of the Rotator Cuff

Shane A. Barwood and Ian K.Y. Lo
Department of Orthopedic Surgery, The University of Calgary, Calgary, Alberta, Canada

INTRODUCTION

Arthroscopic evaluation of the rotator cuff not only enables a complete assessment of both the articular and bursal surfaces of the rotator cuff, but also increases the surgeon's "window of visualization." Although traditional open surgical management has been restricted by a limited anterolateral exposure, arthroscopy allows assessment of the rotator cuff from a multitude of angles and perspectives with minimal disruption to the overlying deltoid. This expanded window of visualization has refuted routine medial to lateral repair of the torn rotator cuff and has emphasized the importance of understanding and recognizing rotator cuff tear patterns.

Arthroscopy allows formal assessment of the natural mobility of the rotator cuff, prior to any surgical releases, which subsequently dictates the appropriate repair configuration. By repairing the tear according to this natural mobility, one may successfully repair more tendon tears, create a mechanically sound construction, minimize repair tension and tension overload, and optimize the results of treatment (1). In this chapter we describe the techniques used to enable accurate tear pattern recognition and how this dictates repair methods. Our assessment of the posterosuperior rotator cuff (i.e., supraspinatus, infraspinatus, and teres minor) is separated from the assessment of the subscapularis tendon that is described later.

POSTEROSUPERIOR ROTATOR CUFF

In general, the posterosuperior rotator cuff tears may be divided into:

- Crescent-shaped tears
- U-shaped tears
- L-shaped tears
- Reverse L-shaped tears
- Massive, contracted, immobile tears.

The key to accurately identify these rotator cuff tear patterns is a complete assessment of the natural mobility of the rotator cuff tear. Prior to any surgical release, the natural mobility of the rotator cuff tear margin is assessed in a precise and stepwise manner (Table 1). By assessing the mobility of the tear in a medial to lateral and an anterior to posterior direction, rapid and reproducible tear pattern recognition may be obtained and subsequent repair may be performed with minimal repair tension.

ASSESSMENT OF MEDIAL TO LATERAL MOBILITY—CRESCENT-SHAPED TEARS

Following complete bursectomy and debridement of overlying fibrofatty tissue but prior to any surgical releases (Fig. 1A), initial assessment of the rotator cuff tear is performed in a medial to lateral direction. We perform this assessment using a tendon grasper introduced through a lateral portal while viewing through a posterior portal (Fig. 1B). The medial aspect of the

---

Please refer to pages 204–209 for the figures in this chapter.

TABLE 1 Stepwise Assessment, Tear Pattern Recognition, and Repair Configuration of Posterosuperior Rotator Cuff Tears

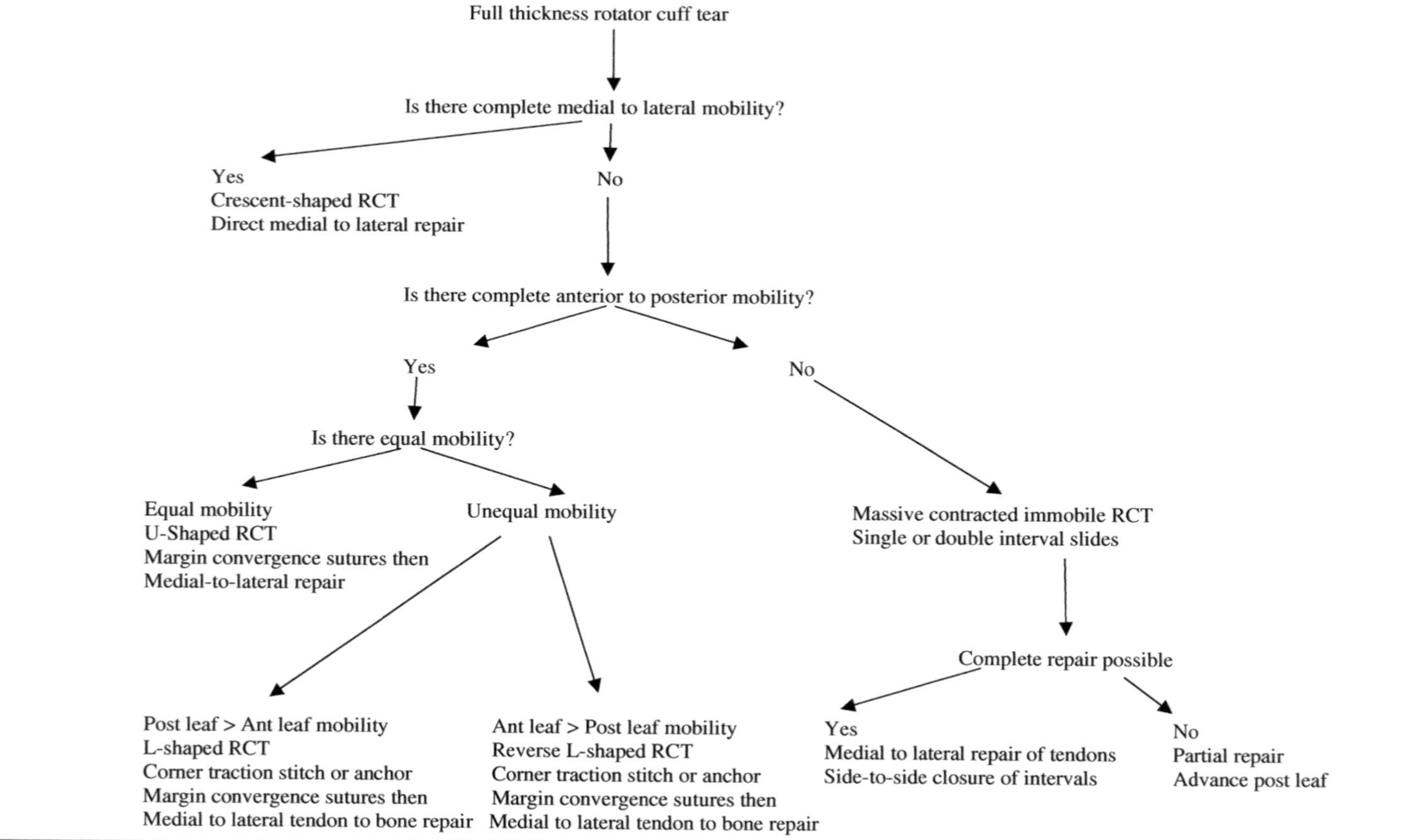

rotator cuff tendon tear is then grasped and pulled to the bone bed laterally (Fig. 1C). If the rotator cuff tendon tear is reducible under minimal tension to or close to the lateral aspect of the footprint, then this represents a crescent-type rotator cuff tear. Crescent-type rotator cuff tears may be repaired anatomically due to the medial to lateral mobility, by direct tendon to bone repair. Even some massive tears may have significant mobility in a medial to lateral direction and may represent massive, crescent-shaped tears. Crescent-shaped tears are highly amenable to a double-row rotator cuff repair, to reconstruct the rotator cuff footprint (2).

When a crescent-type rotator cuff tear is large it may be difficult to reduce using a single tendon grasper. In this situation, we use traction sutures, placed along the margin of the rotator cuff, to assist in tendon reduction and assessment of mobility along the entire length of the tendon margin (Fig. 1D). It is important to place traction sutures evenly along the edge of the tendon and to retrieve them out the appropriate portal, to ensure tension is applied in the proper direction (Fig. 1E). In large chronic crescent-shaped rotator cuff tears, supplemental capsular releases may be performed with an arthroscopic elevator blade to ensure complete tendon reduction under minimal tension.

Assessment of Anterior to Posterior Mobility—U-Shaped, L-Shaped, and Reverse L-Shaped Tears

If the tear is not completely reducible under minimal tension in a medial to lateral direction, then the anterior to posterior mobility of the tendon tear is assessed. We assess the anterior to posterior mobility while viewing through a lateral "50-yard line" portal. While viewing through this portal the tendon grasper is introduced through the posterior portal and grasps along the anterior leaf of the rotator cuff tear (Fig. 2A). Traction is applied posteriorly to determine the posterior mobility of the anterior leaf of the rotator cuff tear (Fig. 2B). To determine the anterior mobility of the posterior leaf, a tendon grasper is introduced through an anterior portal and the posterior leaf of the rotator cuff tear is grasped (Fig. 2C). Traction is then applied anteriorly along the posterior margin of the rotator cuff tear to determine the anterior mobility of the posterior leaf (Fig. 2D)

If there is significant and equal mobility of the tendon margins in both an anterior and posterior direction, then this represents a U-shaped rotator cuff tear (Fig. 3). These tears are amenable to initial side-to-side suturing of the anterior and posterior leafs of the rotator cuff. These side-to-side sutures (margin convergence sutures), when tied, converge the margin of the rotator cuff laterally toward the bone bed (3). Following margin convergence, tendon to bone fixation may be performed. These tears are also commonly amenable to a double row repair, however, placement of the medial row can be difficult if margin convergence sutures have already been placed and tied. We, therefore, place our medial row suture anchors and complete medial row suture passage after side-to-side margin convergence suture placement, but prior to tying the margin convergence sutures.

If there is significant but unequal anterior to posterior mobility then this represents an L-shaped or reverse L-shaped rotator cuff tear. L-shaped rotator cuff tears demonstrate significant anterior mobility of the posterior leaf and commonly have a longitudinal split between the leading edge of the supraspinatus and the rotator interval, whereas reverse L-shaped tears demonstrate significant posterior mobility of the anterior leaf and have a longitudinal split between the supraspinatus and infraspinatus tendons. In both these situations, it is very important to determine the apex of the L- or reverse L-shaped tear. For an L-shaped tear, this is usually best determined while viewing through the lateral portal (Figs. 4A–F) and using a tendon grasper introduced through an anterior or accessory anterolateral portal. The posterior edge of the rotator cuff is grasped (Fig. 4C) and pulled anteriorly and laterally toward the bone bed (Fig. 4D). Different areas along the posterior margin are evaluated for their anterolateral mobility to determine the point with the most mobility (i.e., the apex of the tear), to allow anatomic reconstruction. We find it helpful to place a traction stitch at the apex of the tear (Fig. 4E) and to reduce the tear so that placement of anchors and suture passage may be performed accurately (Fig. 4F). These tears are also amenable to double row repair. Similarly, if the tear is a reverse L-shaped tear then the tendon grasper is introduced through a posterior portal (Fig. 5) and the anterior edge of the rotator cuff is grasped and pulled posteriorly and laterally toward the bone bed.

Minimal or No Mobility—Immobile Contracted Massive Tears

If there is minimal medial to lateral and anterior to posterior mobility of the tendon tear then this represents a massive, contracted, immobile rotator cuff tears (Fig. 6). These tears represent less than 10% of all massive rotator cuff tears and historically were considered irreparable rotator cuff tears. These tears are not amenable to direct medial to lateral repair or a margin convergence repair, even after capsular releases have been performed. These tears are usually only amenable to repair using interval slide techniques (4). With development of the interval slide, particularly the double interval slide, very few rotator cuff tears are not amenable to repair. The double interval slides involve release of the anterior interval (i.e., between the supraspinatus and rotator interval anteriorly) and the posterior interval (i.e., between the supraspinatus and infraspinatus posteriorly). Although rotator cuff repair is possible using these techniques, a double row repair may not be achievable. By using the double interval slide, irreparable tears are distinctly unusual and the indications for partial repair are diminishing. The most common scenario for a partial repair occurs when despite an anterior and posterior interval slide; the supraspinatus tendon is still not amenable to repair and cannot be brought to the bone bed laterally. In this situation, the posterior cuff (that is the infraspinatus and teres minor), which is almost always amenable to repair, is advanced superiorly and laterally to a more biomechanically favorable position by tendon to bone repair.

EVALUATION OF THE SUBSCAPULARIS TENDON

Traditional open surgical approaches to the subscapularis provide only a limited window of the subscapularis. Delto-pectoral incisions are restricted medially by the coracoid and conjoint tendon, whereas anterolateral or mini-open incisions provide limited exposure of the inferior and medial portion of the tendon. In both these open approaches, articular-sided pathology is commonly neglected and difficult to identify. Even full thickness and retracted tendons may appear normal to the unwary eyes, due to a large thickened bursa that may initially appear to insert into the lesser tuberosity. However, closer inspection usually demonstrates that this tissue is merely a "bursal leader" and drapes over the lesser tuberosity without inserting into it (leaving a bare lesser tuberosity).

Arthroscopy of the glenohumeral joint provides an inside-out view of the subscapularis tendon, allowing accurate visualization of the subscapularis tendon and its insertion into the lesser tuberosity. The evaluation of the subscapularis tendon and its insertion is performed through a standard posterior portal. The key to accurate and proper assessment is the arm position of abduction and internal rotation. This maneuver lifts the fibers of the intact portion of the subscapularis away from the footprint, allowing excellent visualization of its insertion (Fig. 7). A 70° arthroscope or an anterosuperolateral viewing portal may also be helpful to the complete assessment of the subscapularis insertion.

PARTIAL SUBSCAPULARIS TENDON TEARS

Since the vast majority of degeneration of the subscapularis begins on the articular side of the upper portion of the subscapularis, partial tears are easily diagnosed by observing a "bare footprint" on the lesser tuberosity revealed by tearing of the fibers (Fig. 8). Estimation of the extent of tearing is performed by relating the size of the observed bare area to the known mean dimensions of the subscapularis footprint (mean tendinous insertion: 2.5 cm; range: 1.5–3.0 cm).

COMPLETE AND RETRACTED SUBSCAPULARIS TENDON TEARS

In full thickness, complete subscapularis tears with lesser tuberosity will appear bare (Fig. 9), and the subscapularis tendon stump may be difficult to identify, particularly in chronic tears.

This difficulty occurs since the tendon is commonly retracted medially and may be found at, or medial to, the glenoid. The situation is further compounded if the tendon is scarred to the inner deltoid fascia or to the coracoid, as this further obscures the tendon edges. In order to identify the retracted tendon edge, one must first understand the relationship between the subscapularis tendon and the humeral insertions of the superior glenohumeral and medial coracohumeral ligament.

Due to their close proximity, as these three structures insert into the humerus, their fibers interdigitate. Thus, when the subscapularis tendon is torn from the humerus, the entire complex is torn collectively from the humerus and their relationship remains intact. This key anatomical relationship forms a "comma-shaped" arc (called the "comma sign") just above the superolateral corner of the subscapularis and provides a marker for the subscapularis tendon (Fig. 10A) (5). We identify and follow the comma sign inferomedially to lead us to the superolateral border of the subscapularis tendon. Following visual identification of the superolateral corner of the subscapularis tendon, we use a tendon grasper from an anterosuperolateral portal to pull the medially retracted tissues laterally until we can definitively identify the upper border of the subscapularis (Fig. 10B).

Chronic subscapularis tears often have reduced mobility and require formal release to enable accurate repair under minimal tension. After the lateral edge of the tendon is identified using the comma sign, a traction suture is passed through the superolateral corner of the subscapularis to allow continuous traction on the lateral edge, during the subsequent medial release. We then perform a three-sided release of the subscapularis. This is performed using a posterior viewing portal and a combination of the anterolateral and anterior working portals. After soft tissue release, we usually perform a subcoracoid decompression in order to facilitate repair under minimal tension (6,7). After completion of these releases, many chronic-retracted subscapularis tears are amenable to double row repairs (2).

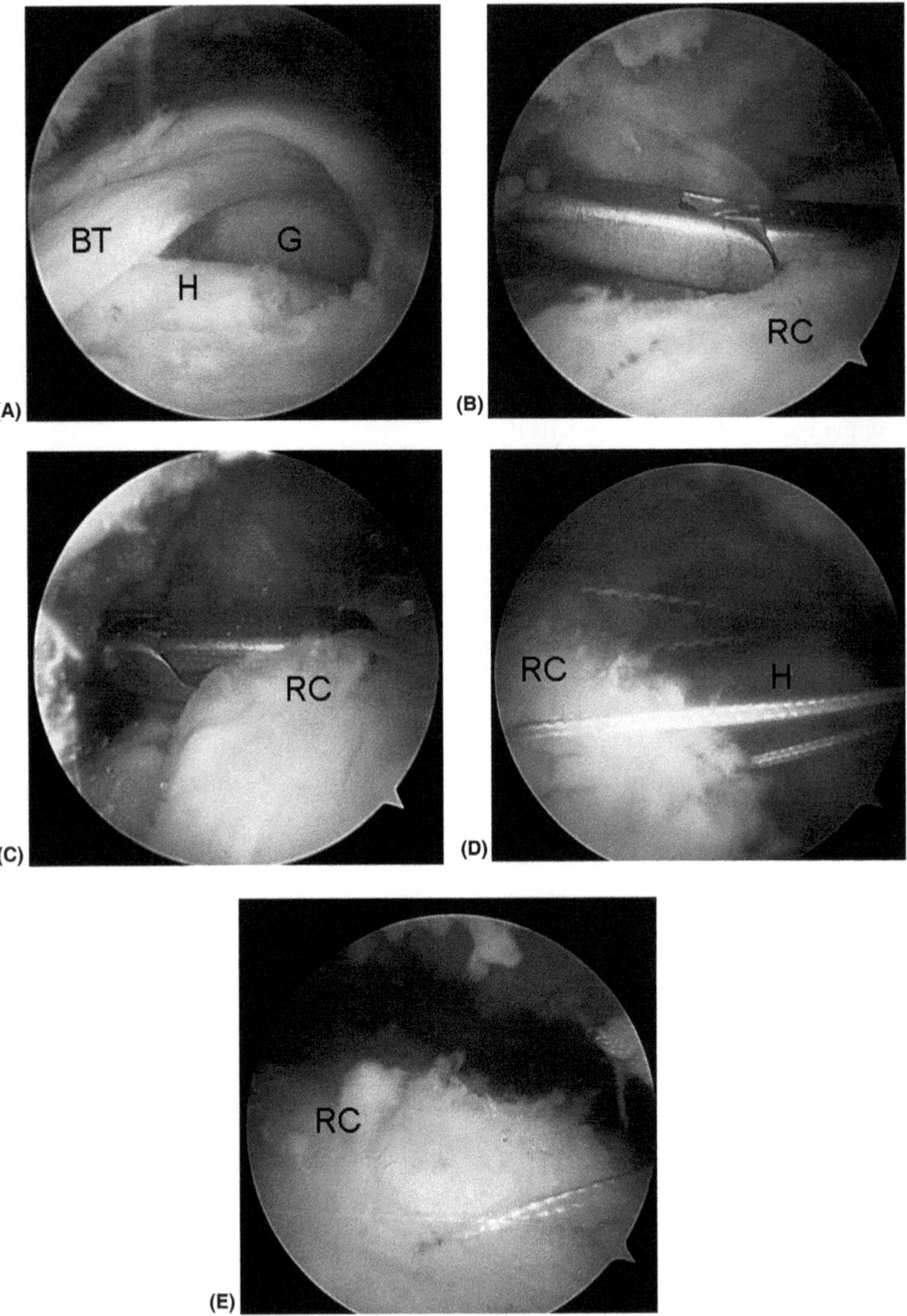

FIGURE 1 Assessment of medial to lateral mobility. (**A**) Initial arthroscopic view through a lateral subacromial portal of a small crescent-shaped rotator cuff tear in a left shoulder. (**B**) While viewing through a posterior subacromial portal, a tendon grasper is introduced through a lateral portal and is used to grasp the medial aspect of the rotator cuff tendon tear. (**C**) The rotator cuff tendon tear is then pulled laterally toward the bone bed, and the medial to lateral mobility of the tendon is assessed. Complete reduction of the rotator cuff tear is obtained to the lateral bone bed, indicating that this represents a small crescent rotator cuff tear. (**D**) Large crescent-shaped rotator cuff tear of a right shoulder. Arthroscopic views through a posterior subacromial portal. Traction sutures are placed along the medial margin of the rotator cuff tear. (**E**) Lateral traction allows reduction of the tendon margin toward the bone bed and assessment of mobility. *Abbreviations*: BT, biceps tendon; G, glenoid; H, humeral head; RC, rotator cuff.

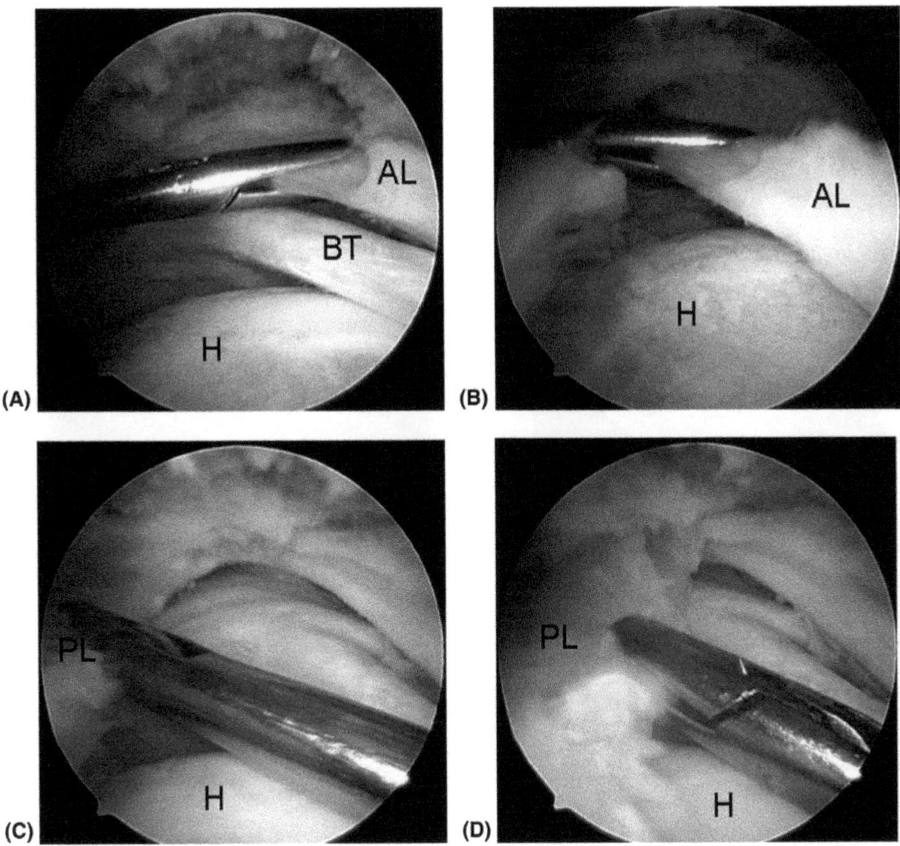

FIGURE 2 Assessment of anterior to posterior mobility. Arthroscopic views through a lateral subacromial portal of a right shoulder. (**A**) A tendon grasper is introduced through the posterior portal and grasps along the anterior leaf of the rotator cuff tear. (**B**) Traction is applied in a posterior direction to determine the posterior mobility of the anterior leaf. (**C**) Anterior mobility of the posterior leaf. A tendon grasper is introduced through an anterior portal and grasps along the posterior leaf of the rotator cuff tear. (**D**) Traction is applied is an anterior direction to determine the anterior mobility of the posterior leaf. *Abbreviations*: AL, anterior leaf of the rotator cuff; BT, biceps tendon; H, humeral head; PL, posterior leaf of the rotator cuff.

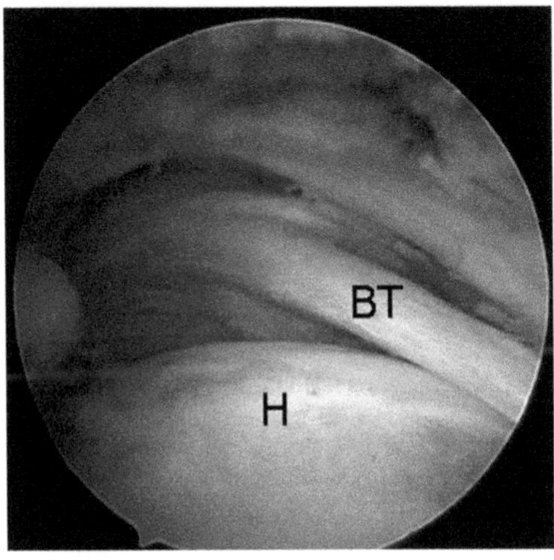

FIGURE 3 U-shaped rotator cuff tear. Arthroscopic view through a lateral subacromial portal. Note how the tear is massive in size but relatively narrow with the medial aspect of the rotator cuff tear, adjacent to the glenoid margin. Same tear as in Figure 2. *Abbreviations*: BT, biceps tendon; H, humeral head.

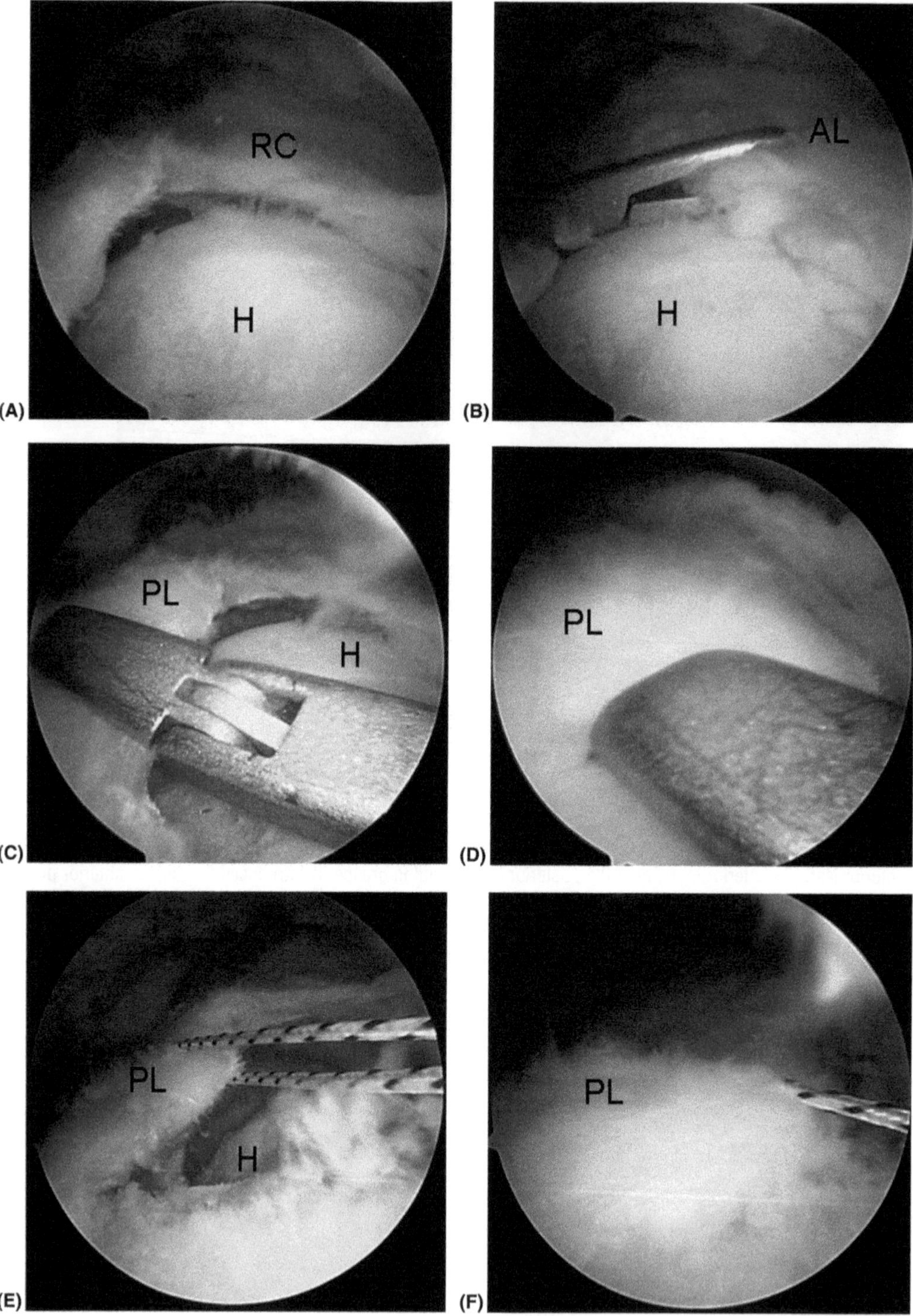

FIGURE 4 L-shaped rotator cuff tear. (**A**) Initial view through a lateral subacromial portal of an L-shaped rotator cuff tendon tear in a right shoulder. (**B**) A tendon grasper is introduced through a posterior portal and grasps the anterior leaf of the rotator cuff. Minimal mobility is noted. (**C**) A tendon grasper is then introduced through the anterior portal and grasps the posterior edge of the rotator cuff tendon tear. (**D**) The tendon margin can be pulled anteriorly and laterally toward the bone bed, reducing the tear. (**E**) A traction stitch is placed at the apex of the tear to temporarily reduce tension during formation of the rotator cuff repair construct (**F**). *Abbreviations*: AL, anterior leaf of the rotator cuff; H, humeral head; PL, posterior leaf of the rotator cuff; RC, rotator cuff.

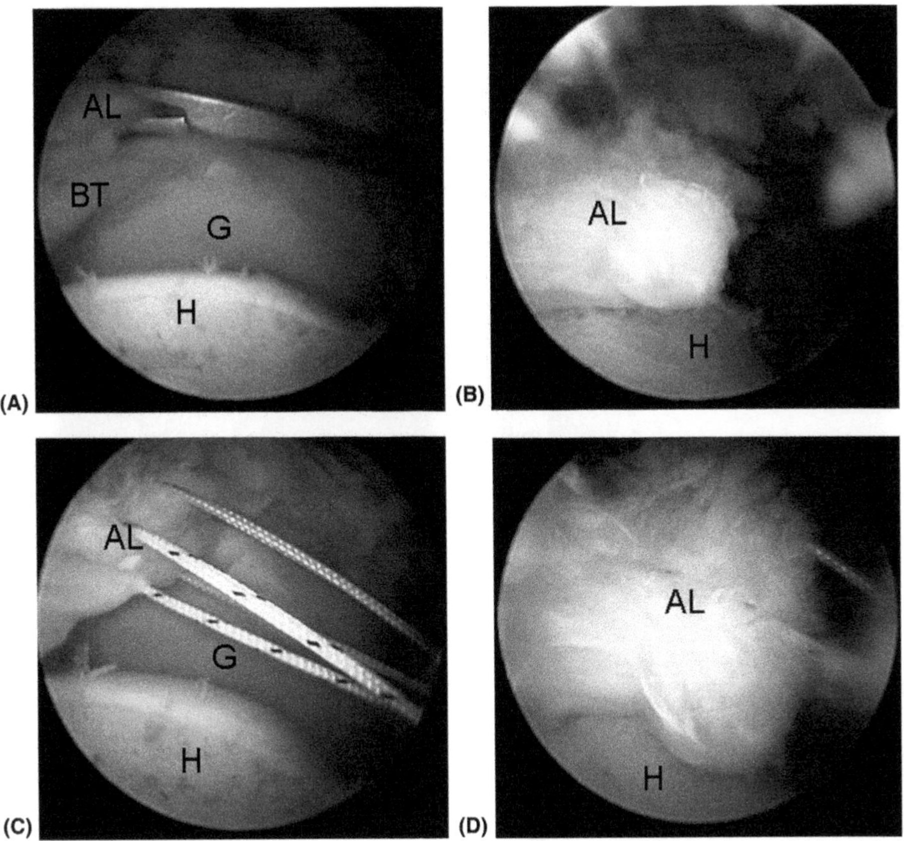

FIGURE 5 Reverse L-shaped rotator cuff tear. Arthroscopic views through a lateral subacromial portal of a right shoulder. (**A**) A tendon grasper is introduced through the posterior portal and grasps the anterior leaf of the rotator cuff tear. (**B**) The tendon margin can be pulled posteriorly and laterally toward the bone bed reducing the tear. (**C**) Traction stitches are placed at the apex of the tear to reduce the tendon during formation of the rotator cuff repair construct (**D**). *Abbreviations*: AL, anterior leaf of the rotator cuff; BT, biceps tendon; G, glenoid; H, humeral head.

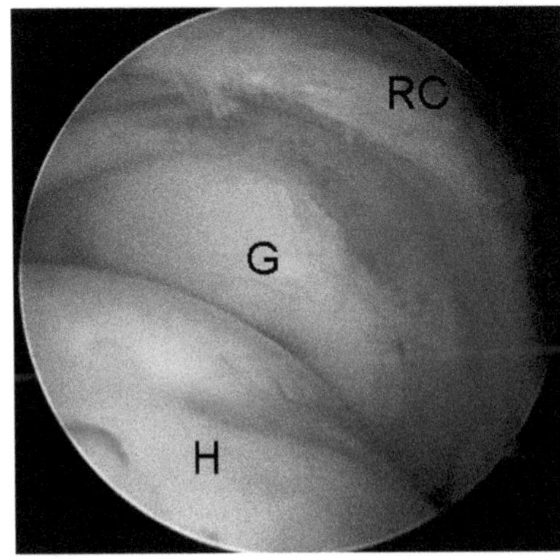

FIGURE 6 Massive, contracted, immobile rotator cuff tear. Arthroscopic view through a lateral subacromial portal of a typical massive, contracted immobile rotator cuff tear with minimal mobility from a medial to lateral and an anterior to posterior direction. *Abbreviations*: G, glenoid; H, humeral head; RC, rotator cuff.

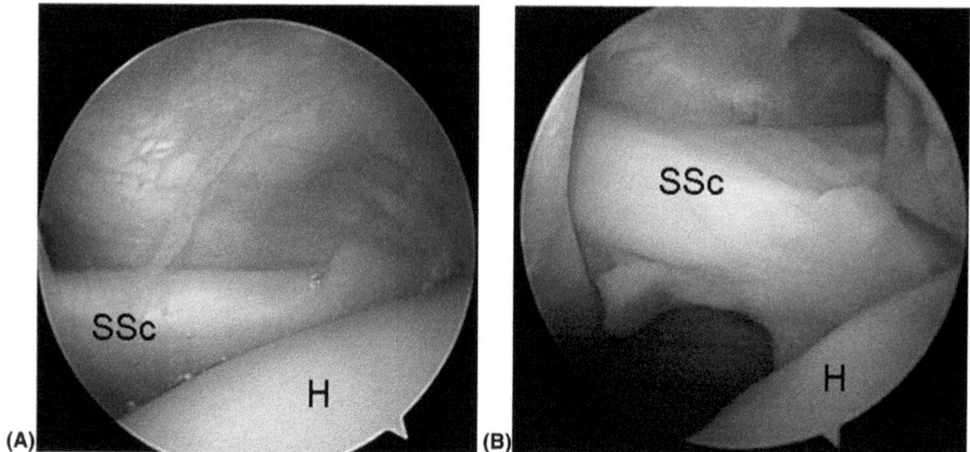

FIGURE 7 Arthroscopic view of the subscapularis insertion of a right shoulder from the posterior portal, using a 30° arthroscope with the arm in 30° of abduction: (**A**) neutral rotation and (**B**) internal rotation. Note how internal rotation slackens the overlying subscapularis fibers and reveals the intact subscapularis insertion. *Abbreviations*: H, humeral head; SSc, subscapularis tendon.

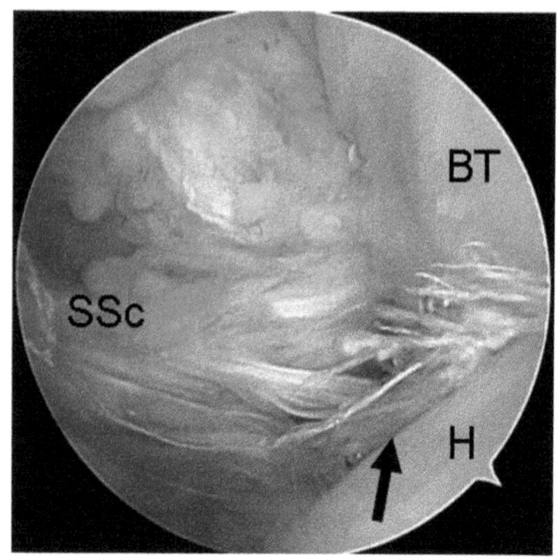

FIGURE 8 Arthroscopic view of the subscapularis insertion of a right shoulder from a posterior portal with the arm in 30° of abduction and internal rotation demonstrating a partial tear of the subscapularis tendon. Note how the tearing of the fibers exposes the underlying footprint of the subscapularis insertion (*arrow*). *Abbreviations*: BT, biceps tendon; H, humeral head; SSs, subscapularis.

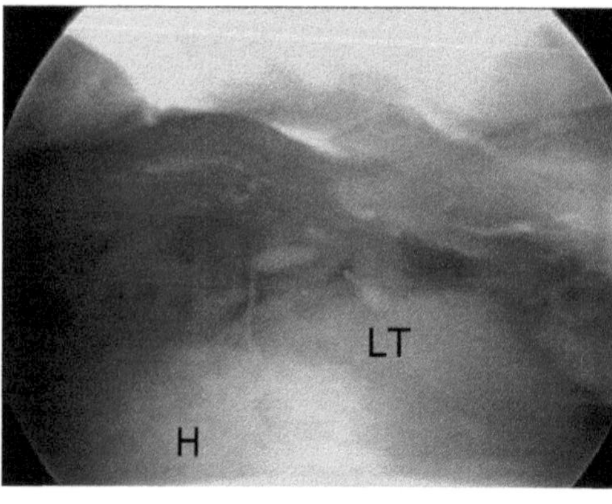

FIGURE 9 Arthroscopic "aerial" view of a right shoulder from a posterior portal using a 70° arthroscope, demonstrating a full-thickness tear of the subscapularis tendon with exposed lesser tuberosity. *Abbreviations*: H, humeral head; LT, lesser tuberosity.

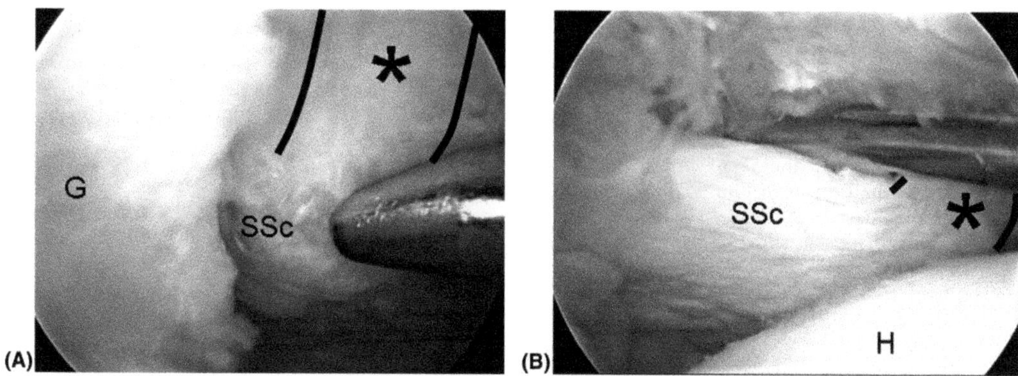

FIGURE 10 The comma sign. Arthroscopic views through a posterior portal using a 30° arthroscope. (**A**) The comma sign is formed by the comma-shaped arc of a portion of the superior glenohumeral ligament/coracohumeral ligament complex (*), which has torn off the humerus. The comma-shaped arc (*) extends to the superolateral corner of the subscapularis tendon. Arthroscopic views of a right shoulder demonstrating a subscapularis tendon tear retracted to the glenoid. (**B**) Traction on the comma sign and the superolateral border of the subscapularis tendon reveals the true borders of the subscapularis. The subscapularis tendon had been significantly retracted, medially and inferiorly. *Abbreviations*: G, glenoid; H, humeral head; SSs, subscapularis.

REFERENCES

1. Burkhart SS, Johnson TC, Wirth MA, Athanasiou KA. Cyclic loading of transosseous rotator cuff repairs: tension overload as a possible cause of failure. Arthroscopy 1997; 13(2):172–176.
2. Lo IK, Burkhart SS. Double-row arthroscopic rotator cuff repair: re-establishing the footprint of the rotator cuff. Arthroscopy 2003; 9(9):1035–1042.
3. Burkhart SS. The principle of margin convergence in rotator cuff repair as a means of strain reduction at the tear margin. Ann Biomed Eng 2004; 32(1):166–170.
4. Lo IK, Burkhart SS. Arthroscopic repair of massive, contracted, immobile rotator cuff tears using single and double interval slides: technique and preliminary results. Arthroscopy 2004; 20(1):22–33.
5. Lo IK, Burkhart SS. The comma sign: An arthroscopic guide to the torn subscapularis tendon. Arthroscopy 2003; 19(3):334–337.
6. Lo IK, Burkhart SS. Arthroscopic coracoplasty through the rotator interval. Arthroscopy 2003; 19(6):667–671.
7. Lo IK, Parten PM, Burkhart SS. Combined subcoracoid and subacromial impingement in association with anterosuperior rotator cuff tears: an arthroscopic approach. Arthroscopy 2003; 19(10): 1068–1078.

20 Arthroscopic Rotator Cuff Repair Instruments and Equipment: Setting Yourself Up for Success

A. Martin Clark, Jr.
The CORE Institute, Sun City West, Arizona, U.S.A.

Peter J. Millett
The Steadman-Hawkins Clinic, Vail, Colorado, U.S.A.

The purpose of this chapter is to discuss the tools, instruments, and equipments that are available for arthroscopic rotator cuff repair. Once a determination has been made that the patient has a reparable rotator cuff tear, having the appropriate set up and equipment available to fix the tear is essential. The authors describe the key instruments needed and how they influence the key steps of the procedure. An improved understanding of the instruments and equipments available for arthroscopic rotator cuff repair and how to use them properly will help make the procedures easier and more efficient, and this in turn will result in improved clinical outcomes for patients.

POSITIONING

The authors prefer to use the beach-chair position as described in chapter 1. An operating table that allows good exposure to the entire shoulder and does not limit arm positioning is a must. The medial border of the scapula must be free so that there is room to pass instruments at the necessary angles. The authors also recommend the use of a mechanical arm holder, such as the Spider limb positioner (Tenet Medical Engineering; Calgary, Canada) or the McConnell arm holder (McConnell Orthopedic Manufacturing Company; Greenville, Texas, U.S.A.), in order to position the arm appropriately during different parts of the case. The arm holder is one of the most important pieces of equipment that facilitates arthroscopic rotator cuff repair—it allows the surgeon to apply traction to the arm, which opens the subacromial space and thus improves visualization; it allows the tear to be rotated into the optimal position; and it obviates the need to have an assistant for arm positioning. Surgeons may also choose to position the patient in the lateral decubitus position, which necessitates the use of lateral traction to place the arm with the appropriate amount of traction and abduction. However, in the authors' opinion, this position does not allow dynamic inspection and movement as readily as the beach chair with an arm holder.

INSTRUMENTATION

There have been great advances in the last few years in arthroscopic shoulder instrumentation. The advent of procedure-specific instruments has greatly facilitated arthroscopic rotator cuff repair.

The basic instruments should include a 30° arthroscope (a 70° can be helpful at times), a motorized shaver, a radiofrequency tissue ablation device, and basic open retractors (particularly, if the rotator cuff repair procedure is converted to open procedure or if an open biceps tenodesis is planned). The authors prefer to use an arthroscopic pump for fluid management, as this allows the surgeon to control the pressure as needed. The authors also use epinephrine in the saline, as this has been shown to decrease bleeding. It is helpful to keep the pump

Please refer to pages 215–218 for the figures in this chapter.

pressure as low as possible so that extravasation of the fluid does not occur. Standard arthroscopic instruments should include an arthroscopic probe, scissors, various graspers, switching sticks, and tissue punches.

The procedure-specific instruments for arthroscopic rotator cuff repairs include instruments, such as crochet hooks, suture retrievers, and tissue graspers (Fig. 1) designed to mobilize the rotator cuff tendons, elevators to mobilize and release tissues, knot pushers, and guillotine knot cutters (which are essential if high-strength sutures are used). Penetrating direct suture passers, such as the Penetrator and BirdBeaks (Arthrex; Naples, Florida, U.S.A.) should also be in this set (Figs. 2 and 3). Depending on the surgeon's preference, reusable suture passers may also be utilized. Examples include the Viper, Needle punch, Scorpion (Arthrex; Naples, Florida, U.S.A.), ExpresSew (Surgical Solutions; Valencia, California, U.S.A.), and Spectrum and Caspari punch suture passers (CONMED Linvatec; Largo, Florida, U.S.A.) (Figs. 4–7).

DISPOSABLES

Disposable single use items include the appropriate clear cannulae, which will be needed, disposable suture passers or shuttling devices, free sutures, and anchors. While it is possible to perform the entire procedure percutaneously without the use of cannulae, the authors always recommend tying the sutures through cannulae to avoid entangling the sutures in the soft tissues of the deltoid and its deep fascia. The cannulae can also aid in suture management by simply parking unwanted sutures outside the working cannula (Fig. 8).

Other items that should be readily available include a burr that can be used to perform the acromioplasty, a full radius shaver, and the appropriate radiofrequency ablation wand (Figs. 9–11). The authors prefer to use 4.5 mm shavers and burrs, as this diameter decreases the turbulence seen with larger diameter shavers. The authors also prefer variable intensity bipolar radiofrequency ablation, as this effectively removes unwanted soft tissue and cauterizes tissues as needed. Suture passers and the surgeon's preferred anchors should also be available.

Once the surgeon has the appropriate items available, the surgery becomes more efficient since the circulating nurse and surgeon will spend less time looking for the desired tools and more time focusing on the procedure at hand.

Surgical Steps

The surgery can be divided into five steps and a review of the steps with the instruments needed at each step will make it easier for the surgeons to make sure that they have the equipment they desire. The stages are exposing the rotator cuff, mobilizing the cuff, placement of suture anchors, passing the sutures, and tying the sutures.

EXPOSURE

Exposure requires a thorough subacromial decompression. This typically takes place after the glenohumeral arthroscopy, during which the cuff is visualized from its articular side. While some surgeons have described waiting until the rotator cuff is repaired to perform the acromioplasty, in most instances, the authors prefer to perform the acromioplasty first, as this creates more room to work and prevents inadvertent damage to any sutures or repaired tendons. Inferior traction is applied with the arm holder, and visualization is initially achieved by placing the arthroscope directly behind the coracoacromial (CA) ligament. For resection of the bursa, the authors use a combination of the 4.5 mm shaver and an ablation device in the subacromial space.

The authors prefer to make the skin portals small so that fluid does not leak out and there is less turbulence. Four portals, widely spaced, are used for all routine cuff repairs. The authors resect all bursa from the lateral gutter and posterior recess of the subacromial space. Failure to do so will result in problems with visualization at later stages of the repair. The deep deltoid fascia should be preserved to prevent the deltoid muscle from imbibing water and swelling, as this will encroach upon visualization. The authors' preference is to use one 6 mm clear screw-in cannula through which the authors pass the anchors and tie the sutures. Smooth push-in cannulae are also available. These are useful for intra-articular work, as they will slide with the shaver as it is passed into deeper areas of the joint; however, smooth cannulae in the subacromial space may fall out with frequent instrument passing. The authors typically place a single cannula anterolaterally, while the remainder of the portals is used for percutaneous instrument passage. This set up minimizes incision size and trauma to the deltoid muscle, yet allows excellent visualization and permits flexible angles for instrument passage.

For debridement of the soft tissue, there are various types of shavers. The authors prefer a full radius shaver with suction. A less aggressive full-radius resector is preferred so that only bursal tissue is resected without harming the underlying rotator cuff or the overlying deltoid fascia. A burr (oval, round, or tapered) should be available to perform the acromioplasty. There are also devices that cut both soft tissue and bone, and the authors prefer this type of resector, as it is more efficient than switching back and forth between shaver and burr as one alternates between bone and soft tissue resection (Fig. 9). Again, the 4.5 mm size is quite effective because the pump can keep up with the outflow generated through the shaver, with subsequently less turbulence and less bone debris. Better visualization once again means better efficiency.

The radiofrequency ablation devices are helpful because they debride tissue without causing much bleeding. The authors prefer a bipolar device with suction in the head. The bipolar devices may generate more heat than the monopolar devices, but seem to allow for more efficient tissue ablation with clear visualization. The authors also prefer variable intensity energy and try to use the ablation device at low power, only when needed for cauterization. The mechanical shaver is the authors' preferred method of tissue resection. Indiscriminant use of radiofrequency may lead to thermal injury to nerves, chondral surfaces, bones, and tendons.

MOBILIZATION

Once the subacromial bursa has been debrided and the tear is identified, the cuff may need to be mobilized. Soft tissues are removed from the tuberosity, but the cortical bone is preserved. Again, the arm holder can be used to rotate the arm so that the tear is in perfect view. Because mobilization of the tear is frequently required, it is imperative that the shoulder repair set includes rotator cuff graspers, basket punches, and soft tissue elevators. The graspers are used like forceps in open surgery—to put traction on the cuff while releases are performed, and to determine tear morphology, the punches are used to freshen the tear edges and the elevators are used to mobilize retracted tendons by developing the necessary anatomic intervals. The shaver and ablation devices will also be used to mobilize the cuff, if the tear is chronic.

ANCHOR PLACEMENT

Next, the suture anchors are placed. If bioabsorbable anchors are to be used, then the appropriate drills, punches, and taps must be available. Either metal anchors or resorbable anchors are acceptable, and there are different designs with fully threaded or partially threaded screws. Screw-in absorbable anchors that are double-loaded are the authors' preference for most tears when bone quality is good. The surgeon should choose an anchor with an eyelet that maximizes sliding and minimizes abrading, as this has been shown to be a weak link in some earlier designs. Under cyclic loading, some sutures may fail at the eyelet due to abrasion. Most modern anchors have good resistance to bone pull-out. The new fully threaded designs may offer better purchase in the dense cortical rim of the tuberosity, and these designs may have some advantages in osteopenic bone. The authors prefer using high-strength sutures, as these are more resistant to breakage and damage during suture retrieval and tying. Most anchors come preloaded with sutures, although it is possible to reload anchors if desired. Suture type depends on surgeon preference, and there are many different commercially available and acceptable types. Most surgeons prefer high-strength sutures [Fiberwire by Arthrex, Herculine by CONMED Linvatec, Orthocord by DePuy Mitek (Rayndaam, Massachusetts, U.S.A.), and others] (Fig. 12).

SUTURE PASSAGE

For passing the sutures through the rotator cuff tendon, there are many different techniques that can be used. Passing can be divided into direct and indirect (shuttling) techniques. With direct suture passage, a sharp device is passed directly through the tendon and then one limb of suture from the anchor is retrieved and passed through the tendon in one step. With indirect techniques, two steps are required. In the first step, a device is passed through the tendon and then a "shuttle" made of wire or suture is passed through the tendon. The shuttle is then retrieved and the final suture is connected to the shuttle. In the second step, the final suture is passed or "shuttled" through the tendon. Direct passage is faster, but sometimes is not practical due to the angles that are needed. Shuttling, although requiring a second step, allows more flexibility in the angles needed and, in some instances, may permit smaller instruments to be passed through the cuff tissue with less damage to the tendon.

The devices for suture passage can also be classified into direct-passing devices or indirect-passing devices. The direct devices include such products as BirdBeaks and Penetrators, which are reusable. There are also needle-based devices, such as the ExpresSew, Needle Punch, Viper, and Scorpion, which allow suture passage through the cuff tendon directly from a lateral portal. These devices allow for a fixed bite of tissue (usually around 12–15 mm of tissue).

The indirect suture-passing devices that require two steps to shuttle the sutures include simple spinal needles that can be used with a polydioxanone suture (PDS) (Ethicon Inc., Somerville, New Jersey, U.S.A.) as the shuttle, Suture Lassos (Arthrex; Naples, Florida, U.S.A.), which uses a wire as the shuttle, the Caspari punches/Spectrum curved passers, which use PDS or a specially designed shuttle known as the "shuttle relay" to shuttle sutures, and the Accupass disposable passers, which come in various angles (Smith and Nephew; Andover, Massachusetts, U.S.A.) and use a loop of monofilament to act as the shuttle.

The proficient arthroscopic surgeon should become familiar with both direct and indirect suture-passing techniques and should be facile with one or two of these devices, in order to increase one's skill and ability to repair complex tears. Sometimes, one technique or device may allow a better angle or more efficient way of passing the suture. Understanding the different techniques will improve efficiency and efficacy of the repairs.

For the vast majority of cases, the authors prefer to use an indirect shuttling technique with a disposable passer, as this allows the most flexibility in positioning of the sutures and in the size of suture bite, permits the most reliability in instrument function, and creates the least damage to the tissue with a very small perforation.

TYING THE SUTURES

For retrieving the sutures, suture retrievers and crochet hooks are essential. Several manufacturers have these available. Sutures should be handled gently, and instruments that retrieve them should be smooth so as not to damage or fray them. A crochet hook is easy to use because it does not require space to open the jaws. It is better to use a crochet hook through a cannula to avoid getting its hook caught in the soft tissues of a percutaneous incision. A suture retriever, because of its tapered design, can be used percutaneously, although sometimes in tight spaces or inside of a cannula it may be difficult to open the jaws of the device. Some new types of retrievers have teeth at the tip, and thus they can be used to grasp tissues or sutures using the teeth or they can be used to retrieve sutures in an atraumatic way by grasping more proximally in the jaws so that the suture can slide as it is retrieved.

For tying and cutting the sutures, the surgeon must be well practiced at arthroscopic tying techniques and should have a knot pusher (either open or closed) and arthroscopic suture cutter in the repair set (Fig. 13).

Arthroscopic rotator cuff repair techniques may seem complex at first. However, having the appropriate equipment and tools is the first step toward increasing the efficiency of the procedure and optimizing the outcome for our patients.

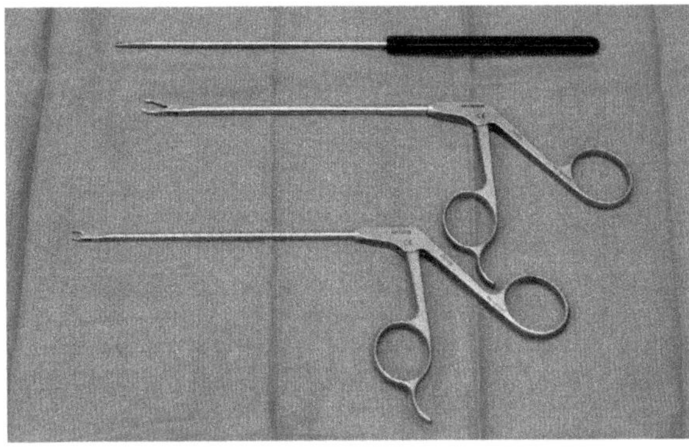

FIGURE 1 Various types of suture retrievers. (*Top*): Crochet hook (Linvatec). (*Middle*): Kingfisher (Arthrex) allows for grasping tissue/suture and atraumatic suture retrieval. (*Bottom*): Crab claw (Arthrex) atraumatic suture retriever. Atraumatic suture handling prevents damage to the suture that could compromise the repair strength.

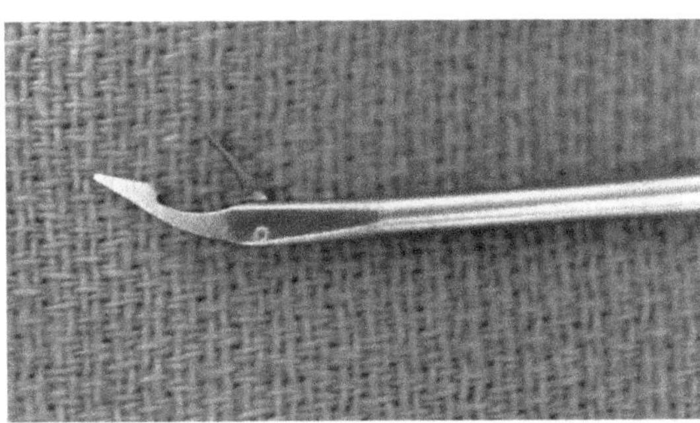

FIGURE 2 Close-up of tip of BirdBeak (Arthrex) suture retriever. This is a direct-passing device.

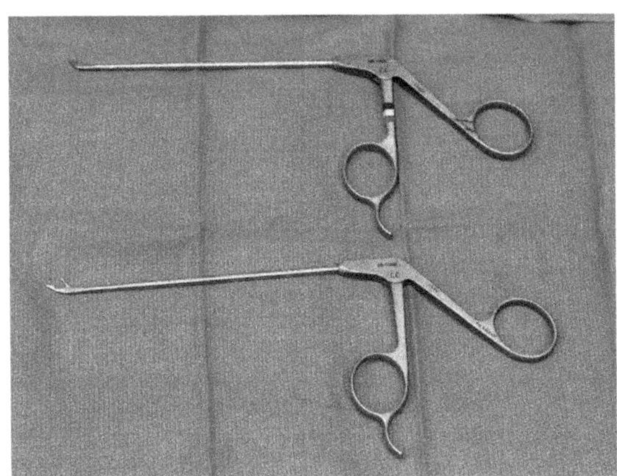

FIGURE 3 Variable angles of BirdBeak (Arthrex) suture retrievers. These devices are passed directly through the tissue, and then the sutures are grasped in the mouth of the instrument and pulled through the tissue.

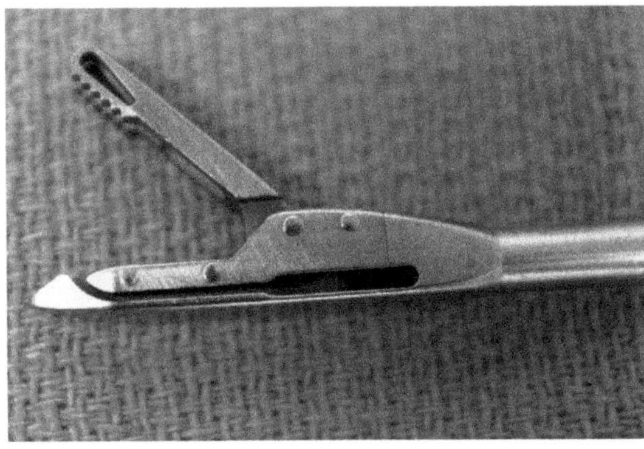

FIGURE 4 Needle punch tip (close-up) (Arthrex). This device requires a special needle, which is loaded into the tip. The tissue is grasped and then the needle with attached suture is passed through the tendon and retrieved on the opposite side.

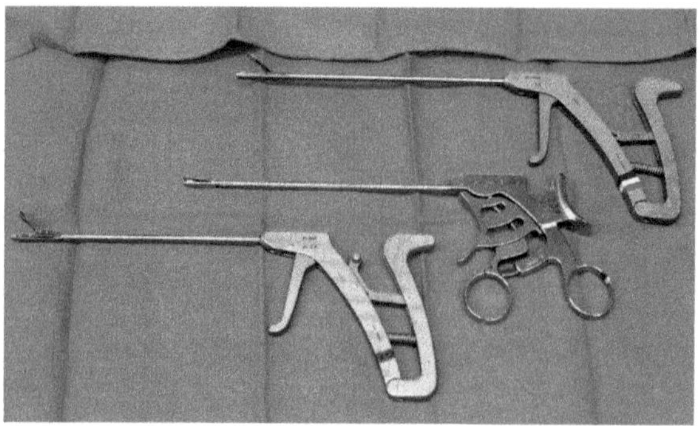

FIGURE 5 Direct suture-passing devices. (*Top*): Scorpion (Arthrex). (*Middle*): ExpresSew (Surgical Solutions). (*Bottom*) Needle punch (Arthrex). These devices rely on specially designed needles, which are passed through the rotator cuff tissue. They are also designed to allow for adequate bites of tissue, usually around 15 mm of tissue.

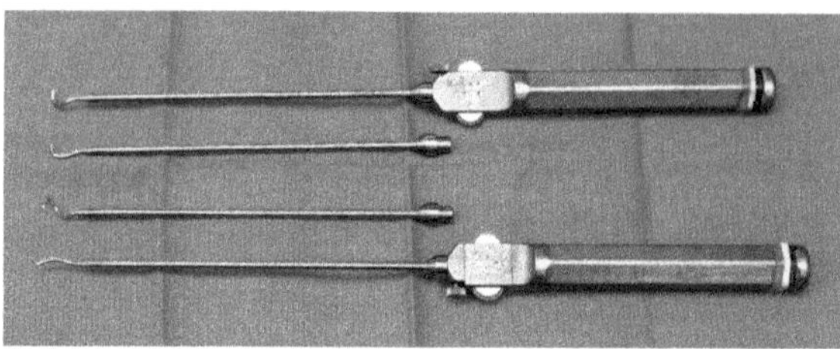

FIGURE 6 Spectrum suture passers with various angled tips (Linvatec). These are shuttling devices that require either monofilament suture or a "shuttle relay" (Linvatec) to pass sutures through tissue. The small diameter and variable angles make these devices very useful.

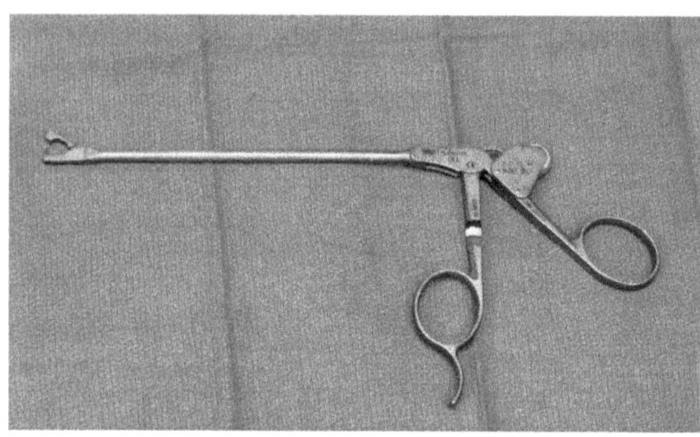

FIGURE 7 Caspari suture punch (Linvatec); this was the original arthroscopic suture-passing device. This is a shuttling device that relies on two wheels to push a monofilament suture through the needle tip, after the needle tip has been passed through the tissue. The monofilament is then used to shuttle the final suture through the tissue. There are modified designs with longer needles for the rotator cuff.

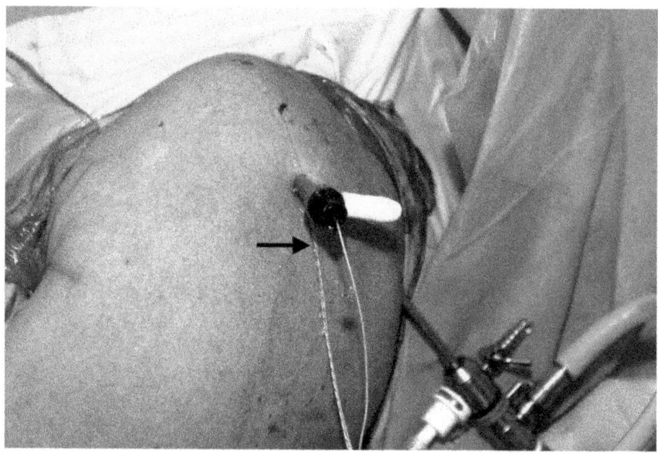

FIGURE 8 Technique for suture management using one portal: an anchor can be placed through the cannula. This prevents the anchor from getting caught in the soft tissues. Once the anchor is securely placed, the cannula can be removed. The sutures will now be exiting through the skin portal. The cannula is then replaced in the same skin portal. In this way, the sutures are now outside the cannula. The desired suture can then be retrieved in the cannula and either shuttled or tied. The steps can then be repeated for each suture coming from the anchor as needed. This simple sequence of steps helps tremendously with suture management and obviates the need for accessory portals and minimizes the risk of tangling.

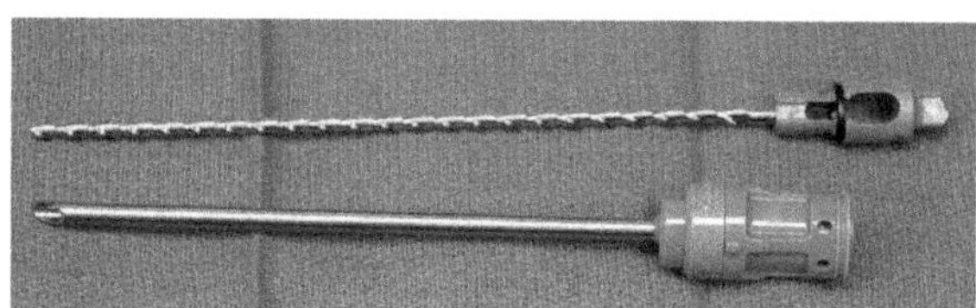

FIGURE 9 Helicut shaver (Smith and Nephew). Allows removal of both soft tissue and bone with same device. Flutes help prevent clogging.

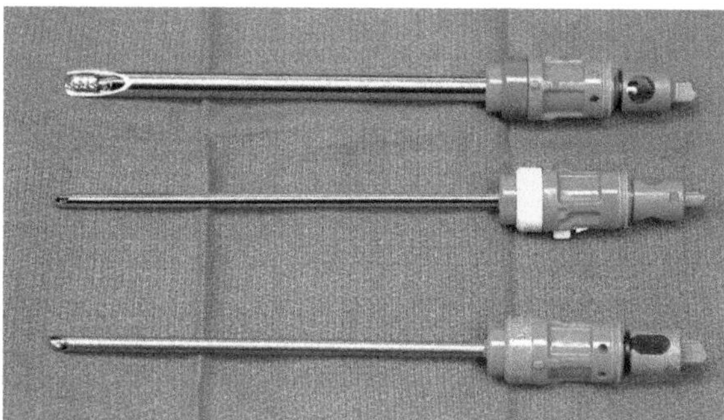

FIGURE 10 Various types of shavers and burrs. (*Top*): Acromionizer high-speed burr for bone resection (Smith and Nephew). (*Middle*): A 4.5 mm full radius shaver for soft tissue resection (Smith and Nephew). (*Bottom*): Helicut 4.5 mm high-speed resector for bone and soft tissue resection (Smith and Nephew).

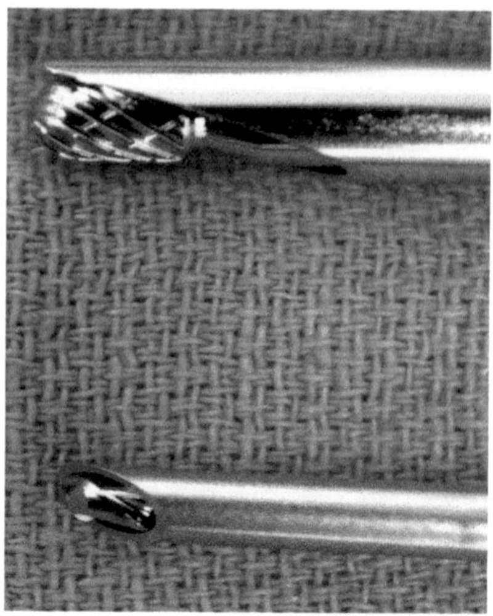

FIGURE 11 Close-up views of shaver tips. (*Top*): A 5.5 mm acromionizer (Smith and Nephew). (*Bottom*): A 4.5 mm helicut burr (Smith and Nephew).

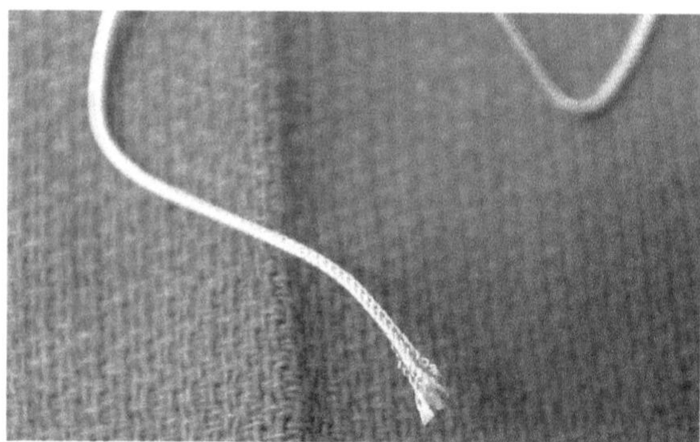

FIGURE 12 Fiberwire (Arthrex) #2 size—high-strength suture materal. High-strength sutures have become the standard in arthroscopic rotator cuff repair.

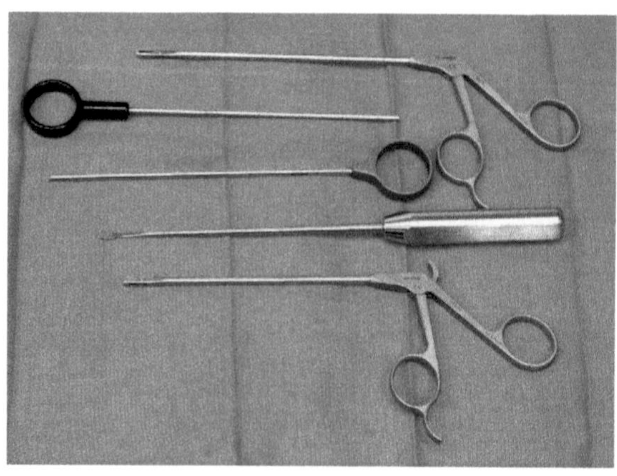

FIGURE 13 Miscellaneous arthroscopic instruments (from Top): Tissue grasper (Arthrex), closed-loop knot pusher (Linvatec), closed-loop knot pusher (Arthrex), knife rasp 15° angled elevator (Arthrex), and closed guillotine knot cutter (Arthrex).

21 Arthroscopic Releases for Rotator Cuff Repair

Kenneth J. Accousti and Evan L. Flatow
Department of Orthopedic Surgery, Mount Sinai Medical Center, New York, New York, U.S.A.

INTRODUCTION

Since the advent of arthroscopic rotator cuff surgery, surgeons have been repairing larger and larger tears arthroscopically. Arthroscopic repair of massive rotator cuff tears (tear diameter greater than 5 cm) has been associated with results comparable to massive tears treated by open methods (1). In addition, arthroscopic repair of large or massive rotator cuff tears preserves the deltoid with less morbidity than an open approach (2,3).

As more and more large and massive tears are repaired arthroscopically, it has become essential to properly mobilize the torn tendons allowing a repair without undo tension (4,5). Open techniques have been modified to arthroscopic approaches to release the contracted tendons from the surrounding tissues. One must understand the arthroscopic anatomy to properly release the rotator cuff muscles and tendons and prevent injury to the surrounding neurovascular structures.

ANATOMY

The tendons of the supraspinatus, infraspinatus, and teres minor form a continuous cuff of tissue that insert onto the greater tuberosity. There is slight thinning of the tendon insertion between the supraspinatus and infraspinatus. The rotator interval separates the supraspinatus tendon from the subscapularis, which inserts anteriorly on the lesser tuberosity. The long head of the biceps brachii tendon runs in the bicipital groove between the greater and lesser tuberosities (6).

Most tears initially involve the supraspinatus tendon. It is important to recognize tear configuration to properly plan reconstruction (see chap. 20 for more in-depth details). If the anterior portion of the supraspinatus is torn, the posterior corner of the tendon will still be tethered to the infraspinatus, creating an L-shaped tear (Fig. 1). The converse is true with a posterior supraspinatus tear, with the anterior supraspinatus tethered to the rotator interval producing a reverse L-shaped tear (Fig. 2). Crescent tears are smaller, more mobile tears involving the supraspinatus tendon, while U-shaped tears are large retracted tears, which may extend into the infraspinatus and subscapularis (Fig. 3A and B). Large L-shaped tears may appear as a U-shaped tear, but it is important to make this distinction because the repair and release will be different for each tear configuration.

The rotator interval is comprised of the coracohumeral ligament, superior glenohumeral ligament, and glenohumeral joint capsule. The coracohumeral ligament originates from the lateral border of the coracoid and inserts onto both the greater and lesser tuberosities of the humerus surrounding the bicipital groove. It divides into an intra- and extra-articular component, which surrounds the long head of the biceps tendon. It is a primary restraint to humeral external rotation when the arm is adducted. Tetro et al. (7) showed that arthroscopic release of the rotator interval completely resected the coracohumeral ligament.

Please refer to pages 222–228 for the figures in this chapter.

INDICATIONS AND CONTRAINDICATIONS

Mobile tears that can be fixed in a medial–lateral direction (crescent-shaped and U-shaped) or in a side-to-side direction (massive U-shaped) do not typically require releases. Indications for releases include tear patterns that are not mobile despite testing in medial–lateral and antero-posterior directions. Glenohumeral capsular releases, anterior interval slide, and the posterior interval slide are the releases necessary dependent on the specific tear pattern as discussed subsequently. Subacromial releases need to be performed in most revision cases, as well, as there is often subacromial scarring directly to the torn cuff tissue.

SURGICAL TECHNIQUE

The patient is placed in the beach chair (author's preference) or in the lateral decubitus position depending on surgeon's preference after interscalene regional block and/or general anesthesia has been administered. We routinely use interscalene block without general anesthesia and have reported a low rate of problems (8). A standard posterior arthroscopic portal is made 2 cm inferior and 1 cm medial to the posterior lateral corner of the acromion. A standard glenohumeral diagnostic arthroscopy and subacromial decompression is performed.

For massive tears, preservation of the coracoacromial (CA) arch during acromioplasty is vital to prevent anterosuperior escape of the humeral head. A more "minimal" acromioplasty is performed, leaving the anterolateral falx of the coracoacromial ligament in continuity with the lateral deltoid fascia. Occasionally, if the leading edge of the coracoacromial ligament is detached during removal of a spur, it is repaired with sutures to the anterior acromion. (Fig. 4A–C) Bleeding is meticulously controlled with electrocautery.

It is very important to then remove the subacromial bursa and free the lateral gutter between the deltoid fascia and humerus/rotator cuff to provide adequate visualization in the subacromial space for tendon mobilization and repair. The footprints on either the greater or lesser tuberosity where the tendons are to be reattached are debrided of all soft tissue. Large excrescences are usually present on the greater tuberosity in patients with massive rotator cuff tears. These should be burred down to prevent further impingement under the acromion and to protect the tendon repair. The tendon edges are also debrided to create a fresh edge for tendon to bone healing.

At this time, tendon mobility of the torn rotator cuff is assessed with an atruamatic tissue grasper through the lateral portal. Depending on the chronicity of the tear, some large, retracted tears may still be very mobile and require only a small release if the tear is addressed early. Long-standing chronic tears with retraction will usually be less mobile and require an adequate release to help repair the tendon to the greater tuberosity without undue tension. Subscapularis tendon mobility can also be assessed either with a tissue grasper through the lateral or anterior portal. It is also important to understand tear configuration and orientation to properly plan the release and repair. Isolated supraspinatus tears may be U-shaped, L-shaped, or crescent-shaped.

The superior glenohumoral joint capsule is first released. A 30° arthroscope is placed in the posterior portal in either the subacromial space or within the glenohumeral joint depending on the size of the tear. An arthroscopic scissors or cautery (via the lateral portal) is used to incise the joint capsule over the superior aspect of the glenoid (Fig. 5). It is important to preserve the superior labrum and biceps anchor during this release. The suprascapular nerve lies approximately 1 cm medial to the glenoid rim as it passes from the supraspinatus to the infraspinatus via the spinoglenoid notch (9).

If more mobility is needed, an anterior interval slide is performed next. The anterior interval slide releases the anterior edge of the supraspinatus from the coracohumeral ligament and rotator interval (10,11). This is performed with either the arthroscope in the posterior or lateral portal. Lo and Burkhart (14) prefer the standard lateral portal for viewing with an accessory lateral "working" portal for instrumentation. For isolated supraspinatus tears, the rotator interval is completely released starting from the lateral rotator interval, which is just anterior to the biceps tendon, down to the coracoid base (Fig. 6). A traction suture is placed through the anterior half of the supraspinatus to help stabilize the tendon once released as well as to facilitate visualization of the apex of the release. The cut is started at the anterior leading edge of the biceps root and continues anteromedially to the base of the coracoid, releasing the coracohumeral ligament. An arthroscopic scissors or cautery is then used to separate the supraspinatus from the interval consisting of glenohumeral joint capsule and any adhesions to the coracoid.

It is important not to dissect medial and inferior to the coracoid to prevent injury to the neurovascular bundle. Release of either the superior capsule or coracohumeral ligament alone reduces tension by an average of 25% on the repaired supraspinatus tendon. Release of both the superior capsule and coracohumeral ligament reduces the tension on the repaired supraspinatus by 40% to 60% (12).

A posterior interval release can also be performed if more mobilization is needed or if there is a reverse-L tear configuration in which the posterior supraspinatus is retracted (13–15). It is difficult to locate the interval between the infraspinatus and supraspinatus tendons laterally, because the tendons converge to form a continuous cuff of tendon. Therefore, the posterior interval must first be localized between the muscle bellies of the supraspinatus and infraspinatus, medially. The landmark is the spine of the scapula that separates these two muscles. First, the fibrofatty tissue that lies medially in the subacromial space must be resected to visualize the spine as it rises to form the acromial arch. This is a highly vascularized tissue and bleeding is very common and can become problematic if not controlled once it is recognized. We prefer to resect this tissue using the electrocautery. Once the lateral border of the spine is visualized, the posterior interval can then be determined. One traction suture is placed into the posterior supraspinatus tendon and another traction suture is placed into the anterior border of the infraspinatus tendon. An arthroscopic scissor is used via an accessory lateral portal, which is placed posterior to the standard lateral portal. While viewing from the lateral portal, with traction on both sutures, the release is started laterally between the sutures and progresses in a medial direction toward the scapular spine. It is extremely important to lift the blades of the scissors upwards to avoid injury to the suprascapular nerve as it passes around the base of the scapular spine in the spinoglenoid notch (Fig. 7). A combined anterior and posterior interval slide can provide 5 cm of lateral mobility to the supraspinatus tendons.

If there is a concomitant subscapularis tear, Lo and Burkhart (16) described an interval slide "in continuity". This is similar to the standard anterior interval slide except that the lateral-most bridge ("comma") of rotator interval tissue connecting the anterior supraspinatus and superior subscapularis is left intact (Fig. 8). By preserving this connection between the supraspinatus and subscapularis, the tendons are more stable during the repair and once the tendon edges are pulled back down below the humeral head, the resultant hoop stresses help to maintain the reduction of the supraspinatus laterally.

Isolated retracted subscapularis tears are much more uncommon than supraspinatus tears or combined supraspinatus and subscapularis tears. One should have a heightened index of suspicion for a subscapularis tear if subluxation of the long head of the biceps tendon is noted. A "360°" release commonly used in open surgery is harder to perform arthroscopically. The axillary nerve passes inferior to the lower border of the subscapularis and arthroscopic release of this portion of the tendon places the nerve and posterior humeral circumflex artery at risk. Adequate mobilization, in most cases, can be obtained with a "270°" release from the eight to four o'clock position thus decreasing the risk to the axillary nerve (Fig. 9).

A traction suture is placed into the upper one-third of the subscapularis via a spinal needle with a polydioxanone (PDS) suture. This suture is then retrieved through a small stab incision and suture retriever on the anterior lateral shoulder. The traction suture allows the surgeon to maintain adequate tension on the free tendon edge during the release, helping to stabilize the tendon as well as improve visualization of the apex of the release. The upper border of the subscapularis tendon is identified by the "comma sign" that represents the confluence of the superior glenohumeral ligament, the coracohumeral ligament, and the upper border of the subscapularis tendon (17,18). The coracoid tip is located by palpation with a probe. The coracoid tip is cleaned of soft tissue using the electrocautery, and a coracoplasty is performed with an arthroscopic burr. The subscapularis is then released from the rotator interval and coracohumeral ligament with either a scissors or electrocautery.

With combined tears of the subscapularis and supraspinatus, an interval slide in continuity is performed, keeping the lateral cuff of rotator interval tissue between the supraspinatus and subscapularis intact. For isolated subscapularis tears, the entire rotator interval should be released if the tendon edge is retracted. The posterior border of the tendon is also released from the anterior joint capsule using the scissors to tease of the capsule from the undersurface of the subscapularis. The anterior surface of the tendon is also freed of any soft tissue adhesions and bursa. The axillary nerve can be visualized inferiorly and anterior to the subscapularis tendon. This "270°" release is usually adequate to achieve enough mobilization of the tendon edge back to the lesser tuberosity. Arthroscopic release of the inferior edge of the subscapularis has been reported (L. Lafosse, personal communication, 2004) but should only be attempted by experienced surgeons due to the close proximity of the axillary nerve. We have only had to perform this dissection occasionally, and have found cautery helpful as there will be a warning twitch of the deltoid as the cautery comes near to the nerve. The repair can be medialized 5 mm, if necessary, to decrease the tension on the repair.

PEARLS AND PITFALLS

Repairs of large and massive rotator cuff tears are now possible with results comparable to those of open repairs (1). The advantages of arthroscopic rotator cuff repair include decreased deltoid morbidity, shorter hospital stay, and cost. Arthroscopy allows for better visualization of the rotator cuff and allows for a better appreciation of tear morphology.

An adequate tendon release is important to allow for proper mobilization and tension free repair of the torn rotator cuff. One must first properly recognize the tear configuration to help plan the release. A thorough understanding of the anatomy is important to prevent injury to the neurovascular structures, including the suprascapular, axillary, and musculocutaneous nerves. For some massive, retracted tears with severe muscle atrophy, mobilization and repair may be impossible. For those cases, partial repair with debridement may be all that can be accomplished.

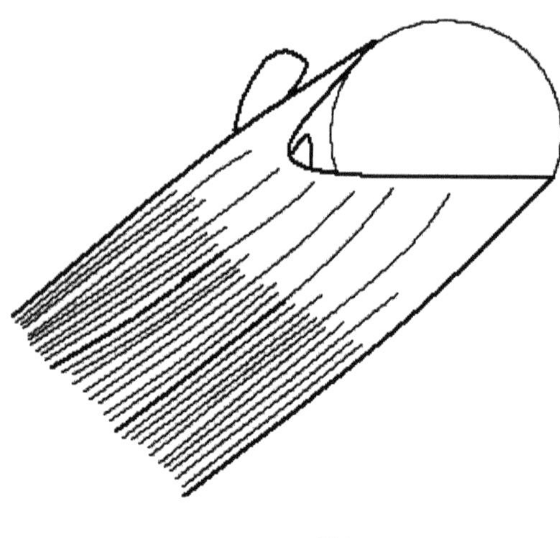

FIGURE 1 L-shaped rotator cuff tear.

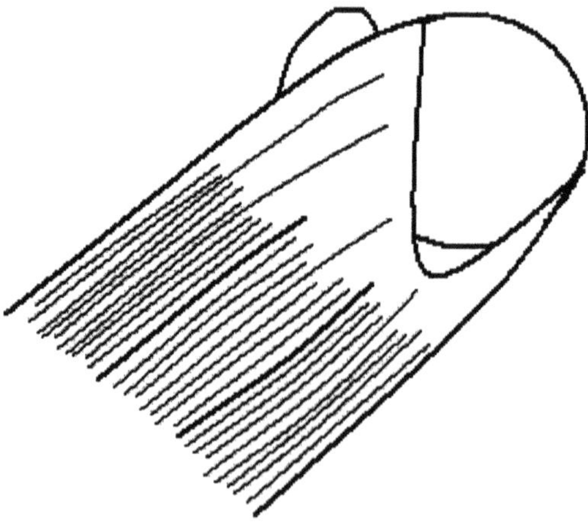

FIGURE 2 Reverse L-shaped rotator cuff tear.

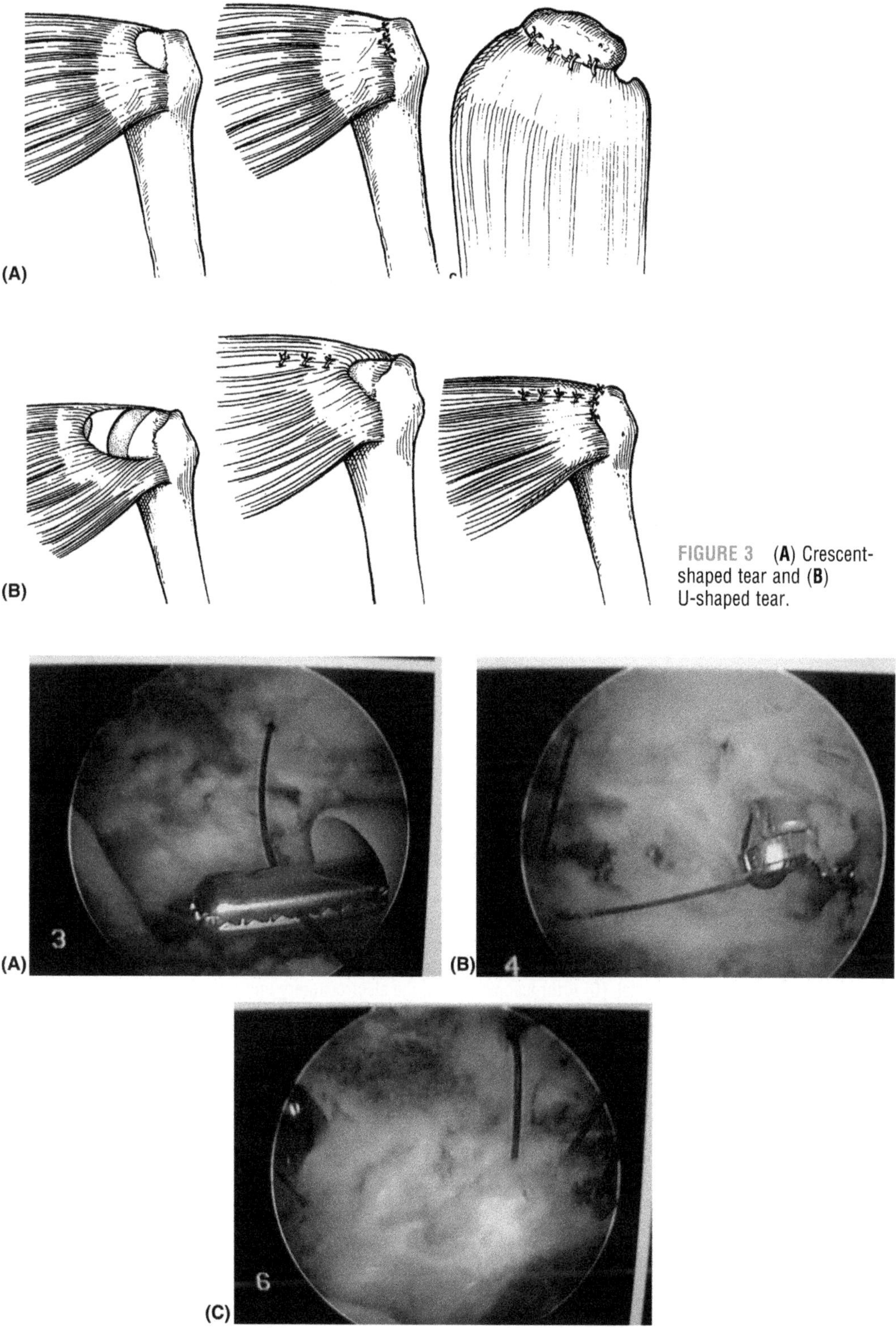

FIGURE 3 (**A**) Crescent-shaped tear and (**B**) U-shaped tear.

FIGURE 4 (**A**) Arthroscopic view of right shoulder in upright position, passing a polydioxanone (PDS) suture just anterior to leading edge of acromion with a spinal needle. (**B**) After passing the suture through the coracoacromial ligament (*bottom left*), the other suture end is fed into the subacromial space via a knot pusher and retrieved out the lateral canula (*right*). (**C**) Final repair of coracoacromial (CA) ligament to anterior lateral acromion. *Abbreviations*: PDS, polydioxanone suture; CA, coracoacromial arch.

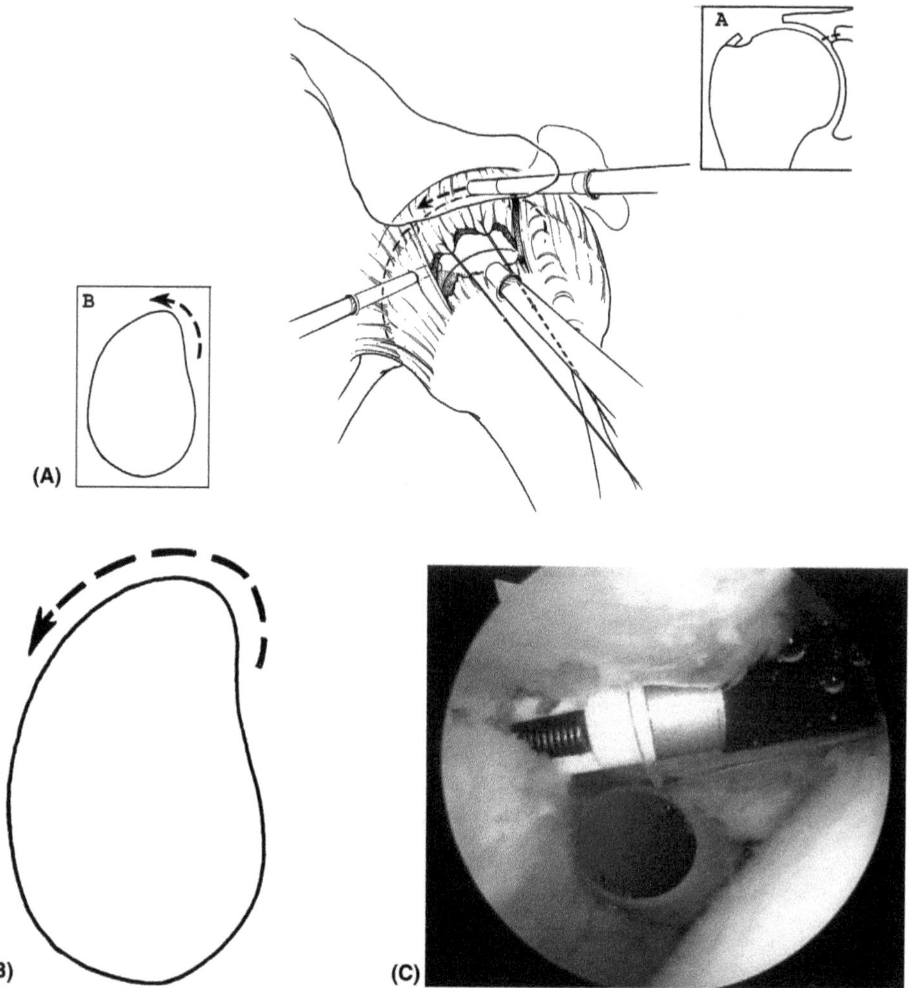

FIGURE 5 Diagram of the continuation of the anterior release over the superior aspect of the glenoid rim to perform a capsular resection (inset A). Again note the relative position of the release to the glenoid (inset B). The release is carried as far posteriorly as possible. (**A**) Drawing of capsular release performed superior to the glenoid rim. (**B**) Diagram of the capsular release performed over the superior aspect of the glenoid rim with the electrocautery unit now placed through the lateral portal. (**C**) Arthroscopic view of the electrocautery unit placed superior to the glenoid rim followed by elevator placement to remove any final adhesions. The traction sutures are used to pull the cuff laterally during this procedure to evaluate for excursion.

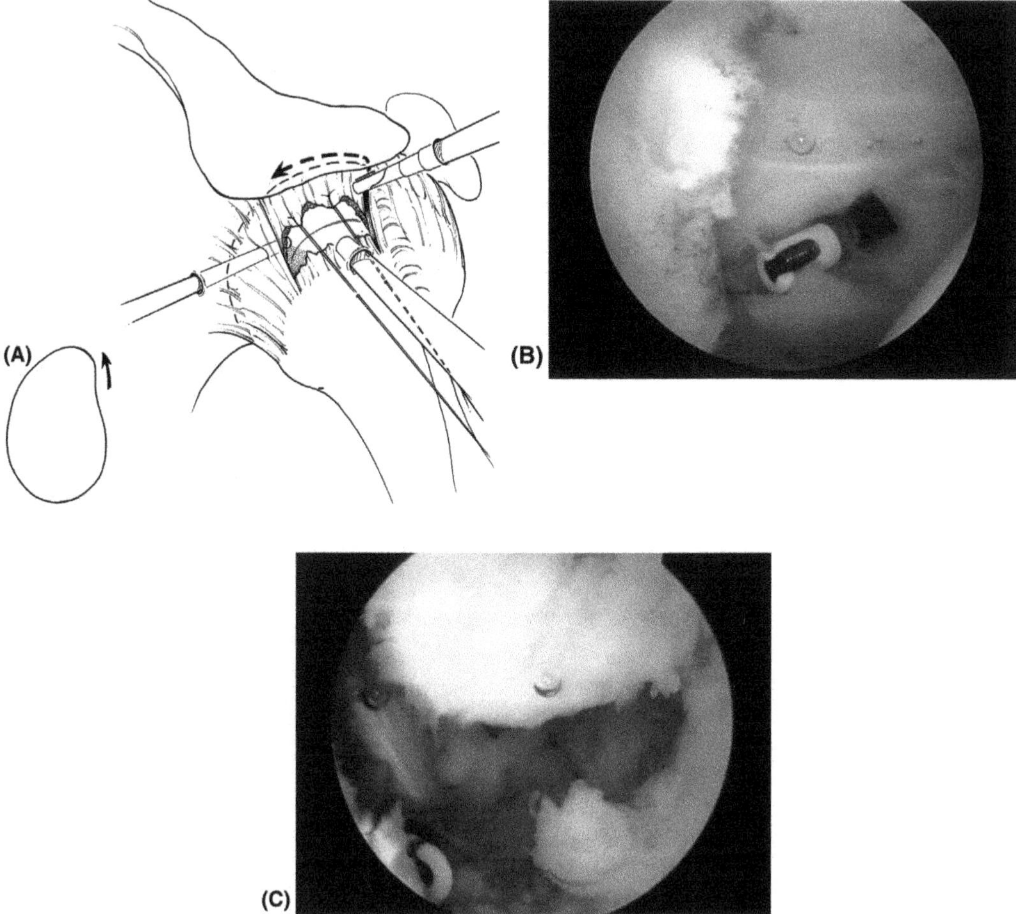

FIGURE 6 (**A**) Diagram of initiation of anterior release through the anterior portal along the rotator interval using the electrocautery device. Note the relative position of the release to the glenoid as it extends medially (inset). Arthroscopic view of anterior release performed through the anterior cannula (**B**) until the CA ligament is exposed and (**C**) seen as a shiny, white band in the right portion of the arthroscopic image. *Abbreviation*: CA, coracoacromial arch.

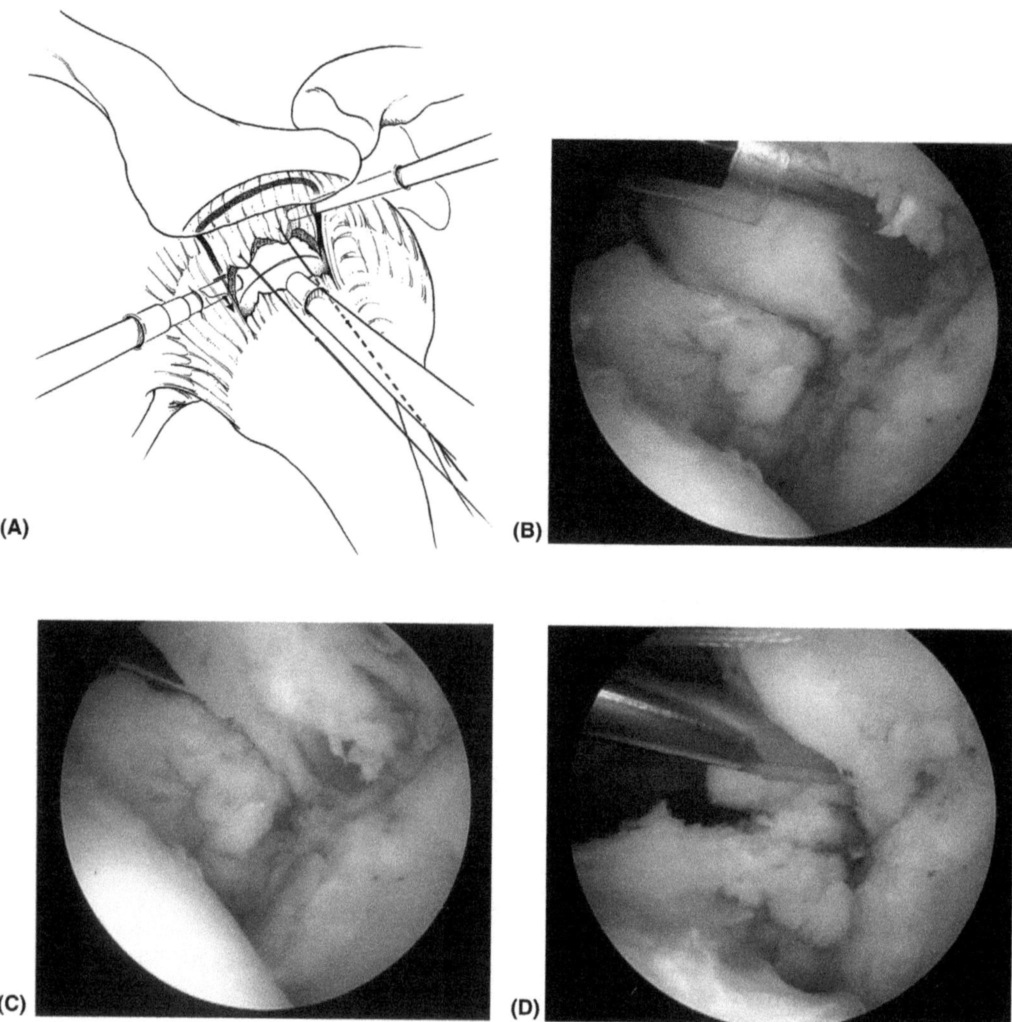

FIGURE 7 (**A**) Diagram of the posterior release with the arthroscope now placed through the anterior portal and the electrocautery unit placed posteriorly. (**B**) The posterior release is begun at the apex of the cuff tear along the glenoid rim and extended laterally (**C**). (**D**) An elevator is used to release any final adhesions.

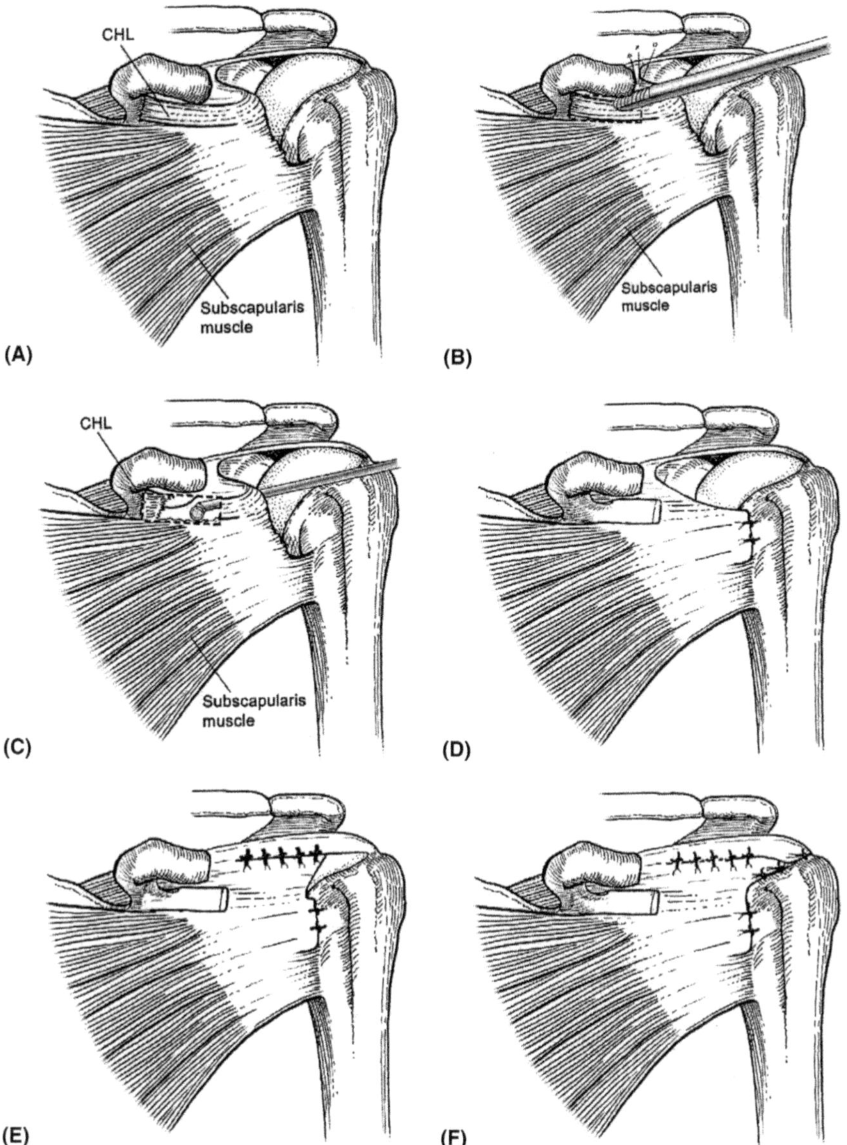

FIGURE 8 Diagram representing an interval slide in continuity. Anterior view of the left shoulder. (**A**) Rotator cuff tear involving the upper 50% of the subscapularis as well as the supraspinatus and infraspinatus tendons. (**B**) Coracoplasty using a burr from the anterior lateral portal. (**C**) The interval slide is begun by exposing the base of the coracoid using a shaver placed in the anterior lateral portal, releasing the coracohumeral ligament. The lateral margin of the rotator cuff is left intact (thus interval slide "in continuity"). (**D**) The subscapularis tendon is then repaired first, followed by the margin convergence of the U-shaped tear (**E**) and, finally, the supraspinatus and infraspinatus tendon edge to bone (**F**).

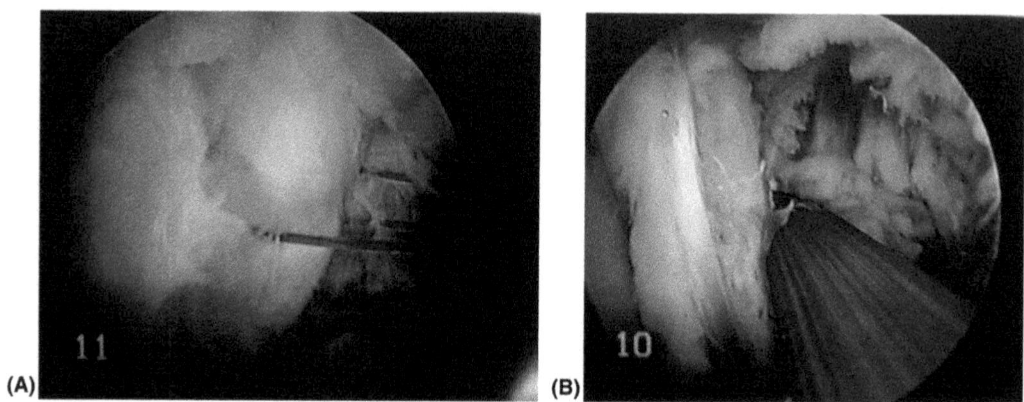

FIGURE 9 (**A**) Arthroscopic picture of right shoulder in beach-chair position looking from posterior portal showing traction sutures in free edge of subscapularis tendon. (**B**) Arthroscopic view from anterior lateral portal of a right shoulder in the beach-chair position with the cautery device releasing the anterior border of the subscapularis from the coracoid. The axillary nerve lies inferiorly (not shown in the picture) and care must be taken not to transect the nerve during the release.

REFERENCES

1. Burkhart SS. Arthroscopic treatment of massive rotator cuff tears. Clin Orthop 2001; 390:107–118.
2. Gartsman GM, Khan M, Hammerman SM. Arthroscopic repair of full-thickness tears of the rotator cuff. J Bone Joint Surg Am 1998; 80:832–840.
3. Tauro JC. Arthroscopic rotator cuff repair: analysis of techniques and results 2- and 3-year follow-up. Arthroscopy 1998; 14:45–51.
4. Burkhart SS, Diaz-Pagan JL, Wirth MA, et al. Cyclic loading of anchor based rotator cuff repairs: confirmation of the tension overload phenomenon and comparison of suture anchor fixation with transosseous fixation. Arthroscopy 1997; 13:720–724.
5. Burkhart SS, Johnson TC, Wirth MA, et al. Cyclic loading of transosseous rotator cuff repairs: tension overload as a possible cause of failure. Arthroscopy 1997; 13:172–176.
6. Klein JR, Burkhart SS. Identification of essential anatomic landmarks in performing arthroscopic single- and double-interval slides. J Arthroscopic Relat Surg 2004; 20(7):765–770.
7. Tetro AM, Bauer G, Hollstein SB, Yamaguchi K. Arthroscopic release of the rotator interval and coracohumeral ligament: an anatomic study in cadavers. J Arthroscopic Relat Surg 2002; 18 (2): 145–150.
8. Bishop JY, Sprague M, Gelber J, et al. Interscalene regional anesthesia for shoulder surgery. J Bone Joint Surg Am 2005; 87(5):974–979.
9. Warner JP, Krushell RJ, Masquelet A, Gerber C. Anatomy and relationships of the suprascapular nerve: anatomical constrains to mobilization of the supraspinatus and infraspinatus muscles in the management of massive rotator-cuff tears. J Bone Joint Surg Am 1992; 74-A(1):36–45.
10. Tauro JC. Arthroscopic "interval slide" in the repair of large rotator cuff tears. J Arthroscopic Relat Surg 1999; 15(5):527–530.
11. Tauro JC. Arthroscopic repair of large rotator cuff tears using the interval slide technique. J Arthroscopic Relat Surg 2004; 20(1):13–21.
12. Hatakeyama Y, Itoi Eiji, Urayama M, Pradhan R, Sato K. Effect of superior capsule and coracohumeral ligament release on strain in the repaired rotator cuff tendon. Am J of Sports Med 2001; 29(5):633–640.
13. Miller SL, Gladstone JN, Cleeman E, Klein MJ, Chiang AS, Flatow EL. Anatomy of the posterior rotator interval: Implications for cuff mobilization. Clin Orthop 2003; 408:152–156.
14. Lo I, Burkart SS. Arthroscopic repair of massive, contracted, immobile rotator cuff tears using single and double interval slides: technique and preliminary results. J Arthroscopic Relat Surg 2004; 20(1):22–33.
15. Codd TP, Flatow EL. Anterior acromioplasty, tendon mobilization, and direct repair of massive rotator cuff tears. In: Burkehead WZ Jr, ed. Rotator Cuff Disorders. Baltimore: Williams & Wilkins, 1996:303–334.
16. Lo I, Burkart SS. The interval slide in continuity: a method of mobilizing the anterosuperior rotator cuff without disrupting the tear margins. J Arthroscopic Relat Surg 2004; 20(4):435–441.
17. Lo I, Burkart SS. The comma sign: an arthroscopic guide to the torn subscapularis tendon. J Arthroscopic Relat Surg 2003; 19(3):334–337.
18. Richards DP, Burkart SS, Lo I. Subscapularis tears: arthroscopic repair techniques. Orthop Clin North Am 2003; 34:485–498.

22 Single-Row Arthroscopic Rotator Cuff Repair

Sara Edwards and Theodore A. Blaine
Center for Shoulder, Elbow, and Sports Medicine, Department of Orthopedic Surgery, Columbia Presbyterian Medical Center, New York, New York, U.S.A.

INTRODUCTION

With the advent of arthroscopic instruments and implantation devices, techniques to repair the rotator cuff arthroscopically have been further refined in the past decade. The most commonly performed technique of arthroscopic rotator cuff repair involves using a single row of implants to reattach the tendon to the rotator cuff footprint. While open repair is still the gold standard, the clinical outcomes of arthroscopic single-row repair have been comparable to open repair. Potential advantages of arthroscopic technique are smaller incisions and less injury to the deltoid origin. In this chapter, the authors describe their preferred technique for single-row arthroscopic rotator cuff repair.

INDICATIONS

Currently, due to increasing data that rotator cuff tears can worsen over time, there is a trend toward surgical fixation of rotator cuff tears to avoid the late development of irreparable rotator cuff tears or rotator cuff arthropathy. However, as these data are further analyzed and compared to the results of surgical fixation, traditional principles for the treatment of rotator cuff tears should be applied. Because rotator cuff tears can be present in the general population in the absence of symptoms or functional deficits, the presence of a documented rotator cuff tear alone does not require surgery. However, when a rotator cuff tear is identified in combination with pain or functional deficit that is not responsive to conservative treatment, surgery is indicated. Nonoperative treatment, consisting of nonsteroidal anti-inflammatory drugs (NSAID) use, physical therapy, and cortisone injection, is typically continued for three to six months prior to surgery. More urgent surgery may be indicated in young patients with acute tears and in older patients with acute or acute extensions of chronic tears. The ability to repair the cuff may be improved in these patients when surgery is performed within the first three weeks of injury.

CONTRAINDICATIONS

In the authors' practice, the size and nature of the rotator cuff tear does not preclude arthroscopic fixation. However, the authors recommend that surgeons perform the rotator cuff repair surgery to the best of their ability, even if that is an open procedure. The potential benefits of arthroscopic fixation are diminished, if the repair is inadequate. Visualization in the subacromial space is also necessary for full-thickness rotator cuff repair. As a result, prolonged arthroscopic decompression can lead to infiltration of the deltoid with fluid, compromising visualization and the repair.

SURGICAL TECHNIQUE

Preoperative planning should begin with the appropriate imaging studies. Routine radiographs are useful to assess underlying arthritis, acromial morphology, and the presence of an acromial spur. In both acute and chronic tears, documentation is recommended by use of magnetic resonance imaging (MRI) (Fig. 1). The MRI is important to assess the size and

---

Please refer to pages 235–242 for the figures in this chapter.

nature of the tear (partial vs. full-thickness), as well as the amount of fatty atrophy present in the rotator cuff muscle, as seen on the sagittal oblique views through the scapula. It also is useful to assess any other pathology, from the biceps tendon to the labrum. Finally, MRI can help to identify cystic changes within the greater tuberosity that may affect the ability to perform suture anchor fixation.

The patient is positioned in either the beach-chair or lateral decubitus position, based on surgeon familiarity and preference. In the authors' experience, they prefer the beach-chair position, which is referenced in the rest of this chapter. In addition, the authors use a hydraulic arm positioner that helps to pull traction when working in the subacromial space without requiring an assistant (Fig. 2). Regional anesthesia using an interscalene block is given, if possible. The authors prefer gravity inflow with epinephrine in the first three bags of irrigation.

The anatomic landmarks of the coracoid, clavicle, acromioclavicular joint, and acromion are marked on the skin (Fig. 3). The posterior inferior portal is made approximately 2 cm inferior and 1 to 2 cm medial to the posterolateral corner of the acromion. The anterior portal is made using an outside-in technique just lateral to the coracoid through the rotator interval. If an acromioclavicular joint resection is planned, this portal can be placed slightly superior.

Routine examination of the glenohumeral joint should be performed with notation of the condition of the cartilage on the humerus and glenoid, biceps tendon, labrum, and the presence of loose bodies. Intra-articular pathology should be addressed in an expeditious manner. Inspection of the rotator cuff should be performed from the articular side of the cuff, with care taken to examine the subscapularis first, followed by the supraspinatus and infraspinatus. If a subscapularis lesion is identified, this should be repaired.

Most rotator cuff lesions will be identified at the leading edge of the supraspinatus (Fig. 4). Using a full-radius shaving instrument, it is useful to debride any frayed tendon at this location to assess the size and thickness of the tear. Occasionally, the rotator cuff tissue will need to be probed to identify the full-thickness tear. If a partial tear originating from the articular surface is identified, intra-articular instruments, such as the shaver or probe, can be used to estimate the depth of the tear. Typically, a partial tear that involves less than 7 mm of the footprint can be debrided, while a tear of $\geq$7 mm (>50% of the tendon) should be repaired. This will be discussed in Chapter 24 in detail. If there is any question as to the continuity or condition of the rotator cuff, a marking suture of 0 or #1 monofilament absorbable suture can be passed through a spinal needle inserted into the area to assist in bursal side identification. For large retracted tears, intra-articular releases of adhesions on the undersurface of the rotator cuff can be performed using an electrocautery device in the space between the rotator cuff tissue and superior labrum.

Full-Thickness Rotator Cuff Repair

Following glenohumeral inspection, the trochar should be introduced into the subacromial space from posterior. The trochar can be swept in a medial to lateral direction underneath the acromion to clear bursa and adhesions. A lateral portal is established 2 cm lateral to the acromion, with the anterior edge of the portal at the level of the posterior border of the clavicle. A thorough bursectomy is performed, alternating between electrocautery and an aggressive 5.5 mm shaver. The bursa within the lateral gutter should be removed as well. Acromial spur and coracoacromial ligament resection is performed as necessary.

Attention is then focused on the tear. The tear morphology (crescent, L-shaped, and V-shaped) should be assessed from both the posterior and lateral portal (Fig. 5). A soft tissue grasper should be used to assess the tear mobility, and additional subacromial releases can be performed if the tear does not mobilize to the footprint (Fig. 6). Awareness of associated neurologic structures is critical and dissection more than 2 cm medially, especially posteromedially should be avoided to prevent injury to the suprascapular nerve. The footprint is identified and debrided using an aggressive shaver to remove the soft tissue and denude the bone over the greater tuberosity (Fig. 7). Suture anchor fixation is dependent on the cortical bone. While preparation to obtain a bleeding surface is typical, it is important to avoid aggressive decortication. Partially threaded 7 mm cannulas are placed into the anterior and lateral portals to allow the surgeon to easily access the tear from all directions.

Depending on tear morphology, marginal convergence sutures can be placed into the apex of a large, V-shaped tear or an L-shaped tear. This is best done by switching one of the 7 mm cannulas to the posterior portal and visualizing the tear from the lateral portal. A free #2 braided nonabsorbable suture is placed into a penetrating grasper to pierce the tissue on one side of the tear, and then passed to a reciprocal penetrating grasper on the opposite side (Fig. 8). Alternatively, there are multiple suture lassos that can be used to penetrate the cuff tissue that require subsequent shuttle of the suture. Sutures are then tied to reduce the size of the tear (Fig. 9).

Once the marginal convergence sutures are placed or if the tear does not require marginal convergence, the authors prefer to repair the tendon to the greater tuberosity using commercially available suture anchors. These anchors come in various sizes and compositions (bioabosorbable vs. metal). The choice as to size and type can be made based on bone quality and number of anchors needed to repair the tendon. The authors' current preference for a simple single-row repair is to use fully threaded bioabsorbable anchors (Biocorkscrew, Arthrex, Naples, Florida, U.S.A.). These may be placed directly through the cannula by rotating the arm, or may be placed through a percutaneous technique. A spinal needle is placed along the anterolateral edge of the acromion to the footprint. Once satisfied with the angle, a 15-blade scalpel is used to create an accessory portal in a vertical direction (Fig. 10). An appropriate tap is used to create a hole in the bone at approximately a 45° angle, followed by placement of the anchor. The anchor should be tested by pulling firmly on the attached suture to make sure it does not pull out. If the anchor fails, a larger diameter anchor can be placed in the hole without further tapping.

Once the anchor is placed, there are multiple devices used to pass the sutures through the tendon. From the lateral portal, one limb of suture from the anchor should be retrieved, with care taken to prevent unloading the suture from the anchor. This can be done by having an assistant grasp the complementary limb of suture from the accessory portal and by watching the anchor while pulling the free limb to make sure that the suture is not unloading from the eyelet. Once out of the cannula, care should also be taken not to let the cannula back out of the subacromial space, as soft tissue can get interposed between the cannula and suture. A suture-passing device, such as a Viper, Scorpion (Arthrex, Naples, Florida, U.S.A.), can be used (Fig. 11A and B). Alternatively, or in addition, a suture shuttling device can be introduced and used to pass suture through the cuff tissue. Traditionally, this technique has been used through Neviasier's portal, just medial to the acromion, although Blaine has also found a percutaneous technique posterior to the acromion to be particularly useful for more posterior tears. One limb of the suture can be placed to create a simple suture construct, or both limbs can be passed to create a mattress suture.

It is the authors' routine to place the anchor, pass the sutures, and then shuttle the sutures anteriorly, outside of the cannula. The sutures are passed from the portal (anterior, lateral, or posterior) that facilitates the best tendon purchase and reduction. Once all of the anchors are placed and sutures passed, the sutures are tied starting posterior, advancing anterior (Fig. 13). Meticulous suture management is required for this, and the anchors should be visualized as the suture limbs are shuttled out to avoid unloading the anchors. The sutures should be tied from a cannula that permits the most direct route for tying. The authors routinely use a sliding knot with three alternating half-hitches, alternating the post.

Small Full-Thickness Tear, Crescent Shaped

For small, single anchor repairs, the authors prefer to pass both limbs of one suture to create a mattress, followed by a single limb from the other suture more medial to the mattress configuration to perform a "cruciate-footprint" or Mason-Allen type repair. Both limbs of each suture are sequentially brought out of the lateral portal (mattress suture first) and tied using a low-profile sliding knot, followed by alternating half-hitches.

L-Shaped Tear

Margin convergence stitches are placed at the medial apex as described earlier. The first anchor should be placed at the lateral base of the "L," with the stitches placed in a simple pattern. This will reduce the tear anatomically. If possible, another lateral anchor is placed to fix more tissue to the tuberosity using simple sutures (Figs. 15A and B).

V-Shaped Large Crescent Tear

Margin convergence sutures are placed as described earlier (Fig. 16A and B). The authors recommend passing all sutures of the first anchor before placing the second. Once the first anchor sutures are passed, they are removed from the cannulas to prevent confusion. The second anchor can then be placed, followed by suture passage. The posterior sutures are tied first, followed by the sutures from the first anterior anchor (Fig. 17). Following fixation of the tear, the camera should be placed back into the glenohumeral joint to confirm adequate coverage of the humeral head.

SUBSCAPULARIS TEARS

The overall incidence of subscapularis tears is low compared to supraspinatous and infraspinatous tears. The location of these tears can make visualization difficult, particularly if significant swelling has occurred. These tears should therefore be addressed first in patients with multiple tendon tears.

Subscapularis repair is typically performed through three portals: anterior, anterolateral, and posterior. Portal sites are localized with a spinal needle, prior to placing cannulas. Partial subscapularis tears involving the superior one-third or one-half of the tendon are usually less retracted and more readily reduced. Complete tears with retraction can be adherent to the anterior capsule requiring mobilization (Fig. 18). Positioning the arm in flexion and internal rotation improves visualization of the lesser tuberosity footprint. The footprint is prepared with a burr, and the first suture anchor is placed inferiorly into the lesser tuberosity via the anterior portal. One limb of the suture is brought out of the anterolateral cannula. A Birdbeak or suture lasso (Arthrex, Naples, Florida, U.S.A.) is passed from the anterior cannula through the subscapularis tendon at the inferior aspect of the tear (Fig. 19). The nitinol loop is used to shuttle the suture limb through the tendon and out of the anterior cannula (Fig. 20). The same technique is repeated for other suture limb to create a mattress suture (Fig. 21). Additional anchors are placed, as dictated by the size of the tear. Following completion of the repair (Fig. 22), the arm is gently rotated to evaluate security of repair and limits for postoperative range of motion. External rotation is usually limited to 40° for four to six weeks postoperatively.

Rehabilitation

Despite the smaller incision used in arthroscopic rotator cuff repair, it is important to remember that the same length of postoperative protection and therapy is required to ensure tendon healing. Patients will frequently need to be reminded of the postoperative restrictions in rehabilitation because they may have less pain from surgery.

The rehabilitation begins with passive-assisted range of motion exercises on the first postoperative day; and, the program is tailored to the degree of rotator cuff injury and repair. Patients with small to medium size tears undergo a modified Neer phase I protocol for six weeks that includes pendulum exercises, passive-assisted forward elevation to 140°, and passive-assisted external rotation (supine) to 30° tears. In patients with large to passive tears, no physical tear is performed on the shoulder for four to six weeks. Pulley exercises are avoided for the first six weeks, in order to protect the cuff repair. Strengthening with isometric exercises is initiated at six weeks, accompanied by active-assisted range of motion. Use of weights is avoided for at least three months in the rehabilitation period to avoid re-tear. Resistance exercises with lightweights (1–3 pounds) can be initiated at 12 weeks, progressing to dynamic strengthening exercises at six to eight months. Patients should be aware that full return of strength might require 12 to 18 months.

For subacromial decompression only, the rehabilitation program is accelerated. The sling can be removed within the first one to two weeks, and the patient may use the arm for routine ADLs immediately. Return to athletics, particularly, overhead sports, however, should be delayed until 6 to 12 weeks to prevent the development of a postoperative bursitis.

Pearls and Pitfalls

1. A hydraulic arm positioner is useful to position the arm in space without the need of an assistant; traction may be applied, if necessary.
2. Avoid "suture madness" by placing anchors and sutures in small accessory portals. Only the suture limbs that are actively being shuttled or tied should be in the working cannula.
3. Cannulas should be used to avoid soft tissue interposition.
4. When a sliding knot does not slide easily, it should not be forced, as this can cause suture cut-out of the soft tissue. A simple knot may be used consisting of alternating half-hitches, instead.
5. The limb of suture that passes through the rotator cuff tissue should be the post for knot tying. This will help prevent tissue cut-out.

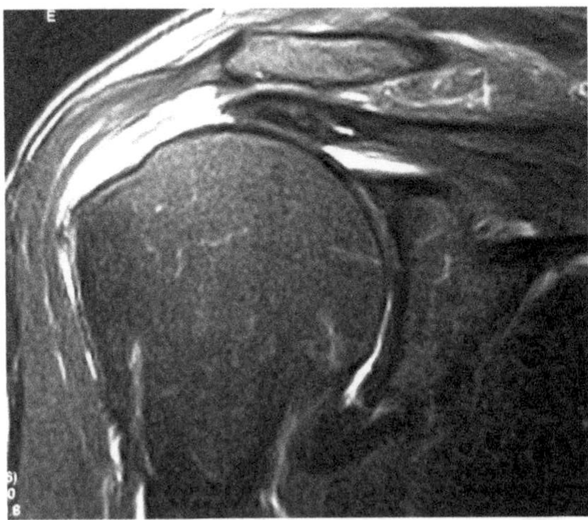

FIGURE 1 Coronal magnetic resonance imaging scan demonstrating a large full thickness rotator cuff tear.

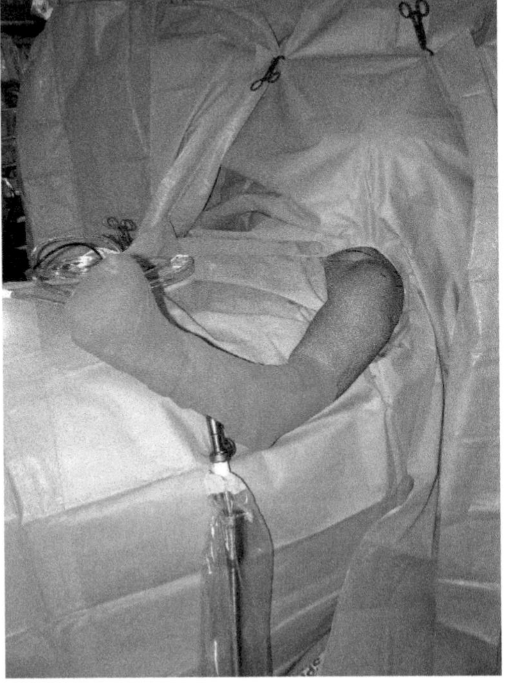

FIGURE 2 Hydraulic arm positioner used to position the arm with patient in the beach-chair position.

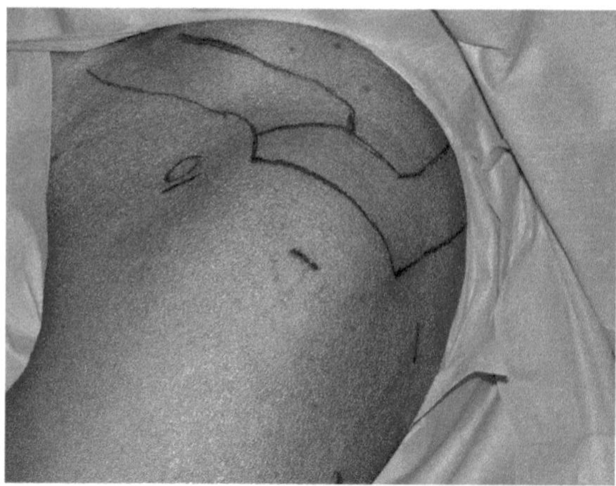

FIGURE 3 A left shoulder prepped and draped in the beach-chair position. The commonly used portals are shown (posterior, mid-lateral, anterior).

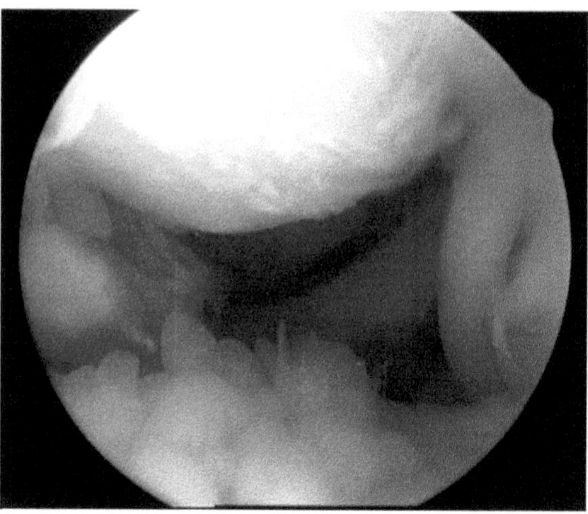

FIGURE 4 Arthroscopic view from posterior portal of the left shoulder. A full thickness tear of the supraspinatus tendon is seen.

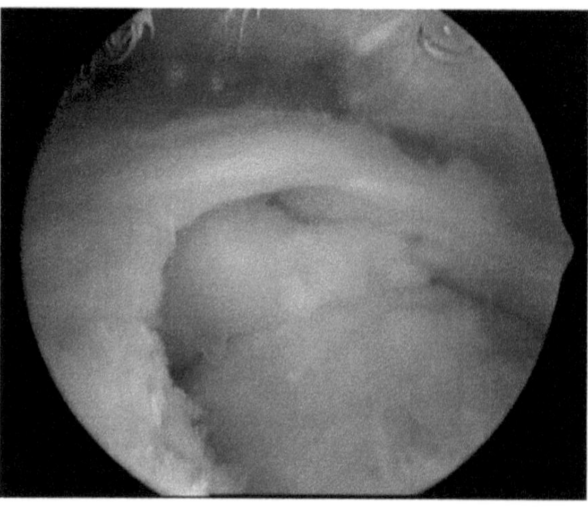

FIGURE 5 Arthroscopic view from posterior portal of the right shoulder. There is a large rotator cuff tear present which is in a "u-shaped" configuration.

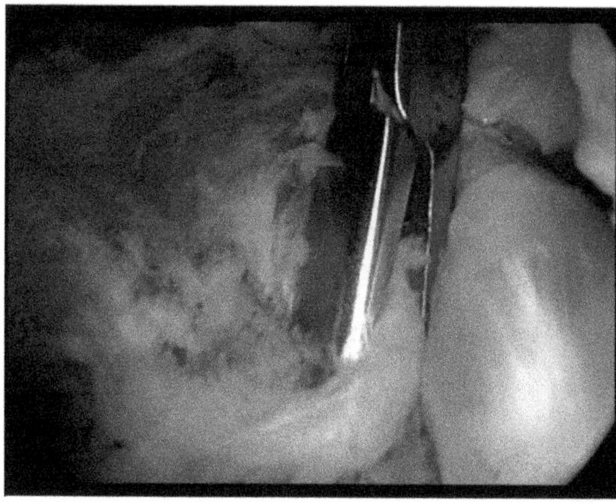

FIGURE 6 Arthroscopic view from posterior portal of the right shoulder. A soft tissue grasper is used to assess the mobility of the tear and plan for the repair.

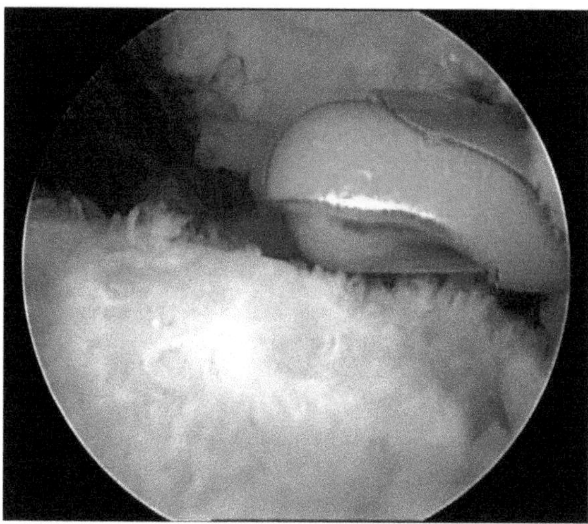

FIGURE 7 Arthroscopic view from posterior portal of the right shoulder. A motorized burr/ shaver is used to debride and abrade the greater tuberosity to stimulate a healing response.

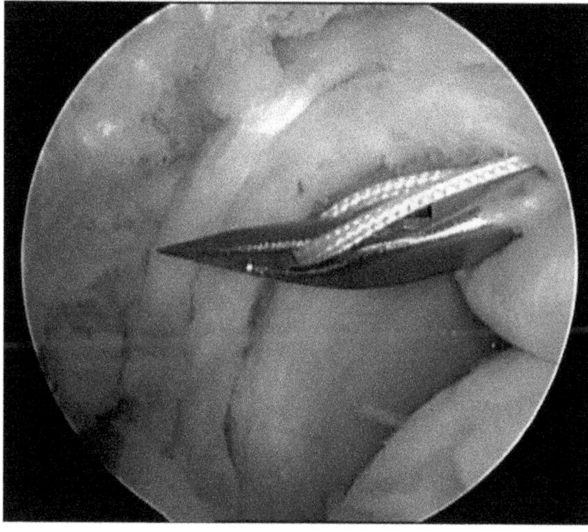

FIGURE 8 Arthroscopic view from lateral portal of the right shoulder. A blue fibrewire suture has been passed through the anterior edge of the u-shaped tear using a penetrator to perform margin convergence but has not yet been tied.

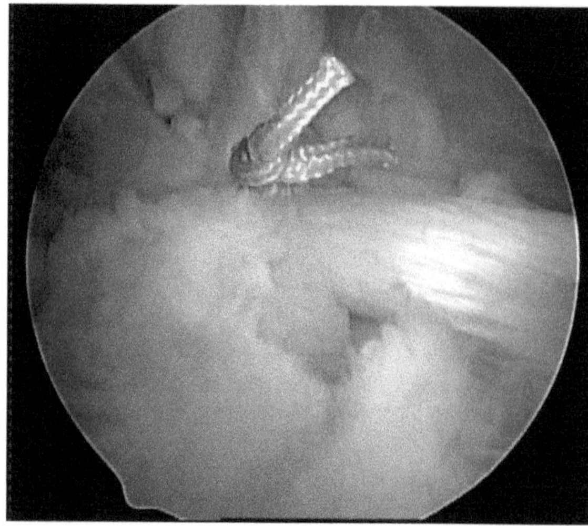

FIGURE 9 Arthroscopic view from lateral portal of the right shoulder. A blue fibrewire suture has been passed through the anterior and posterior edges of the u-shaped tear to perform margin convergence and has been tied.

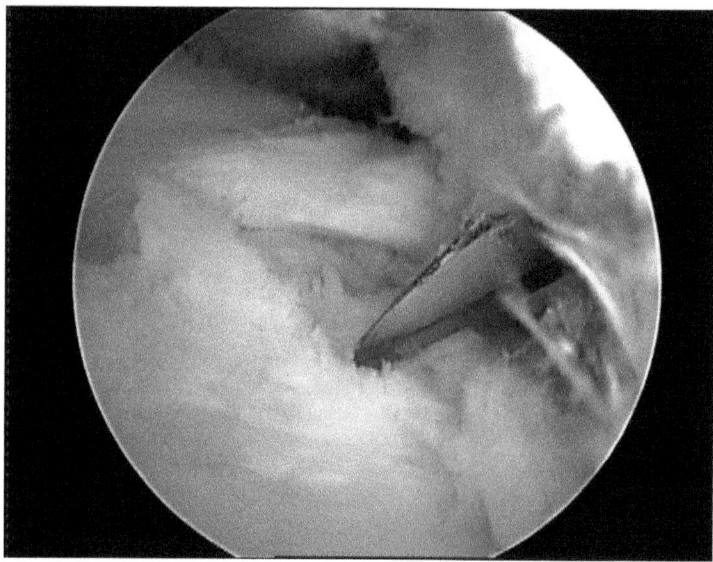

FIGURE 10 Arthroscopic view from posterior portal of the right shoulder. An eleven blade knife has been passed through rotator cuff longitudinally to allow for percutaneous placement of a suture anchor.

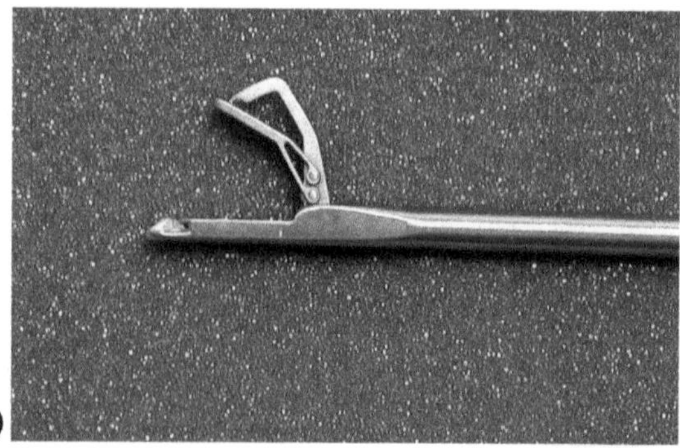

(A)

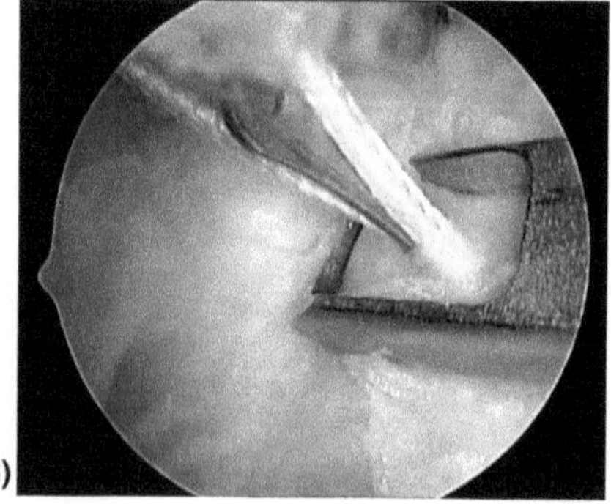

(B)

FIGURE 11 Photograph of a viper suture passing instrument used in rotator cuff repair. (**A**) Arthroscopic view of another suture passing instrument (scorpion) used to pass sutures through the rotator cuff tendon edge (**B**).

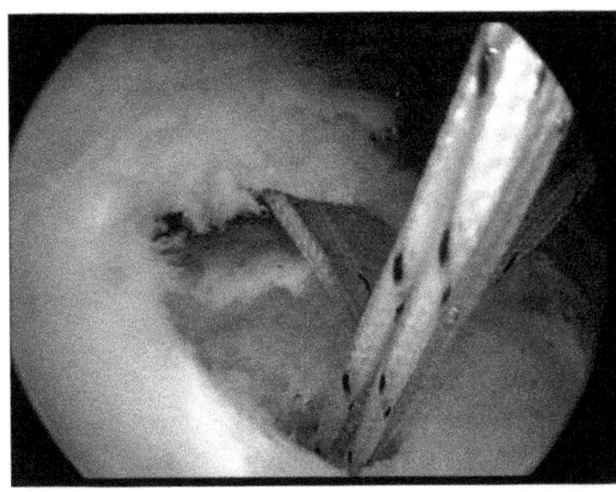

FIGURE 12 Arthroscopic view from posterior portal of the right shoulder. Two suture anchors have been placed into the tuberosity. Posterior anchor sutures (*double loaded blue and striped*) are exiting the lateral portal, while the more anterior sutures have been passed through the tendon edge but have not yet been tied.

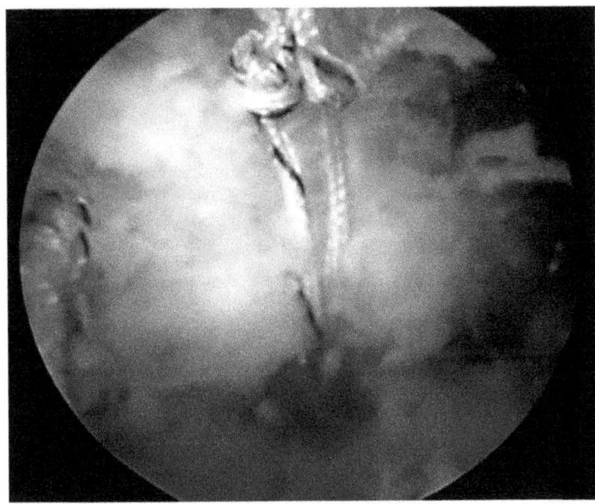

FIGURE 13 Arthroscopic view from lateral portal of the right shoulder. Sutures have been passed through the lateral tendon edge, tied and cut, to achieve water-tight repair.

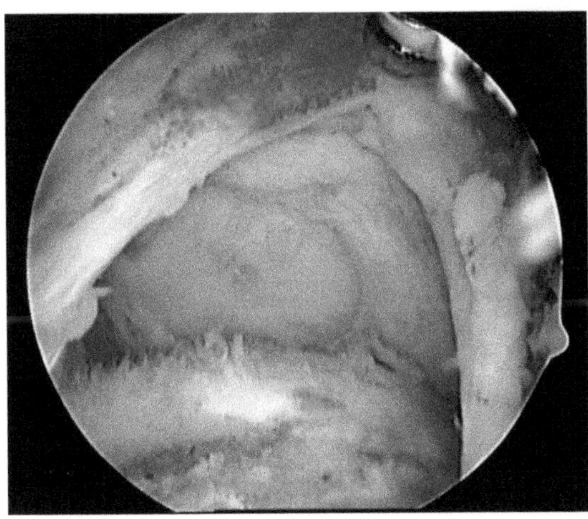

FIGURE 14 Arthroscopic view from lateral portal of the right shoulder. There is a large rotator cuff tear present which is in a "v-shaped" configuration.

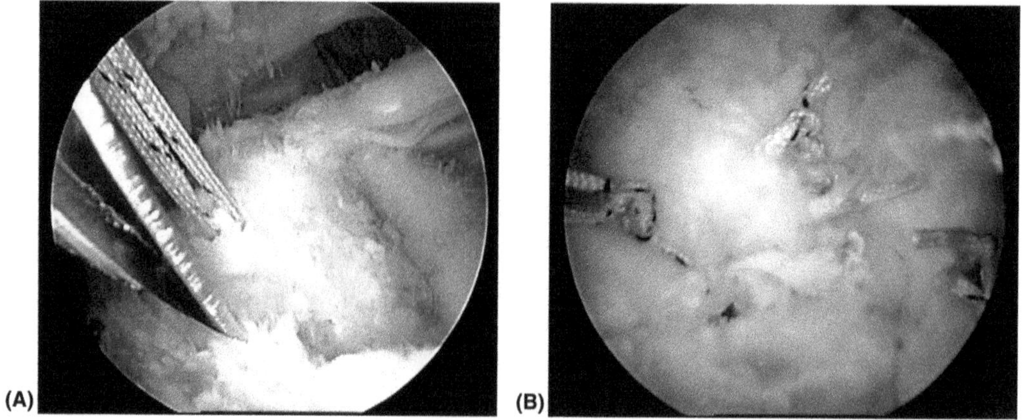

FIGURE 15 Arthroscopic view from posterior portal of the left shoulder. An anterior suture anchor has been placed into the greater tuberosity double loaded with fiberwire sutures. A second more posterior will be placed after creating a path through the deltoid with an eleven blade knife to allow for percutaneous placement (**A**). The arthroscope is now moved to the lateral portal. Sutures have been tied and cut to complete the rotator cuff repair (**B**).

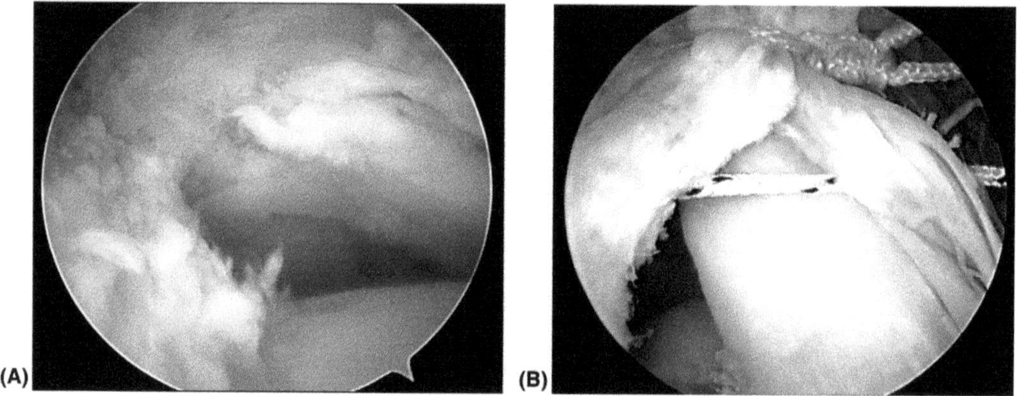

FIGURE 16 Arthroscopic view from lateral portal of the right shoulder. There is a large u-shaped tear of the supraspinatus tendon (**A**). A margin convergence suture has been tied and cut, while a second more lateral margin convergence suture has been placed but not yet tied (**B**).

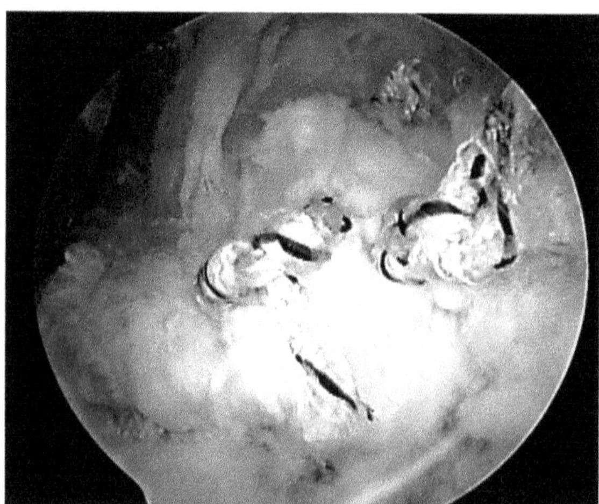

FIGURE 17 Arthroscopic view from lateral portal of the right shoulder. The lateral edge of the supraspinatus tendon has now been repaired to the greater tuberosity with two suture anchors (striped sutures attached).

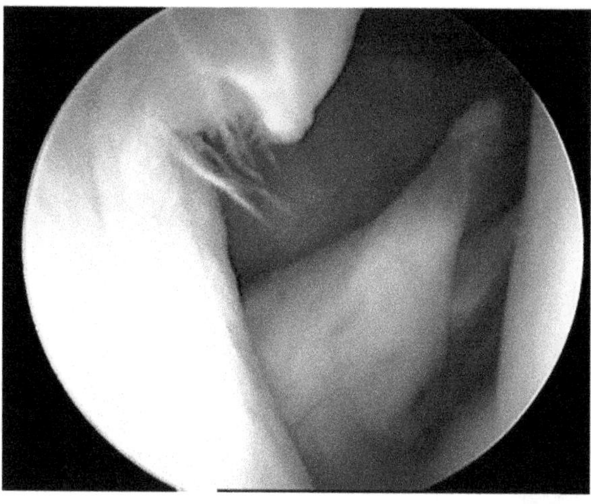

FIGURE 18 Arthroscopic view from posterior portal of the right shoulder, demonstrating complete tear of the subscapularis tendon with detachment from the lesser tuberosity.

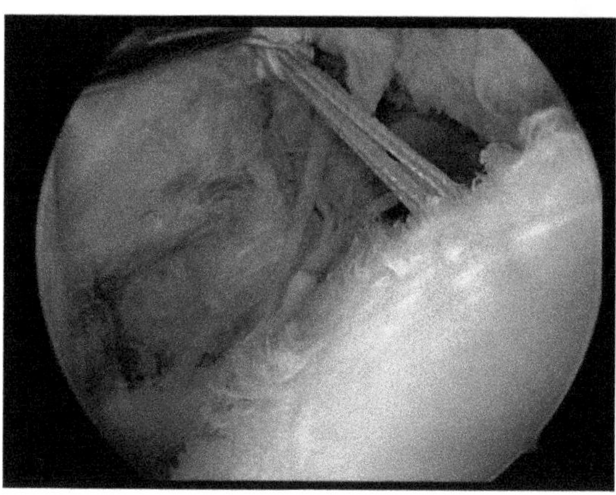

FIGURE 19 Arthroscopic view from posterior portal of the right shoulder. A suture anchor has been placed into the lesser tuberosity double loaded with sutures (*striped and blue*).

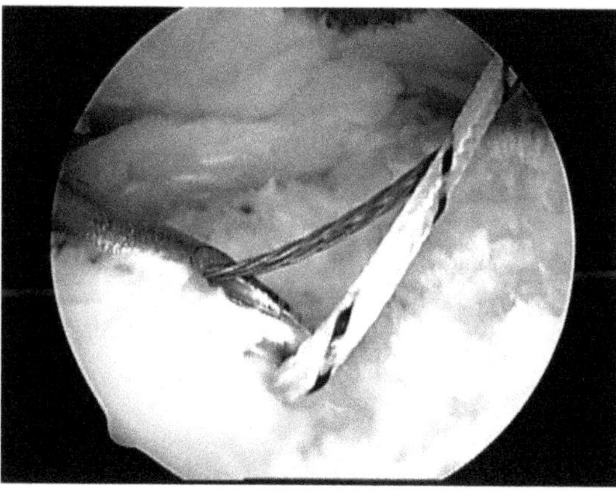

FIGURE 20 Arthroscopic view from lateral portal of the right shoulder. A lasso type suture passing instrument is used to penetrate the torn subscapularis tendon. The striped suture which is attached to underlying anchor is then shuttled through the subscapularis tendon and tied.

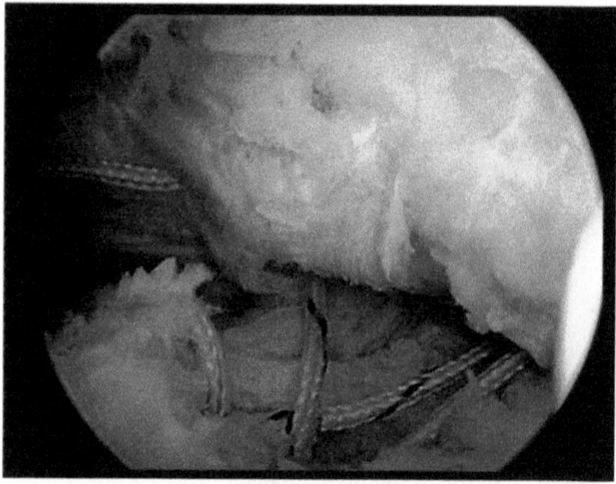

FIGURE 21 Arthroscopic view from posterior portal of the right shoulder. The sutures have been passed through the subscapularis tendon but not yet tied.

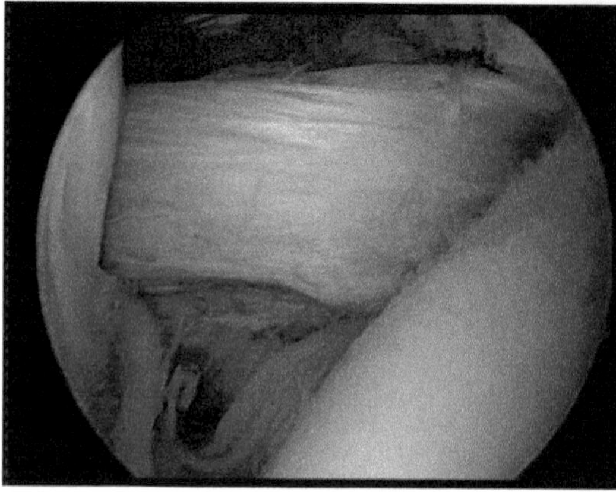

FIGURE 22 Arthroscopic view from posterior portal of the right shoulder. The sutures have been tied and the subscapularis tendon is securely repaired to the lesser tuberosity.

BIBLIOGRAPHY

Ahmad CS, Levine WN, et al. Arthroscopic rotator cuff repair. Orthopedics 2004; 27(6):570–574.

Ahmad CS, Stewart AM, et al. Tendon-bone interface motion in transosseous suture and suture anchor rotator cuff repair techniques. Am J Sports Med 2005; 33(11):1667–1671.

Baker CL, Whaley AL, et al. Arthroscopic rotator cuff tear repair. J Surg Orthop Adv 2003; 12(4):175–190.

Baysal D, Balyk R, et al. Functional outcome and health-related quality of life after surgical repair of full-thickness rotator cuff tear using a mini-open technique. Am J Sports Med 2005; 33(9):1346–1355.

Bennett WF. Arthroscopic repair of full-thickness supraspinatus tears (small-to-medium): a prospective study with 2- to 4-year follow-up. Arthroscopy 2003; 19(3):249–256.

Bennett WF. Arthroscopic repair of isolated subscapularis tears: a prospective cohort with 2- to 4-year follow-up. Arthroscopy 2003; 19(2):131–143.

Bigliani LU, Ticker JB, et al. The relationship of acromial architecture to rotator cuff disease. Clin Sports Med 1991; 10(4):823–838.

Blaine TA, Kim YS, et al. The molecular pathophysiology of subacromial bursitis in rotator cuff disease. J Shoulder Elbow Surg 2005; 14(1 suppl S):84S–89S.

Blevins FT, Warren RF, et al. Arthroscopic assisted rotator cuff repair: results using a mini-open deltoid splitting approach. Arthroscopy 1996; 12(1):50–59.

Bokor DJ, Hawkins RJ, et al. Results of nonoperative management of full-thickness tears of the rotator cuff. Clin Orthop Relat Res 1993; (294):103–110.

Boszotta H, Prunner K. Arthroscopically assisted rotator cuff repair. Arthroscopy 2004; 20(6):620–626.

Buess E, Steuber KU, et al. Open versus arthroscopic rotator cuff repair: a comparative view of 96 cases. Arthroscopy 2005; 21(5):597–604.

Burkhart SS. Arthroscopic treatment of massive rotator cuff tears. Clin Orthop Relat Res 2001; (390): 107–118.

Burkhart SS. The principle of margin convergence in rotator cuff repair as a means of strain reduction at the tear margin. Ann Biomed Eng 2004; 32(1):166–170.

Burkhart SS, Athanasiou KA, et al. Margin convergence: a method of reducing strain in massive rotator cuff tears. Arthroscopy 1996; 12(3):335–358.

Burkhart SS, Danaceau SM, et al. Arthroscopic rotator cuff repair: analysis of results by tear size and by repair technique-margin convergence versus direct tendon-to-bone repair. Arthroscopy 2001; 17(9):905–912.

Codman E. Complete rupture of the supraspinatus tendon: operative treatment with report of two successful cases. Boston Med Surg J 1911; 164:708–710.

Codman EA. Rupture of the supraspinatus tendon. 1911. Clin Orthop Relat Res 1990; (254):3–26.

Dalton SE. The conservative management of rotator cuff disorders. Br J Rheumatol 1994; 33(7):663–667.

Demirhan M, Atalar AC, et al. Arthroscopic-assisted mini-open rotator cuff repair. Acta Orthop Traumatol Turc 2002; 36(1):1–6.

Demirhan M, Esenyel CZ. All arthroscopic treatment of rotator cuff tears. Acta Orthop Traumatol Turc 2003; 37(suppl 1):93–104.

Duralde XA, Bair B. Massive rotator cuff tears: the result of partial rotator cuff repair. J Shoulder Elbow Surg 2005; 14(2):121–127.

Esch JC, Ozerkis LR, et al. Arthroscopic subacromial decompression: results according to the degree of rotator cuff tear. Arthroscopy 1988; 4(4):241–249.

Fealy S, Kingham TP, et al. Mini-open rotator cuff repair using a two-row fixation technique: outcomes analysis in patients with small, moderate, and large rotator cuff tears. Arthroscopy 2002; 18(6):665–670.

Fischmeister MF. Functional and anatomical results after rotator cuff repair. Clin Orthop Relat Res 1995; (315):285.

Fuchs B, Gilbart MK, et al. Clinical and structural results of open repair of an isolated one-tendon tear of the rotator cuff. J Bone Joint Surg Am 2006; 88(2):309–316.

Galatz LM, Ball CM, et al. The outcome and repair integrity of completely arthroscopically repaired large and massive rotator cuff tears. J Bone Joint Surg Am 2004; 86-A(2):219–224.

Galatz LM, Griggs, et al. Prospective longitudinal analysis of postoperative shoulder function: a ten-year follow-up study of full-thickness rotator cuff tears. J Bone Joint Surg Am 2001; 83-A(7):1052–1056.

Gartsman GM, Milne JC. Articular surface partial-thickness rotator cuff tears. J Shoulder Elbow Surg 1995; 4(6):409–415.

Gazielly, DF, Gleyze P et al. Functional and anatomical results after rotator cuff repair. Clin Orthop Relat Res 1994; (304):43–53.

Gleyze P, Thomazeau H, et al. Arthroscopic rotator cuff repair: a multicentric retrospective study of 87 cases with anatomical assessment. Rev Chir Orthop Reparatrice Appar Mot 2000; 86(6):566–574.

Goldberg BA, Lippitt SB, et al. Improvement in comfort and function after cuff repair without acromioplasty. Clin Orthop Relat Res (390):142–150.

Goutallier D, Postel JM, et al. Tension-free cuff repairs with excision of macroscopic tendon lesions and muscular advancement: results in a prospective series with limited fatty muscular degeneration. J Shoulder Elbow Surg 2006; 15(2):164–172.

Grana WA, Teague B, et al. An analysis of rotator cuff repair. Am J Sports Med 1994; 22(5):585–588.
Gschwend N, Bloch HR, et al. Long-term results of surgical management of rotator cuff rupture. Orthopade 1991; 20(4):255–261.
Gupta R, Leggin BG, et al. Results of surgical repair of full-thickness tears of the rotator cuff. Orthop Clin North Am 1997; 28(2):241–248.
Habernek H, Schmid L, et al. Five year results of rotator cuff repair. Br J Sports Med 1999; 33(6):430–433.
Hattrup SJ. Rotator cuff repair: relevance of patient age. J Shoulder Elbow Surg 1995; 4(2):95–100.
Hawkins RH, Dunlop R. Nonoperative treatment of rotator cuff tears. Clin Orthop Relat Res 1995; (321):178–188.
Hersch JC, Sgaglione NA. Arthroscopically assisted mini-open rotator cuff repairs. Functional outcome at 2- to 7-year follow-up. Am J Sports Med 2000; 28(3):301–311.
Ide J, Maeda S, et al. A comparison of arthroscopic and open rotator cuff repair. Arthroscopy 2005; 21(9):1090–1098.
Klepps S, Bishop J, et al. Prospective evaluation of the effect of rotator cuff integrity on the outcome of open rotator cuff repairs. Am J Sports Med 2004; 32(7):1716–1722.
Kreuz PC, Remiger A, et al. Isolated and combined tears of the subscapularis tendon. Am J Sports Med 2005; 33(12):1831–1837.
Levy HJ, Gardner RD, et al. Arthroscopic subacromial decompression in the treatment of full-thickness rotator cuff tears. Arthroscopy 1991; 7(1):8–13.
Levy HJ, Uribe JW, et al. Arthroscopic assisted rotator cuff repair: preliminary results. Arthroscopy 1990; 6(1):55–60.
Lindblom K. On pathogenesis of ruptures of the tendon aponeurosis of the shoulder joint. Acta Radiol 1939; 20:563–577.
Liu SH, Baker CL. Arthroscopically assisted rotator cuff repair: correlation of functional results with integrity of the cuff. Arthroscopy 1994; 10(1):54–60.
Lo IK, Burkhart SS. Double-row arthroscopic rotator cuff repair: re-establishing the footprint of the rotator cuff. Arthroscopy 2003; 19(9):1035–1042.
Lo IK, Burkhart SS. Arthroscopic repair of massive, contracted, immobile rotator cuff tears using single and double interval slides: technique and preliminary results. Arthroscopy 2004; 20(1):22–33.
Lo IK, Burkhart SS. Arthroscopic revision of failed rotator cuff repairs: technique and results. Arthroscopy 2004; 20(3):250–267.
Lo IK, Burkhart SS. Transtendon arthroscopic repair of partial-thickness, articular surface tears of the rotator cuff. Arthroscopy 2004; 20(2):214–220.
Lyons RP, Green A. Subscapularis tendon tears. J Am Acad Orthop Surg 2005; 13(5):353–363.
Mansat P, Frankle MA, et al. Tears in the subscapularis tendon: descriptive analysis and results of surgical repair. Joint Bone Spine 2003; 70(5):342–347.
Mazoue CG, Andrews JR. Repair of full-thickness rotator cuff tears in professional baseball players. Am J Sports Med 2006; 34(2):182–189.
Mazzocca AD, Millett PJ, et al. Arthroscopic single-row versus double-row suture anchor rotator cuff repair. Am J Sports Med 2005; 33(12):1861–1868.
McBirnie JM, Miniaci A, et al. Arthroscopic repair of full-thickness rotator cuff tears using bioabsorbable tacks. Arthroscopy 2005; 21(12):1421–1427.
McCallister WV, Parsons IM, et al. Open rotator cuff repair without acromioplasty. J Bone Joint Surg Am 2005; 87(6):1278–1283.
McConville OR, Iannotti JP. Partial-thickness tears of the rotator cuff: evaluation and management. J Am Acad Orthop Surg 1999; 7(1):32–43.
McLaughlin H. Lesions of the musculotendinous cuff of the shoulder: I. The exposure and treatment of tears with retraction. J Bone Joint Surg 1944; 26:31–51.
McLaughlin HL. Repair of major cuff ruptures. Surg Clin North Am 1963; 43:1535–1540.
McLaughlin HL. Lesions of the musculotendinous cuff of the shoulder. The exposure and treatment of tears with retraction. 1944. Clin Orthop Relat Res 1994; (304):3–9.
Meyer A. Further observations on use-destruction in joints. J Bone and Joint Surg 1922; 4:491–511.
Miller SL, Hazrati Y, et al. Failed surgical management of partial thickness rotator cuff tears. Orthopedics 2002; 25(11):1255–1257.
Millett PJ, Mazzocca A, et al. Mattress double anchor footprint repair: a novel, arthroscopic rotator cuff repair technique. Arthroscopy 2004; 20(8):875–879.
Morrison DS, Frogameni AD, et al. Non-operative treatment of subacromial impingement syndrome. J Bone Joint Surg Am 1997; 79(5):732–737.
Murray TF Jr, Lajtai G, et al. Arthroscopic repair of medium to large full-thickness rotator cuff tears: outcome at 2- to 6-year follow-up. J Shoulder Elbow Surg 2002; 11(1):19–24.
Norberg FB, Field LD, et al. Repair of the rotator cuff. Mini-open and arthroscopic repairs. Clin Sports Med 2000; 19(1):7799.
Park JY, Chung KT, et al. A serial comparison of arthroscopic repairs for partial- and full-thickness rotator cuff tears. Arthroscopy 2004; 20(7):705–711.

Park MC, Cadet ER, et al. Tendon-to-bone pressure distributions at a repaired rotator cuff footprint using transosseous suture and suture anchor fixation techniques. Am J Sports Med 2005; 33(8):1154–1159.

Paulos LE, Kody MH. Arthroscopically enhanced "miniapproach" to rotator cuff repair. Am J Sports Med 22(1):19–25.

Posada A, Uribe JW, et al. Mini-deltoid splitting rotator cuff repair: do results deteriorate with time? Arthroscopy 2000; 16(2):137–141.

Rebuzzi E, Coletti N, et al. Arthroscopic rotator cuff repair in patients older than 60 years. Arthroscopy 2005; 21(1):48–54.

Richards DP, Burkhart SS. Margin convergence of the posterior rotator cuff to the biceps tendon. Arthroscopy 2004; 20(7):771–775.

Richards DP, Burkhart SS, et al. Subscapularis tears: arthroscopic repair techniques. Orthop Clin North Am 2003; 34(4):485–498.

Roddey TS, Cook KF, et al. The relationship among strength and mobility measures and self-report outcome scores in persons after rotator cuff repair surgery: impairment measures are not enough. J Shoulder Elbow Surg 2005; 14(1 suppl S):95S–98S.

Romeo AA, Hang DW, et al. Repair of full thickness rotator cuff tears. Gender, age, and other factors affecting outcome. Clin Orthop Relat Res 1999; (367):243–255.

Romeo AA, Mazzocca A, et al. Shoulder scoring scales for the evaluation of rotator cuff repair. Clin Orthop Relat Res 2004; (427):107–114.

Sauerbrey AM, Getz CL, et al. Arthroscopic versus mini-open rotator cuff repair: a comparison of clinical outcome. Arthroscopy 2005; 21(12):1415–1420.

Savoie FHIII, Field LD, et al. Costs analysis of successful rotator cuff repair surgery: an outcome study. Comparison of gatekeeper system in surgical patients. Arthroscopy 1995; 11(6):672–676.

Severud EL, Ruotolo C, et al. All-arthroscopic versus mini-open rotator cuff repair: a long-term retrospective outcome comparison. Arthroscopy 2003; 19(3):234–238.

Shinners TJ, Noordsij PG, et al. Arthroscopically assisted mini-open rotator cuff repair. Arthroscopy 2002; 18(1):21–26.

Skutek M, Fremerey RW, et al. Outcome analysis following open rotator cuff repair. Early effectiveness validated using four different shoulder assessment scales. Arch Orthop Trauma Surg 2000; 120(7–8):432–436.

Sperling JW, Cofield RH, et al. Rotator cuff repair in patients fifty years of age and younger. J Bone Joint Surg Am 2004; 86-A(10):2212–2215.

Spielmann AL, Forster BB, et al. Shoulder after rotator cuff repair: MR imaging findings in asymptomatic individuals—initial experience. Radiology 1999; 213(3):705–708.

Stollsteimer GT, Savoie FHIII. Arthroscopic rotator cuff repair: current indications, limitations, techniques, and results. Instr Course Lect 1998; 47:59–65.

Sugaya H, Maeda K, et al. Functional and structural outcome after arthroscopic full-thickness rotator cuff repair: single-row versus dual-row fixation. Arthroscopy 2005; 21(11):1307–1316.

Tashjian RZ, Henn RF, et al. Effect of medical comorbidity on self-assessed pain, function, and general health status after rotator cuff repair. J Bone Joint Surg Am 2006; 88(3):536–540.

Tauro JC. Arthroscopic rotator cuff repair: analysis of technique and results at 2- and 3-year follow-up. Arthroscopy 1998; 14(1):45–51.

Travis RD, Burkhead WZ Jr, et al. Technique for repair of the subscapularis tendon. Orthop Clin North Am 2001; 32(3):495–500.

Uhthoff HK, Hammond DI, et al. The role of the coracoacromial ligament in the impingement syndrome. A clinical, radiological and histological study. Int Orthop 1988; 12(2):97–104.

Uhthoff HK, Sano H, et al. Early reactions after reimplantation of the tendon of supraspinatus into bone. A study in rabbits. J Bone Joint Surg Br 2000; 82(7):1072–1076.

Uhthoff HK, Sarkar K. Surgical repair of rotator cuff ruptures. The importance of the subacromial bursa. J Bone Joint Surg Br 1991; 73(3):399–401.

Uhthoff HK, Trudel G, et al. Relevance of pathology and basic research to the surgeon treating rotator cuff disease. J Orthop Sci 2003; 8(3):449–456.

Van Linthoudt D, Deforge J, et al. Rotator cuff repair. Long-term results. Joint Bone Spine 2003; 70(4):271–275.

Vives MJ, Miller LS, et al. Repair of rotator cuff tears in golfers. Arthroscopy 2001; 17(2):165–172.

Warner JJ, Tetreault P, et al. Arthroscopic versus mini-open rotator cuff repair: a cohort comparison study. Arthroscopy 2005; 21(3):328–332.

Watson EM, Sonnabend DH. Outcome of rotator cuff repair. J Shoulder Elbow Surg 2002; 11(3):201–211.

Wilson F, Hinov V, et al. Arthroscopic repair of full-thickness tears of the rotator cuff: 2- to 14-year follow-up. Arthroscopy 2002; 18(2):136–144.

Wirth MA, Basamania C, et al. Nonoperative management of full-thickness tears of the rotator cuff. Orthop Clin North Am 1997; 28(1):59–67.

Wolf EM, Pennington WT, et al. Arthroscopic rotator cuff repair: 4- to 10-year results. Arthroscopy 2004; 20(1):5–12.

Wolf EM, Pennington WT, et al. Arthroscopic side-to-side rotator cuff repair. Arthroscopy 2005; 21(7):881–887.
Yel M, Shankwiler JA, et al. Results of decompression and rotator cuff repair in patients 65 years old and older: 6- to 14-year follow-up. Am J Orthop 2001; 30(4):347–352.
Youm T, Murray DH, et al. Arthroscopic versus mini-open rotator cuff repair: a comparison of clinical outcomes and patient satisfaction. J Shoulder Elbow Surg 2005; 14(5):455–459.
Zandi H, Coghlan JA, et al. Mini-incision rotator cuff repair: a longitudinal assessment with no deterioration of result up to nine years. J Shoulder Elbow Surg 2006; 15(2):135–139.
Zvijac JE, Levy HJ, et al. Arthroscopic subacromial decompression in the treatment of full thickness rotator cuff tears: a 3- to 6-year follow-up. Arthroscopy 1994; 10(5):518–523.

23 Arthroscopic Rotator Cuff Repair: Double-Row Repair

David P. Huberty and Stephen S. Burkhart
The San Antonio Orthopedic Group, San Antonio, Texas, U.S.A.

INTRODUCTION

Over the past decade, arthroscopic treatment of rotator cuff tears has become a well-established technique gaining widespread acceptance due to the favorable patient outcomes and minimal patient morbidity. Clinical results have been reported as comparable or superior to open-repair techniques. However, the ideal technique and fixation construct continues to be an area of great interest and study. In this chapter we will review the relevant literature regarding rotator cuff footprint reconstruction and describe our technique to optimize the repair construct.

OPTIMIZING THE REPAIR

Healing of the rotator cuff tendon to bone depends largely on three variables: the surgical fixation of tendon to bone; the postoperative stresses/rehabilitation; and the natural biological response. The focus of this chapter is on fixation of the rotator cuff tendon to bone, the one variable entirely controlled by the surgeon. Recently, a great deal of research has been directed to facilitate an understanding of the rotator cuff insertion and how we can best recreate this insertion in a manner that will lead to durable healing of the tendon to bone.

With regard to fixation of the tendon to bone, three factors should be considered: the restoration of the anatomical insertion (the footprint); the strength of the repair; and the elimination of interface motion between tendon and bone. Optimization of these three factors will best allow for the natural biologic healing response to occur. Failure of rotator cuff repair surgery to facilitate healing of tendon to bone can, at least in part, be attributed to failure of the fixation. Many current techniques such as transosseous fixation of tendon to bone are not sufficiently strong (fail by suture cutting through cancellous bone), while single-row suture anchor-repair techniques do not adequately restore the anatomic insertion (1,2). A relatively novel technique of double-row tendon fixation has been suggested as a means of improving fixation (3). First row (or line) of anchors is placed medially at the articular margin, and a subsequent row of anchors is placed at the lateral margin of the greater tuberosity (Fig. 1). This method of repair has greater strength, reconstructs the anatomic rotator cuff tendon insertion more accurately, and minimizes interface motion between the tendon and bone, allowing more predictable healing.

To optimize rotator cuff tendon healing to bone, it is important to first consider the anatomical dimensions of the tendon insertion site or footprint. Despite many traditional assumptions about this anatomy, the insertion footprint of the supraspinatus tendon is almost twice the width of the actual tendon (Fig. 2). The supraspinatus, (the most commonly torn tendon) has an average insertion width of 14.7 mm from medial to lateral (4–6) with the medial most fibers starting less then 1 mm from the articular margin and the lateral most fibers originating along the lateral ridge of the greater tuberosity. A recent cadaveric study by Tuoheti et al. (7) demonstrated that the double-row suture anchor repair technique produced a tendon to bone contact area that was 42% and 60% greater than that achieved with transosseous repair and single-row suture anchor-repair techniques, respectively. A similar cadaveric study by Meier et al. (8) demonstrated that a double-row repair technique restored 100% of the supraspinatus native footprint while transosseous and single-row repair reconstituted only 71% and 46% of the footprint, respectively.

Please refer to pages 251–256 for the figures in this chapter.

Finally, to optimize the biologic conditions for tendon to bone healing to occur, the interface motion between tendon and bone should be minimized (9,10). Therefore, with the goal being to eliminate interface motion between the tendon and bone during the healing phase of a rotator cuff repair, there are several points to consider. First, both suture loop and knot security are essential to maintain solid fixation of the tendon to bone. Loss of loop security will allow gap formation and interface motion between tendon and bone. Loss of knot security (unraveling) will lead to catastrophic failure of fixation. Lo et al. have determined that a static knot (as opposed to sliding knot) backed up with three alternating post half hitches yields the optimal balance of loop and knot security (14). Finally, early postoperative active motion protocols must be discouraged because they certainly risk creation of interface motion between tendon and bone, or worse, tensile failure of the construct.

INDICATIONS AND TECHNIQUE: DOUBLE-ROW REPAIR

At our institution we attempt to maximize footprint reconstruction by performing a double-row repair for all rotator cuff tears (regardless of size) so long as there is sufficient mobility of the tendons to achieve such a repair (12).

The patient is placed in the lateral decubitus position following induction with general anesthesia. The Star Sleeve Traction System (Arthrex, Naples, Florida, U.S.A.) is used to maintain balanced suspension in approximately 30° of abduction and 20° forward flexion. Diagnostic arthroscopy is performed from the posterior portal with an arthroscopic pump, maintaining 60 mmHg pressure. Subacromial decompression, rotator cuff margin debridement, and bone bed preparation are completed. Medial to lateral and anterior to posterior mobility of the rotator cuff tear margins are evaluated and the rotator cuff tear is classified as crescent-shaped, U-shaped, L-shaped, or massive contracted. If the rotator cuff margin demonstrates excursion to the lateral aspect of the bone bed, then it is amenable for double-row repair (Fig. 3A and B). We have found most small to large tears (<5cms), as well as some massive tears, sufficiently mobile to allow double-row repair. However, massive contracted immobile tears require interval slides to achieve tendon excursion to bone and, rarely, in these cases will double-row repair be possible (13).

When the rotator cuff tendons show adequate mobility to allow double-row repair, we proceed with placement of two rows of suture anchors. The medial row anchors are inserted first, right at the articular margin of the greater tuberosity (Fig. 4A and B). An 18-gauge spinal needle is used as a guide for anchor insertion so that anchors are inserted at a "deadman's" angle (8) of approximately 45°. The bone punch alone (no tap) is used in preparation for insertion of the suture anchor (5.5 mm BioCorkscrew FT; Arthrex, Inc. Naples, Florida, U.S.A.), which is double loaded with No. 2 Fiberwire (Arthrex, Inc. Naples, Florida, U.S.A.). If the tear is larger than 1 cm in the anterior to posterior dimension, then we prefer to use the "double pulley" technique of medial row fixation. With this technique, the medial-row sutures from the anteromedial and posteromedial anchors are tied together to create a horizontal mattress-type stitch that uses the eyelets of the two anchors as pulleys to compress the tendon to bone.

The repair of a large crescent-shaped tear is described in order to illustrate our double-row repair technique with double-pulley medial-row fixation. After placement of the anterior and posterior medial row anchors, the tendon grasper placed through the lateral portal is utilized to assess tendon mobility and to plan the location of medial-row suture passage. We prefer to use an antegrade method of suture passage with a modified shuttling technique for the medial-row sutures. First an 8.25 mm clear cannula is placed in the lateral portal. The Scorpion suture passer (Arthrex, Inc. Naples, Florida, U.S.A.) is loaded with a fiberwire suture loop (Fig. 5). The Scorpion suture passer allows up to a 20 mm depth of "bite," which is important for medial-row suture passage, considering that the average tuberosity footprint measures 15 mm from medial to lateral (4–6). Beginning anteriorly, the scorpion is used to pass the suture loop from joint to bursal side at approximately a 15 mm "bite" depth (Fig. 6). The suture is retrieved from the bursal side out the anterior cannula. The loop portion of the suture loop remains out the lateral cannula, and next all four suture limbs from the anterior anchor are retrieved out the lateral cannula. These four suture strands are passed through the looped end of the suture loop (Fig. 7) and by pulling on the free end of the suture loop (out anterior cannula), the four sutures are shuttled through the cuff and out the anterior cannula (Fig. 8). All four sutures are passed, simultaneously, through the same site in the cuff tissue. This same process is repeated in order to pass the sutures from the posterior medial row. Alternatively, in some instances it is easier to pass the posterior sutures in a retrograde fashion while viewing from lateral. A Penetrator (Arthrex, Inc. Naples, Florida, U.S.A.) is placed through the posterior portal and passed through the cuff tissue. The four strands from the posterior medial anchor are grasped and retrieved out the posterior portal. Next, with passage of medial-row sutures completed, attention is turned to the lateral row fixation.

The lateral-row anchors are inserted at the lateral aspect of the footprint just medial to the "drop-off" of the greater tuberosity (Fig. 9). When planning the location of the medial and lateral row anchors with respect to one another, care must be taken to preserve an adequate bone bridge between anchors (8 to 10 mm will usually prevent fracture and preserve pull-out strength). The size and configuration of the tear will obviously determine the number and location of lateral-row anchors. If the lateral footprint is too small for two anchors, we will often place one triple loaded 5.0 mm BioCorkscrew anchor (Arthrex, Inc. Naples Florida, U.S.A.).

Typically, we prefer to pass and tie the lateral-row sutures prior to tying the medial-row sutures. This is important for two reasons. First, this ensures that we will be able to get under the cuff margin to obtain a good "bite" (5–10 mm of tissue for lateral row). Second, the lateral-row sutures are tied first to establish the rotator cuff length tension relationship. The lateral-row sutures are also generally passed in an antegrade fashion with the Viper suture passer (Arthrex, Inc. Naples, Florida, U.S.A.) (Fig. 10A and B). The lateral-row sutures are passed with the Viper in the lateral working portal while viewing from the posterior. Suture passage proceeds from front to back in simple suture fashion. To avoid difficulty with the suture jungle that has been created (Fig. 11), one set of lateral-row sutures is retrieved one at a time, out of the lateral portal for tying. We always use a clear cannula for tying (helps eliminate soft tissue interposition in knots) and proceed from back to front so that there is an unobstructed view from the posterior portal. To optimize both loop and knot security, we prefer to tie static knots with a double-diameter knot pusher (Surgeon's Sixth Finger, Arthrex, Inc., Naples, Florida, U.S.A.) (Fig. 12). Once all lateral-row sutures have been tied, the lateral edge of the repair is assessed for integrity by rotating the arm. It is interesting, at this point, to place the scope back intraarticularly to evaluate the extent of footprint coverage prior to medial-row sutures being tied. While the repair often looks quite satisfactory from the subacromial space, one will often find that there is a great deal of uncovered footprint at the articular margin (Fig. 13A and B).

Next, the medial-row fixation is achieved by first retrieving one blue suture from the anterior and posterior medial anchors out the clear cannula in the lateral portal. These two suture strands are hand tied together over a rigid post with six alternating throws (Fig. 14). Tension is placed on the other two blue suture strands in order to pull this knot down into the cannula and onto the cuff tissue. These two blue tensioning sutures are then retrieved out the lateral clear cannula, and tied securely over the cuff tissue as a static nonsliding knot with the double-diameter knot pusher. This construct compresses a horizontal band of cuff tissue against the bone bed by using the anchor eyelets as pulleys. Anterior and posterior Tigerwire (black and white) sutures are tied together in the same fashion outside of the lateral cannula and this knot is pulled down onto the cuff tissue (Fig. 15). The remaining Tigerwire strands are tensioned and tied against the cuff tissue to complete the medial-row repair. Again the completed repair is evaluated for security during internal and external rotation of the arm. It is our routine to again view from intraarticular to assess footprint coverage. The surgeon will now usually find complete coverage of the prepared bone bed (Fig. 16).

PEARLS AND PITFALLS

1. Understand footprint anatomy to accurately reconstruct the rotator cuff.
2. Double-row fixation more closely recreates footprint anatomy compared to single-row fixation.

3. There are many novel approaches to double-row fixation with little long-term clinical follow-up studies but biomechanical studies almost universally have demonstrated superior strength, decreased motion interface, and improved biomechanics.
4. Suture placement and management is critical to avoid suture entanglement, increased operative time, and surgeon frustration.
5. Appropriate loop and knot security are critical elements to assure appropriate tendon to footprint apposition and decreased bone–tendon interface motion (14).
6. While it still remains to be seen, it is hoped that optimized biomechanical properties will yield improved biologic healing of the rotator cuff.
7. Avoid overaggressive early rehabilitation to improve biologic healing and potential early retearing.

REHABILITATION

Following the operation, the patient is placed in a sling with a small pillow. For the first 6 post-operative weeks the patient wears the sling continuously, except for shower and exercises. During this time the patient is instructed to perform active elbow, wrist, and hand motion and 60° of passive external rotation with the arm at the side is encouraged, assuming that the subscapularis did not require repair. Beginning at six weeks postoperatively, patients use rope and pulley to establish passive forward flexion and internal rotation behind the back, and a cane is used to regain normal passive external rotation. Isotonic strengthening with thera-band is started at 12 weeks following surgery with focus on rehabilitation of the rotator cuff, deltoid, and scapular stabilizers. Progressive activities are incorporated as strength allows. However, return to labor or sporting activity is delayed until at least six months, postoperatively. This rehabilitation protocol was developed as a result of our belief that early aggressive motion and strengthening negatively impact the healing of tendon to bone.

CONCLUSIONS

Research will continue to be directed at identifying the superior rotator cuff repair constructs as we strive for optimum surgical outcomes. Currently, we believe that the double-row repair method of rotator cuff footprint reconstruction makes the most sense, has yielded the best results, and the technique outlined earlier is used whenever possible. The double-row repair technique most closely restores the anatomic footprint, has the greatest strength against tensile failure, and most effectively resists interface motion between tendon and bone. There are several factors that affect the ultimate healing of the rotator cuff. Considering the one factor entirely under the surgeon's control (fixation of tendon to bone), we believe that a double-row fixation technique gives the greatest chance for a successful outcome. There is no doubt that, performing an arthroscopic double-row rotator cuff repair requires more from the surgeon in terms of surgical time and effort, and also more from the medical system in terms of expense. Improved clinical outcomes will serve as justification for this technique despite these disadvantages.

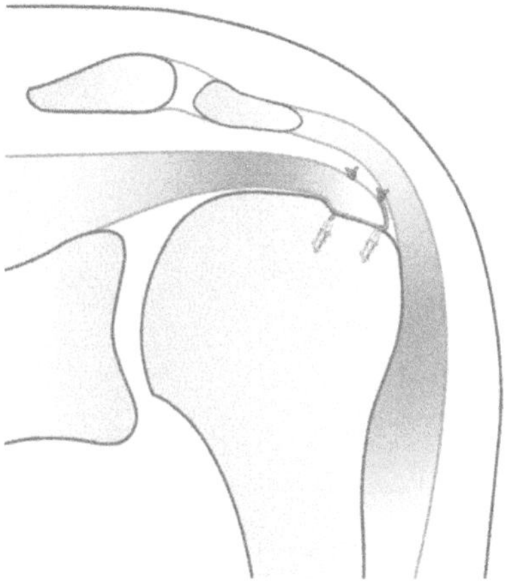

FIGURE 1 The double-row method of rotator cuff repair utilizes suture anchors placed medially adjacent to the articular margin and laterally just proximal to the tuberosity drop off. With this anchor configuration, the rotator cuff tendon can be compressed to the bone bed across the entire anatomic footprint.

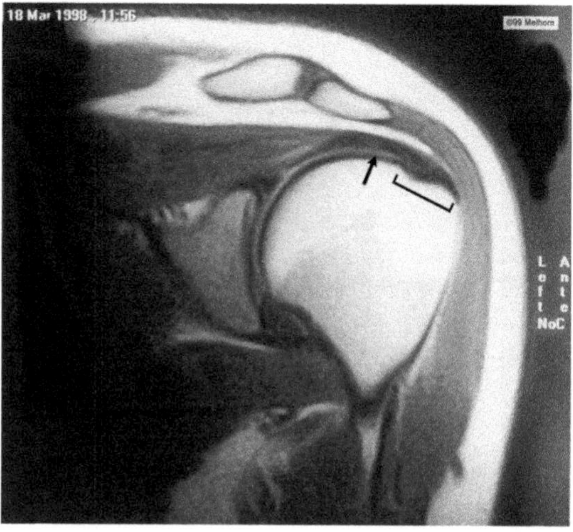

FIGURE 2 This coronal oblique MRI image of the left shoulder demonstrates the normal width of the rotator cuff insertion. Note the width of the insertion (*bracket*) compared to the width of the tendon just proximal to the insertion (*arrow*).

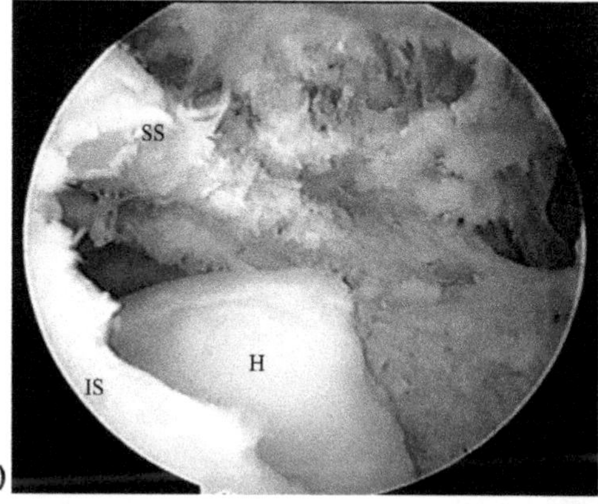

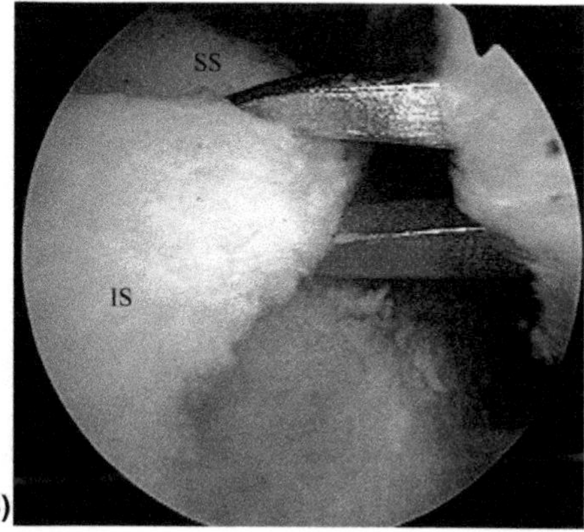

FIGURE 3 (**A**) Arthroscopic view of the right shoulder from the posterior viewing portal demonstrating a large crescent shaped tear involving the supraspinatus (SS) and infraspinatus (IS) tendons. The articular margin of the humeral head (H) is visible and the bone bed has been prepared. (**B**) Arthroscopic tendon grasper placed through the lateral portal is used to assess excursion of the tendon. In this case the tendon will easily reach the lateral aspect of the bone bed, confirming that this is an ideal tear for a double-row repair.

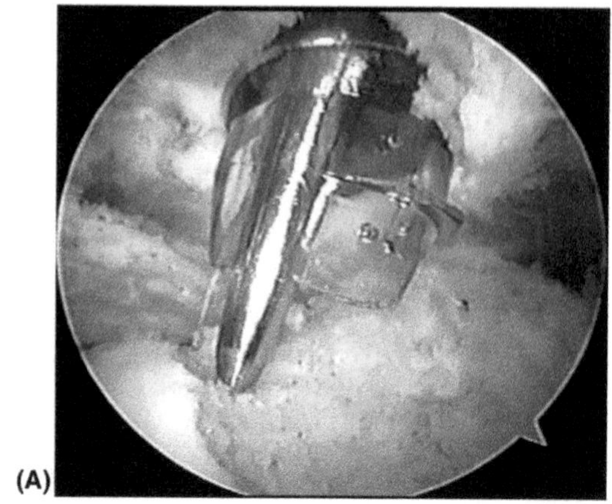
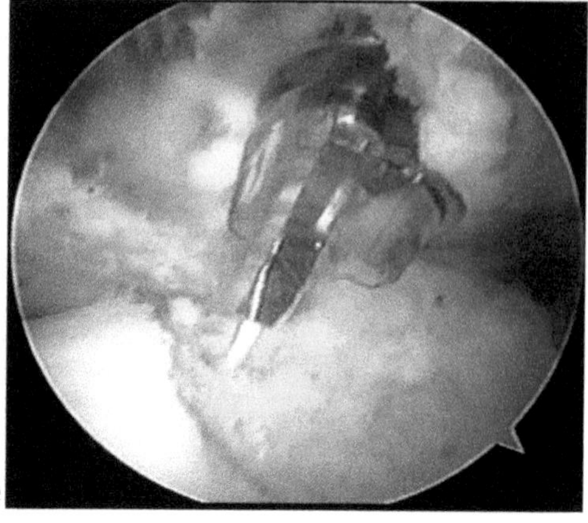

FIGURE 4 (**A**) The 5.5 mm bone punch for the Bio-Corkscrew FT suture anchor is positioned directly adjacent to the articular margin at the anterior aspect of the tear. The punch is impacted to the laser mark depth. (**B**) The anterior medial-row anchor is inserted at approximately a 45° angle to the bone surface without having tapped the hole. *Source*: courtesy of Arthrex, Inc. Naples, Florida, U.S.A.

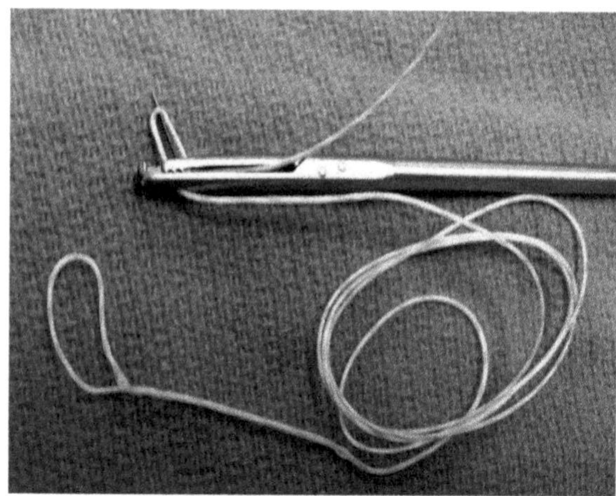

FIGURE 5 The Scorpion suture passer is loaded with a #2 Fiberwire suture snare loop. This suture loop will be passed through the cuff tissue and used to shuttle the medial-row sutures. *Source*: courtesy of Arthrex, Inc. Naples, Florida, U.S.A.

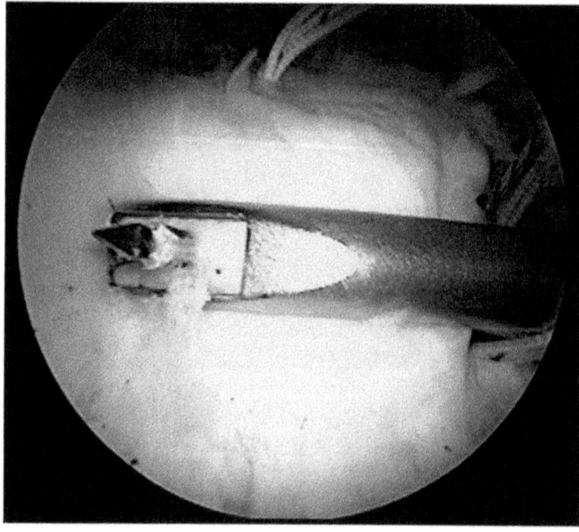

FIGURE 6 Arthroscopic view of the right shoulder from the posterior portal. The Scorpion suture passer is placed through the lateral portal and is used to pass the suture snare loop. The suture share loop will be used to shuttle the medial-row sutures.

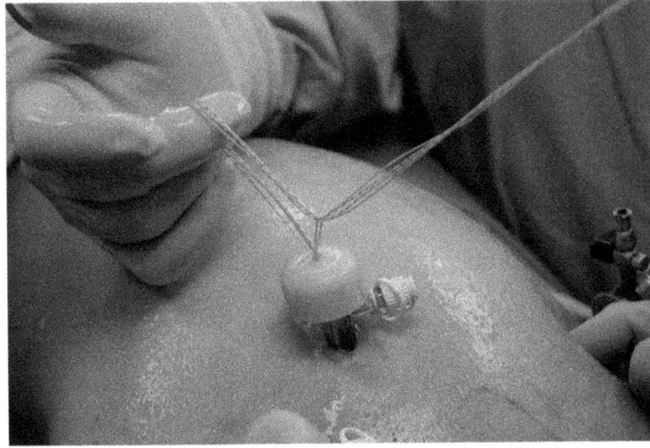

FIGURE 7 All four suture strands from the anterior medial anchor are passed through the suture snare loop. As the free end of the suture share loop is pulled out the anterior cannula, an assistant guides the looped end (and four suture strands) into the lateral cannula to avoid tangling and friction build up during passage.

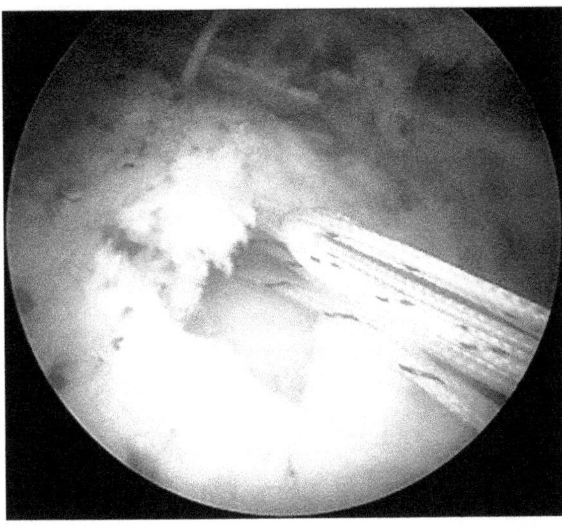

FIGURE 8 Arthroscopic view of the right shoulder posterior viewing portal. The suture snare loop is used to shuttle all four-suture limbs through the supraspinatus tendon and out the anterior cannula.

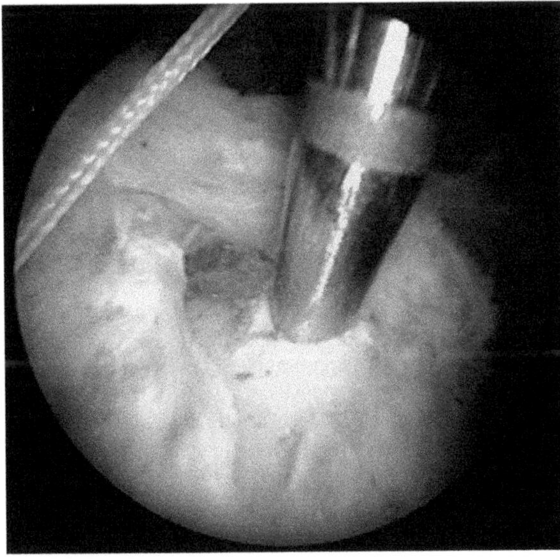

FIGURE 9 Arthroscopic view of the right shoulder posterior viewing portal. The bone punch is placed just medial to the drop off of the greater tuberosity in preparation for lateral-row anchor insertion.

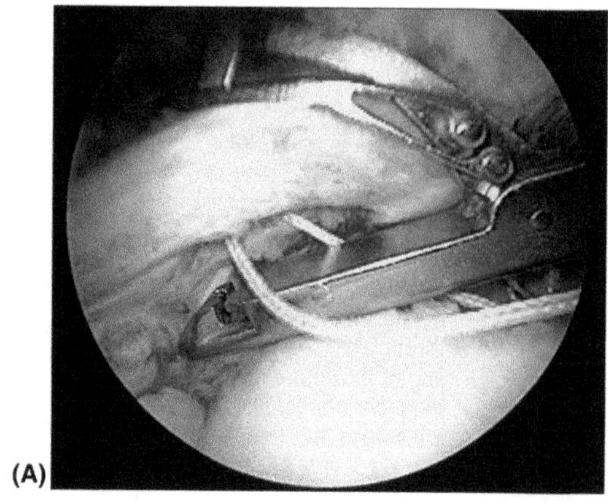

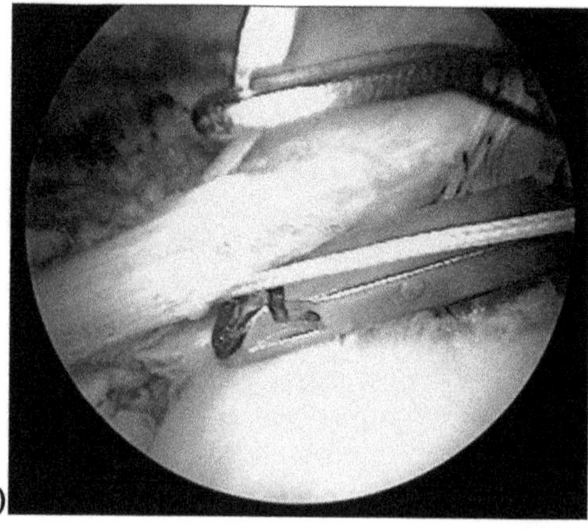

FIGURE 10 (**A** and **B**) Arthroscopic views of the right shoulder from the posterior viewing portal. These images demonstrate the technique of antegrade suture passage with the Viper suture passer. This technique is very effective for passage of lateral-row sutures (ideal bite depth is 5–8 mm). *Source*: courtesy of Arthrex, Inc. Naples, Florida, U.S.A.

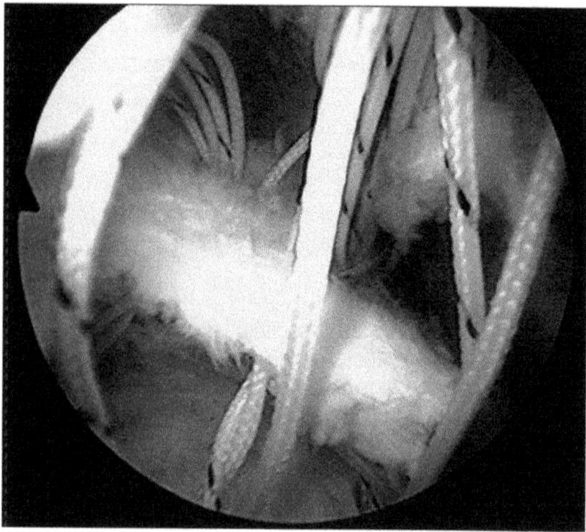

FIGURE 11 Arthroscopic view of the right shoulder from a lateral viewing position with a double-row repair in progress. Careful suture management becomes critical to avoid frustration.

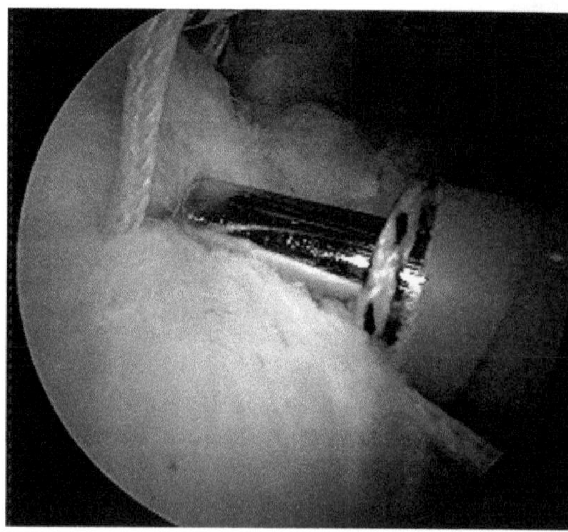

FIGURE 12 Arthroscopic view of the right shoulder from a posterior portal. The double diameter knot pusher is used to tie one of the lateral-row knots. Note how the knot pusher is used to manipulate the tissue over the anchor prior to pressing the knot down onto the tissue. This helps prevent the suture from cutting through the tendon as the knot is being tightened over the anchor.

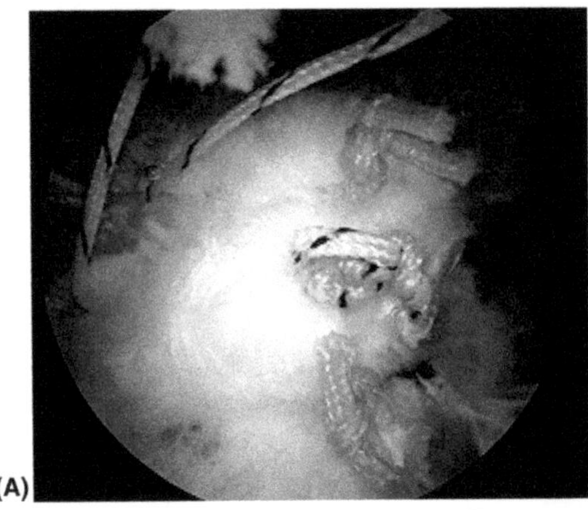

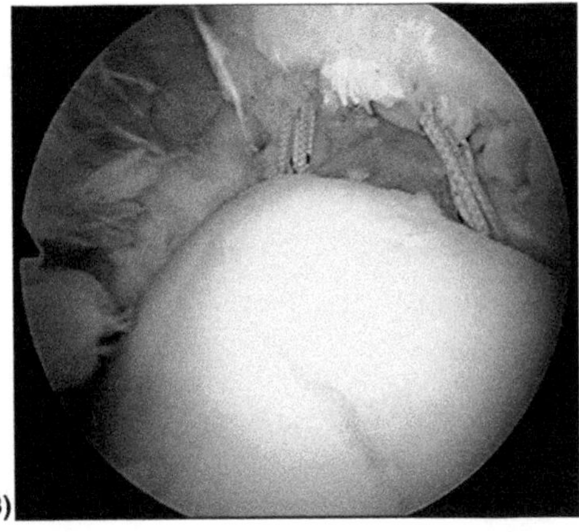

FIGURE 13 (**A**) Arthroscopic view of the right shoulder from the posterior portal. The security of the repair is evaluated after the lateral-row repair is completed. The tendon appears to cover the footprint well. The medial-row sutures have been passed but are not yet tied. (**B**) Arthroscopic joint side view of the right shoulder from posterior portal. Note the extent of uncovered footprint prior to the medial-row sutures being tied.

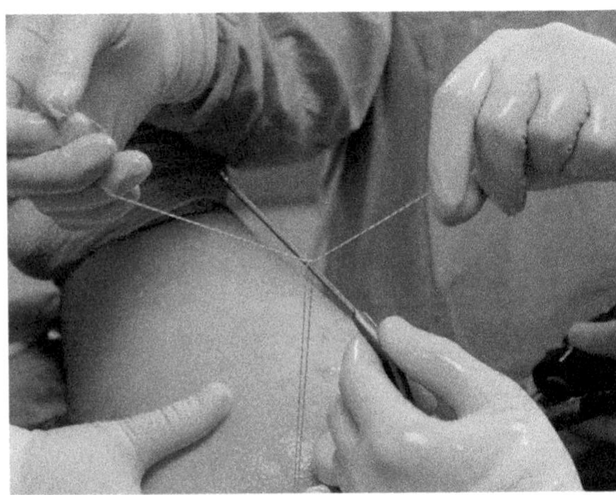

FIGURE 14 One blue suture from each of the medial-row anchors has been retrieved out the lateral cannula. The sutures are tied together over a post with a 6-throw square knot.

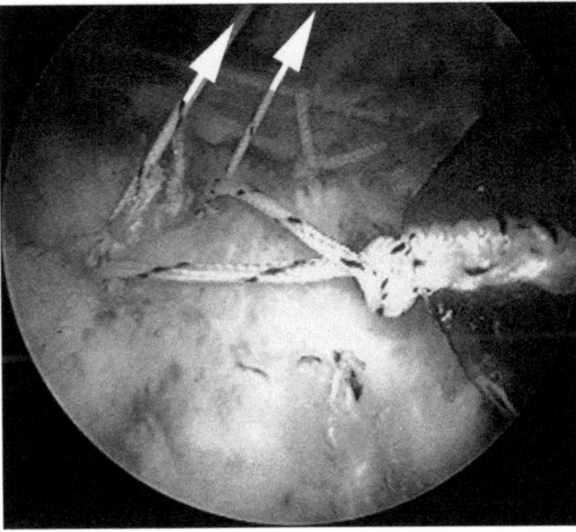

FIGURE 15 Arthroscopic view of the right shoulder from the posterior viewing portal. The remaining Tigerwire sutures (*yellow arrows*) are tensioned from the anterior cannula in order to draw the medial-row stitch down onto the cuff tissue. These tensioning strands will then be tied against the cuff tissue with the double-diameter knot pusher in order to complete the medial-row repair.

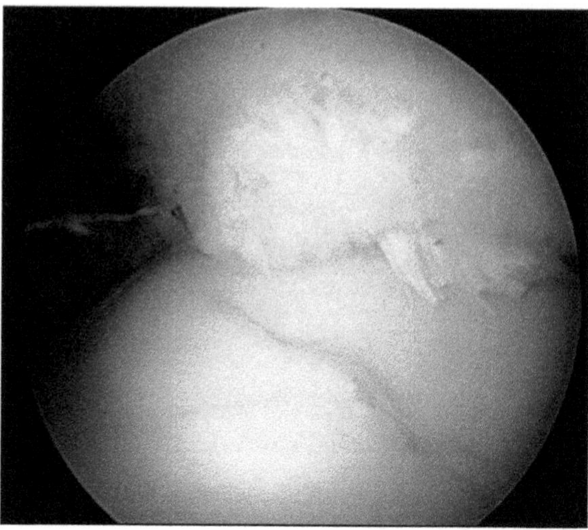

FIGURE 16 Arthroscopic intraarticular view of the right shoulder from the posterior portal (same view and same shoulder as Figure 13B). The medial-row sutures have just been tensioned and tied and the double-row repair is complete. Note how the bone bed has been completely covered at this time.

REFERENCES

1. Burkhart SS, Diaz Pagan JL, Wirth MA, Athanasiou KA. Cyclic loading of anchor-based rotator cuff repairs: confirmation of the tension overload phenomenon and comparison of suture anchor fixation with transosseous fixation. Arthroscopy 1997; 130:720–724.
2. Mazzocca AD, Millett PJ, Guanche CA, Santangelo SA, Arciero RA. Arthroscopic single-row versus double-row suture anchor rotator cuff repair. Am J Sports Med 2005; 33(12):1861–1868.
3. Lo IK, Burkhart SS. Double-row arthroscopic rotator cuff repair: re-establishing the footprint of the rotator cuff. Arthroscopy 2003; 19:1035–1042.
4. Dugas JR, Campbell DA, Warren RF, Robie BH, Millett PJ. Anatomy and dimensions of rotator cuff insertions. J Shoulder Elbow Surg 2002; 11(5):498–503.
5. Ruotolo C, Fow JE, Nottage WM. The supraspinatus footprint: an anatomic study of the supraspinatus insertion. Arthroscopy 2004; 20(3):246–249.
6. Tierney JJ, Curtis AS, Kowalk DL, et al. The footprint of the rotator cuff. Arthroscopy 1999; 15: 556–557.
7. Tuoheti Y, Itoi E, Yamamoto N, et al. Contact area, contact pressure, and pressure patterns of the tendon-bone interface after rotator cuff repair. Am J Sports Med 2005; 33(12).
8. Meier SW, Meier JD, Levy AS. Rotator cuff repair: the effect of double-row fixation versus single-row fixation on three-dimensional repair site. Arthroscopy 2004; 20:E2.
9. Ahmad CS, Stewart AM, Izquierdo R, Bigliani LU. Tendon-bone interface motion in transosseous suture and suture anchor rotator cuff repair techniques. Am J Sports Med 2005; 33:1667–1671.
10. Apreleva M, Ozbaydar M, Fitzgibbons PG, Warner JJP. Rotator cuff tears: the effect of the reconstruction method on three-dimensional repair site area. Arthrosocopy 2002; 18:519–526.
11. Lo IK, Burkhart SS, Chan KC, et al. Arthroscopic knots: determining the optimal balance of loop security and knot security. Arthroscopy 2004; 20:489–502.
12. Brady PC, Arrigoni P, Burkhart SS. Arthroscopic rotator cuff repair: establishing the footprint. Tech Shoulder Elb Surg 2005; 6(4).
13. Burkhart SS. The deadman theory of suture anchors: observations along a South Texas fence line. Arthroscopy 1995; 11:119–123.
14. Lo IK, Burkhart SS. Arthroscopic repair of massive, contracted, immobile rotator cuff tears using single and double interval slides: technique and preliminary results. Arthroscopy 2004; 20(1):22–33.

24 Arthroscopic Subscapularis Repair

David P. Huberty and Stephen S. Burkhart
The San Antonio Orthopedic Group, San Antonio, Texas, U.S.A.

INTRODUCTION

Subscapularis function and the clinical relevance of subscapularis pathology have recently received significant attention. A heightened awareness of subscapularis injury, refined clinical exam tests, and increasing familiarity with arthroscopic inspection of the subscapularis tendon have led to more frequent diagnosis of subscapularis tendon tears (1–4). Advanced arthroscopic techniques now allow accurate identification of subscapularis pathology and reliable treatment (1,2,4–8). The subscapularis, however, remains the most difficult of the rotator cuff tendons to repair arthroscopically for several reasons. The subcoracoid space is significantly constrained making visualization and manipulation of instruments here challenging. The completely torn subscapularis tends to retract and scar far medially in a position where visualization and manipulation of the tendon is even further compromised. Finally, the subscapularis tends to scar to the coracoid in close proximity to important neurovascular structures making mobilization a particularly daunting task. It is clear that subscapularis tendon tears can occur in isolation or as part of the continuum of large and massive anterosuperior rotator cuff tears (1,2,9–11).

The subscapularis muscle originates from the anterior scapula, courses laterally below the coracoid, becomes tendinous near the glenoid rim, and inserts into the lesser tuberosity of the proximal humerus. The tendinous insertion is roughly trapezoidal in shape and has a superior to inferior length of approximately 2.5 cm. The subscapularis tendon, the largest rotator cuff tendon, is considered primarily an internal rotator of the glenohumeral joint and a constraint against anterior instability. It is often underappreciated however, that the subscapularis is an essential component of the transverse plane force couple (Fig. 1A and B). Any major disruption of the subscapularis tendon leads to a relative deficiency of the anterior cuff and the anterior moment leading to an unbalanced force couple. The result is an unstable fulcrum for glenohumeral motion and potential for superior migration of the humeral head. The diagnosis and treatment of the isolated subscapularis tear will be the focus of this chapter.

ETIOLOGY

We believe that subcoracoid stenosis and subcoracoid impingement may contribute to and exacerbate subscapularis tendon degeneration and tearing (7,12,13). When subcoracoid stenosis and impingement occur the subscapularis tendon drapes across the prominent coracoid. As the coracoid presses into the anterior surface of the subscapularis tendon, the tensile forces at the under (articular) surface of the tendon insertion are increased (Fig. 2A and B).

PREOPERATIVE PLANNING

History and Physical Examination

Patients frequently will give a history of a traumatic episode (forced external rotation) with resultant loss of arm strength and function in front of the body. The classic exam findings are those of decreased internal rotation strength and increased passive external rotation compared to the normal side. There are several special physical exam tests that are useful in making the diagnosis of subscapularis injury. The lift-off test is classically described, however, we have not found this test positive until at least three-fourths of the tendon is torn. The Napoleon or

---

Please refer to pages 265–271 for the figures in this chapter.

belly press test can aid in predicting the amount of subscapularis torn (14). The senior author has found the "Bear Hug" test to be the most sensitive test for subscapularis injury, particularly, a partial tear involving only the upper tendon (14). In this test the patient places the hand of the affected extremity on the opposite shoulder with the fingers extended and the elbow elevated to a forward position. The physician then tries to pull the patient's hand away from the shoulder while the patient resists (Fig. 3). If the physician is able to lift the patient's hand away from the shoulder this is a positive test.

Imaging

We routinely obtain five radiographic views of the shoulder to assess for proximal humeral migration and for early signs of arthritis. Evidence of early proximal humeral migration is not necessarily a contraindication to rotator cuff repair surgery as this has been predictably reversed after subscapularis repair (2). MRI evaluation will give important information regarding location and extent of injury and will help rule out other concomitant pathology (ganglion cyst, labral tears). The axial plane images give the best appreciation of the subscapularis insertion (Fig. 4).

INDICATIONS FOR SURGERY

Patients with documented subscapularis tears who have functional disability and pain are the usual indications for surgery. Contraindications include fixed proximal migration with massive three tendon tear and grade IV Goutallier stage atrophy.

RECOGNIZING THE PATHOLOGY

Arthroscopic Evaluation

Following administration of general anesthesia, the patient is positioned in the lateral decubitus position on a beanbag and a warming blanket is placed to prevent hypothermia. Five to ten pounds of balanced suspension is used with the arm in 30° of abduction and 20° of forward flexion (Star Sleeve Traction System, Arthrex, Inc., Naples, Florida, U.S.A.). Diagnostic arthroscopy is performed through a standard posterior viewing portal with an arthroscopic pump maintaining 60 mm Hg of pressure. The subscapularis insertion is best visualized with the arm abducted and internally rotated. In this position the insertional fibers are oriented nearly perpendicular to the lesser tuberosity allowing a clear view of the footprint. A 70° scope is frequently employed at this time to gain the best view of the tendon insertion (Fig. 5A–C). The tear size is estimated by comparing the bare area of footprint to that of the known average dimensions of the subscapularis footprint.

The Working Portals

If subscapularis pathology is confirmed arthroscopically, this is dealt with first, as working in this confined area is very technically challenging. Soft-tissue swelling that occurs as the case proceeds will make work in this area increasingly difficult. The first critical step is in establishing well-placed working portals. In addition to the posterior viewing portal, the anterior and anterosuperolateral portals are created (Fig. 5D). The primary working portal for subscapularis repair is the anterosuperolateral portal and this is established first. An 18-gauge spinal needle is inserted into the glenohumeral joint from just off the anterolateral tip of the acromion. It is directed into the joint to make a 10° angle of approach to the lesser tuberosity. This angle will allow for ease of preparation of the lesser tuberosity bone bed and also a near parallel angle of approach to the subscapularis tendon for lysis of adhesions and antegrade suture passage. An 8.25 mm clear cannula is inserted into this portal.

The anterior portal is established next. This portal is located more medially on the skin than the standard anterior portal. The 18-gauge spinal needle enters the glenohumeral joint space just off the lateral tip of the coracoid with the goal being to hit the lesser tuberosity at a 45° angle. This portal is used primarily for anchor placement and as a holding cannula for sutures. Occasionally this portal is used for retrograde suture passage. An 8.25 mm clear cannula is inserted into this portal as well.

Identifying the Torn Subscapularis Tendon Edge

In complete and chronic subscapularis tears, the lesser tuberosity will be bare and the leading edge of the subscapularis tendon can be difficult to delineate. The tendon will often retract to the level of the glenoid and become scarred to the inner deltoid fascia and to the coracoid making its distinction difficult. The key for locating the leading edge of the torn and retracted subscapularis tendon lies in understanding the "comma sign." When the upper subscapularis tears off the humerus, the medial-biceps sling, which is composed of a portion of the superior glenohumeral ligament and the medial head of the coracohumeral ligament is pulled off along with the subscapularis tendon as one collective unit. This occurs because of their close approximation and interdigitation at their insertions. This avulsed medial sling forms a "comma" shaped arc of tissue that leads directly to the superolateral corner of the subscapularis tendon (Fig. 6A and B). By grasping this confluence of tissue and pulling the retracted tissue laterally, one can definitively identify the superior border of the subscapularis tendon.

PREPARATION FOR REPAIR

The Biceps Tendon

Before proceeding to repair the subscapularis, the biceps tendon should be carefully examined. Subluxation and fraying of the biceps tendon is commonly found in association with subscapularis tears. The insertion of the medial-biceps sling lies directly adjacent to the upper subscapularis insertion and when the upper subscapularis tears, the medial-biceps sling usually becomes disrupted as well. Biceps subluxation out of the groove can be visualized with internal and external rotation of the arm. A proximal biceps tendon that lies posterior to the plane of the projected fibers of the subscapularis tendon is diagnostic of medial subluxation (Fig. 7). Fraying on the medial edge of the biceps tendon is also usually a sign that indicates that subluxation is occurring. Biceps tenodesis or tenotomy is indicated if the biceps tendon is felt to be subluxing or is significantly frayed and degenerated. Just tenotomy alone is performed rarely and only in elderly patients with low demands and poorly defined upper arm musculature. In preparation for biceps tenodesis, two half racking sutures are placed through the intra articular portion of the biceps and the tendon is tenotomized at its root. The tendon is then pulled out the anterosuperolateral portal (elbow is flexed to gain length) and a running whip stitch is placed. The tendon is then held in the anterosuperolateral portal outside the cannula for later tenodesis with a Biotenodesis screw (Arthrex, Inc., Naples, Florida, U.S.A.) after the subscapularis repair is completed. Visualization and working space around the subscapularis is improved following tenotomy of the biceps tendon. It is critical to treat biceps pathology when repairing the subscapularis. Persistent biceps subluxation will cause failure of the subscapularis repair.

Subcoracoid Space and The Coracoplasty

After identification of the subscapularis tendon edge and appropriate treatment of biceps pathology, attention is shifted to the subcoracoid space. The subcoracoid space is the interval between the tip of the coracoid and the humeral head (coracohumeral interval). This space must accommodate the subscapularis tendon, the subscapularis bursa, the rotator interval tissue, and a small amount of the insertions of the coracoacromial ligament and conjoint tendon. Anatomic and imaging studies have established the normal coracohumeral interval to be between 8.4 and 11.0 mm (15–18). The senior author has previously defined subcoracoid stenosis as a coracohumeral interval of less then 6 mm (18). While MRI examination gives a good estimation of the coracohumeral interval, it is clearly most accurate to measure this interval intraoperatively.

When the subscapularis is intact or only partially torn, the coracoid can be located in the soft tissues just anterior to the upper border of the subscapularis tendon (Fig. 8). In the case of a complete, retracted subscapularis tear, the coracoacromial ligament serves as a useful guide to the coracoid tip. It is best to confirm the coracoid's location by palpation of the boney prominence with an instrument. Next, a window is created in the rotator interval tissue just above the subscapularis tendon with the electrocautery device. In creating this window, the medial sling of biceps and superior glenohumeral ligament should be preserved. With the tip of the coracoid identified, the coracohumeral interval is measured by placing an instrument of known width through the anterosuperolateral cannula and placing it between the coracoid and humerus (Fig. 9). This measurement is made with gentle distraction on the arm to remove the effect of proximal humeral migration. We have encountered instances where this space was so tight that a 5 mm shaver would not fit between the coracoid and humerus. If the subcoracoid space is 6 mm or less then a diagnosis of subcoracoid stenosis is made. Impingement can be confirmed by placing the arm in the provocative position of flexion, adduction, and internal rotation and visualizing if the coracoid contacts the lesser tuberosity or sharply indents into the subscapularis tendon. If a diagnosis of subcoracoid stenosis and impingement are made in combination with a partial or complete subscapularis tear, then we routinely perform a coracoplasty.

In performing a coracoplasty, our goal is to create an 8 to 10 mm space between the humerus and the reshaped coracoid tip. This is accomplished by first skeletonizing the posterolateral surface of the coracoid by using an electrocautery device and motorized shaver (Fig. 10). Care is taken not to release the conjoint tendon from the under surface of the tip. The coracoacromial ligament can be released from the coracoid if necessary. With the tip exposed, a high-speed burr is placed through the anterosuperolateral cannula and used for coracoplasty (Fig. 11). The plane of the coracoplasty is parallel to the subscapularis tendon. This is easily possible because of the precise location and angle of the working portal. This subcoracoid decompression improves the space available for repair and will prevent abrasive effect of the coracoid on the subscapularis repair.

Improving the Space for Repair

There are several tricks one can use to improve anterior visualization and to gain space for work in these tight confines. The use of a 70° scope can dramatically improve visualization when working at the level of the glenoid, at the coracoid tip, and further medial around the coracoid base (lysis of adhesions). However, we do not recommend the use of this scope during the initial identification and dissection around the coracoid as it is easy to become disoriented. If dissection strays inferior or inferomedial to the coracoid base there is significant risk of neurological injury. It can occasionally become difficult to visualize the subscapularis footprint on the lesser tuberosity even with the use of the 70° scope. In this situation we have found the "posterior lever push" to be helpful in gaining extra subcoracoid space and a better view. To perform the maneuver, a second assistant, positioned anterior to the patient, levers the humeral head posterior by placing a posterior force on the proximal humerus while simultaneously pulling the distal humerus forward (Fig. 12).

SUBSCAPULARIS REPAIR

Mobilization

In the case of a complete subscapularis tear with retraction, a three-sided release is performed. It is critical to understand the anatomy around the coracoid, as it is this aspect of the subscapularis repair where risk of neurovascular injury is the highest. The structures most at risk include the axillary nerve, axillary artery, musculocutaneus nerve, and lateral cord of the brachial plexus. These structures are all located greater than 25 mm from the coracoid base on anatomic cadaver dissection (18). Release of the anterior, superior, and posterior surfaces of the subscapularis tendon is facilitated by placing a traction suture at the superolateral corner of the tendon (at the junction with the comma tissue). The Viper suture passer (Arthrex, Inc., Naples, Florida, U.S.A.) loaded with a free number 2 Fiberwire suture (Arthrex, Inc., Naples, Florida, U.S.A.) is used through the anterosuperolateral cannula to place this suture. The suture limbs are then held in the anterosuperolateral portal (but outside the cannula) so as not to obstruct the instrument passage through this working portal.

It is generally easiest to perform the anterior release first. Here, it is necessary to release the scar tissue that binds the subscapularis to the posterolateral aspect of the coracoid. The electrocautery and shaver are used to dissect and essentially skeletonize the posterolateral surface of the coracoid. The dissection begins at the previously identified coracoid tip and proceeds medially along the posterolateral surface of the coracoid until the subscapularis muscle belly is visible passing freely beneath the coracoid neck and base (Fig. 13).

Natural progression leads one directly to the superior release. Scar tissue binding the superior surface of the subscapularis to the under surface of the coracoid base is released with the use of a 30° arthroscopic elevator. It is very risky to continue the dissection medial past the coracoid base and so our dissection is stopped at the mid-point of the base of the coracoid.

Finally, the posterior release is performed. It is helpful to maintain tension on the traction suture throughout the releases, but especially during the posterior release. A 15° arthroscopic elevator is generally used to severe any adhesions between the posterior surface of the subscapularis and the glenoid neck (Fig. 14). There is virtually no risk of nerve injury during this portion of the release as the muscle belly of the subscapularis serves as protection from the neurovascular structures, which lie more anterior.

Bone Bed Preparation

Next it is important to prepare the subscapularis bone bed to optimize conditions for tendon to bone healing. Again the anterosuperolateral portal is the main working portal. The electrocautery is used to remove fibrous and granulation tissue from the lesser tuberosity. A ring curette is used to remove soft tissue very precisely up to the articular margin. The burr is used to lightly dust the bone surface removing a very fine layer of bone to prepare a bleeding surface without completely decorticating the bone (Fig. 15). In rare chronic contracted cases the footprint will be medialized by 5 mm to create a larger footprint and to reduce the tension in the repair. The senior author has not found this to negatively impact the functional recovery.

Anchor Insertion

The superior to inferior length of the subscapularis footprint measures 2.45 cm on an average. We prefer to use one double loaded suture anchor for each linear centimeter of tendon detachment. If a complete tear of the subscapularis is encountered, we will generally use two double loaded anchors. Occasionally, there exists enough lateral excursion of the tendon to perform a double-row repair. However this is very difficult and is not routinely performed. In general, the clinical results have been very acceptable after a single-row repair of the subscapularis.

The anterior portal was specifically placed to allow an appropriate angle of approach for anchor insertion. The bone punch is generally placed through this portal. When the correct angle of approach is achieved with the bone punch the surgeon will find that his hand is very near the patient's jaw and face (Fig. 16). Because of this our anesthesiologist routinely places eye protection on the patient (plastic goggles) to avoid inadvertent eye injury during anchor insertion.

Suture Passage

It is important to realize that in dealing with the subscapularis, retrograde passage of sutures is very difficult because the coracoid blocks access to the tendon from the necessary angle. Hence, antegrade suture passage is preferred, in this case. We generally prefer to use the Viper suture passer (Arthrex, Inc., Naples, Florida, U.S.A.). After inferior anchor placement through the anterior cannula, one strand of suture is retrieved out the anterosuperolateral cannula and loaded into the Viper. Tension is maintained on the previously placed traction suture (out the anterosuperolateral portal but outside the cannula) while the Viper is used to obtain a 10 mm bite inferiorly along the lateral margin of the tendon. The process is repeated for the second suture for the same anchor. These sutures are tied prior to placement of the superior anchor so as to minimize problems with suture management in these tight confines. When passing sutures from the superior anchor, we prefer to obtain a bite of tissue along the superolateral border of the tendon just medial to the comma tissue (Fig. 17). The comma tissue has fibers running perpendicular to the subscapularis fibers and we believe this tissue serves as a "rip stop" to prevent suture cutout.

Knot Tying

Knots are tied through the anterosuperolateral clear cannula with a double diameter knot pusher (Surgeon's Sixth Finger; Arthrex, Inc., Naples, Florida, U.S.A.) Use of this knot pusher allows one to manipulate the tissue over the anchor while securing the knot (Fig. 18). We do not use a sliding knot, but rather tie a static knot with three stacked half hitches followed by three throws with a consecutively reversed post. When tested in the lab, this knot has been found to offer the best combination of loop and knot security (19). With the completed repair there should be secure apposition of the tendon to bone as visualized during internal and external rotation of the arm (Fig. 19).

Pearls and Pitfalls

1. Establishing precise portals including the anterosuperolateral portal is critical to the success of this operation.
2. Identification of the "comma sign" helps to identify, release, and mobilize the medially retracted subscapularis tendon.
3. Coracoplasty is recommended when the coracohumeral interval is <6 mm.
4. Care must be taken to stay lateral to the coracoid process to avoid inadvertent neurovascular injury.
5. Care must be taken when mobilizing the subscapularis to avoid axillary nerve and musculocutaneous nerve injury.

REHABILITATION

A consistent rehabilitation protocol is recommended following subscapularis repair regardless of whether or not there has been concomitant repair of the posterosuperior rotator cuff. The patient is placed in a sling with a small pillow after the operation and this sling is worn for six weeks. During this time, the patient is instructed to remove the sling daily for active wrist and elbow motion and for passive shoulder external rotation to neutral only. No overhead motion is allowed during the first six weeks. The sling is discontinued at six weeks and a passive stretching program is initiated (passive external rotation with cane to 45°, overhead and internal rotation stretch with rope and pulley). At 12 weeks postoperatively, a strengthening program is initiated with elastic bands and progression to lightweights is allowed, based on patient progress. Return to unrestricted activity is delayed for 6 to 12 months postoperatively depending on the size of the repair and patient's rehabilitation progress.

CONCLUSION

Advances in arthroscopic shoulder surgery have lead to an increased awareness of subscapularis tendon injury, its causes, and refined minimally invasive treatments. The arthroscopic subscapularis repair is a safe and effective procedure that has produced consistently gratifying results for both the patient and surgeon.

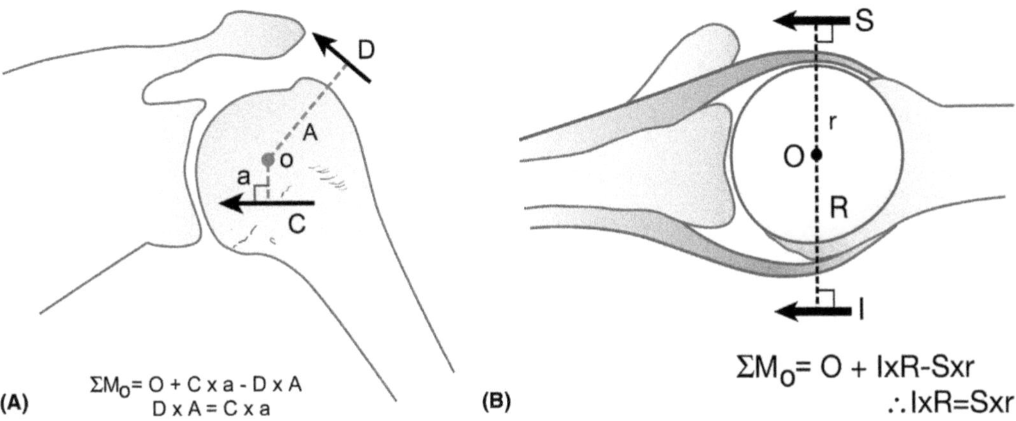

FIGURE 1 (**A**) The coronal plane force couple. The inferior portions of the anterior and posterior rotator cuff (below the center of rotation) must create a moment that will counteract and balance the moment created by the deltoid. (**B**) The transverse plane force couple. The subscapularis anteriorly is balanced against the infraspinatus and teres minor posteriorly. *Abbreviations*: A, moment arm of the deltoid; a, moment arm of the inferior portion of the rotator cuff; C, resultant of rotator cuff forces; D, deltoid force; I, infraspinatus; O, center of rotation; r, moment arm of the subscapularis; R, moment arm of the infraspinatus and teres minor; S, subscapularis.

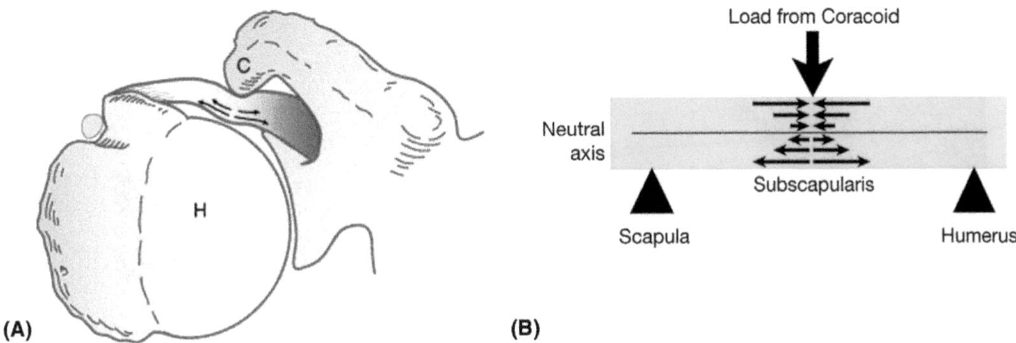

FIGURE 2 (**A**) When subcoracoid impingement occurs, the prominent coracoid presses into the anterior surface of the subscapularis tendon. This creates an increased tensile force on the convex (articular) surface of the subscapularis tendon, which commonly leads to tendon fiber failure (joint sided subscapularis insertional tears). (**B**) This schematic diagram illustrates the effect of subcoracoid impingement. In this scenario, the subscapularis is supported on ends by the scapula and humerus respectively. The coracoid imparts a force perpendicular to the subscapularis, which results in compressive forces on the superficial side and tensile forces on the deep convex side of the tendon.

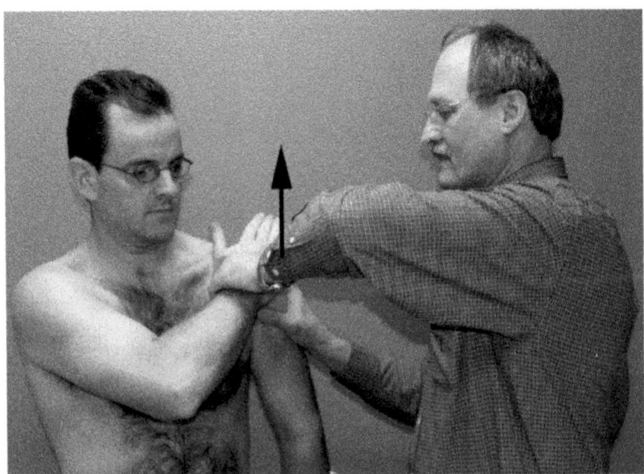

FIGURE 3 The bear hug test for subscapularis tendon injury. Patients with a partial or complete subscapularis tear will not be able to maintain their hand apposed to their opposite shoulder in this position when the examiner attempts to lift the hand away.

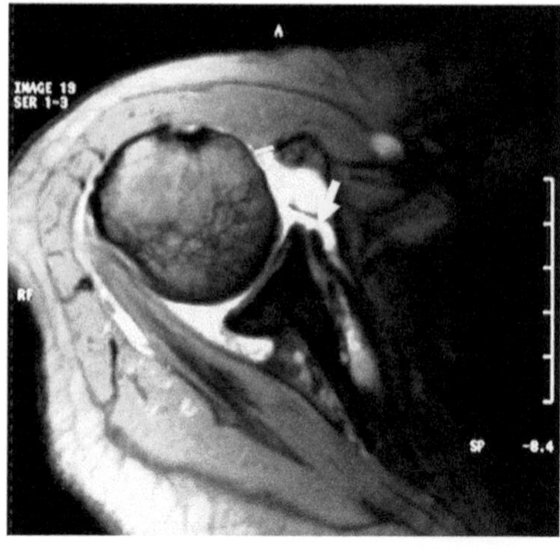

FIGURE 4 Axial plane MRI image demonstrating a full thickness, retracted, subscapularis tear (yellow arrow), and a narrow coraco-humeral interval.

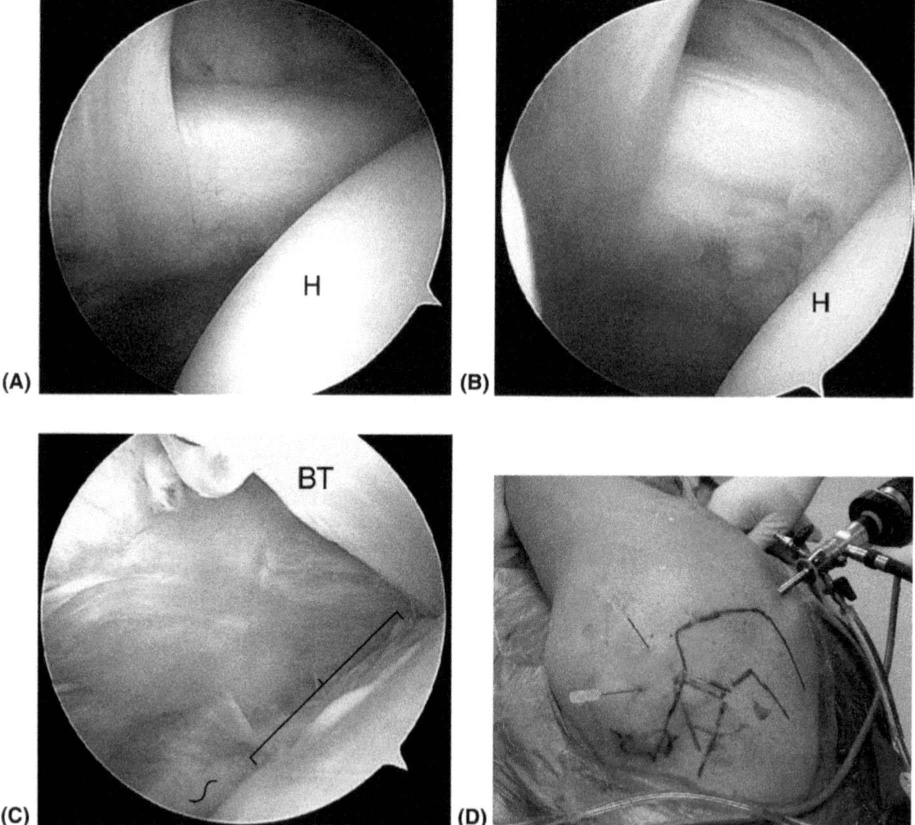

FIGURE 5 (**A**) Arthroscopic view of the right shoulder. The subscapularis insertion is visualized from the posterior viewing portal with a 30° scope while maintaining neutral arm rotation. It is difficult to assess the subscapularis footprint in this manner. (**B**) Arthroscopic view of the right shoulder with the same scope position, however, the view is now through a 70° scope and the arm has been positioned in internal rotation. This arm position brings the subscapularis tendon more perpendicular to the bone at the insertion while this scope allows an excellent view of the footprint. (**C**) Arthroscopic view of a right shoulder with a 70° scope through the posterior portal demonstrating a full thickness tear of the upper portion of the subscapularis tendon. Note the bare area of footprint (bracket) and the intact inferior most portion of the subscapularis insertion (~). (**D**) There are two standard working portals for an arthroscopic subscapularis repair (see the two spinal needles). The anterosuperolateral portal is used for bone bed preparation, coracoid exposure and coracoplasty, lysis of adhesions, and suture passage. The Anterior portal is used primarily for anchor insertion and for suture management.

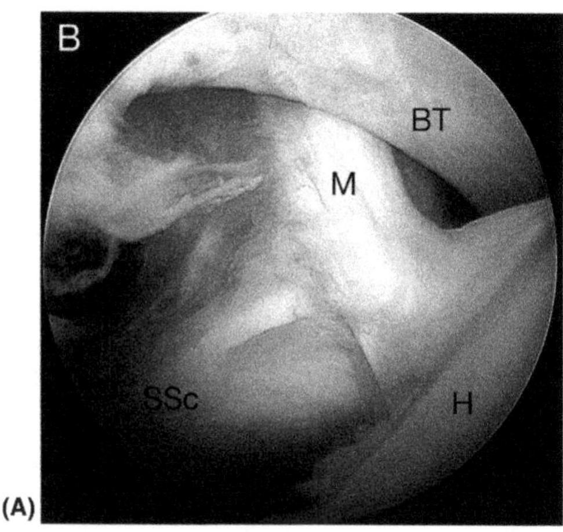

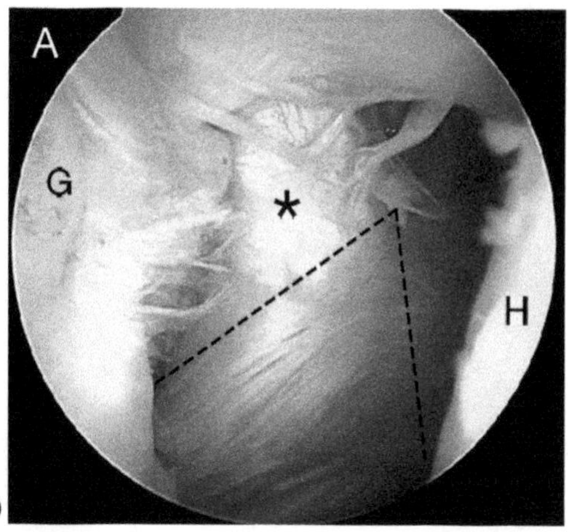

FIGURE 6 (**A**) Arthroscopic view of the right shoulder from the posterior portal with a 70° scope demonstrating the normal anatomic relationship of the subscapularis insertion (SSc), the medial-biceps sling (M), and the biceps tendon (BT). Note how the insertions of the medial-biceps sling and subscapularis tendon are adjacent and interdigitate. (**B**) Arthroscopic view of the right shoulder posterior viewing portal demonstrating the "comma sign"(*). This comma shaped arc of tissue will always lead the surgeon to the superolateral corner of the torn subscapularis tendon. *Abbreviations*: G, glenoid; H, humeral head.

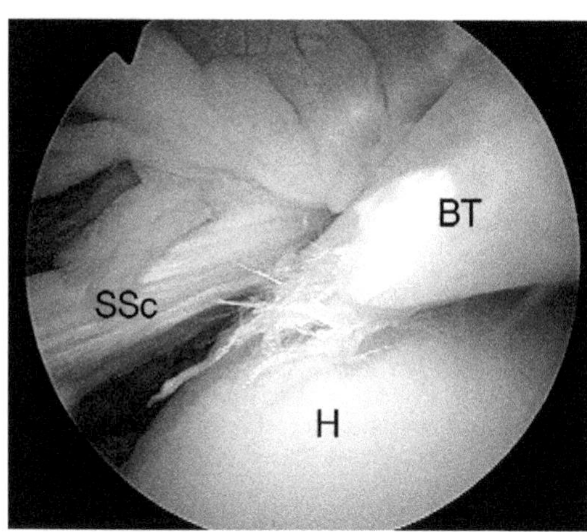

FIGURE 7 Arthroscopic view of the right shoulder from the posterior portal demonstrating an upper subscapularis tendon (SSc) tear. Fraying on the biceps tendon (BT) in this location suggests failure of the medial-biceps sling and that biceps subluxation is occurring. The biceps tendon lies posterior to the projected plane of the subscapularis fibers indicating that the upper subscapularis has torn from its insertion. *Abbreviation*: H, humeral head.

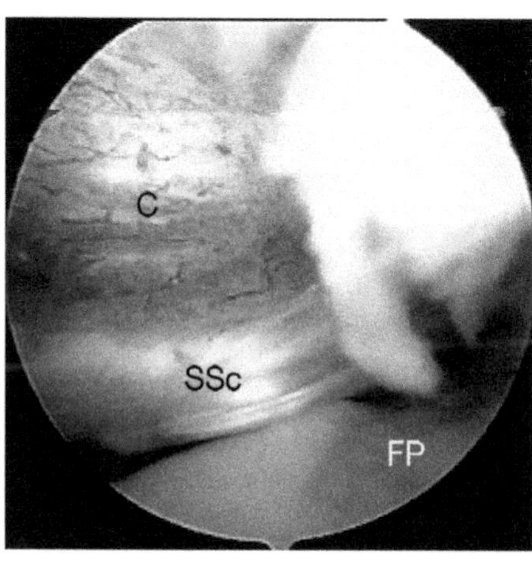

FIGURE 8 Arthroscopic view of the right shoulder from the posterior portal in which the coracoid tip (C) is identified as a bulge in the soft tissues anterosuperior to the subscapularis tendon (SSc). *Abbreviation*: FP, uncovered upper subscapularis footprint.

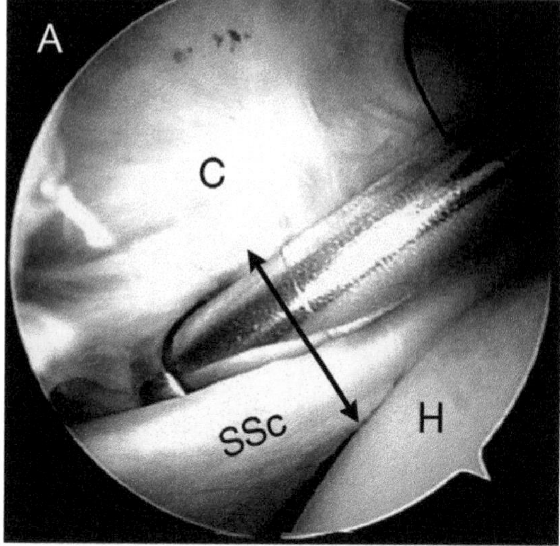

FIGURE 9 Arthroscopic view of the right shoulder, in which the coraco-humeral interval width can be estimated by the use of an instrument of known size (this shaver tip width is 4.5 mm). Borderline subcoracoid stenosis exists in this case as the coraco-humeral interval is estimated at 7 to 8 mm. *Abbreviation*: H, humeral head.

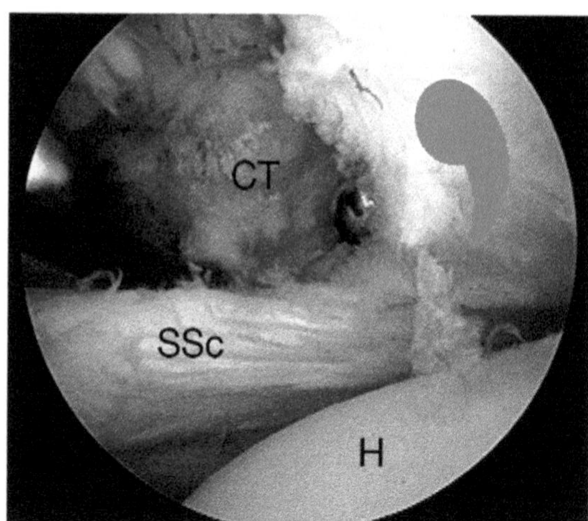

FIGURE 10 Arthroscopic view of the right shoulder demonstrating an upper subscapularis (SSc) tear. The comma tissue is evident (,) and the rotator interval tissue has been resected with an electrocautery device exposing the coracoid tip (CT) just anterosuperior to the subscapularis tendon.

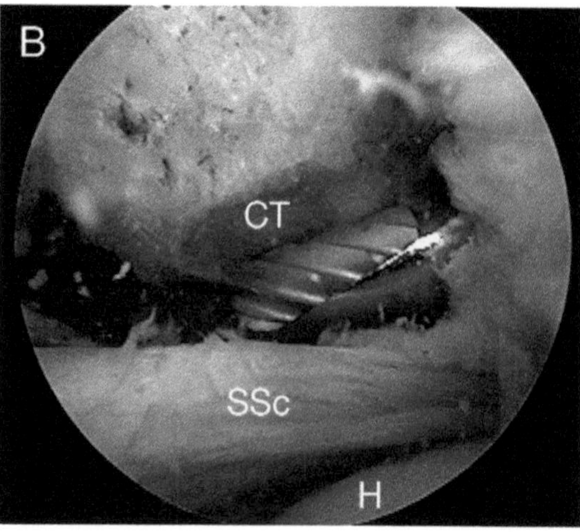

FIGURE 11 Arthroscopic view of the right shoulder, in which the coracoplasty is performed with a high-speed bur. Resection of bone is performed in a plane parallel to the subscapularis so as to create a coraco–humeral interval of 8 to 10 mm. *Abbreviations*: CT, coracoid tip; SSc, subscapularis tendon; H, humeral head.

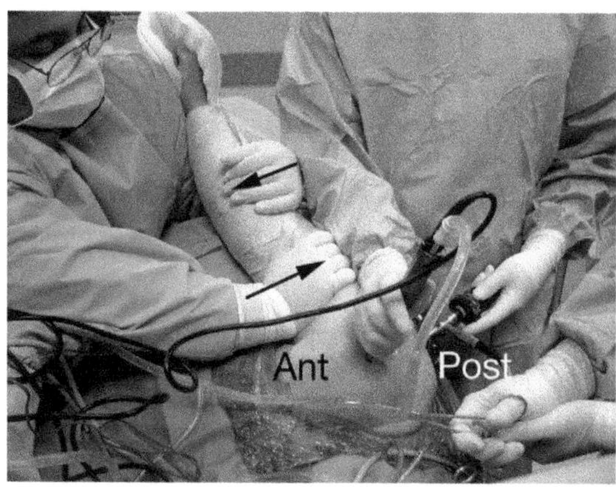

FIGURE 12 The "posterior lever push" is performed by an assistant who stands anterior to the patient who is in the lateral decubitus position.

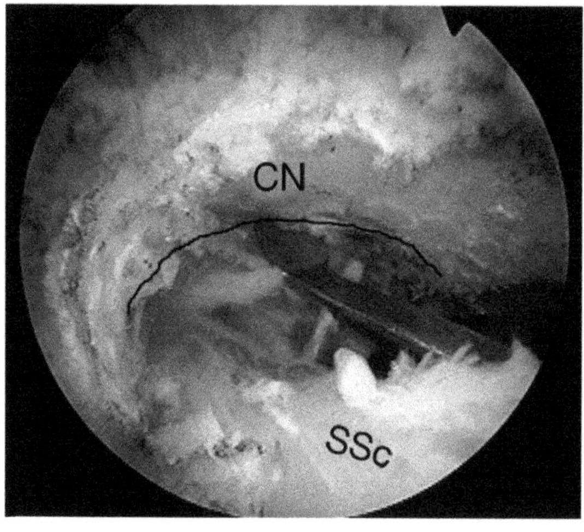

FIGURE 13 Arthroscopic view of the right shoulder from a posterior viewing portal with a 70° scope. The posterolateral surface of the coracoid has been skeletonized and adhesions to the anterior and superior surface of the subscapularis tendon have been released. Subscapularis muscle belly is visible passing beneath the coracoid neck (CN). *Abbreviation*: SSc, subscapularis tendon.

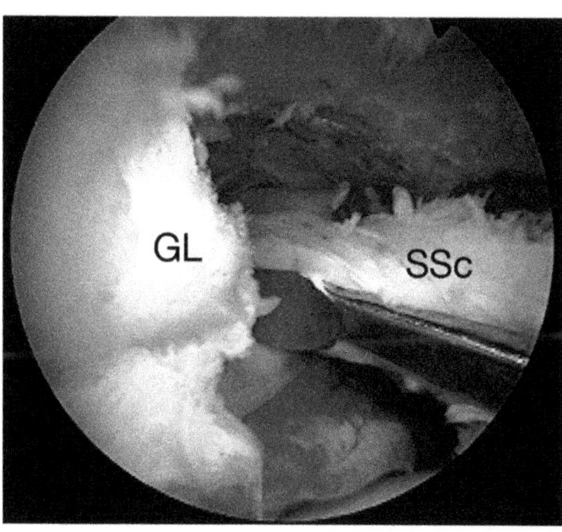

FIGURE 14 Arthroscopic view of the right shoulder from a posterior viewing portal with a 70° scope. The 15° arthroscopic elevator is placed through the anterosuperolateral cannula and is used to sever adhesions along the posterior surface of the subscapularis tendon (SSc). *Abbreviation*: GL, glenoid labrum.

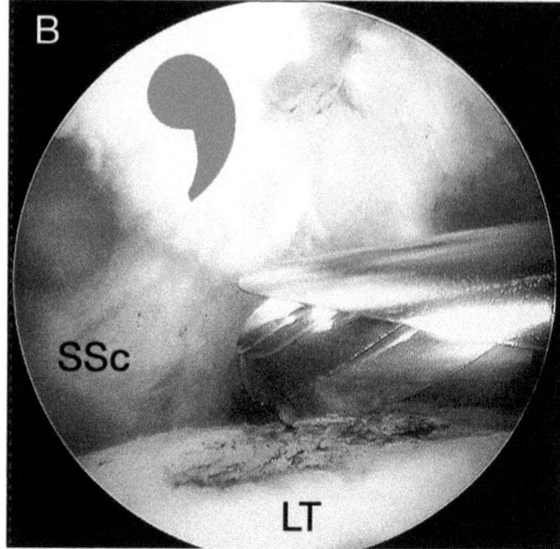

FIGURE 15 Arthroscopic view of the right shoulder from the posterior viewing portal. The high-speed bur is placed through the anterosuperolateral portal. This portal was created to have a 10° to 15° angle of approach to the footprint of the subscapularis which is ideal for preparation of the bone bed. Fibrous tissue has been removed from the footprint with the electrocautery. *Abbreviations*: SSc, subscapularis tendon; LT, lesser tuberosity of the humerus.

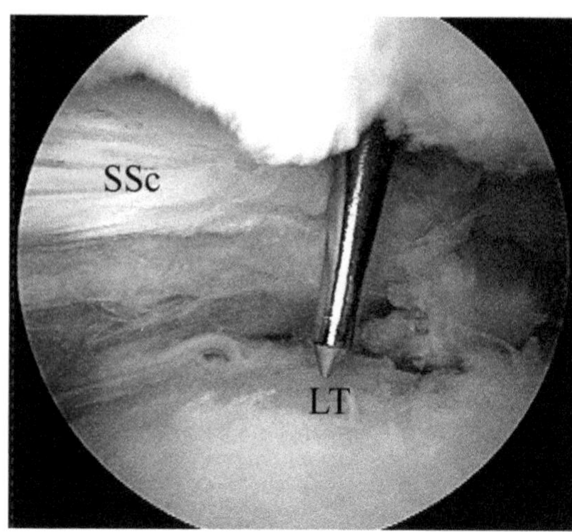

FIGURE 16 Arthroscopic view of the right shoulder from the posterior viewing portal with a 70° scope. The bone punch is brought through the anterior portal and will be positioned in the superolateral corner of the footprint entering at a 30° to 60° angle to the bone bed. In this case the upper 50% of the subscapularis tendon (SSc) has torn from the insertion. *Abbreviation*: LT, lesser tuberosity of the humerus.

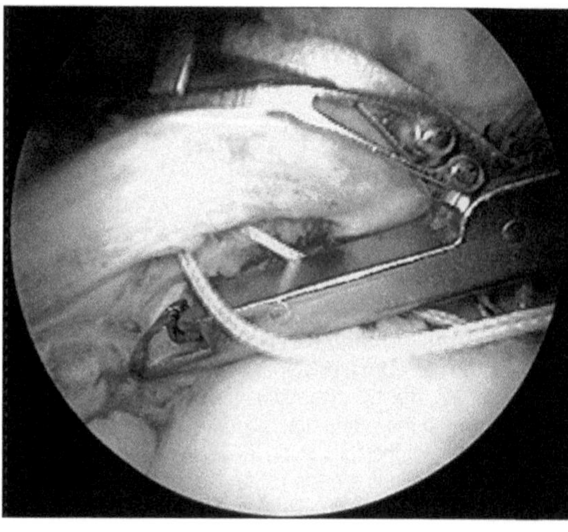

FIGURE 17 Arthroscopic view of the right shoulder posterior viewing portal. The Viper suture passer (Arthrex, Inc., Naples, Florida, U.S.A.), introduced through a clear cannula in the anterosuperolateral portal, is used to pass suture in an antegrade direction through the superolateral corner of the subscapularis tendon (SSc).

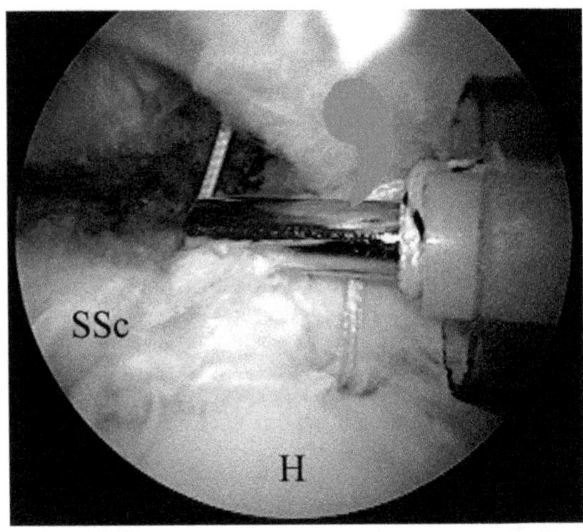

FIGURE 18 Arthroscopic view of the right shoulder posterior viewing portal. The double diameter knot pusher is used to hold the tendon over the anchor while tying the knot, (placed through a clear cannula in the anterosuperolateral portal). *Abbreviations*: SSc, subscapularis tendon; H, humeral head.

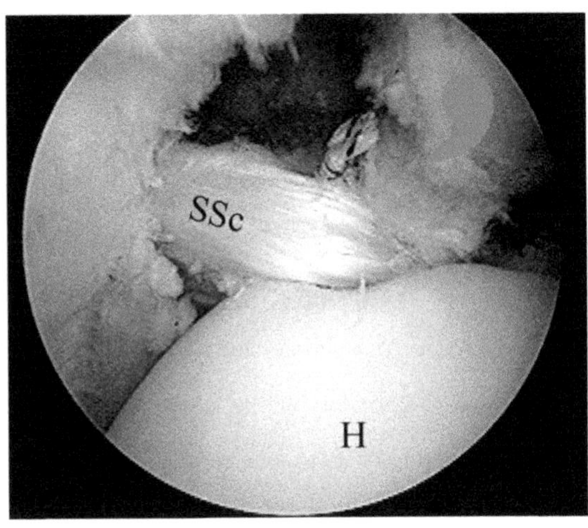

FIGURE 19 Arthroscopic view of the right shoulder posterior viewing portal. The subscapularis (SSc) repair has been completed. Good compression of the tendon into the bone bed has been achieved and the comma tissue (,) remains intact. *Abbreviation*: H, humeral head.

REFERENCES

1. Bennett WF. Arthroscopic repair of isolated subscapularis tears: a prospective cohort with 2- to 4-year follow-up. Arthroscopy 2003; 19(2):131–143.
2. Burkhart SS, Tehrany AM. Arthroscopic subscapularis tendon repair: technique and preliminary results. Arthroscopy 2002; 18(5):454–463.
3. Kim TK, Rauh PB, McFarland EG. Partial tears of the subscapularis tendon found during arthroscopic procedures on the shoulder: a statistical analysis of sixty cases. Am J Sports Med 2003; 31:744–750.
4. Lo IK, Burkhart SS. Subscapularis tears: arthroscopic repair of the forgotten rotator cuff tendon. Tech Shoulder Elbow Surg 2002; 3:282–291.
5. Kim SK, Oh I, Park J, et al. Intra-articular repair of an isolated partial articular-surface tear of the subscapularis tendon. Am J Sports Med 2005; 33(12):1825–1830.
6. Lo IK, Burkhart SS. The comma sign: an arthroscopic guide to the torn subscapularis tendon. Arthroscopy 2003; 19(3):334–337.
7. Lo IK, Burkhart SS. The etiology and assessment of subscapularis tendon tears: a case for subcoracoid impingement, the roller-wringer effect, and TUFF lesions of the subscapularis. Arthroscopy 2003; 19(1):1142–1150.
8. Lo IK, Burkhart SS. The interval slide in continuity: a method of mobilizing the anterosuperior rotator cuff without disrupting the tear margins. Arthroscopy 2004; 20(4):435–441.
9. Gerber C, Hersche O, Farron A. Isolated rupture of the subscapularis. Results of operative repair. J Bone Joint Surg Am 1996; 78:1015–1023.
10. Gerber C, Krushell RJ. Isolated rupture of the tendon of the subscapularis muscle. Clinical features in 16 cases. J Bone Joint Surg Br 1991; 73:389–394.
11. Lo IK, Parten PM, Burkhart SS. Combined subcoracoid and subacromial impingement in association with anterosuperior rotator cuff tears: an arthroscopic approach. Arthroscopy 2003; 19(10):1068–1078.
12. Dines DM, Warren RF, Inglis AE, Pavlov H. The coracoid impingement syndrome. J Bone Joint Surg Br 1990; 72:314–316.
13. Ferrick MR. Coracoid impingement: a case report and review of the literature. Am J Sports Med 2000; 28:117–119.
14. Barth JRH, Burkhart SS, DeBeer JF. The bear hug test: a new and sensitive test for diagnosing a subscapularis tear. Arthroscopy 2006; 22:1076–1084.
15. Friedman RJ, Bonutti PM, Genez B. Cine magnetic resonance imaging of the subcoracoid region. Orthopedics 1998; 21:545–548.
16. Gerber C, Terrier F, Ganz R. The role of the coracoid process in the chronic impingement syndrome. J Bone Joint Surgy Br 1985; 67:703–708.
17. Gerber C, Terrier F, Zehnder R, Ganz R. The subcoracoid space. An anatomic study. Clin Orthop 1987; 215:132–138.
18. Lo IK, Burkhart SS. Arthroscopic coracoplasty through the rotator interval. Arthroscopy 2003; 19(6):667–671.
19. Lo IK, Burkhart SS. Arthroscopic knots: determining the optimal balance of loop and knot security. Arthroscopy 2004; 20:489–502.

25 Arthroscopic Partial Rotator Cuff Repair—Convert to Full Tear

Christopher S. Ahmad
Center for Shoulder, Elbow, and Sports Medicine, Department of Orthopedic Surgery, Columbia Presbyterian Medical Center, New York, New York, U.S.A.

Neal S. ElAttrache
Kerlan-Jobe Orthopedic Clinic and Department of Orthopedic Surgery, University of Southern California School of Medicine, Los Angeles, California, U.S.A.

INDICATIONS/CONTRAINDICATIONS

Partial thickness rotator cuff tears are extremely common in both younger and older patients with shoulder pain. Patients with symptomatic partial thickness rotator cuff tears who fail nonoperative treatment, including physical therapy, nonsteroidal anti-inflammatory drugs (NSAIDs), cortisone injections, and rest, are candidates for surgery. Many surgical options exist for managing partial thickness rotator cuff tear (PTRCT), including debridement of rotator cuff tear, subacromial decompression, arthroscopic in situ repair, or completion of the tear followed by open, mini-open, or all arthroscopic repair. Tears are classified according to the percent of thickness of tear, number of tendons involved, and whether it involves the bursal or articular side. Partial articular supraspinatous tendon avulsion (PASTA) lesions refer to partial articular supraspinatous tendon avulsions. While a consensus has not been established for treatment, the authors have created general guidelines. If 25% of cuff is torn, rotator cuff debridement and subacromial decompression is performed. If 50% of cuff is torn, an in situ all-arthroscopic repair to footprint is performed without completing the tear. If ≥75% of cuff is torn, the tear is completed and all-arthroscopic rotator cuff repair is performed. Bursal-sided tears have superior results when an acromioplasty is performed. For intratendinous laminar tears, intratendinous repair is performed. In younger throwing athletes, the authors favor intratendinous repairs and avoid acromioplasty.

When tear completion is performed, the authors prefer all-arthroscopic rotator cuff repair compared to mini-open for several reasons. The techniques for arthroscopic rotator cuff repair techniques have evolved from single-row suture anchors to double rows of suture anchors in the greater tuberosity with increased strength of fixation and restoration of insetional footprint (1,2). Research studies have also shown that transosseous tunnel repair techniques provide improved footprint coverage (3), pressurized contact area at the footprint (4), and reduced motion at the footprint tendon-bone interface (5). It is believed that improved contact characteristics will help maximize healing potential between repaired tendons and the greater tuberosity. The most recent techniques developed in all-arthroscopic double-row rotator cuff repair now replicate transosseous tunnel techniques and create tissue compression against the tuberosity to enhance healing (6). These new techniques have been referred to as suture bridge techniques.

SURGICAL TECHNIQUE

Anesthesia and Positioning

Surgeon, anesthesiologist, and patient preferences determine the type of anesthesia administered and regional, general, or a combination may be used. The patient may be positioned in either the beach-chair or the lateral decubitus position. Beach chair is more familiar to many

---

Please refer to pages 275–278 for the figures in this chapter.

surgeons and is often easier to convert to an open procedure. Lateral decubitus position provides traction on the arm, which enhances visualization in the subacromial space.

Diagnostic arthroscopy is performed to determine the rotator cuff involved, the magnitude of partial thickness tear, and whether the tear is bursal of articular. Standard anterior, posterior, and lateral portals are used. Diagnostic arthroscopy is performed with the camera introduced through a standard posterior working portal. Glenohumeral diagnositic is performed with specific emphasis on the evaluating undersurface rotator cuff tears. An anterior working portal is established, and undersurface tears are gently debrided with a motorized shaver. Figure 1 demonstrates a typical PTRCT articular-sided tear. The degree of partial thickness tear is estimated based on the amount of tendon detached from the greater tuberosity. Percent involvement may be calculated assuming a tendon attachment of 12 mm. A spinal needle may be used to percutaneously penetrate the tear and shuttle monofilament suture. The camera is then placed in the subacromial space and the bursal surface of the tear is inspected (Fig. 2).

For tears greater than 75% with existing tendinosis in the remaining attached tendon, the authors recommend completion of the tear with arthroscopic repair. With the camera in the subacromial space, a bursectomy is performed, and if a curved acromion exists, an acromioplasty is performed. The tear is then completed with either a beaver blade, shaver, or ablation device. Figure 3 demonstrates a high percentage bursal-sided partial thickness tear, and Figure 4 demonstrates a crescent-shaped tear created with a sharp beaver blade and shaver.

The lateral mobility of the tear is assessed by grasping the tear edge and pulling laterally (Fig. 5). These tears usually mobilize easily to the lateral aspect of the greater tuberosity footprint with minimal tension and do not require releases or mobilization techniques. The greater tuberosity footprint is debrided with removal of soft tissue, and the cortical bone is abraded to stimulate healing. Decortication is avoided since it may compromise suture anchor fixation strength.

STANDARD DOUBLE-ROW REPAIR

The repair sequence involves placing a medial row of suture anchors, followed by suture passing through the tendon in a mattress fashion. The medial row anchors are positioned as medial as possible adjacent to the articular surface of the humeral head. For a typical crescent-shaped supraspinatous tear, two anchors are placed; one in the anterior one-third and one in the posterior one-third of the footprint. For larger tears, more anchors are placed as necessary. Suture anchors that are double loaded with two sutures are preferred.

Medial suture anchor passing is then performed creating medial mattress suture configurations, ideally 10 to 12 mm medial to the lateral edge of the rotator cuff tear. Passing the suture far medial maximizes the tendon available for contact with the footprint. Suture-passing instrumentation that will facilitate far medial placement of the suture in the tendon is preferred (Fig. 6). The second suture from the anchor, if it is double-loaded, may also be placed as a second mattress suture.

Next, the lateral row of suture anchors is placed. On the basis of the size of the footprint repair site, one or two lateral suture anchors are placed. The anchors are placed lateral to the lateral edge of the footprint to fully maximize the tendon to footprint contact. For nonsuture bridge double-row repair, the lateral sutures are placed in a simple fashion using surgeon-preferred suture-passing devices. Typically, 5 to 8 mm of tissue is captured in the simple sutures.

Knot tying is typically performed in the following sequence. Lateral sutures working from posterior to anterior. Medial sutures working from posterior to anterior. Figure 7 demonstrates a completed double-row repair.

Suture Bridge Repair Technique

Techniques have been developed to create suture bridges that are equivalent to transosseous tunnel compression stitches. New implants have been developed to greater facilitate placement of compression sutures and reduce knot tying. For the Push Lock (Arthrex; Naples, Florida, U.S.A.) device, the medial suture anchors and suture passing is performed, as previously described for the double-row repair technique. A hole is then punched at the intended site for the lateral implant, just lateral to the lateral edge of the tuberosity. The medial sutures to be used for compression (one suture from the anterior medial anchor and one suture from the posterior medial anchor) are then passed through the eyelet of the implant outside the cannulae. Manual tension is then applied to the suture bridge sutures as they are delivered into the tunnel to achieve the desired compression. The implant is then advanced over the inserter and captures the eyelet, which fixes the sutures in place and eliminates need for knot tying (Fig. 8). The sutures are then cut without knot tying. Figure 9 demonstrates a crescent-shaped tear repaired with a single medial anchor with double-loaded sutures passed medially in a horizontal mattress fashion in combination with a single push loc implant.

PEARLS AND PITFALLS

Pearls for management of partial thickness rotator cuff tears treated with completion of the tear and repair involve proper patient selection. Throwing athletes often have partial thickness rotator cuff tears, but takedown of the tear with repair should be avoided because of poor clinical results in this population. The goal for the surgery is to obtain tendon healing, minimize complications, and achieve improvement in pain and function. The authors also believe that several factors can improve healing, including avoidance of NSAIDs and smoking, during the healing process and less aggressive early physical therapy.

REHABILITATION

Patients are placed in a sling with a small abduction pillow. The sling is worn continuously for six weeks except for bathing. During the first six weeks, active elbow, wrist, and hand exercises are performed. From 6 to 12 weeks, passive range and active-assisted range of motion is initiated. After 12 weeks, active motion and gentle strengthening is initiated. More aggressive strengthening is initiated at four months.

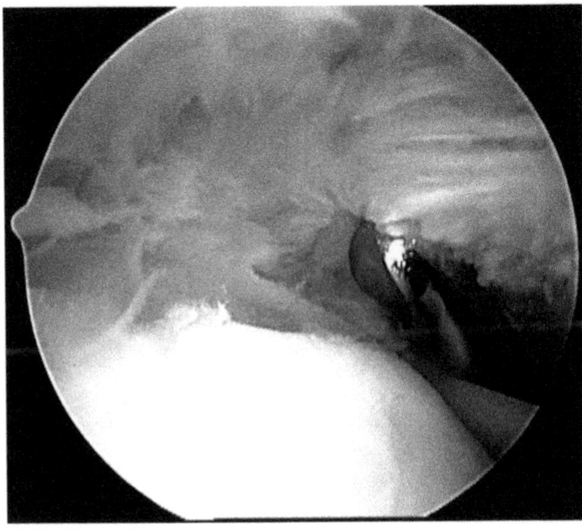

FIGURE 1 Articular-sided partial thickness rotator cuff tear. A 3.5 mm shaver assists in determining the number of millimeters that rotator cuff is detached from tuberosity.

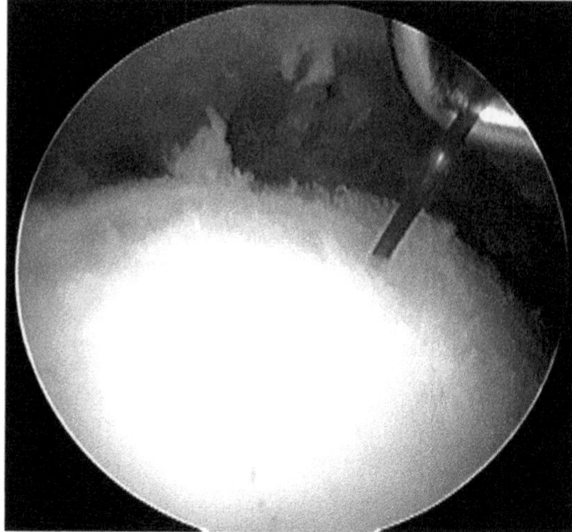

FIGURE 2 Suture passed percutaneously to locate bursal rotator cuff corresponding to articular-sided tear. No corresponding tear is observed on the bursal side.

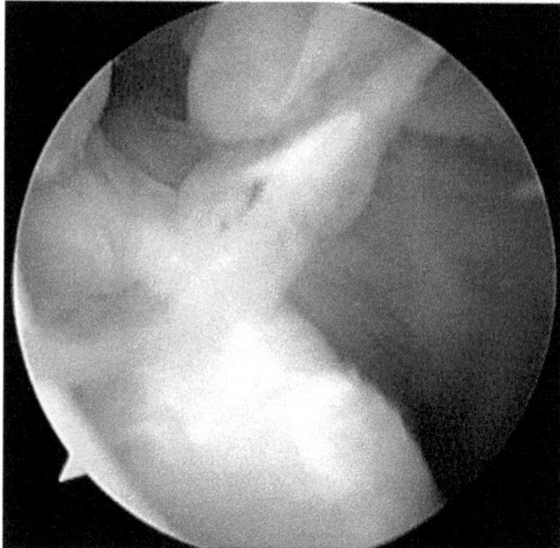

FIGURE 3 High percentage bursal-sided partial thickness supraspinatous cuff tear.

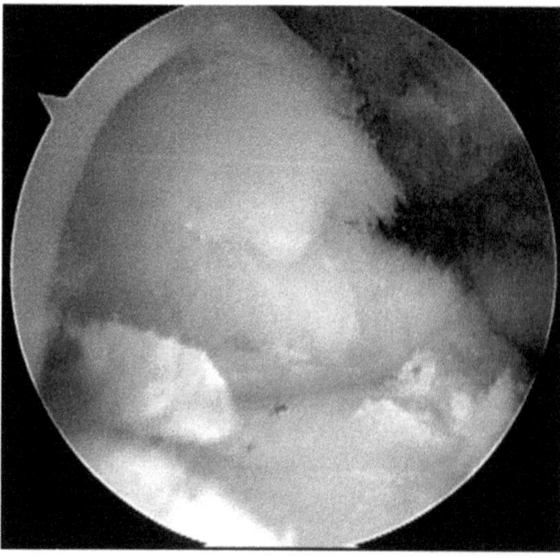

FIGURE 4 Partial tear converted to complete crescent-shaped tear.

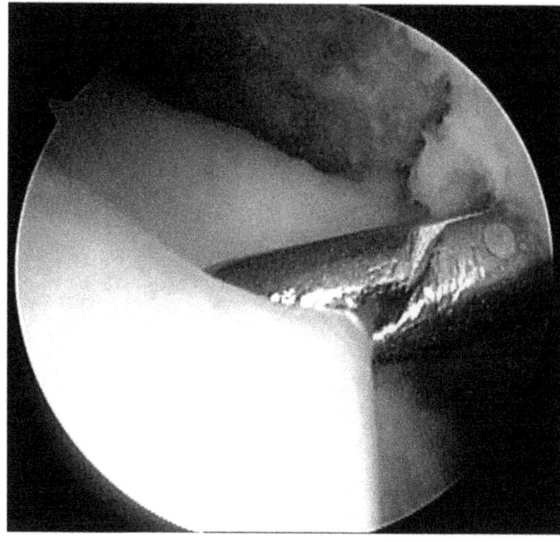

FIGURE 5 Grasper used to reduce tear to greater tuberosity footprint.

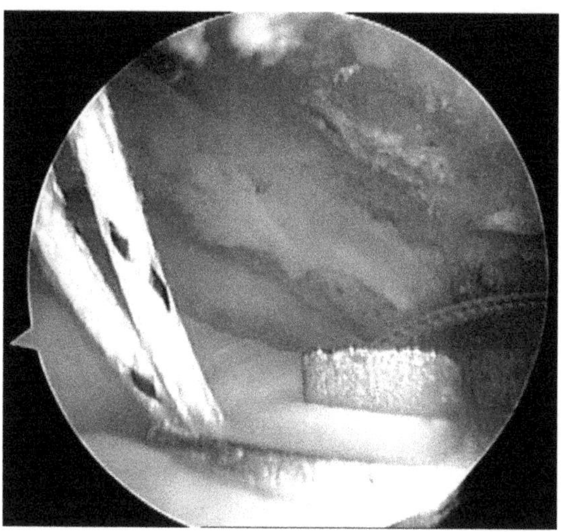

FIGURE 6 Medial sutures passed 10 to 12 mm medially using suture passer.

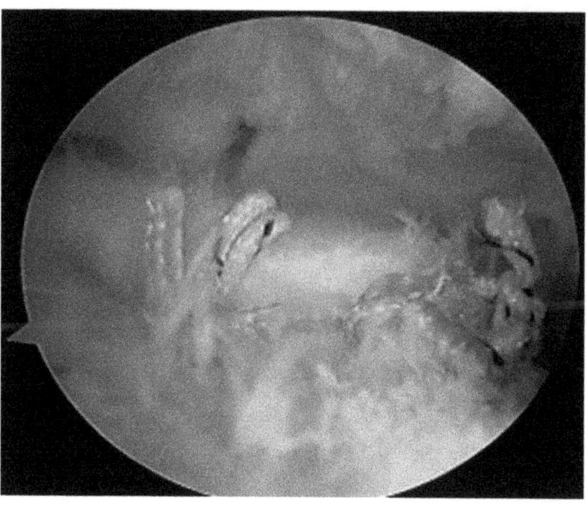

FIGURE 7 Double-row repair with medial horizontal mattress sutures and lateral simple sutures.

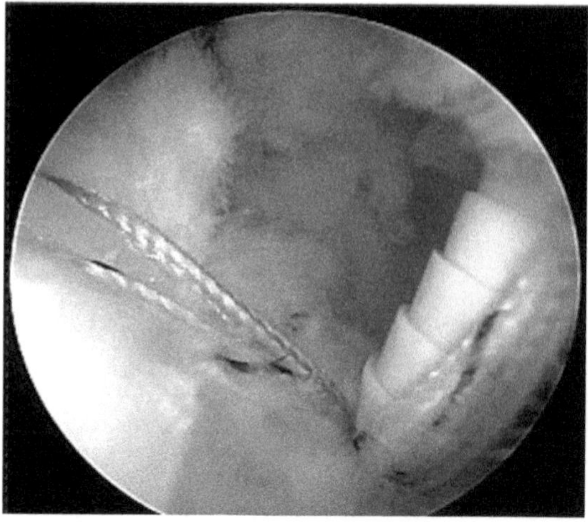

FIGURE 8 Push loc inserted at lateral aspect of greater tuberosity to create suture bridge.

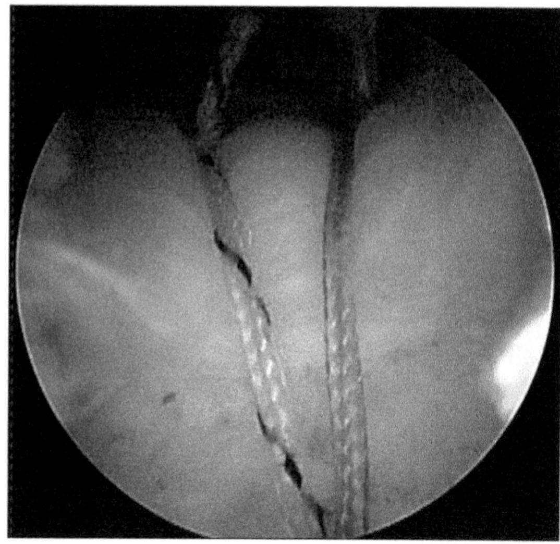

FIGURE 9 Completed repair viewed from lateral portal.

REFERENCES

1. Kim DH, Elattrache NS, Tibone JE, et al. Biomechanical comparison of a single-row versus double-row suture anchor technique for rotator cuff repair. Am J Sports Med 2006; 34(3):407–414.
2. Ma CB, Comerford L, Wilson J, Puttlitz CM. Biomechanical evaluation of arthroscopic rotator cuff repairs: double-row compared with single-row fixation. J Bone Joint Surg Am 206; 88(2):403–410.
3. Apreleva M, Ozbaydar M, Fitzgibbons PG, Warner JJ. Rotator cuff tears: the effect of the reconstruction method on three-dimensional repair site area. Arthroscopy, 2002; 18(5):519–526.
4. Park MC, Cadet ER, Levine WN, Bigliani LU, Ahmad CS. Tendon-to-bone pressure distributions at a repaired rotator cuff footprint using transosseous suture and suture anchor fixation techniques. Am J Sports Med 2005; 33(8):1154–1159.
5. Ahmad CS, Stewart AM, Izquierdo R, Bigliani LU. Tendon-bone interface motion in transosseous suture and suture anchor rotator cuff repair techniques. Am J Sports Med 2005; 33(11):1667–1671.
6. Park M, ElAttrache N, Tibone J, Ahmad C, Jun B, Lee T. Footprint contact biomechanics for a new arthroscopic transossesous-equivalent rotator cuff repair technique compared to a double-row technique arthroscopic rotator cuff repair. American Shoulder and Elbow Surgeons Specialty Day Meeting. Edited, Chicago, IL, 2006.

26 Arthroscopic Repair of Partial Thickness Rotator Cuff Tears—Repair In Situ

Eric H. Gordon
Arkansas Specialty Orthopaedics, Little Rock, Arkansas, U.S.A.

Stephen J. Snyder
Southern California Orthopaedic Institute, Van Nuys, California, U.S.A.

INDICATIONS FOR SURGERY

The appropriate treatment of partial-thickness rotator cuff tears (PTRCT) can be rather confusing. First of all, once a PTRCT is found in a symptomatic patient, the clinician must decide if the tear is the cause of the patient's symptoms. It has been well documented in the literature that PTRCT are often found in asymptomatic shoulders based on MRI and cadaveric studies (1–7). Therefore, the prudent physician will use physical examination and appropriate radiographic studies to identify any associated pathology such as subacromial impingement or instability before determining that all of the patient's symptoms are due to the PTRCT. Unfortunately, the full natural history of these lesions is not completely known. Generally, a trial of physical therapy is recommended. However, when doing this, the patient and physician must realize that studies have found that these tears do not heal on their own, and in fact, may progress to full-thickness tears (7–11).

The next challenge arises when a patient fails nonoperative treatment and requires surgical intervention. At the time of surgery, how should the tear be treated? Should the tear be repaired or is debridement adequate? Unfortunately, there are no prospective randomized trials to guide us in a definitive direction. A major limiting factor in creating a definitive treatment algorithm is the fact that not every PTRCT is the same. It can vary not only in location (articular or bursal), size, and chronicity but also in the type of patient who sustains such an injury. For example, the treatment of PTRCT in an elderly patient may require different treatment than the same lesion in an athlete. Given the wide array of tear configurations and clinical scenarios, it is difficult to obtain a large enough clinical sample to study and draw definitive conclusions about specific lesions. Most authors have, therefore, treated these lesions with a common-sense type approach with support from several case series that have been published.

Most treatment recommendations are based on tear thickness. Ellman proposed a classification system based on tear location and tear thickness (13). Tear location can be described either as articular, bursal, or intratendinous. Tear thickness is graded one to three with a grade 1 tear being less than 3 mm thick, grade 2 tear being 3 to 6 mm thick and grade 3 tear greater than 6 mm thick. It has been recommended that grade 1 and 2 tears can be treated with debridement and grade 3 tears treated with repair. In our practice, we use a classification that can describe not only partial-thickness tears but also full-thickness tears (14) (Table 1). For simplification, the five categories of partial tears can be divided into two main categories with those classified as grades 0, 1, and 2 being relatively minor and grade 3 and 4 tears being more severe and therefore requiring more involved treatment. An easy way to approach these tears is that any tear that is greater than 50% of the tendon thickness should be repaired.

From anatomic studies, we know that the average medial to lateral footprint of the supraspinatus insertion is 12 mm and the footprint begins about 1 mm lateral to the edge of the articular cartilage of the humeral head. Therefore, when viewing the supraspinatus tendon from within the glenohumeral joint, one should see less than 1 mm of exposed bone

---

Please refer to pages 285–288 for the figures in this chapter.

TABLE 1 Classification of Rotator Cuff Tears

Location of Tear	
A	Articular side
B	Bursal side
C	Complete tear
Tear Severity (A or B Partial Tears)	
0	Normal cuff
1	Minimal, superficial bursal/synovial irritation or minimal capsular fraying in small area less than 1 cm
2	Actual fraying and failure of some rotator cuff fibers usually less than 2 cm
3	More severe rotator cuff injury including fraying and fragmentation of tendon fibers, usually less than 3 cm
4	Very severe tear that contains a sizeable flap and often encompasses more than one tendon
Classification of Complete Tears (C)	
C1	Small complete tear like a puncture
C2	Moderate tear less than 2 cm involving only one muscle tendon of the cuff and without retraction
C3	A large complete tear with minimal retraction, usually 3 to 4 cm
C4	Massive rotator cuff tear involving two or more tendons, often retracted

lateral to the cartilage (15,16). When an articular-sided tear of the supraspinatus is present, more exposed bone will be seen. The amount of bone visualized can help determine the thickness of the tear. A significant lesion of 50% or more of the tendon being torn will result in greater than 6 mm of exposed bone, lateral to the articular cartilage (Fig. 1). These would be classified as grade 3 in the Ellman classification, and as grade 3 or 4 in our classification system. These are the tears that should be repaired. Lesser tears can often be treated with debridement alone. In addition, one must always be cognizant that a lesion on the bursal surface might also exist. For this reason, we always mark the location of any articular-sided tear with a marker stitch before placing the arthroscope into the subacromial space. Then, during subacromial evaluation, we closely inspect the bursal surface of the cuff looking for any evidence of tearing, particularly in the area of the marker suture that corresponds to the location of the articular-sided tear that is present. In addition, tear thickness can often be estimated based on the preoperative MRI, especially if gadolinium is used (Fig. 2). This information should be considered prior to making a final treatment decision.

CONTRAINDICATIONS

Contraindications for repairing in situ include tears that involve too much of the footprint and would instead benefit from conversion to a full-thickness tear with standard repair. While there are no concrete guidelines available to make this determination, we have arbitrarily chosen tendon remaining that is greater than 30% to proceed with repair in situ. However, if less than 30% of the tendon remaining is intact, we would convert to takedown of the remaining cuff and repair in a standard fashion (see chap. 25).

TECHNIQUE OF ARTHROSCOPIC IN SITU REPAIR OF PARTIAL THICKNESS ROTATOR CUFF TEARS

Once it has been determined that the tear is significant for the patient and warrants repair, the decision then has to be made as to how the repair should be carried out. Repair can be done using either a transtendinous technique or by taking down the remaining cuff, thereby creating a full-thickness tear. To make this determination, the surgeon has to consider the cuff attachment that remains and decide if it is worth saving. Obviously, there are benefits in saving the remaining cuff as it helps decrease stress on the repair, thereby shortening the required immobilization. Our cutoff for saving the cuff is greater than 30% of the cuff thickness remaining. If less than this thickness remains, then we would proceed with takedown of the bursal side of the tear and repair the tear like a full-thickness tear.

Besides the size of the tear, another important factor for the surgeon to consider and correct, if possible, is the etiology of the tear. Often this may consist of multiple factors. These etiologic factors can broadly be classified as traumatic, extrinsic, or intrinsic to the rotator cuff. Extrinsic causes include subacromial impingement (17), shoulder instability (18), or repetitive microtrauma such that they might occur with internal impingement (19–25). On the other hand, intrinsic factors, or changes within the tendon substance itself, can also contribute to these tears. As the rotator cuff tendons age, they develop changes like fascicular thinning and formation of granulation tissue and dystrophic calcification. In addition, the relative hypovascularity of the articular side of the rotator cuff is worsened with aging (26–30). The physical examination and radiographic work up should attempt to identify a suspected etiology, with particular attention given to identifying any extrinsic causes that also need to be addressed at the time of surgery not only to alleviate symptoms but also to prevent recurrence.

TECHNIQUE OF REPAIR

1. Carry out a thorough diagnostic arthroscopic examination of the shoulder utilizing the posterosuperior (PSP) and anterosuperior (ASP) portals.
2. Identify articular-sided cuff tear.
3. Debride torn cuff as needed using a motorized shaver and make assessment of remaining cuff thickness by evaluating the exposed footprint as seen in Figure 1.
4. Insert a spinal needle percutaneously so that it pierces the rotator cuff in the area of the articular-sided tear.
5. Pass a no. 1 polydioxanone (PDS) stitch through the spinal needle (Fig. 3). Feed enough of the suture into the joint so that it will remain in place after removing the spinal needle. Remove the spinal needle.
6. Change the arm position and proceed with subacromial arthroscopy.
7. Establish a lateral acromial portal (LAP). Resect bursa to provide adequate visualization and identify marker stitch. Evaluate bursal side of cuff for any evidence of tearing.
8. Evaluate the coracoacromial ligament for fraying. After using this information in combination with preoperative history, physical exam findings, and X-ray findings, proceed with subacromial decompression, as needed.
9. Based on the perceived amount of remaining rotator cuff thickness and integrity, proceed with repair. In general, if remaining cuff tissue is deemed greater than 30% but less than 50% of normal cuff thickness, proceed with repair utilizing the transtendinous technique. If it is less than 30%, then proceed with takedown of the cuff and routine repair.
10. Place the arm back into position for glenohumeral arthroscopy. Re-establish glenohumeral arthroscopy with the camera in the PSP. Place a crystal cannula (Arthrex) into the ASP.
11. Using the motorized shaver, debride the humeral head bone of any remaining soft tissue in the area of the footprint defect just lateral to articular cartilage. Take care not to injure the remaining cuff attachment. Create a fresh bony surface to optimize healing of the cuff back to its insertion site similar to what is seen in Figure 4.
12. Insert a spinal needle percutaneously through the partial-thickness tear onto the prepared bony surface. Use the needle to plan insertion of the first anchor and assess for the appropriate angle for insertion. If the patient is in the lateral position, decreasing the amount of abduction on the traction tower can help to obtain a "tent peg" angle for anchor insertion.
13. Incise the skin at the proposed site and screw the anchor through the bursal side of the cuff. As seen in Figure 5, the anchor should be placed just off the articular cartilage edge at a 45° angle to the bone. Of course, one should follow the appropriate procedure of punching and tapping, as the selected anchor requires. The anchor can be loaded with one, two, or even three sutures depending on the situation and the surgeon's skill in suture management. We prefer to use a double-loaded Super-Revo anchor (Linvatec) loaded with no. 2 nonabsorbable suture of different colors.
14. When placing the anchor, use the laser-etched lines on the insertion handle to make sure the sutures are properly aligned. For example, if simple stitches are to be placed, the sutures should exit the eyelet perpendicular to the torn cuff edge. If a mattress stitch is to be used, make sure the sutures are exiting parallel to the torn cuff edge.
15. Remove the insertion handle and pull on the sutures to assure adequate stability of the anchor within the bone.
16. Insert a crochet hook from the ASP and take out the limb of the anterior most suture that is closest to the torn cuff edge, that is, most medial. To assist in differentiating the two limbs of suture, one side can be colored with a purple surgical marker prior to insertion. The

anchor can then be inserted with the purple side either toward the cuff or away. By convention, we use one white no. 2 Ethibond and one green no. 2 Ethibond. We mark one side of each with the purple marker. When the anchor is inserted, the purple side is placed so that it faces the cuff with the green suture being the most anterior. Therefore, we take out the green/purple limb first (Fig. 6).

17. Insert an 18-gage spinal needle percutaneously through the bursal side of the torn cuff, approximately 5 mm anterior to the suture anchor and 5 mm medial to the torn edge of the cuff. Pass a Shuttle-Relay Suture Passer (Linvatec) down the needle and into the joint. Using a grasper from the ASP, grab the Shuttle. Make sure to grab the Shuttle on the anterior side of the white sutures so as not to tangle the sutures, once the Shuttle is brought back into the joint. Remove the needle and pull the Shuttle out from the Crystal cannula in the ASP (Fig. 7).
18. Load the green/purple suture limb into the Shuttle. Pull the Shuttle back, thereby pulling the green/purple suture limb back through the torn cuff edge, deltoid muscle, and then the skin. Put a hemostat on both limbs of the green suture.
19. If a second suture has been used, retrieve the medial-most limb (white/purple) out from the ASP using the crochet hook. Be careful not to tangle it around the green sutures.
20. Insert the spinal needle again. This time, aim 5 mm posterior to the anchor. Pass the Shuttle down the needle and into the joint. Insert the grasper from the ASP and grasp the Shuttle. Once again, make sure to take the Shuttle out in the appropriate path to avoid tangling it with the green sutures. Remove the spinal needle and pull the Shuttle out from the Crystal cannula in the ASP.
21. Load the white/purple limb of suture in the Shuttle. Pull the Shuttle back, thereby pulling the white/purple suture limb back through the torn cuff edge, deltoid muscle, and then the skin. Place a hemostat on both limbs of the white suture.
22. If additional anchors are needed, repeat the steps 12 to 21.
23. Reposition the patient's arm for subacromial burscoscopy. Re-establish the arthroscope in the PSP to view the subacromial space and outflow via the ASP. Reinsert the Crystal cannula into the LAP.
24. Locate the sutures. Using the crochet hook, pull both the green sutures out from the Crystal cannula. Pull on the suture limbs to make sure they slide. Tie the knot. We prefer an Samsung Medical Center (SMC) sliding-locking knot followed by three additional half hitches. If the suture limbs do not slide, then use a Revo knot (Fig. 8).
25. Repeat the step 24 for the white suture.
26. To view the repair, reinsert the arthroscope back into the shoulder joint (Fig. 9).

Note: In order to create a horizontal mattress suture configuration, you can pass both limbs of the same suture via the above noted technique with the spinal needle and Shuttle.

PEARLS AND PITFALLS

1. Determine the thickness of articular sided PTRCT by understanding anatomic landmarks as described earlier—footprint starts 1 mm lateral to articular cartilage and on average is 12 mm medial to lateral. Any time 6 mm of footprint is exposed, consider this a "high-grade" PTRCT and repair should be performed.
2. If enough bursal side attachment is intact, proceed with in situ repair as outlined earlier.
3. Anchor placement and suture passage are critical in successfully repairing the articular side anatomically.
4. Suture management is critical—consider performing the subacromial bursectomy prior to anchor placement and suture passage to facilitate suture retrieval in the subacromial space later in the case.
5. Prior to tying the arthroscopic knots, place the scope in the glenohumeral joint and pull up on all four limbs of the suture pairs and visualize the anatomic reduction of the articular side of the supraspinatus to the footprint; if you do not see the cuff anatomically, assume the sutures have not been appropriately placed and should be revised prior to knot tying.

POSTOPERATIVE CARE

Postop care for a repair of a partial thickness tear of the rotator cuff is similar to that of a normal rotator cuff repair. However, since a portion of the cuff is left intact, the required immobilization is less. Normally, we leave these patients in an Ultra Sling [dj (Don Joy) Ortho] for only four weeks. Rehabilitation then follows the normal course for a full thickness tear.

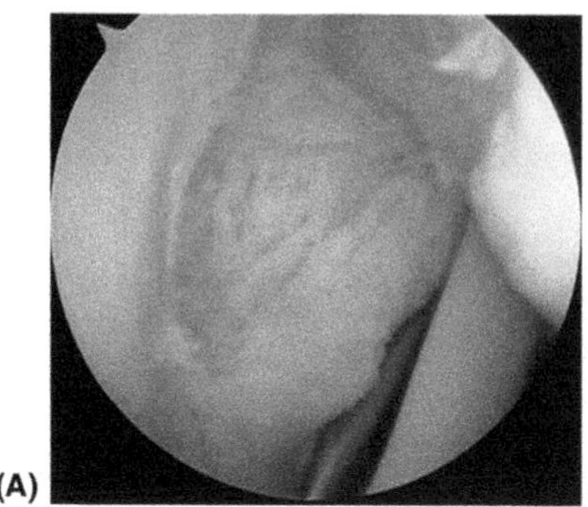
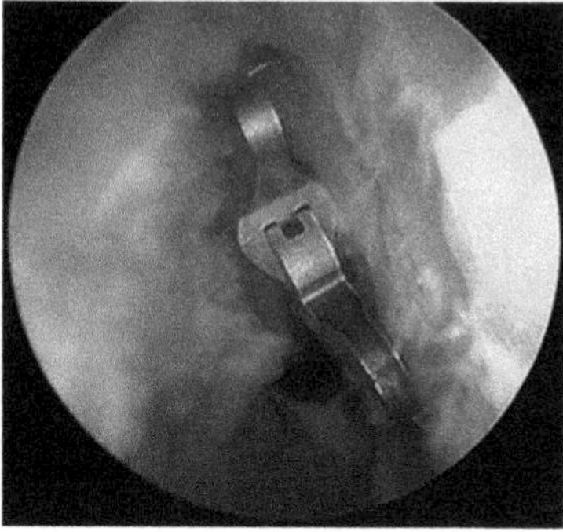

FIGURE 1 (**A**) Exposed bone lateral to articular cartilage of the humeral head after debridement. (**B**) Measuring the distance from articular cartilage to intact rotator cuff tissue.

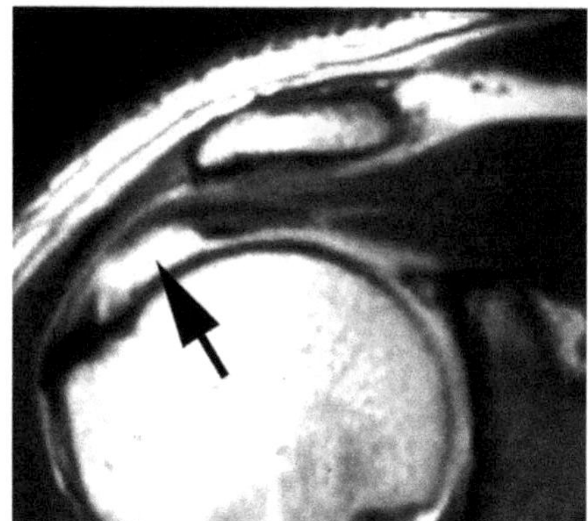

FIGURE 2 Coronal T2 MRA of the shoulder displaying an articular-sided partial thickness tear of the supraspinatus.

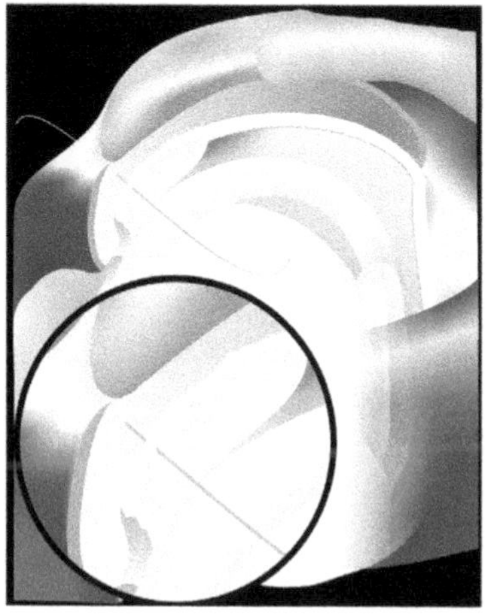
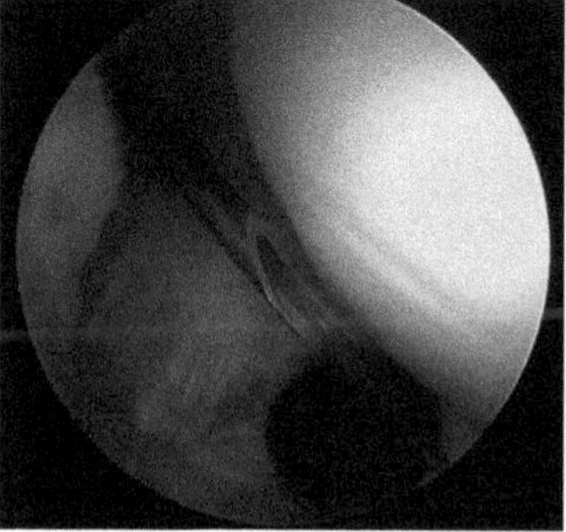

FIGURE 3 A no. 1 Prolene or polydioxanone stitch can be inserted to mark the area of rotator cuff fraying or tearing.

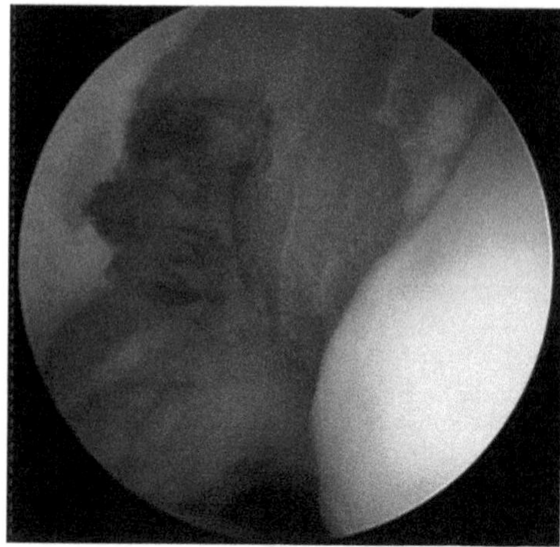

FIGURE 4 The bony surface is prepared on the rotator cuff footprint to optimize healing.

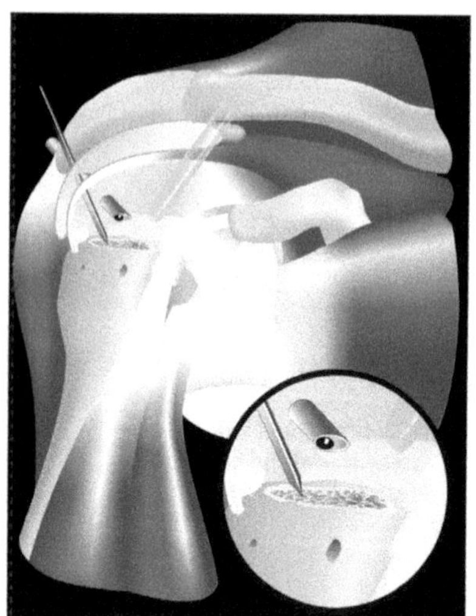

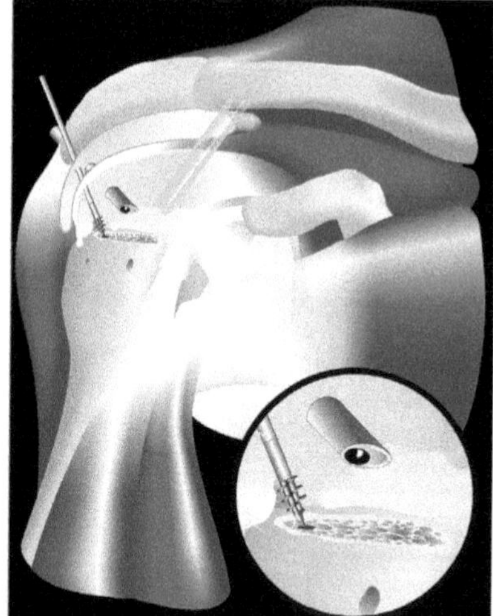

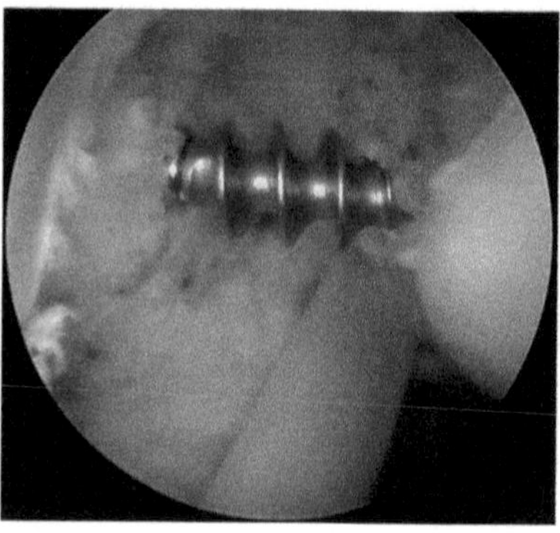

FIGURE 5 The anchors are inserted via a transtendinous technique as shown.

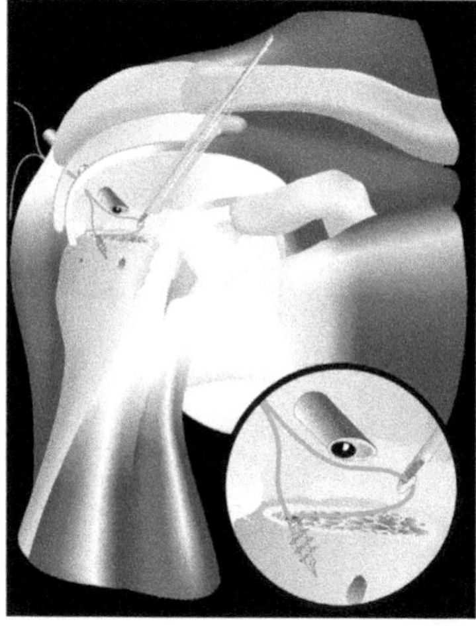
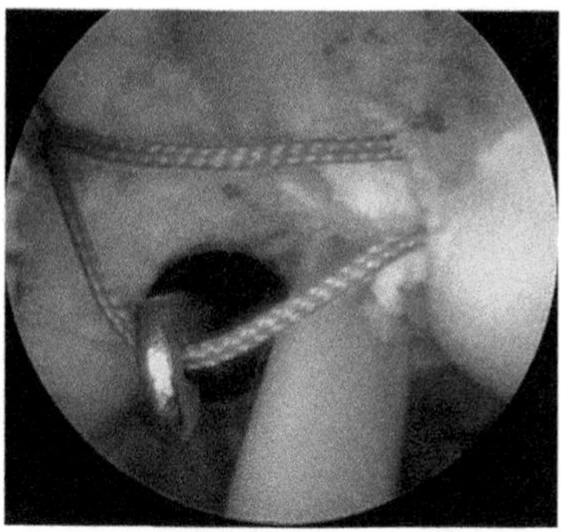

FIGURE 6 The medial-most suture of the pair of sutures to be passed is taken out the anterior superior portal with a crochet hook.

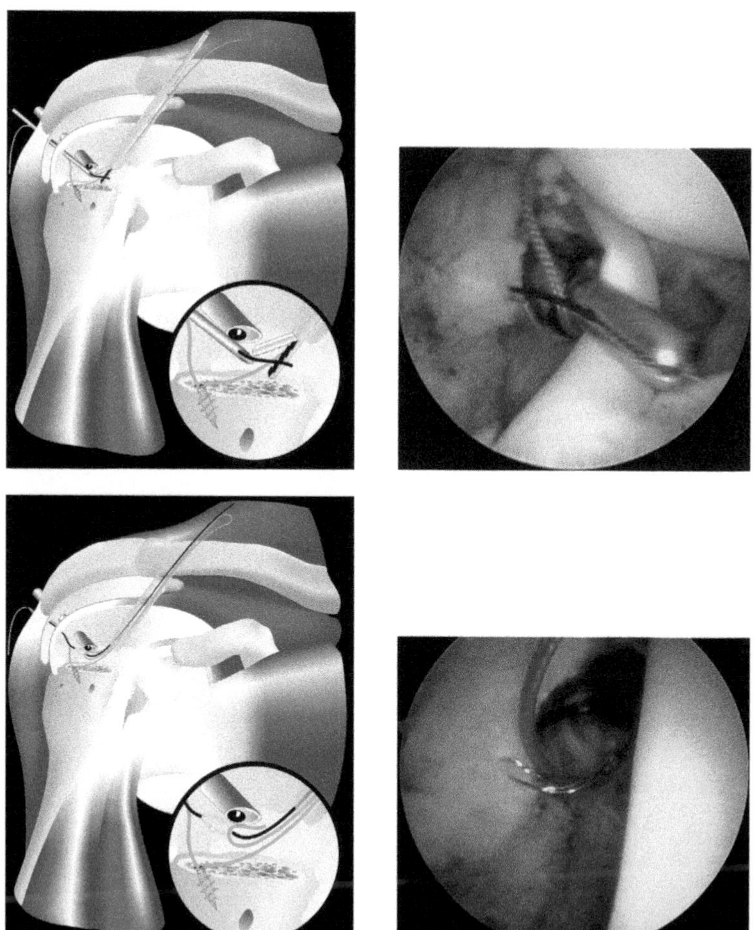

FIGURE 7 An 18-gage spinal needle is inserted through the torn edge of rotator cuff and a shuttle relay is manually fed down the needle. A grasper inserted via the anterior superior portal is used to take the shuttle out. The suture is then loaded and brought back through the cuff.

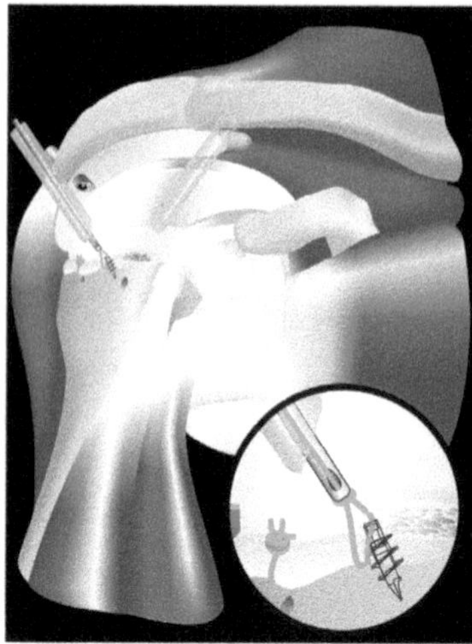

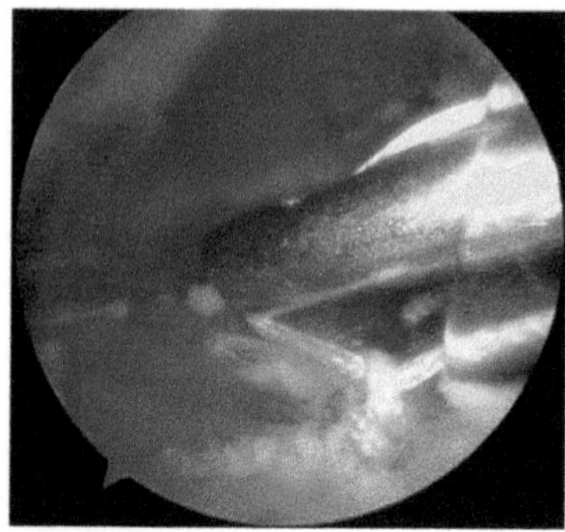

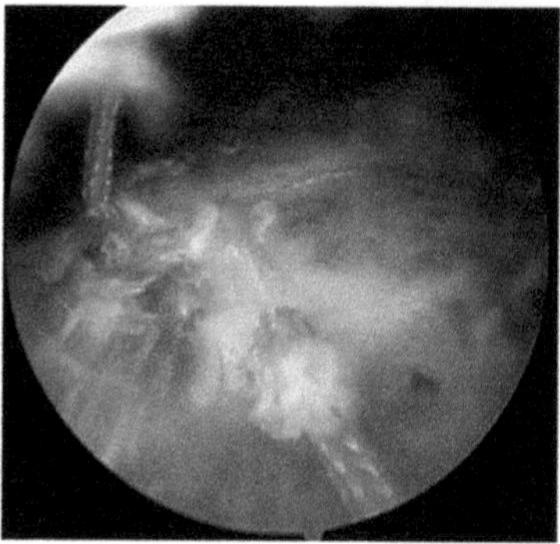

FIGURE 8 The scope is repositioned in the subacromial space from the posterior portal. The suture pairs are taken out the lateral portal and tied on top of the cuff.

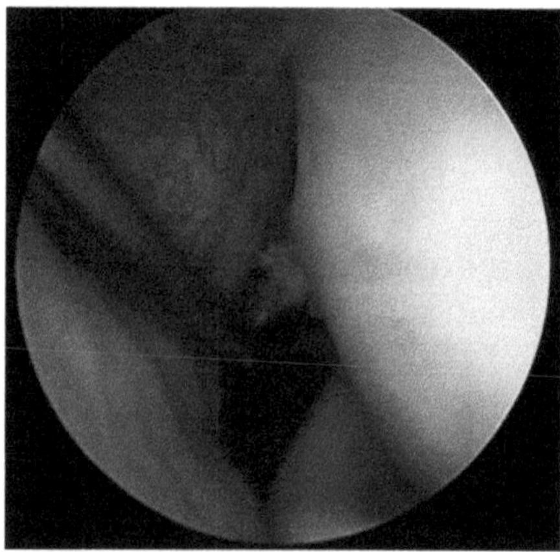

FIGURE 9 Once the sutures have been tied on the bursal side, the scope can be reinserted into the joint to inspect the completed repair.

REFERENCES

1. Lohr JF, Uhtoff HK. The pathogenesis of degenerative rotator cuff tears. Orthop Trans 1987; 11:237.
2. Yamanaka K, Fukuda H. Pathologic studies of the supraspinatus tendon with reference to incomplete partial-thickness tear. In: Takagishi N, ed. The Shoulder. Tokyo, Japan: Professional Postgraduate Services, 1987:247–258.
3. Fukuda H, Mikasa M, Yamanaka K. Incomplete thickness rotator cuff tears diagnosed by subacromial bursography. Clin Orthop 1987; 223:51–58.
4. Chandnani V, Ho C, Gerharter J, et al. MR findings in asymptomatic shoulders: a blind analysis using symptomatic shoulders as controls. Clin Imaging 1992; 16:25–30.
5. Connor PM, Banks DM, Tyson AB, Coumas JS, D'Alessandro DF. MRI of the asymptomatic shoulder of overhead athletes: a 5-year follow-up study. Am J Sports Med 2003; 31:724–727.
6. Miniaci A, Dowdy PA, Willits KR, Vellet AD. MRI evaluation of the rotator cuff tendons in the asymptomatic shoulder. Am J Sports Med 1995; 23:142–145.
7. Sher JS, Uribe JW, Posada A, Murphy BJ, Zlatkin MB. Abnormal findings on MRI of asymptomatic shoulders. J Bone Joint Surg Am 1995; 77:10–15.
8. Fukuda H, Hamada K, Nakajima T, Tomonaga A. Pathology and pathogenesis of the intratendinous tearing of the rotator cuff viewed from en bloc histologic sections. Clin Orthop 1994; 304:60–67.
9. Fukuda H, Hamada K, Nakajima T, Yamada N, Tomonaga A, Goto M. Partial-thickness tears of the rotator cuff: a clinicopathological review based on 66 surgically verified cases. Int Orthop 1996; 20:257–265.
10. Fukuda H, Hamada K, Yamanaka K. Pathology and pathogenesis of bursal-side rotator cuff tears viewed from en-bloc histologic sections. Clin Orthop 1990; 254:75–80.
11. Hamada K, Tomonaga A, Gotoh M, Yamanaka H, Fukuda H. Intrinsic healing capacity and tearing process of torn supraspinatus tendons: in situ hybridization study of alpha 1 procollagen mRNA. J Orthop Res 1997; 15:24–32.
12. Hyvonen P, Lohi S, Jalovaara P. Open acromioplasty does not prevent the progression of an impingment syndrome to a tear: nine year follow-up of 96 cases. J Bone Joint Surg Br 1998; 80-B:813–816.
13. Ellman H. Diagnosis and treatment of incomplete rotator cuff tears. Clin Orthop 1990; 254:64–74.
14. Snyder SJ. Rotator cuff lesions. In: Snyder SJ, ed. Shoulder Arthroscopy. 2nd ed. Van Nuys, CA: Lippincott William & Wilkins, 2003:203–207.
15. Dugas JR, Campbell DA, Warren RF, Robie BH, Millett PJ. Anatomy and dimensions of rotator cuff insertions. J Shoulder Elbow Surg 2002; 11:498–503.
16. Ruotolo C, Fow JE, Nottage WM. The supraspinatus footprint: an anatomic study of the supraspinatus insertion. Arthroscopy 2004; 20:246–249.
17. Neer CS II. Impingement lesions. Clin Orthop 1983; 173:70–77.
18. Myers JB, Ju YY, Hwang JH, McMahon PJ, Rodosky MW, Lephart SM. Reflexive muscle activation alterations in shoulders with anterior glenohumeral instability. Am J Sports Med 2004; 32:1013–1021.
19. Fleisig GS, Andrews JR, Dillman CJ, Escamilla RF. Kinetics of baseball pitching with implications about injury mechanisms. Am J Sports Med 1995; 23:233–239.
20. Davidson PA, ElAttrache NS, Jobe CM, Jobe CW. Rotator cuff and posterior-superior glenoid labrum injury associated with increased glenohumeral motion: a new site of impingement. J Shoulder Elbow Surg 1995; 4:384–390.
21. Jobe CM. Posterior superior glenoid impingement: expanded spectrum. Arthroscopy 1995; 11:530–536.
22. Jobe CM. Superior glenoid impingement: current concepts. Clin Orthop 1996; 330:98–107.
23. Meister K, Seroyer S. Arthroscopic management of the thrower's shoulder: internal impingement. Orthop Clin North Am 2003; 34:539–547.
24. Paley KJ, Jobe FW, Pink MM, Kvitne RS, ElAttrache NS. Arthroscopic findings in the overhand throwing athlete: evidence for posterior internal impingement of the rotator cuff. Arthroscopy 2000; 16:35–40.
25. Walch G, Boileau P, Noel E, Donell ST. Impingement of the deep surface of the supraspinatus tendon on the posterosuperior glenoid rim: an arthroscopic study. J Shoulder Elbow Surg 1992; 1:238–245.
26. Kumagai J, Sarkar K, Uhthoff HK. The collagen types in the attachment zone of the rotator cuff tendons of the elderly: an immunohistological study. J Rheumatol 1994; 21:2096.
27. Lohr JF, Uhthoff HK. The microvascular pattern of the supraspinatus tendon. Clin Orthop 1990; 254:35–38.
28. Rothman RH, Parke W. The vascular anatomy of the rotator cuff. Clin Orthop 1965; 41:176–186.
29. Sano H, Ishii H, Yeadon A, Backman DS, Brunet JA, Uhthoff HK. Degeneration at the insertion weakens the tensile strength of the supraspinatus tendon: a comparative mechanical and histologic study of the bone-tendon complex. J Orthop Res 1997; 15:719–726.
30. Yamanaka K, Fukuda H. Ageing process of the supraspinatus with reference to rotator cuff tears. In: Watson MS, ed. Surgical Disorders of the Shoulder. Edinburgh, Scotland: Churchill Livingstone, 1991:247–258.

27 Conversion to Mini-Open Rotator Cuff Repair Following Attempted Arthroscopic Repair

Michael Q. Freehill
Sports and Orthopedic Specialists, Edina, Minnesota, U.S.A.

INTRODUCTION

The technique of arthroscopic repair has progressed significantly over the past few years largely due to improved suture anchor design and suture passing instrumentation. These elements, combined with more available knowledge regarding arthroscopic repairs and a broader educational system, allow arthroscopic rotator cuff repairs to no longer be a cutting edge procedure, but an approach used by many orthopedists. Recent literature has transitioned from arthroscopic assisted mini-open rotator cuff-repair technique to an all-arthroscopic rotator cuff repair (1–3). The major focus has been to develop surgical strategy allowing orthopedists to gradually change from a mini-open approach that was arthroscopically assisted, to an all-arthroscopic approach incorporating techniques used in traditional- or mini-open procedures. The advantages of arthroscopic repairs have been widely publicized including less postoperative pain, theoretically easier rehabilitation, and decreased postoperative stiffness. Indications for all arthroscopic repair have evolved secondary to the improved technical considerations. Arthroscopic methods have improved in terms of mobilization of the tendons, ability to place sutures within the tendon, and surgical technique. Double-row fixation and modified suture-passing techniques such as the modified Mason Allen and the Mac stitch have allowed for arthroscopic indications to include larger, complex tears.

Conversion to a mini-open repair following an arthroscopic attempt has been presented recently. Kim et al. (4) described an arthroscopic versus mini-open salvage repair of the rotator cuff. The study concluded that an arthroscopic repair of medium to large full-thickness rotator cuff-tears repaired through a mini-open technique had an equal outcome to those reconstructed with a complete arthroscopic approach. The surgical outcome in this study was dependent upon the size of the tear rather than the specific method utilized.

Recent studies comparing all-arthroscopic repair/arthroscopic-assisted repairs or mini-open repair, demonstrates few differences in the ultimate outcome with regards to motion and patient satisfaction (5–9). The mini-open approach has been demonstrated to provide excellent outcome with 89% to 100% patient satisfaction based upon studies utilizing single-row transosseous tunnels, single-row suture anchor fixation and more recently, two-row fixation technique (10–14).

This chapter will provide detailed elements of the arthroscopic repair that may potentially require conversion to a mini-open approach allowing for a successful rotator cuff repair. The focus will be on rationale for conversion, intra-operative decision making, and methods for transition to a mini-open approach.

INDICATIONS FOR CONVERSION TO MINI-OPEN REPAIR

Failure of Fixation

Multiple successful interfaces are required during an all-arthroscopic repair to ensure that appropriate tissue-to-tissue reconstruction is achieved in addition to the more vital tendon-to-bone repair. Regardless of the surgeon's implant preference, the ability to maintain fixation within the bone is an utmost priority. Anchor devices include bio-absorbable tack fixation,

---

Please refer to pages 296–299 for the figures in this chapter.

suture loop fixation in a bio-absorbable corkscrew anchor, and metal corkscrew anchors. Failure at the anchor-bone interface may be more prevalent in osteoporotic bone, however, this is not currently a contraindication to arthroscopic repair. Disengagement of the anchor is most likely to occur when initially tensioning the anchor after placement or during arthroscopic knot tying of the rotator cuff tear (Fig. 1). If such failure occurs, a larger anchor may be placed within the previously drilled hole. This would typically allow for appropriate fixation within the bone. Conversion to metal anchor fixation is more likely to provide implant stability if previous fixation was performed with a bio-absorbable anchor. If a metal anchor cannot be adequately secured within the bone, then conversion to a mini-open approach should be considered to allow for more appropriate anchor placement, in addition to or in combination with transosseous tunnel placement (Fig. 2). The importance of anchor or transosseous tunnel placement is vital to avoid multiple insults that may produce a stress riser within the greater tuberosity and subsequent intra-operative or postoperative fracture in this area.

Additional loss of fixation can be apparent at the suture-tissue interface. This includes the inability to capture delaminated portions of rotator cuff tears (Fig. 3). This is more likely with chronic tears in which atrophic or degenerative tendon is present. With the advancement of suture passing devices such as the Scorpion (Athrex, Naples, Florida, U.S.A.) and the ExpresSew (DePuy Mitek, Raynam, Massachusetts, U.S.A.) (see chap. 20), the ability to pass sutures into all of the tendon has been enhanced. Theoretically, with advanced surgical skills, a surgeon could technically perform a modified Mason Allen suture configuration as described by Gerber et al. (15). In addition, a stitch technique known as the "Mac stitch" has also been described to enhance tissue-grasping ability while using arthroscopic repair methods (16).

If unable to perform such suture configuration techniques or if the tissue is too degenerative to allow for appropriate fixation with a simpler mattress and/or simple suture configuration, a conversion to a mini-open approach should be considered. Mini-open approach allows for a Mason Allen suture configuration or mattress suture configuration using single- or double-row fixation techniques (Fig. 4A–C).

Current suture material, including Fiberwire (Arthrex, Naples, Florida, U.S.A.), Herculine (ConMed Linvatec, Largo, Florida, U.S.A.), and Orthocord (DePuy Mitek, Raynam, Massachusetts, U.S.A.) prevents suture breakage in most cases. In the author's experience, rare instances of suture damage have occurred with the newer suture passing devices, potentially, leading to failure of the suture during the repair. If a portion of the repair has been completed at the time of suture failure, a conversion to mini-open approach may be necessary to avoid further disruption of the repair. This facilitates additional suture anchor placement of transosseous tunnels to augment the repair.

The potential need for tissue augmentation has been discussed when approaching repairs from an arthroscopic viewpoint. Recently, Snyder (17) described a technique of tissue augmentation utilizing the graft jacket, which is applied using arthroscopic suturing techniques prior to a tendon-to-bone fixation. This technique, however, is exceedingly challenging and reserved for very experienced shoulder arthroscopists. The ultimate outcome following tissue augmentation with either a porcine small intestine submucosa or human dermal tissue has yet to be validated, and very limited data is present in the literature to support the use of the augmentation implants. In a six-month follow-up of large to massive tears reinforced with porcine submucosa, Sclamberg and Tibone demonstrated 10 out of 11 tears recurred, indicating that the use in the face of a large to massive tear may not be appropriate (18).

Loss of Visualization

Depending upon the experience of the arthroscopist, the time to complete a rotator cuff repair in appropriate fashion is often dependent upon the size of the tear and the surgeon's ability to mobilize the tissue in an appropriate fashion. With extended time for arthroscopy, tissue distention is evident as fluid extravasation occurs into the surrounding soft tissues. If an inadequate bursectomy was performed, this may further impede the surgeon's ability to perform the rotator cuff repair in a timely and appropriate fashion. Should a loss of visualization occur during the attempt at arthroscopic repair, a conversion to a mini-open approach should be considered. However, with significant fluid extravasation, the deltoid will frequently exhibit moderate swelling, thereby, making a mini-open approach potentially difficult. As such, prevention is the best method to avoid loss of visualization secondary to tissue swelling or bursal distension. It has been recommended that arthroscopic procedures in the shoulder generally should last less than two hours to avoid the potential difficulty with soft tissue distention (19).

Deltoid Detachment

Deltoid detachment with arthroscopic techniques, although rarely reported, has been associated with aggressive arthroscopic acromioplasty, potentially leaving a very thin layer of deltoid attached anteriorly (Fig. 5A and B). With regards to rotator cuff surgery, this is one of the more devastating complications that can occur although traditionally associated with more extensile open approaches. Frequently, this complication will be under-recognized following arthroscopy until the patient presents postoperatively with pain over the anterior acromion and a visible or palpable deltoid defect. Conservative arthroscopic decompression by removing enough acromial undersurface to create a flat undersurface seen in a type I acromial morphology will prevent this complication. If concerned about the integrity of the deltoid origin, the area can be visualized through the lateral portal in the subacromial space to assure that the deltoid fibers are maintained in continuity to the anterior acromion. Typically, a white periosteal layer can be visualized if the deltoid origin has been preserved appropriately, following the acromioplasty.

If deltoid detachment is recognized intra-operatively, conversion to a more extensile open approach with a traditional incision within Langer's lines should be performed. This will allow for an appropriate reconstruction of the deltoid with the underlying coracoacromial ligament to restore the soft tissue constraints of the coracoacromial arch.

Extensive Soft Tissue Injury

Despite the improved sensitivities in MRI, there are occasions the surgeon may discover more extensive soft tissue injury than previously anticipated during pre-operative planning. Such soft tissue injury frequently involves the biceps tendon and the subscapularis. Arthroscopic repair of the subscapularis can be very challenging even for experienced arthroscopists. This tear configuration combined with associated biceps pathology may lead to a more expansive approach than planned pre-operatively. Depending on the surgeon's experience, this situation could yield a combined approach in which the posterior and superior rotator cuff tear could be repaired arthroscopically followed by a conversion to a deltopectoral approach to address the subscapularis and biceps pathology. This combined approach is particularly relevant when considering a tenodesis as opposed to a tenotomy of the biceps.

The deltopectoral approach allows excellent exposure to the anterior shoulder structures, and since it is an intramuscular plane, there is typically minimal morbidity and relatively minor increase in postoperative pain following this approach. However, in the face of an extended arthroscopic procedure the anterior deltoid area can become distended allowing for difficulty in obtaining appropriate visualization through the deltopectoral approach, particularly in muscular or obese individuals.

Contraindications

There are no absolute contraindications to mini-open repair of the rotator cuff tear. However, one should keep in mind that a standard open repair may be more desirable if visualization and mobilization are the factors leading to a conversion to an open procedure. This is especially true when significant fluid extravasation has occurred and a mini-open approach may afford suboptimal visualization and working space as well.

Techniques for Conversion to Mini-Open Repair

This section describes specific approaches once the surgeon has made the decision to convert to a mini-open repair. The specific approaches are based upon the pathologies identified during the arthroscopic portion of the procedure. In rare instances, use of more than one approach may be required depending on the extent of the soft tissue injury and the surgeon's ability to complete portions of the repair arthroscopically (Fig. 6A and B).

LATERAL APPROACH

A direct lateral approach has been the traditional technique used in the previously described mini-open procedures (Fig. 7A). This is initiated with an extension of the lateral portal to approximately 3 cm. The deltoid split is propagated superiorly to permit visualization of the tear within the subacromial space (Fig. 7B). Extension of the deltoid split greater than 3 to 4 cm distally should be avoided to prevent injury to the axillary nerve. If there is a concern with the deltoid split propagating during the procedure due to retraction, a suture can be placed at the inferior apex of the split to prevent propagation. Furthermore, care should be taken during the mini-open approach to avoid excessive traction on the deltoid muscle as this has been proposed as a possible etiologic factor in postoperative stiffness (5). The lateral approach is typically reserved for tears involving the supraspinatus and anterior aspect of the infraspinatus. With rotation of the arm, it is possible for posterior infraspinatus tears to be visualized, and with placement of traction sutures, mobilized to the appropriate area on the greater tuberosity. Tears involving the superior border of the subscapularis can also be visualized through the direct lateral approach, however, this is more difficult and may be significantly impeded if the patient is larger in size. Further mobilization of the rotator cuff can be performed through the mini-open approach followed by placement of either suture anchors, transosseous tunnels, or a combination of fixation methods depending on the surgeon's preference (Fig. 2). Tissue grasping techniques such as the Mason Allen grasping suture can then be performed with relative ease through the mini-open approach.

Deltopectoral Approach

The deltopectoral approach is a conversion typically used to address pathology involving the subscapularis, the adjacent biceps, or pathology within the subcoracoid space. This approach can be used to address concomitant tears involving the anterior distal aspect of the supraspinatus. Following arthroscopy, the anterior portal can be extended 3 to 5 cm to permit the deltopectoral approach (Fig. 8). The cephalic vein is identified and retracted laterally or medially depending on the surgeon's preference. Frequently, after an extensile arthroscopy there can be moderate distension of the subcoracoid bursa throughout this area requiring excision prior to addressing pathologic lesions. The subscapularis can then be addressed and mobilized in an appropriate fashion, including capsular release, if required. The biceps can also be tenodesed if necessary. In addition, a curved or bent chandler placed into the subacromial space will permit exposure of the anterior distal supraspinatus allowing for appropriate repair through the deltopectoral approach. Furthermore, an open coracoplasty can be performed concomitantly, if required.

Anterolateral Approach

A modified approach to supraspinatus and subscapularis pathology can be created using the accessory anterior lateral portal as a basis for the mini-open approach (Fig. 9). The incision is centered over the anterolateral portal, approximately 3 cm in length. The deltoid is maintained on its origin and split along the anterolateral raphe of the deltoid. The split should not be propagated more than 3 to 4 cm distally. This allows for more appropriate exposure of the supraspinatus and any concomitant biceps or subscapularis pathology that may be present. This is particularly helpful in cases where the tear extends through the rotator interval toward the base of the coracoid and requires mobilization in this region. Repair techniques including transosseous tunnels or suture fixation can be used as, previously described.

Posterolateral Approach

Although this approach is rarely required, it is useful in tears that involve the more posterior aspect of the rotator cuff including the infraspinatus and the rarer teres minor tear. This approach is centered over the accessory posterolateral portal based off of the posterolateral corner of the acromion (Fig. 10). This allows for a direct visualization of the posterior aspect of the shoulder, including the infraspinatus and teres minor tendons.

There is, on rare occasion, the need for an extensile approach using a direct lateral in combination with a deltopectoral approach depending on the extent of the rotator cuff tear and the surgeon's ability to achieve repair or releases arthroscopically. For example, if a surgeon is unable to completely arthroscopically repair a supraspinatus and infraspinatus tear and there is a concomitant subscapularis tear, conversion to a traditional open procedure may be necessary. This can be performed with deltoid detachment or possibly using two separate approaches, including the direct lateral for the supraspinatus and infraspinatus pathology and a subsequent deltopectoral approach to address an extensile subscapularis tear or associated long head of the biceps tendon pathology. This approach does allow for preservation of the deltoid origin but does not afford the direct visualization that a complex tear may require.

PEARLS AND PITFALLS

With the advancement of arthroscopic techniques and instrumentation, the need to convert to a mini-open approach has become rarer. A surgeon may encounter cases when the tissue is poor in quality or mobilization cannot be appropriately performed. The surgeon's level of comfort and experience will frequently dictate the need to convert to an open procedure, if the repair cannot be performed in a timely fashion. From a technical standpoint, due to the difficulty with a fluid extravasation and soft tissue swelling following extensive arthroscopic procedures, the need to convert to a mini-open approach should be considered early in the process if it is apparent that the tissue quality is degenerative, bone quality is insufficient to hold suture anchor devices, or if visualization becomes significantly limited during the case.

It is important for the surgeon to base his approach on the focus of greatest pathology. If the infraspinatus and supraspinatus are the primary focus of repair then the direct lateral approach is recommended. However, if the pathology is more apparent in the anterior cuff including the subscapularis with any associated biceps lesions, then a conversion to a deltopectoral approach, whether a mini-open or more traditional extensile approach, can be beneficial to address these specific lesions.

The hybrid anterolateral approach allows for inspection and repair of tears involving the supraspinatus, the rotator interval and the upper subscapularis. If this lesion is identified, it will be beneficial to assess coracoid morphology at the time of surgery to prevent any potential recurrent lesions.

REHABILITATION

Postoperative management of patients following mini-open rotator cuff repair is based on the following factors: Patient age, size of tear, quality of tendons, quality of repair, and patient's compliance capacity. In general, however, all patients wear a sling for four to six weeks postoperatively. Patients with small to medium tears (1–3 cm) will generally begin passive and active assisted range of motion, beginning in the second postoperative week. Guidelines for range of motion restrictions will be based individually in reference to the factors detailed earlier. We typically do not allow active motion to begin until four to six weeks depending on tear size and quality. Light strengthening is introduced in six to eight weeks postoperatively and resistance exercises typically begin in 8 to 12 weeks.

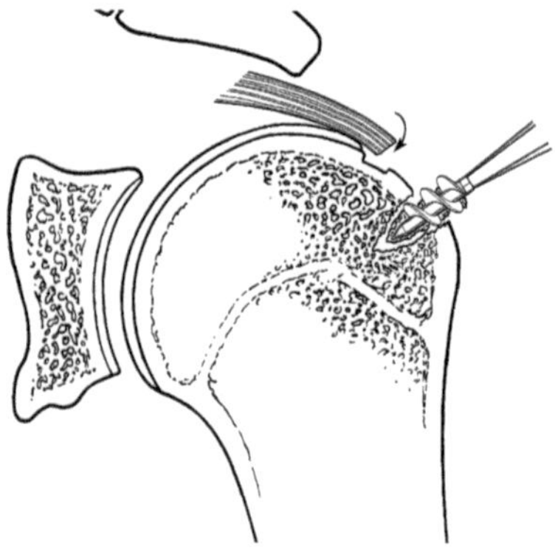

FIGURE 1 Disengagement of anchor from greater tuberosity.

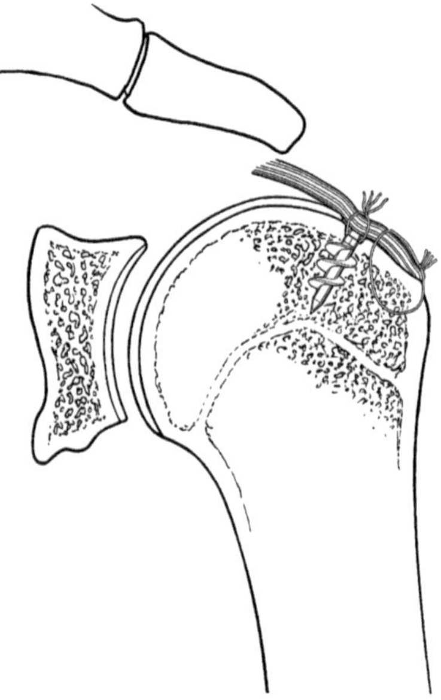

FIGURE 2 Two-row repair using transosseous tunnels for lateral fixation.

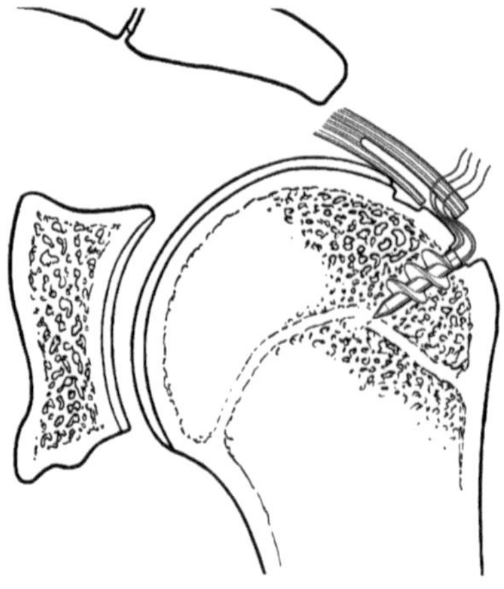

FIGURE 3 Failure to capture delaminated undersurface component of rotator cuff tear.

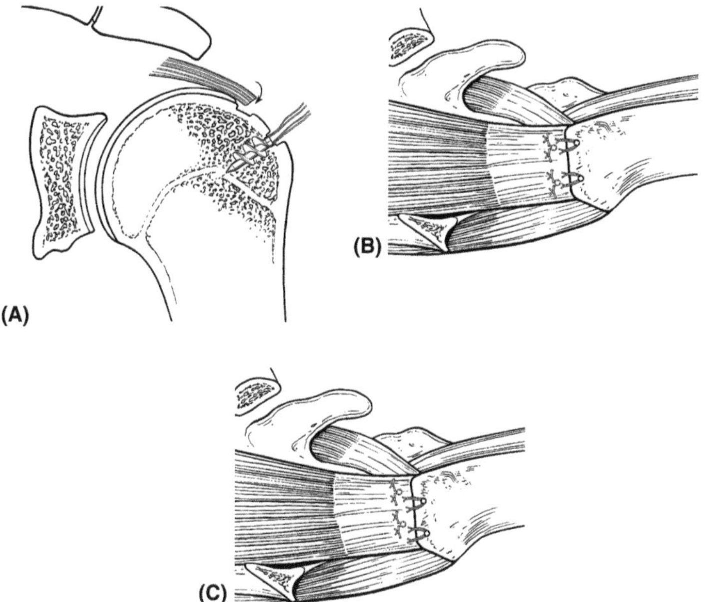

FIGURE 4 (**A**) Traditional single-row repair with anchor placement into lateral aspect of tuberosity, (**B**) parallel suture anchor configuration for two-row repair, and (**C**) offset suture anchor configuration for two-row repair.

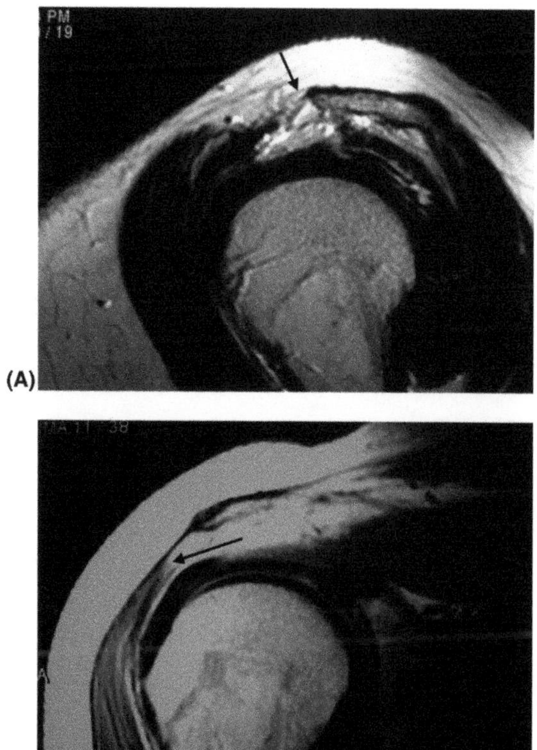

FIGURE 5 (**A**) Coronal MRI view demonstrating deficient deltoid attachment after arthroscopic decompression. (**B**) Sagittal MRI view demonstrating deltoid detachment following arthroscopic decompression.

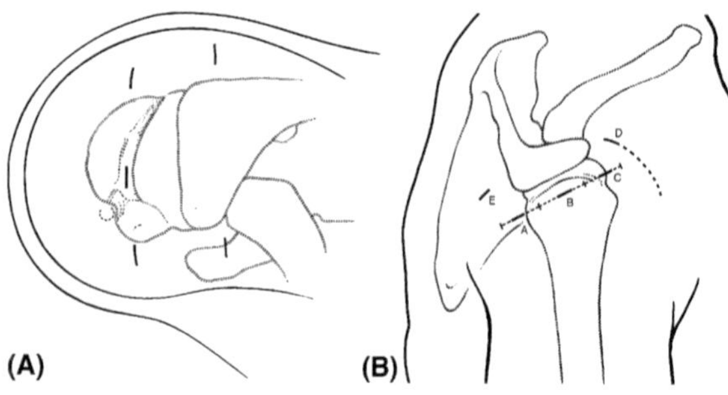

FIGURE 6 (**A**) Superior view demonstrating standard portal placement options for arthroscopic rotator cuff repair. (**B**) Sagittal view demonstrating portal extension options for mini-open repair. *Abbreviations*: A, posterolateral; B, lateral; C, anterolateral; D, deltopectoral.

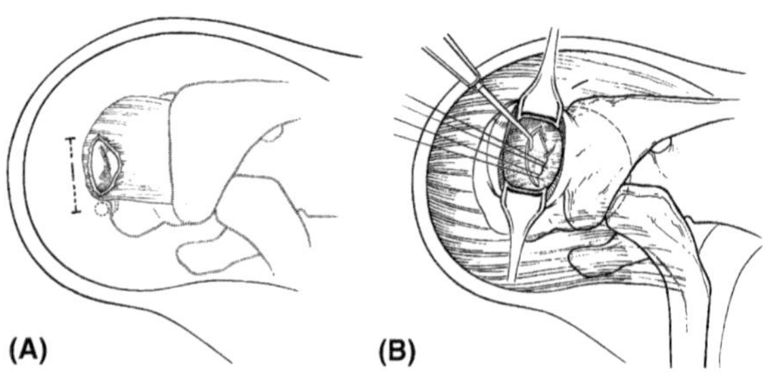

FIGURE 7 (**A**) Traditional lateral portal extension for isolated supraspinatus tear. (**B**) Deltoid retraction in the traditional approach allowing for direct visualization of supraspinatus tear.

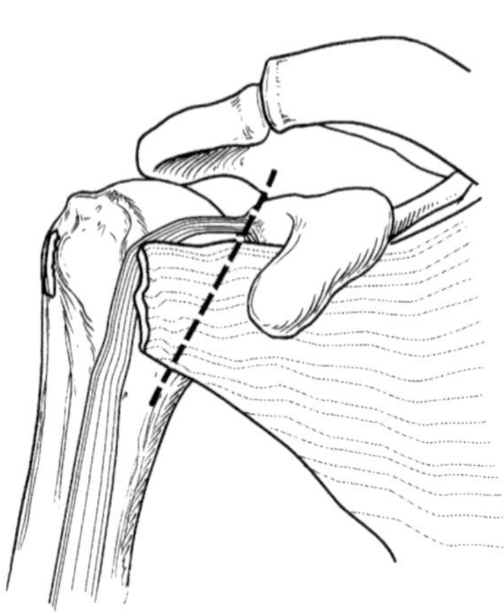

FIGURE 8 Anterior portal extension allowing for deltopectoral approach.

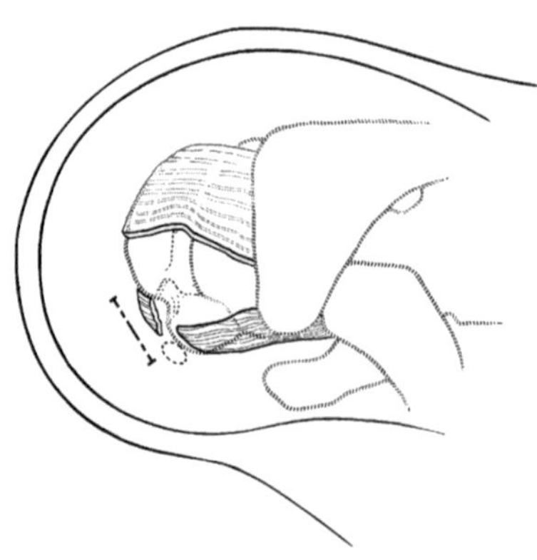

FIGURE 9 Anterolateral portal extension for rotator interval lesions including superior subscapularis, biceps, and anterior supraspinatus.

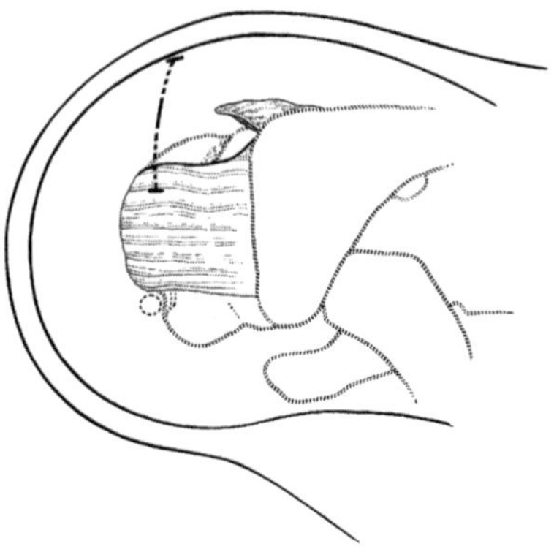

FIGURE 10 Posterolateral portal extension for posterior rotator cuff tears.

REFERENCES

1. Yamaguchi K, Ball CM, Galatz LM. Arthroscopic rotator cuff repair. Clin Orthop 2001; Sep(390):83–94.
2. Yamaguchi K, Levine WN, Marra G, et al. Transitioning to arthroscopic rotator cuff repair: the pros and cons. Instr Course Lect 2003; 52:81–92.
3. Yamaguchi K. Mini-open rotator cuff repair: an updated perspective. Instr Course Lect 2001; 50:53–61.
4. Kim SH, Ha KI, Park JH, et al. Arthroscopic versus mini-open salvage repair of the rotator cuff repair: outcome analysis at 2 to 6 years' follow-up. Arthroscopy 2003; 19(7):746–754.
5. Severud EL, Ruotolo C, Abbott DD, et al. All arthroscopic versus mini-open rotator cuff repair: a long-term retrospective outcome comparison. Arthroscopy 2003; 19(3):234–238.
6. Warner JJ, Tetreault P, Lehtinen J, et al. Arthroscopic versus mini-open rotator cuff repair: a cohort comparison study. Arthroscopy 2005; 21(3):328–332.
7. Ide J, Maeda S, Takagi K. A comparison of arthroscopic and open rotator cuff repair. Arthroscopy 2005; 21(9):1090–1098.
8. Youm T, Murray DH, Kubiak EN, et al. Arthroscopic versus mini-open rotator cuff repair: a comparison of clinical outcomes and patient satisfication. J Shoulder Elbow Surg 2005; 14(5):455–459.
9. Sauerbrey AM, Getz CL, Piancastelli M, et al. Arthroscopic Versus Mini-Open Rotator Cuff Repair: a comparison of clinical outcome. Arthroscopy 2005; 21(12):1415–1420.
10. Paulos LE, Kody MH. Arthroscopically enhanced "mini-approach" to rotator cuff repair. Am J Sports Med 1994; 22(1):19–25.
11. Blevins FT, Warren RF, Cavo C, et al. Arthroscopic rotator cuff repair: results using a mini-open open deltoid splitting approach. Arthroscopy 1996; 12(1):50–59.
12. Pollock RG, Flatow EL. Full-thickness tears: mini-open repair. Orthop Clin North Am 1997; 28:169–177.
13. Fealy S, Kingham TP, Altchek DW. Mini-open rotator cuff repair using two-row fixation technique: outcomes and analysis in patients with small, moderate and large rotator cuff tears. Arthroscopy 2002; 18(6):665–670.
14. Shinner TJ, Noordssij PG, Orwin JF. Arthroscopically assisted mini-open rotator cuff repair. Arhtroscopy 2002; 18(1):21–26.
15. Gerber C, Schneeberger AG, Perren SM, et al. Experimental rotator cuff repair: a preliminary study. J Bone Joint Surg Am 1999; 81(9):1281–1290.
16. MacGillivray JD, Ma CB. An arthroscopic stitch for massive rotator cuff tears: the Mac stitch. Arthroscopy 2004; 20(6):669-671.
17. Snyder SJ. Arthrscopic graft reconstruction for the deficient cuff. 24th Annual Meeting of the Arthroscopy Association of American, Phoenix, AZ, December 1–3, 2005.
18. Sclamberg SG, Tibone JE, Itamure JE, et al. Six-month magnetic resonance imaging follow-up of large and massive rotator cuff repairs reinforced with procine small intestinal submucosa. J Shoulder Elbow Surg 2004; 13(5):538–541.
19. Cowen BS, Hatzidakis AM, Romeo AA. Complications of rotator cuff surgery. In: Norris TR, ed. Orthopaedic Knowledge Update: Shoulder and Elbow. 2nd ed. Rosemont: American Academy of Orthopaedic Surgeons, 2002:181–190.

28 Elbow Arthroscopy: Set-Up, Anatomy, and Portal Placement

Timothy J. Strigenz and April D. Armstrong
Department of Orthopedics and Rehabilitation, Penn State Milton S. Hershey Medical Center, Hershey, Pennsylvania, U.S.A.

INTRODUCTION

Arthroscopy of the elbow was initially described by Burman (1) in 1931 when he described the elbow joint as "unsuitable for examination." A year later, he revised his thoughts, but his initial writings emphasize similar problems that remain for orthopedic surgeons today with elbow arthroscopy, most notably the risk of neurovascular injury and the difficulty examining small spaces within the elbow. Fortunately, our technology has improved as well as our knowledge of relevant anatomy. With these advances, elbow arthroscopy has become more widely accepted. It is currently a viable and effective option for much intra-articular pathology, and indications for this procedure continue to expand. However, the learning curve remains steep. The elbow is a complex articulation and allows for only a small working space. Neurovascular structures are in close proximity and at significant risk for injury. Critically important as knowing the anatomy is also managing arthroscopic operative time efficiently. During this procedure, one is working with a tourniquet, and swelling in an already small space puts a premium on surgical speed. A strong working knowledge of the anatomy of the elbow is crucial so that a safe and efficient procedure can be accomplished.

Proper portal placement is essential both to prevent neurovascular injury and obtain adequate visualization within the joint and will be discussed at length in this chapter. Positioning of the patient as well as the relevant intra-articular anatomy will be highlighted.

ANESTHESIA

A general anesthetic for elbow arthroscopy is preferred as it allows for total muscle relaxation and is the most comfortable option for the patient with a tourniquet on the arm. If the surgical plan involves placing the patient in the prone position, general anesthesia is mandatory in order to protect their airway. Depending on the patient's medical history, however, general anesthesia may not be possible and, in this case, the use of regional blocks have been described (2). Most commonly, an interscalene block is used, although Bier and axillary blocks have also been used to provide intraoperative and postoperative pain control (3,4). The main disadvantage of regional anesthesia is the inability to obtain an accurate neurovascular exam, following the procedure.

INSTRUMENTATION

Similar to arthroscopy in other joints, a variety of commercial systems are available for elbow arthroscopy. Typically, a 4.0 mm, 30° arthroscope is used and offers excellent visualization within the joint. Both 2.7 mm and 70° scopes should also be available, if the surgeon is having difficulty maneuvering and visualizing into the small spaces of the elbow. Interchangeable cannula systems exist for both the 2.7 and 4.0 mm arthroscopes and may be used in order to minimize the number of capsulotomies and also facilitate transfer of the camera and the instruments between portals. This will lessen the chance of damaging neurovascular structures and decrease the amount of fluid extravasation, which could lead to compartment syndrome

---

Please refer to pages 306–311 for the figures in this chapter.

(5). A closed, unfenestrated cannula system should also be used to prevent fluid extravasation into the subcutaneous tissues.

Cannula systems should be blunt rather than sharp ended. These work sufficiently well to traverse the soft tissues and enter the joint and pose less of a risk to the neurovascular structures than the sharp-tipped trocars. The cannulae may be attached either to a pump at low pressure (<30 mmHg) or flow with gravity pressure alone. Other instruments that may be useful include a probe, graspers, forceps, pituitary rongeurs, switching sticks, cannula dilator sets, osteotomes, motorized burrs and shavers, and small biting instruments.

PATIENT POSITIONING

Patient positioning ultimately depends on the experience and comfort level of the surgeon. It is extremely important that the patient be adequately padded over all bony prominences and that the antecubital space of the elbow remain free of constriction to protect the neurovascular structures. Also, the hand and distal forearm should be wrapped to help prevent leakage of fluid down the forearm, which could cause a compartment syndrome. Finally, a tourniquet placed high enough on the arm to prevent constriction of the antecubital space can be used to maintain hemostasis and enhance visualization within the joint.

Supine Position

Andrews and Carson (6) first described elbow arthroscopy with the patient supine. In their description, the affected arm is suspended by an overhead traction system that is connected to the hand and forearm by a prefabricated gauntlet. The shoulder is positioned at the edge of the table and the arm is allowed to hang freely over the operating room table with the elbow flexed at 90°, allowing access to the entire elbow.

One advantage of this position is that the arm is in a flexed position that allows the neurovascular structures around the elbow to be relaxed. This is crucial when working inside the joint and can aid in preventing a neurovascular injury. Also, the elbow is oriented in an anatomic position, which makes the intra-articular anatomy more perceptible when viewing through the arthroscope (3,6). Lastly, this position offers the anesthesiologist easy access to the airway.

One potential disadvantage of the supine position, however, is instability of the arm as it hangs in the traction device. Without an outside stabilizing force or a second person, the arm can swing due to external forces (7). Access to the posterior aspect of the arm is also compromised and working in the posterior compartment of the elbow in this position forces the surgeon to operate in an "uphill" direction. It is not only difficult technically and perceptually, but also allows for potential contamination of the field, as irrigation fluid runs down the arthroscope.

Prone Position

Poehling et al. (8) described the prone position in 1989. In their description, the patient is positioned prone on chest rolls with the affected shoulder abducted to 90° and the arm draped over an arm board or commercial arthroscopic arm holder. The elbow is left in a dependant position and naturally falls into 90° of flexion. Care should be taken to ensure that pressure from the arm board is eliminated from the anterior aspect of the distal arm, as this may compromise joint distension and will place the neurovascular structures at risk (Figs. 1 and 2).

The primary advantages of this position when compared to the supine position are the stability of the arm and the elimination of a traction device. Also, the prone position allows improved access to the posterior compartment and eliminates the need to operate in an upside down manner. Another potential advantage, should the procedure necessitate, is the ability of the surgeon to move to an open procedure, as most approaches are accessible. Finally, and probably most importantly, gravity along with distention of the elbow moves the neurovascular structures away from the joint and from potential danger (9). The primary disadvantage of the prone position is the need to reposition the patient if an open anterior approach is needed (4,7). Also, in this position, the airway access is compromised due to the patient being prone and this position will not be tolerated in a patient who is receiving a regional block.

Lateral Decubitus Position

The lateral position was described by O'Driscoll and Morrey (10). It offers the same advantages of the prone position, but does not compromise access to the airway. The patient is positioned in the lateral decubitus position with the affected side up, ensuring adequate padding of all bony prominences. The shoulder is forward flexed to 90° and internally rotated, the arm is supported on a padded bolster with the elbow flexed to 90°, and the forearm allowed to hang free (Figs. 1 and 2). Again, the antecubital space should be left free of any constriction to avoid neurovascular injury. This position allows the surgeon access to medial, lateral, and posterior aspects of the elbow. The main disadvantage is the need to occasionally reposition the patient if an open procedure is needed (10).

ANATOMY

The three major articulations at the elbow are the ulno-humeral, radio-capitellar, and proximal radioulnar. The distal humerus is defined by its convex trochlea, medially, and the capitellum, laterally. The trochlea articulates with the concave olecranon and coronoid process of the proximal ulna. Laterally, the capitellum freely articulates with the radial head. It is through these two articulations that the elbow flexion and extension arc is obtained. The proximal radioulnar joint articulation allows for pronation and supination.

The bony anatomy of the elbow divides the elbow into three compartments arthroscopically: (*i*) anterior, (*ii*) posterior, and (*iii*) posterolateral. The anterior compartment is composed of the coronoid process, the anterior trochlea, the radial head, the capitellum, and the medial and lateral condyles. The posterior compartment contains the olecranon tip, the olecranon fossa, posterior trochlea, and the medial and lateral gutters. The posterolateral compartment contains the radial head, olecranon, lateral gutter, and capitellum.

Surface Anatomy

Anatomical understanding of the elbow starts with identifying the superficial landmarks. This should be done prior to joint distention, as distension can make palpating the normal landmarks more difficult. The structures that are most readily palpable are the olecranon, the medial and lateral epicondyles, the radial head/capitellum articulation (rotate the forearm to help localize), lateral supracondylar ridge, the medial intermuscular septum, and the ulnar nerve. The ulnar nerve should be palpated while flexing and extending the elbow to determine if it subluxates or dislocates so that it can be protected during the procedure. It may also be helpful to diagram the paths of the radial, ulnar, and median nerves and the brachial artery prior to the procedure.

PORTAL PLACEMENT AND INTRA-ARTICULAR ANATOMY

Joint distension is one of the key aspects in elbow arthroscopy to prevent neurovascular injury when establishing portals. It has been shown that distention provides maximum distance of the nerves from the elbow joint, thereby decreasing their risk of injury (11). (Table 1). However, it is important to realize that distension only increases the distance of nerves and capsule from bone, but does not change the relationship of the nerves to the capsule itself (Figs. 3 and 4). In stiff elbows, it has been shown that capsular compliance may be only 15% of the normal joint, significantly increasing risk of neurovascular injury (4). Positioning the elbow in

TABLE 1 Neurovascular Proximity to Portal Placement Before and After Elbow Distension

	No distension (mm)	Distension (mm)
Median nerve	4	14
Brachial artery	9	17
Radial nerve	4	11

Source: Adapted from Ref. 11.

flexion and distending the joint has been shown to decrease the chance of neurovascular injury to anterior structures when establishing portals (11–14).

The joint is distended by injecting sterile fluid into the joint at the lateral "soft spot" (Fig. 5). The boundaries of the soft spot are usually palpable through the soft tissues and consist of the radial head, lateral humeral epicondyle, and the tip of the olecranon. A needle is directed medially from the soft spot and approximately 30 cc of fluid may be injected with the elbow flexed, and as the joint pressure increases, slight extension of the elbow may be visualized (15). Once the elbow is distended, portal placement is ready to commence.

When making portals, only the skin should be incised with the scalpel. The subcutaneous tissues should be dissected bluntly using either hemostats or a blunt-tipped trocar, in order to protect the superficial nervous structures. The joint itself is also entered using the blunt-tipped trocar and every attempt should be made to create a single puncture rather than making multiple passes through the joint capsule. It is surgeon's preference whether to enter the joint medially or laterally, initially.

Anterior Compartment

The anterior compartment may be visualized by a variety of anterolateral and anteromedial portals. The anterolateral portals consist of the classic anterolateral, the mid anterolateral, and proximal anterolateral portals.

Anterolateral Portals

The classic anterolateral portal is the most distal of the anterolateral portals and was first described by Andrews and Carson (3) in 1985 (Fig. 6). It lies in the sulcus just anterior to the radial head, approximately 1 cm distal and 3 cm anterior to the lateral epicondyle and can be palpated by pronating and supinating the forearm (6). Cadaveric studies have shown that during placement of the classic anterolateral portal, the trocar and arthroscope pass through the extensor carpi radialis brevis and supinator muscle (6) and passes posterolateral to the radial nerve. As the sheath passes through the forearm, the radial nerve has been shown to be as close as 3 mm in distended elbows (16). The most superficial structure, the posterior antebrachial cutaneous nerve, averages about 2 mm from the portal site (11). The posterior interosseus nerve (PIN) is also at risk, with the distance varying between 1 to 13 mm from the portal depending on the degree of forearm pronation, with greater pronation increasing the distance (13). Because of the inherent risks of this portal, its use has fallen out of favor. The mid-anterolateral and proximal anterolateral portals are now the more preferred portals from the anterolateral side.

The mid-anterolateral portal is placed 2 cm directly anterior to the lateral epicondyle in line with the joint, and proximal anterolateral portal is placed approximately 2 cm proximal and 1 cm anterior to the lateral epicondyle (Fig. 6). Stothers et al. (17) compared the proximal anterolateral portal to the classic anterolateral portal in cadavers and found it to be safer and provided improved visualization of the joint. A study by Field et al. (18) compared the classic anterolateral portal, the mid anterolateral portal, and the proximal anterolateral portal. They found that all of these portals provide good visualization of the ulnohumeral articulation, in addition to the radiocapitellar joint. However, they reported that joint visualization was "most complete" and "technically easier" using the proximal anterolateral portal. The proximal anterolateral portal site also allowed for the furthest distance from the radial nerve, making it the safest of the three lateral portals.

The predominant anatomic structures viewed from the anterolateral portals are the coronoid process and the trochlea (Figs. 7 and 8). Flexion and extension of the elbow helps to identify these structures, as they articulate. Also visible more proximally is the coronoid fossa, which accepts the coronoid process at the extreme of flexion and is commonly a site of rest for loose bodies. More distally, the brachialis insertion is covered by a sheath of synovium and can be seen inserting on the coronoid process. By moving the camera medially, the medial capsule can be identified and, occasionally, a thickening can be appreciated, which represents the anterior bundle of the medial collateral ligament.

Anteromedial Portals

The anteromedial and proximal anteromedial portals are the most commonly used medial portals in elbow arthroscopy. The anteromedial portal is placed in line with the joint approximately 2 cm anterior and 2 cm distal to the medial epicondyle and traverses the common flexor origin (6). The proximal anteromedial portal is located approximately 2 cm proximal to the medial epicondyle and 1 to 2 cm anterior to the intermuscular septum (Fig. 9). The main structures at risk are the ulnar nerve, median nerve, brachial artery, and the medial antebrachial cutaneous nerve. The medial intermuscular septum protects the ulnar nerve. The elbow should be maintained at 90° of flexion and the trocar directed toward the center of the joint, in front of the medial intermuscular septum, in order to protect the ulnar nerve. The brachialis on the anterior aspect of the joint acts as a cushion to protect the median nerve and brachial artery. These portals provide excellent visualization of the radiocapitellar and ulnohumeral joints.

Once inside the joint from the anteromedial portal, the radial head serves as the landmark and can be identified as it rotates during pronation and supination. Just proximal to the radial head is the anterosuperior portion of the capitellum and the bare radial fossa. On occasion, a fold of synovium exists between the radial head and capitellum, looking like a thin meniscus. Fibers of the annular ligament may be visible over the radial head. Moving more medially, the coronoid, coronoid fossa, trochlea, and capsule may be visualized (Figs. 10 and 11).

Posterior/Posterolateral Compartments

As with the other compartments of the elbow, a variety of posterior and posterolateral portals have been utilized to view the posterior compartment. The posterior portals include the posterocentral, proximal posterolateral, and distal posterolateral portals and the lateral soft spot (Fig. 12). The posterocentral portal is placed in the midline 3 cm proximal to the olecranon directly through the musculotendinous portion of the triceps. It should be established with the elbow in 20° to 30° of flexion to permit relaxation of the triceps. It provides very good visualization of the posterior compartment of the elbow and is useful in removing loose bodies and osteophytes off the olecranon (19). The main dangers in this portal are the posterior antebrachial cutaneous nerve and the ulnar nerve, both of which pass within 25 mm of the portal (20). These structures should be a little risk, as long as the cannula is maintained lateral at the midline or lateral to the midline.

The proximal posterolateral portal is located anywhere from the lateral tip of the olecranon to 3 cm proximal of this point along the lateral border of the triceps tendon (20). Similar to the direct posterior portal, the portal is established with the elbow in 20° to 30° of flexion with the cannula inserted toward the olecranon fossa. This portal functions as an accessory to the posterocentral portal and allows work to be done on the olecranon tip, olecranon fossa, and posterior trochlea.

When viewed through the arthroscope, the posterior compartment's main anatomic landmark is the tip of the olecranon that can be identified with flexion and extension of the elbow and can be seen seating in the olecranon fossa. The insertion of the triceps can also be used to identify the tip of the olecranon. The olecranon fossa itself is triangular in shape and can have osteophytes growing from it and may hold loose bodies. The posteromedial and posterolateral gutters are best seen in this compartment and can be visualized by directing the camera medially or laterally, respectively. The posterior capsule is also well seen in this compartment and, more medially, the posteromedial aspect of the joint should be accessed, as this shows the vertically oriented fibers of the posterior band of the ulnar collateral ligament. Approximately 50% of the ligament can be visualized and just superficial to this lies the ulnar nerve (21) (Figs. 13 and 14).

The laterally located soft spot, previously discussed as the site used to distend the joint, can also be used as a portal to visualize the posterior compartment of the elbow, mainly the posterolateral aspect. It offers excellent visualization of the inferior-posterior aspect of the capitellum and also the radioulnar articulation (20).

The posterolateral compartment is visualized through the direct lateral portal, or the "soft spot," as described by Poehling et al. (8). Within this compartment, the capitellum is the most obvious structure, and the evaluation of an osteochondritis dissecans lesion is afforded. The radial head is also well visualized by bringing the scope anteriorly. The radial head should be slightly concave on its most proximal surface, whereas the capitellum should be gently convex. The scope can be redirected posteriorly and medially between the olecranon and trochlea. By looking down on the olecranon articular surface, a roughened area that lacks articular cartilage can commonly be observed, which denotes the apophyseal scar or bare area of the olecranon. By turning the scope anteriorly, the underside of the trochlea can be visualized. A distal posterolateral portal can be created along the posterolateral gutter where a portal is needed to facilitate arthroscopic work (Fig. 15).

SUMMARY

Elbow arthroscopy continues to be a challenging procedure for orthopedic surgeons. The space within the elbow joint is small, and visualizing the three compartments of the elbow can be difficult and requires the use of multiple portals. Each of the portals used by the surgeon requires a comprehensive knowledge of elbow anatomy and an ability to relate superficial anatomy to intra-articular anatomy, in order to minimize the risk of neurovascular injury. However, with the proper planning, setup, and foundation of knowledge, elbow arthroscopy can be safely performed for a wide variety of elbow pathologies.

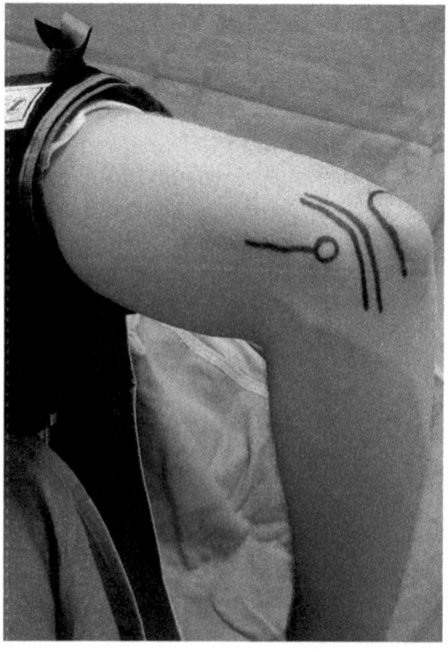

FIGURE 1 Medial aspect of the elbow in the lateral decubitus or prone position. Note that the antecubital space is free of any restriction. The medial epicondyle, path of the ulnar nerve, and olecranon are marked out. This arm position would be similar for the patient in the prone position.

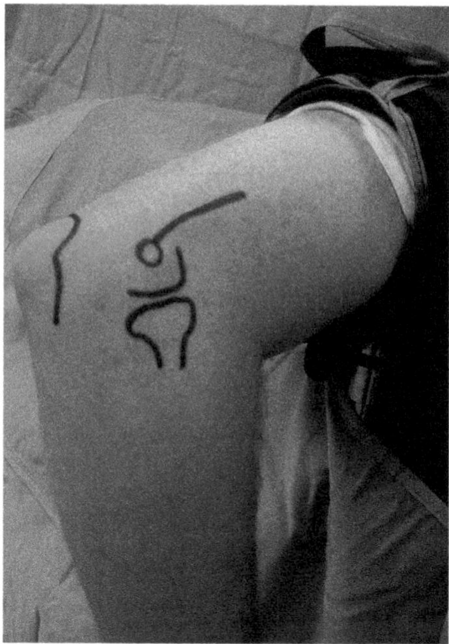

FIGURE 2 Lateral aspect of the elbow in the lateral decubitus or prone position with the lateral epicondyle, lateral supracondylar ridge, capitellum, radial head, and lateral olecranon marked out.

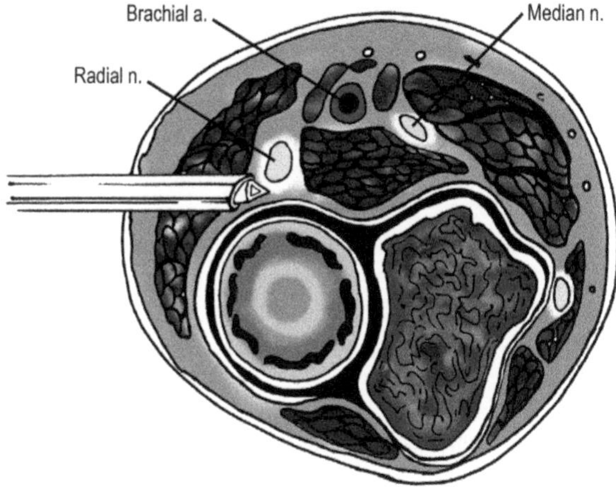

FIGURE 3 The elbow joint is shown prior to distension. Note the proximity of the neurovascular bundles to the joint.

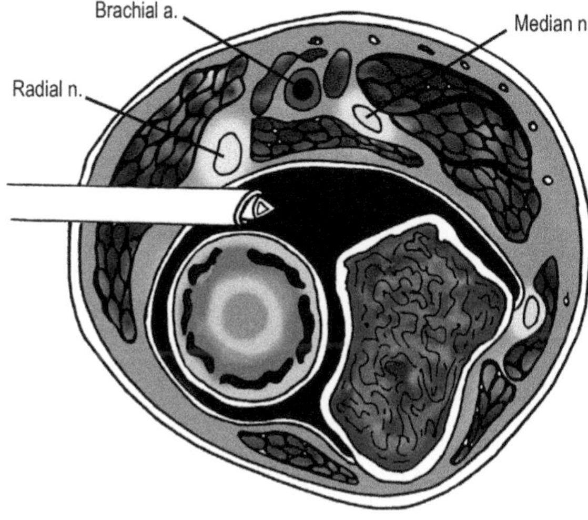

FIGURE 4 The elbow joint after distension. Note the increased distance of the neurovascular bundles to the bone, but that nerves have a similar distance to the joint capsule itself.

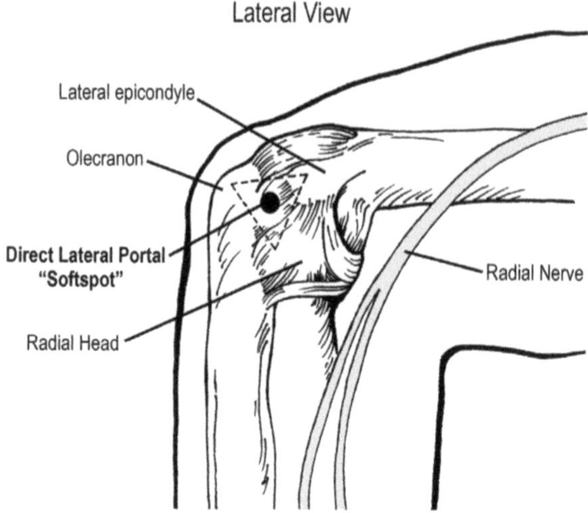

FIGURE 5 The lateral "soft spot" of the elbow between the radial head, lateral epicondyle, and olecranon. This is the site for initial distension of the elbow joint.

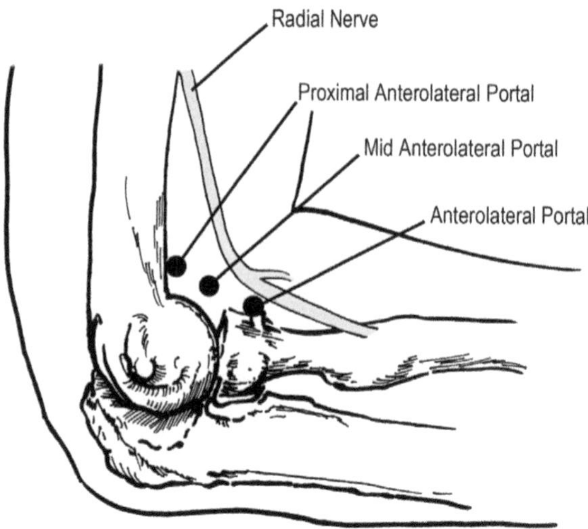

FIGURE 6 The positions of the various anterolateral portals.

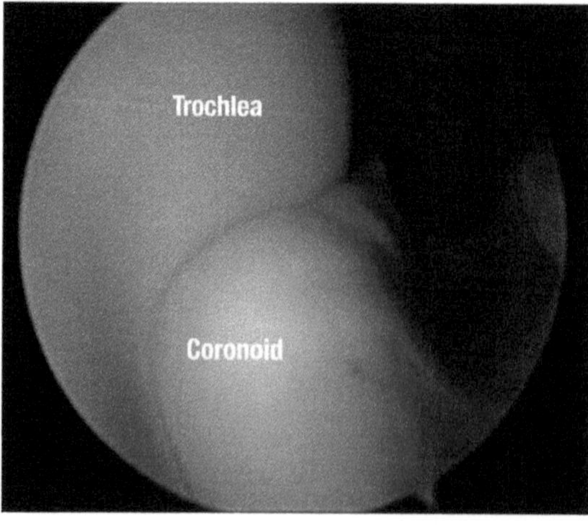

FIGURE 7 The anterior compartment as viewed from the proximal anterolateral portal, with the camera aimed medially.

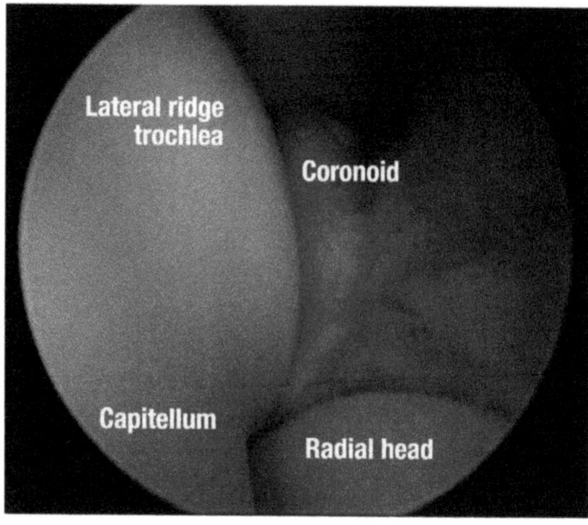

FIGURE 8 The anterior compartment as viewed from the proximal anterolateral portal, with the camera aimed laterally.

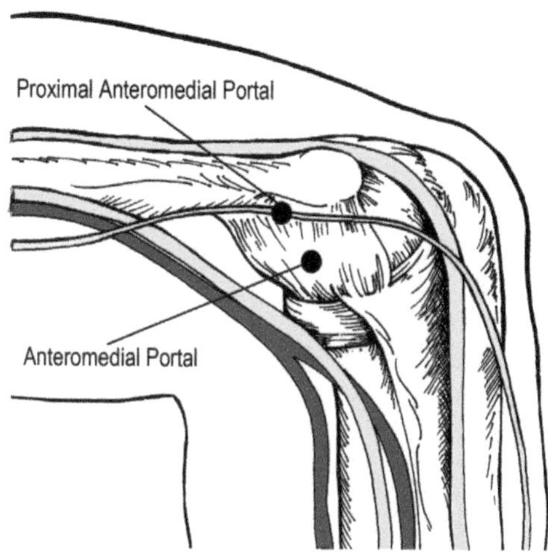

FIGURE 9 The positions of the various anteromedial portals.

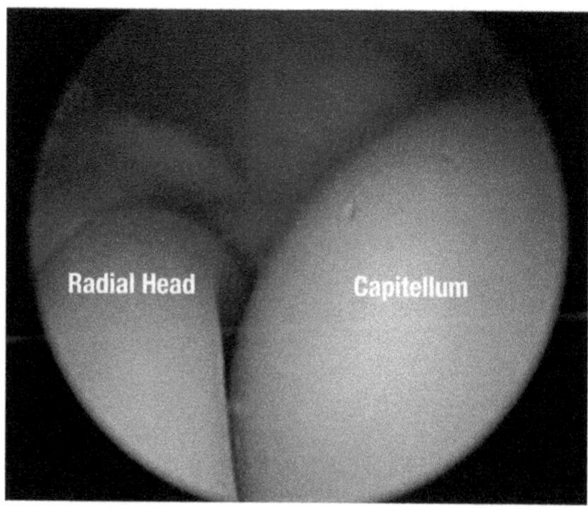

FIGURE 10 The anterior compartment as viewed from the anteromedial portal, with the camera aimed laterally.

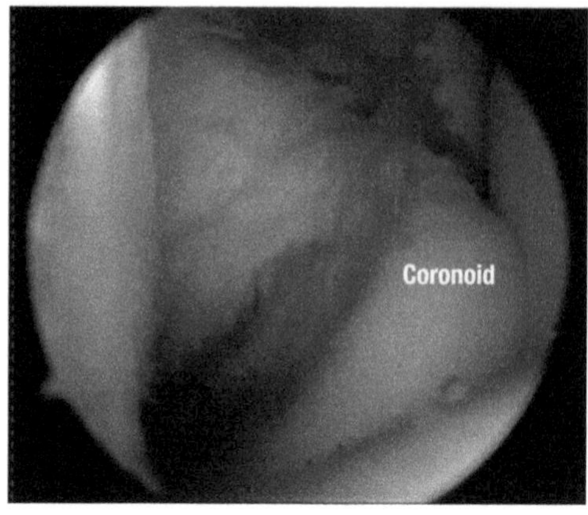

FIGURE 11 The anterior compartment as viewed from the anteromedial portal, with the camera aimed medially.

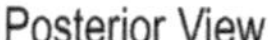

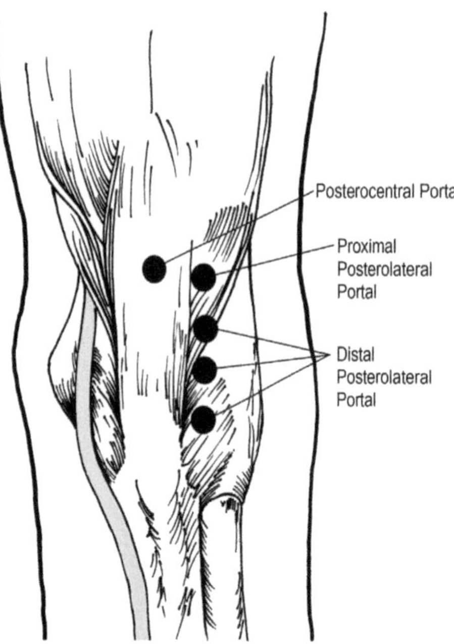

FIGURE 12 The positions of the posterior and posterolateral portals.

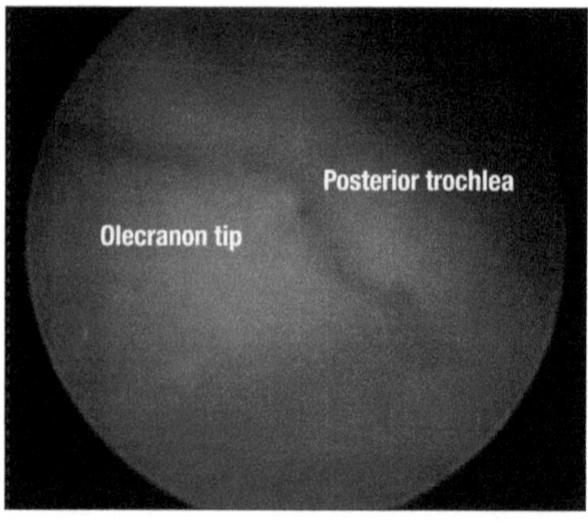

FIGURE 13 Posterior compartment as viewed from posterior portal.

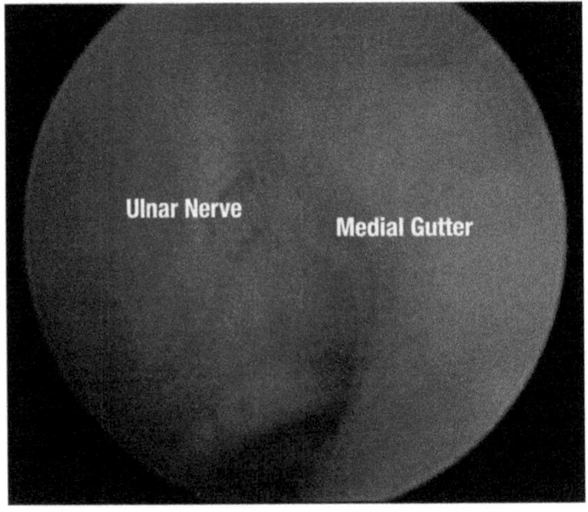

FIGURE 14 The medial gutter as viewed from the posterior portal. The ulnar nerve is located directly posterior to the soft tissues.

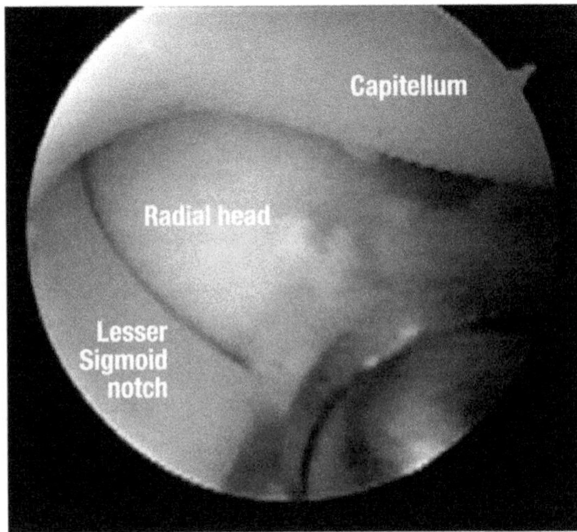

FIGURE 15 Posterolateral compartment as viewed from the posterolateral portal.

REFERENCES

1. Burman MS. Arthroscopy or the direct visualization of joints. J Bone Joint Surg 1931; 13:669–695.
2. Johnson LL. Elbow arthroscopy. Diagnostic and Surgical Arthroscopy. St Louis: C.V. Mosby, 1981:390–399.
3. Carson WG Jr, Meyers JF. Diagnostic arthroscopy of the elbow: supine position surgical technique, arthroscopic and portal anatomy. In: Mcginty JB, Caspari RB, Jackson RW, Poehling GG, eds. Operative Arthroscopy. 2nd ed. Philadelphia: Lippincott-Raven, 1996:851–868.
4. Plancher KD, Peterson RK, Bresenkoff L. Diagnostic arthroscopy of the elbow: set-up, portals and technique. Oper Tech Sports Med 1998; 6:2–10.
5. Angelo RL. Advances in elbow arthroscopy. Orthopedics 1993; 16(9):1037–1046.
6. Andrews JR, Carson WG. Arthroscopy of the elbow. Arthroscopy 1985; 1:97–107.
7. Baker CL Jr. Normal arthroscopic anatomy of the elbow: surgical technique with the patient in prone. In: McGinty JB, Caspari RB, Jackson RW, Poehling GG, eds. Operative Arthroscopy. 2nd ed. Philadelphia: Lippincott-Raven, 1996:869–876.
8. Poehling GG, Whipple TL, Sisco L, et al. Elbow arthroscopy: a new technique. Arthroscopy 1989; 5:222–224.
9. Baker CL Jr, Shalvoy RM. The prone position for elbow arthroscopy. Clin Sports Med 1991; 10:623–628.
10. O'Driscoll SW, Morrey BF. Arthroscopy of the elbow: diagnostic and therapeutic benefits and hazards. J Bone Joint Surg 1992; 74A:84–94.
11. Lynch GJ, Meyers JF, Whipple TL, et al. Neurovascular anatomy and elbow arthroscopy: inherent risks. Arthroscopy 1986; 2:190–197.
12. Adolffson L. Arthroscopy of the elbow joint: a cadaveric study of portal placement. J Shoulder Elbow Surg 1994; 3:53–61.
13. Marshall PD, Fairclough JA, Johnson SR, et al. Avoiding nerve damage during elbow arthroscopy. J Bone Joint Surg 1993; 75B:129–131.
14. Poehling GG, Ekman EF. Arthroscopy of the elbow. Instr Course Lect 1995; 44:217–223.
15. O'Driscoll SW, Morrey BF, An KN. Intra-articular pressure and capacity of the elbow. Arthroscopy 1990; 6(2):100–103.
16. Lindenfield TN. Medial approach in elbow arthroscopy. Am J Sports Med 1990; 18:413–417.
17. Stothers K, Day B, Regan WR. Arthroscopy of the elbow: anatomy, portal sites, and a description of the proximal lateral portal. Arthroscopy 1995; 11:449–457.
18. Field LD, Altchek DW, Warren RF, et al. Arthroscopic anatomy of the lateral elbow: a comparison of three portals. Arthroscopy 1994; 10:602–607.
19. Andrews JR, St. Pierre RK, Carson WG. Arthroscopy of the elbow. Clin Sports Med 1986; 5:653–662.
20. Baker CL Jr, Brooks AA. Arthroscopy of the elbow. Clin Sports Med 1996; 15:261–281.
21. Andrews JR, Baumgarten TE. Arthroscopic anatomy of the elbow. Ortho Clin N Am 1995; 26(4):671–677.

29 Diagnostic Elbow Arthroscopy

Douglass E. Stull and Matthew L. Ramsey
Department of Orthopedic Surgery, University of Pennsylvania School of Medicine, Philadelphia, Pennsylvania, U.S.A.

INTRODUCTION

Arthroscopy is an important tool in the diagnosis and treatment of many conditions that afflict the elbow. Despite the utility of diagnostic arthroscopy, it should not take the place of a good history and physical examination as well as appropriately ordered imaging studies. The value of diagnostic arthroscopy lies in the ability to directly visualize the intra-articular structures of the elbow, confirm suspected diagnoses, and treat confirmed pathology. Elbow arthroscopy is technically demanding. The close proximity of neurovascular structures requires the surgeon to maintain a three-dimensional understanding of elbow anatomy. With this understanding, and with the proper indications, elbow arthroscopy has proven reproducible, safe, and effective.

INDICATIONS

Elbow arthroscopy has value in providing the surgeon direct visualization of the intra-articular structures of the elbow. Assessment of static structures, such as the joint cartilage, synovium, capsule, and the presence or absence of loose bodies, is possible for the purposes of diagnosis. Additionally, dynamic relationships of the highly congruent joint structures can be observed by visualizing their respective relationships with combined range of motion and application of varus, valgus, or rotational forces.

The ideal indication for elbow arthroscopy is a history of mechanical symptoms or pain in the elbow, supported by physical examination and radiographs demonstrating intra-articular pathology. Arthroscopy for patients with pain from injury to the elbow without supporting physical exam findings or radiographs does not typically yield an intra-articular diagnosis and is therefore of limited value (1). Therefore, the value of arthroscopy as a diagnostic tool is the confirmation of suspected pathology and the identification of associated pathology not identified preoperatively. Occasionally, in a small, very select subset of patients, a diagnostic arthroscopy to disprove pathology may prove beneficial.

CONTRAINDICATIONS

There are very few absolute contraindications to elbow arthroscopy. The surgeon should avoid attempted arthroscopy when ankylosis or severe capsular contracture prevents protection of the surrounding neurovascular structures through joint distension, such as in the case of heterotopic ossification (2). Relative contraindications include any condition that alters the normal anatomy so as to make safe portal placement impossible or the risk to neurovascular structures unacceptably high. Examples of such conditions include congenital anomalies (radial head dislocation), post-traumatic deformity, such as after lateral condyle fracture nonunion (cubitus valgus) or supracondylar fracture malunion (cubitus varus), and previous submuscular or subcutaneous ulnar nerve transposition.

Please refer to pages 317–320 for the figures in this chapter.

GENERAL PRINCIPLES

Although there are significant potential benefits to arthroscopic surgery of the elbow, several features of the elbow joint provide unique challenges to the treating surgeon. Additionally, the relative rarity of problems amenable to arthroscopic management in most practices results in a longer learning curve to competency. These features include: (*i*) close proximity of major neurovascular structures (3,4). The ulnar nerve is at risk with posterior compartment surgery, and its close proximity to the posteromedial joint capsule limits medial gutter surgery. It also is at risk with superomedial portal placement, and it is mandatory to identify if the ulnar nerve subluxes anteriorly with elbow flexion. The median nerve and brachial artery are structures at risk during medial portal placement. These structures are protected by the brachialis when working against the anteromedial capsule. However, median nerve transection has been reported with anteromedial surgery unrelated to portal placement (4). The radial nerve is a high-risk structure both when establishing an anterolateral portal and intra-articularly, as the posterior interosseous branch lies in close proximity to the anterolateral joint capsule. (*ii*) The complex nature of the articular anatomy. There are three highly congruent joints (ulnohumeral, radiocapitellar, and radioulnar), which require assessment from multiple portals to visualize them entirely. (*iii*) The elbow has a relatively small working space as it compares to other large joints (shoulder and knee), which are routinely treated arthroscopically. (*iv*) The relative unfamiliarity of many surgeons with the relevant three-dimensional and cross-sectional anatomy. (*v*) A difficulty in gaining necessary case experience, as elbow complaints that meet indications for elbow arthroscopy are not nearly as common as those found in the shoulder or knee. (*vi*) There is a relative premium on surgical speed due to the potential neurovascular complications associated with prolonged arthroscopy of the elbow (5).

SURGICAL TECHNIQUE

While discussed in detail in chapter 28, a brief discussion of patient position, anesthesia, incisions, portal anatomy, and instruments are important to review in any description of diagnostic elbow arthroscopy.

The position of the patient can be supine, prone, or lateral. All three have advantages and disadvantages, as previously discussed in chapter 28. The authors prefer the lateral decubitus position, as it represents a compromise between safe maintenance of the airway and providing an accessible, stable platform for arthroscopy (1,6).

General anesthesia is typically preferred for patients undergoing elbow arthroscopy in the lateral decubitus position. Regional blockade is possible, but some surgeons prefer general anesthesia alone to allow for postoperative neurologic assessment (7). The authors prefer a combination that allows for both intra-operative comfort and postoperative pain control. Neurologic status is assessed after the regional block is no longer in effect. If the surgeon prefers to assess neurologic status postoperatively, local anesthetic in the portal sites is not recommended, as it may cause prolonged cutaneous sensory deficits.

Incisions to establish portals should only be made through the skin. Subcutaneous dissection should proceed with a blunt hemostat to the level of the joint capsule; this technique avoids injury to superficial sensory nerves.

Instrumentation in elbow arthroscopy is very similar to other joints. A standard 4.0 mm, 30° arthroscope provides excellent visualization. Occasionally, a 2.7 mm arthroscope may be required for visualization in the posterolateral gutter or in adolescent patients. All trocars are blunt and conical to avoid neurovascular injury. Inflow cannulas should be devoid of side vents to prevent fluid extravasation into the soft tissues (Fig. 1). Standard arthroscopic instruments, such as grasping forceps, punches, shavers and burrs, are used during elbow arthroscopy (Fig. 2). Specialty instruments for elbow arthroscopy, including portal dilators and intra-articular retractors, have been developed in an attempt to improve the safety of the surgery (Fig. 3).

In no other joint is portal anatomy as critical as in the elbow. This relates again to the close proximity of neurovascular structures. Prior to insufflation of the joint and portal establishment, the topographical anatomy is drawn with a sterile marker on the skin (Fig. 4). The lateral and medial columns with the medial and lateral epicondyles of the humerus are drawn, with the course of the ulnar nerve clearly marked. The radial head and its articulation with the humerus and the olecranon process are all marked as well. Portal placement has previously been discussed, but one principle to remember is in the anterior compartment of the elbow, more proximal portals are generally safer (8).

AUTHORS' PREFERRED TECHNIQUE

After placing a regional blockade of the affected extremity, the patient receives a general anesthesia and is placed in the lateral decubitus position. A tourniquet is placed high on the arm and the arm is placed over a padded bolster at 90° of abduction and with the humerus parallel to the floor (Fig. 5). It is important to ensure that the elbow can be fully extended and, more importantly, flexed beyond 90°.

The extremity is prepped and draped such that the arm can be manipulated intraoperatively. The hand and forearm are wrapped with an elastic bandage to help minimize fluid extravasations into the forearm. Topographical anatomy is clearly identified and marked. An esmarch bandage is used to exsanguinate the limb, and the tourniquet is insufflated to 250 mmHg.

Joint insufflation is performed with an 18-gauge spinal needle directed into the lateral "soft spot" with infusion of around 25 mL of sterile saline (9). The volume of fluid may be greater in inflammatory elbows and less in contracted elbows. Joint distension is an important part of protecting the neurovascular structures during portal placement, in that they are lifted away from the bone, increasing the bone-to-nerve distance (10). It should be noted that the capsule-to-nerve distance does not change, and therefore joint distension does not help protect the nerves when working against the joint capsule.

Regardless of the surgeon's sequence in establishing portals, a consistent systematic approach should be established that allows for visualization of the anterior compartment and the three posterior compartments (the posterior ulnohumeral joint, the posteromedial gutter, and the posterolateral gutter).

The superomedial portal (11) is established 2 cm proximal to the medial epicondyle. The skin is incised with a #11 blade, and subcutaneous dissection is performed with a hemostat. The end of the blunt trocar is used to palpate the intramuscular septum and the trocar is advanced just anterior to the septum, down the anteromedial supracondylar column until a "pop" is felt that signifies the cannula has punctured the distended joint capsule. A 30°, 4.0 mm arthroscope is placed in the cannula, and inflow is established through the arthroscope. Gravity inflow or inflow utilizing a pump set at 50 mm can be performed. Higher pump pressures have been associated with fluid extravasation and loss of joint distension and visualization (9). Initial orientation from the superomedial portal is established by visualizing the radiocapitellar articulation (Fig. 6). Structures that require visualization in the anterolateral aspect of the joint include the articular surface of the radial head, its articulation with the capitellum, and its articular margin. The superior and anterior portions of the capitellum are inspected and, with progressive extension, more visualization of the anterior capitellum is afforded, recalling that, with progressive extension, the working space decreases, as the anterior capsule tightens. The radial fossa just superior to the capitellum is easily seen and inspected for osteophyte formation (Fig. 7). The synovium of the anterolateral joint capsule and, if possible, the annular ligament are also inspected. To assist in visualization of the radial articular margin, the forearm can be pronated and supinated. A varus force with forearm pronated helps to visualize the articular surface of the radial head. As the arthroscope is slowly withdrawn, the anterior aspect of the proximal radioulnar articulation and anterior ulnohumeral articulation can be visualized (Fig. 8). It has to be noted that the lateral ligamentous complex cannot be visualized through the anterior medial portal.

An anterolateral portal is established under direct visualization with use of a spinal needle for localization. A proximal portal is preferred, as the radial nerve is kept at a greater distance from this portal while maintaining excellent visualization (11). This portal allows for instrumentation of the anterolateral compartment of the elbow. Placing the arthroscope in this portal provides excellent visualization of the anterior ulnohumeral articulation and the remainder of the anteromedial compartment of the elbow (Fig. 9). The ulnohumeral articulation provides for initial orientation, and the coronoid process and its fossa should be inspected for osteophytes and loose bodies. The trochlea is viewed and, with flexion and extension, its articular surface can be better visualized. The anterior medial capsule and the anterior portion of the anterior bundle of the medial collateral ligament are visualized (12).

Withdrawing the arthroscope provides visualization of the trochleo-capitellar groove. This completes the diagnostic arthroscopy of the anterior compartment.

Diagnostic arthroscopy of the posterior compartment begins with a posterolateral portal approximately 3 cm proximal to the tip of the olecranon at the lateral border of the triceps tendon (Fig. 10). Frequently, soft tissue obstructs visualization and a second posterocentral working portal is established. The posterior compartment requires thorough inspection, as this is where loose bodies frequently migrate. The posterior aspect of the trochlea, the olecranon fossa, and the tip of the olecranon can all be inspected from the posterolateral or posterocentral portal (Fig. 11). In extension, any bony or soft tissue impingement between the olecranon process and olecranon fossa is seen. Advancement of the arthroscope into the lateral gutter provides for completion of the inspection of the capitellum by viewing its inferior surface. Occasionally, visualization of the inferior surface of the capitellum is difficult from the proximal posterolateral portal. The soft spot or direct lateral portal can assist in better visualization of this portion of the capitellum. The lateral portion of the ulnohumeral joint is also visualized while in the lateral gutter. Switching the arthroscope to the posterocentral portal allows for examination of the posteromedial gutter and the posterior bundle of the medial collateral ligamentous complex (Fig. 12). Just superficial to the posterior bundle of the medial collateral ligamentous complex lies the ulnar nerve. Therefore, caution should be exercised when instrumenting this area.

Completion of diagnostic arthroscopy of the elbow is performed through the direct lateral portal, sometimes referred to as the "soft-spot" portal. It is found in the center of a triangle formed by the tip of the olecranon, the radial head, and the lateral epicondyle, the initial site of joint distension (Fig. 13). The inferior aspect of the capitellum and the undersurfaces of the radioulnar articulation and the radial head articular margin (that portion not visible through the initial anteromedial portal) are inspected. This is another common location for loose bodies and they should be identified and removed. Lastly, with the forearm supinated and a valgus stress applied postero-rotatory, instability can be diagnosed while visualizing the posterior subluxation of the radial head on the capitellum.

This completes the diagnostic arthroscopy of the elbow. All instruments are removed from the joint, and portals are closed using interrupted nylon suture. Closure is particularly important for the direct lateral portal, as little tissue lies between the joint and the skin and synovial fistulas have been reported (1).

COMPLICATIONS

Complications of elbow arthroscopy are relatively rare, ranging from 7% to 11% (1,13,14). Transient as well as permanent injury to all three major nerves around the elbow have been reported and remain the most concerning of complications related to the procedure. Both outside-in injuries (related to portal placement or use of local anesthetics) and inside-out injuries (related to violating the joint capsule or using motorized instruments near the capsule) can occur. Non-neurologic complications are similar to other arthroscopic procedures and include persistent portal drainage (1,14) with possible fistula formation, superficial and deep infection (15), hematoma formation (14), chronic regional pain syndrome (14), and contracture (1,14,16).

CONCLUSIONS

Diagnostic arthroscopy of the elbow has become a valuable tool for surgeons in the evaluation of the patient with elbow pain and mechanical symptoms. It should not replace a thorough history, physical examination, and appropriate imaging, but rather, should extend the focus of these indirect evaluations by its ability to directly visualize the intra-articular structures of the elbow. All three major nerves to the hand are in close proximity during the procedure, and a thorough knowledge and constant awareness of their respective anatomy is paramount. This understanding of anatomy and attention to technical detail will help surgeons to avoid most complications. Finally, complete diagnostic arthroscopy of the elbow is made expeditious, benefits the patient and avoids complications by creating a reproducible systematic routine.

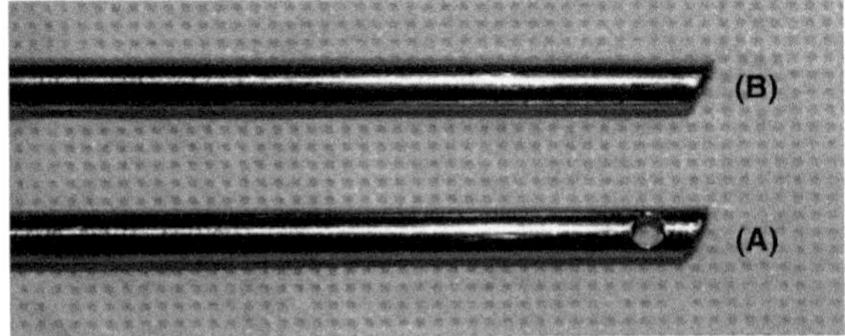

FIGURE 1 Inflow cannula with side vents (**A**) and without side vents (**B**).

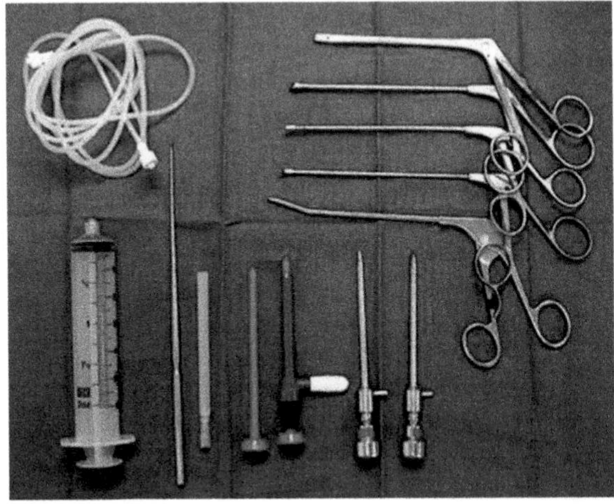

FIGURE 2 Standard arthroscopic instruments used in elbow arthroscopy.

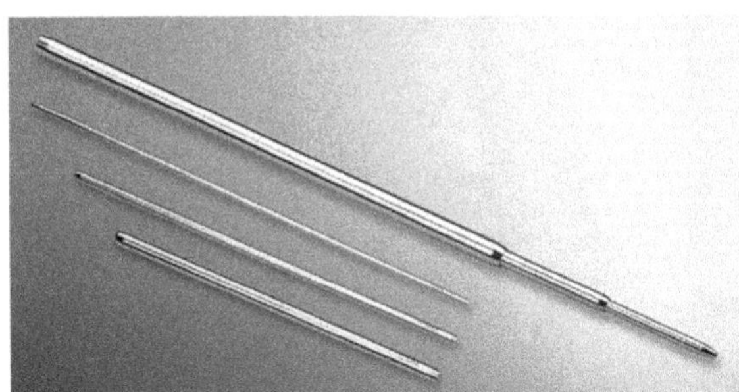

FIGURE 3 Arthroscopic portal dilators. Allow exact placement of portals for elbow arthroscopy, once an initial visualization portal is established.

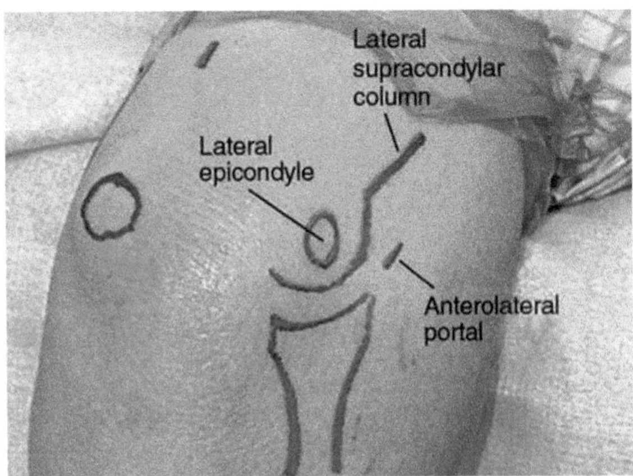

FIGURE 4 Surface landmarks are drawn to facilitate portal placement and avoidance of neurovascular structures.

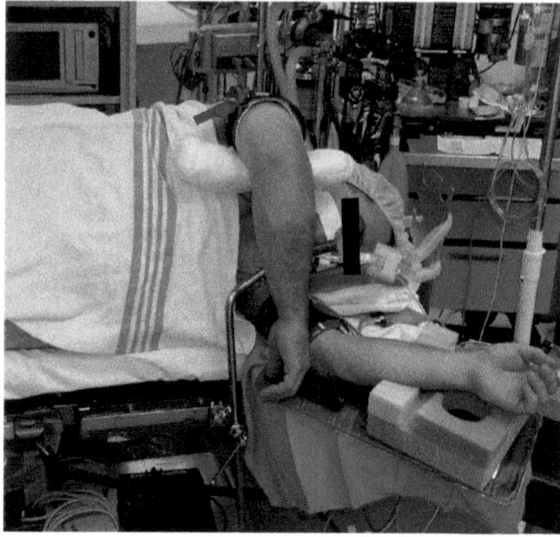

FIGURE 5 Lateral decubitus position. The arm is maintained over a lateral arm support that allows flexion and extension of the arm.

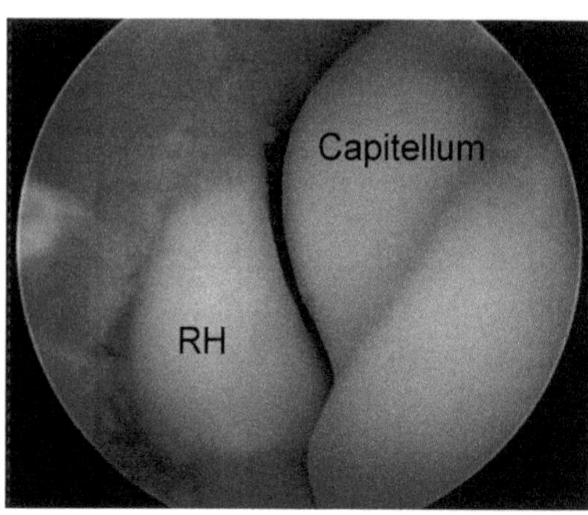

FIGURE 6 View from the superomedial portal. Allows visualization of the radial head, capitellum, and radiocapitellar joint. The capitellar-trochlear groove and the lateral face of the trochlea can be visualized from this portal as well. *Abbreviation*: RH, radial head.

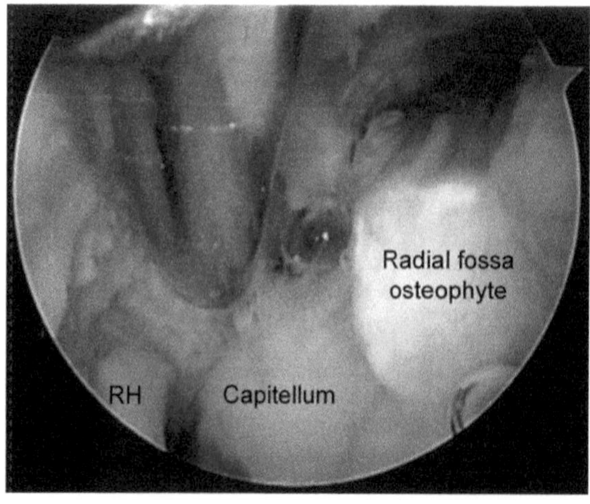

FIGURE 7 View from the superomedial portal of the anterolateral compartment of the elbow. The concavity of the radial fossa is obliterated by an osteophyte that limits flexion due to abutment against the margin of the radial head. *Abbreviation*: RH, radial head.

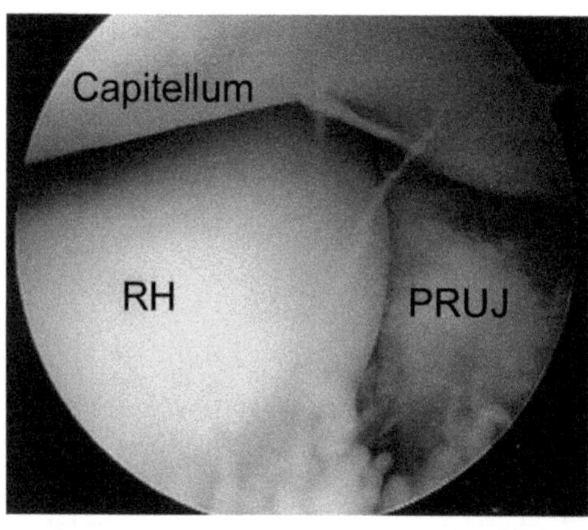

FIGURE 8 The posterior aspect of the radiocapitellar joint. The scope is in the posterocentral portal and advanced into the posterolateral gutter, allowing visualization of the inferior aspect of the radial head, capitellum, and proximal radioulnar joint. *Abbreviations*: PRUJ, proximal radioulnar joint; RH, radial head.

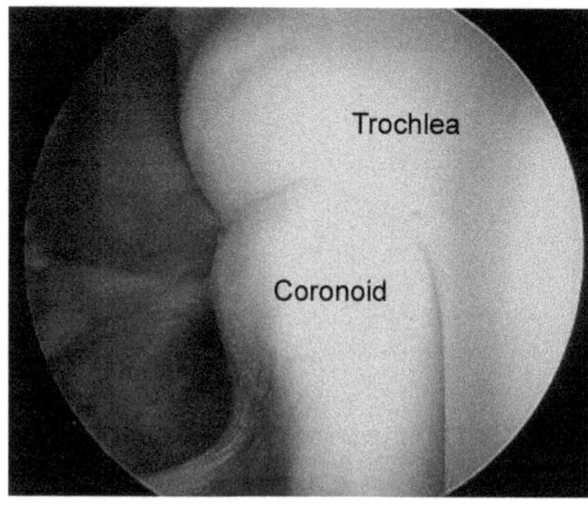

FIGURE 9 View from the proximal anterolateral portal. Allows visualization of the coronoid, trochlea, and anterior ulnohumeral joint.

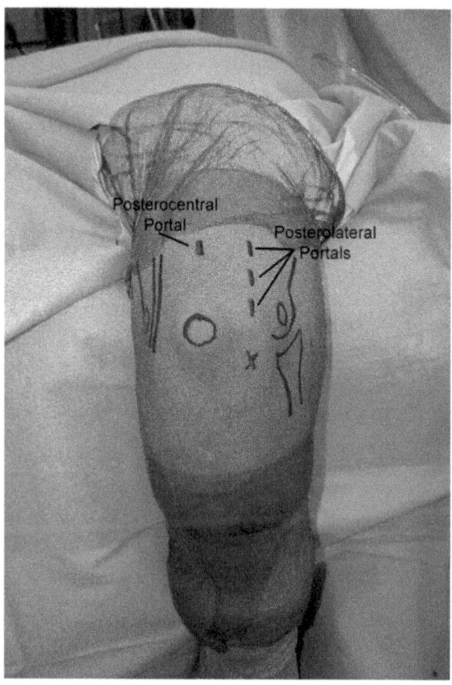

FIGURE 10 Family of posterior portals. The posterocentral portal lies 3 cm proximal to the tip of the olecranon. A series of posterolateral portals along the lateral borders of the triceps allows complete visualization of the posterior compartment of the elbow.

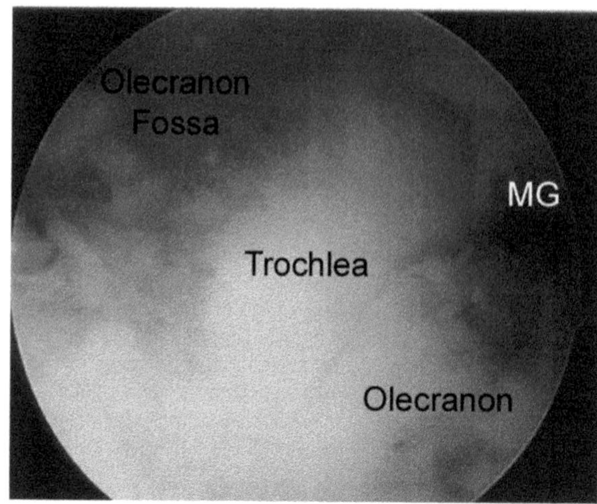

FIGURE 11 View of the posterior compartment from the posterolateral portal. Allows visualization across the posterior compartment of the olecranon tip, the posterior aspect of the trochlea, the olecranon fossa, and the medial gutter. *Abbreviation*: MG, medial gutter.

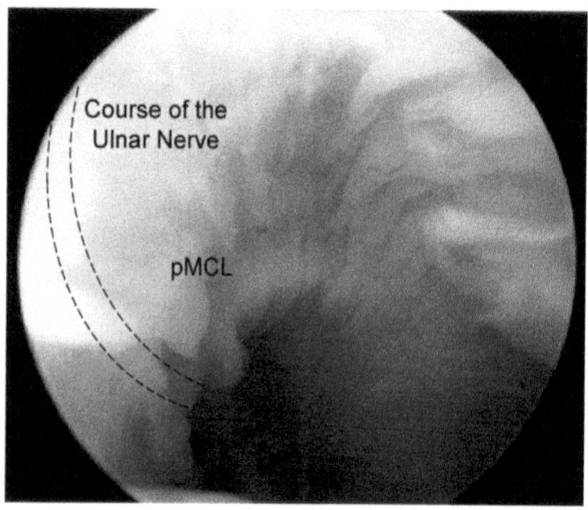

FIGURE 12 The posteromedial gutter viewed from the posterocentral portal. The course of the ulnar nerve in proximity to the posterior bundle of the medial collateral ligament is demonstrated. *Abbreviation*: pMCL, posterior bundle of the medial collateral ligament.

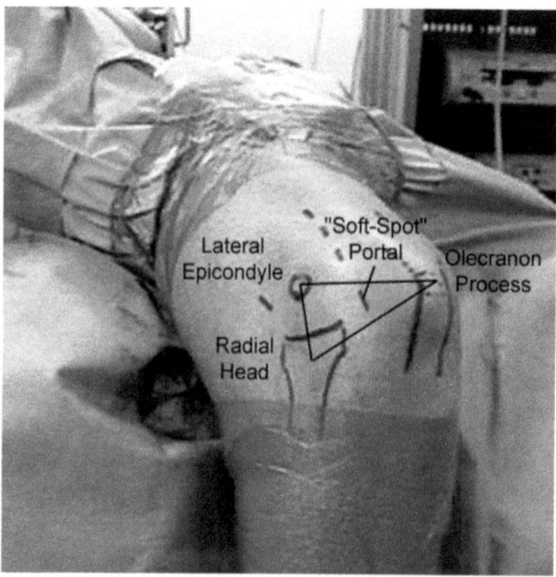

FIGURE 13 Topographical landmarks for the "soft-spot" portal. The portal lies at the center of the triangle formed by the lateral epicondyle, radial head, and olecranon process.

REFERENCES

1. O'Driscoll SW, Morrey BF. Arthroscopy of the elbow. Diagnostic and therapeutic benefits and hazards. J Bone Joint Surg Am 1992; 74:84–94.
2. Baker CL, Brooks AA. Arthroscopy of the elbow. Clin Sports Med 1996; 15:261–281.
3. Lynch GJ, Meyers JF, Whipple TL, Caspari RB. Neurovascular anatomy and elbow arthroscopy: inherent risks. Arthroscopy 1986; 2:190–197.
4. .Miller CD, Jobe CM, Wright MH. Neuroanatomy in elbow arthroscopy. J Shoulder Elbow Surg 1995; 4:168–174.
5. Ogilvie-Harris DJ, Weisleder L. Fluid pump systems for arthroscopy: a comparison of pressure control versus pressure and flow control. Arthroscopy 1995; 11:591–595.
6. Ramsey ML. Elbow arthroscopy: basic set up and treatment of arthritis. Instr Course Lect 2002; 51:69–72.
7. Baker CL Jr, Jones GL. Arthroscopy of the elbow. Am J Sports Med 1999; 27:251–264.
8. Lindenfeld TN. Medial approach in elbow arthroscopy. Am J Sports Med 1990; 18:413–417.
9. O'Driscoll SW, Morrey BF, An KN. Intra-articular pressure and capacity of the elbow. Arthroscopy 1990; 6:100–103.
10. Poehling GG, Whipple TL, Sisco L, Goldman B. Elbow arthroscopy: a new technique. Arthroscopy 1989; 5:222–224.
11. Field LD, Altchek DW, Warren RF, O'Brien SJ, Skyhar MJ, Wickiewicz TL. Arthroscopic anatomy of the lateral elbow: a comparison of three portals. Arthroscopy 1994; 10:602–607.
12. Field LD, Callaway GH, O'Brien SJ, et al. Arthroscopic assessment of the medial collateral ligament complex of the elbow. Am J Sports Med 1995; 23:396–400.
13. Kelly E, O'Driscoll SW, Morrey BF. Complications of elbow arthroscopy. J Bone and Joint Surg Am 2001; 83:25–34.
14. Savoie FH III. Complications. In: Savoie FH III, Field LD, eds. Arthroscopy of the Elbo. New York: Churchill Livingstone, 1996:151–156.
15. Redden JF, Stanley D. Arthroscopic fenestration of the olecranon fossa in the treatment of osteoarthritis of the elbow. Arthroscopy 1993; 9:14–16.
16. Jones GS, Savoie FH III. Arthroscopic capsular release of flexion contractures (arthrofibrosis) of the elbow. Arthroscopy 1993; 9:277–283.

30 Lateral Epicondylitis

R. Vaughan Massie and Champ L. Baker, Jr.
The Hughston Clinic and The Hughston Foundation, Inc., Columbus, Georgia, U.S.A.

BACKGROUND AND INDICATIONS

The term "lawn tennis arm" was coined by Morris (1) in 1882 to describe a condition causing lateral elbow pain in tennis players that is now called "tennis elbow." However, both terms, lateral epicondylitis and tennis elbow, are misnomers. First, the condition is actually one of marked tendinosis; it is not an inflammatory condition, as the term epicondylitis implies. Inflammation and inflammatory cells are only present early in the course of the disease; therefore, researchers have come to prefer the term "tendinosis" (2,3). Histologically, Nirschl noted that the tissue was characterized by disorganized, immature collagen formation with in-growth of immature fibroblastic, vascular, and granulation tissues (3,4). Clinically, the characteristic tissue is noted to be gray and friable with varying degrees of tearing. This abnormal tissue is almost universally found in the tendinous origin of the extensor carpi radialis brevis (ECRB) muscle, but the tendons of the extensor carpi radialis longus (ECRL) and extensor digitorum communis (EDC) may also be involved, albeit much less commonly (5,6).

The second reason the term is somewhat inaccurate is that the vast majority of those with tennis elbow are not tennis players. Several studies have shown that most often the condition is work-related. However, it has been estimated that 10% to 50% of persons who play tennis regularly develop lateral elbow pain at some time during their careers (7). Other suggested causes of tennis elbow, or lateral epicondylitis, include trauma to the lateral region of the elbow, relative hypovascularity of the region, and fluoroquinolone antibiotics.

The average age of a patient with lateral epicondylitis is 42 years, with a bimodal distribution in the general population. An acute onset of symptoms occurs more often in young athletes, and chronic, recalcitrant symptoms typically occur in older patients. Because lateral epicondylitis is believed to be caused by repetitive eccentric or concentric overloading of the extensor muscle mass, any person who participates in such activities, whether occupational or sports-related, is predisposed to develop the condition. Even so, many have the condition in the absence of such risk factors.

DIAGNOSIS: HISTORY, PHYSICAL EXAMINATION, AND RADIOLOGICAL EVALUATION

Patients with lateral epicondylitis typically present with pain primarily located at the lateral aspect of the elbow. Often, patients report that the pain radiates down the dorsal or lateral forearm; less commonly, the pain extends proximally. Patients usually report a gradual, insidious onset of pain, but, occasionally, will report an acute, traumatic event prior to the onset of symptoms. Patients often report weakness in their grip strength or difficulty lifting or carrying items in their hand, especially, when attempting to do so at a distance from their body. Patients should be questioned about other symptoms, such as numbness or tingling, as this may help differentiate this disorder from other conditions.

Examination of a patient with lateral epicondylitis begins with a handshake. Many patients will wince with pain, give minimal effort, or completely avoid the handshake all together. Examination of the cervical spine can exclude the possible diagnosis of radicular arm pain. A thorough shoulder examination is important because increased stresses on the elbow from decreased range of motion can contribute to elbow pain.

Please refer to pages 326–328 for the figures in this chapter.

In these patients, examination of the elbow reveals point tenderness to palpation over the lateral epicondyle and less so over the supinator muscle or radial tunnel. Commonly, three provocative maneuvers are positive. First, patients have reproducible pain at the lateral epicondyle when the examiner tests resisted wrist extension with the elbow in full extension. This maneuver tests ECRB strength and causes pain at the origin of the muscle in an individual with lateral epicondylitis. Pain is also reproduced with maximal passive wrist flexion, again with the elbow in full extension. The second maneuver places the ECRB on maximal stretch, again causing pain at the origin of the muscle. The third provocative maneuver is resisted forearm supination that causes pain. Grip strength should be tested to determine whether it is decreased compared with the unaffected side or whether gripping causes significant discomfort. The neurovascular status of the hand should be fully evaluated, as well.

Routine anteroposterior, lateral, and axial radiographs are obtained, but are frequently normal. Soft tissue calcification adjacent to the lateral epicondyle is present in as many as 25% of patients with lateral epicondylitis (8), especially, if the patient has had previous steroid injections. Magnetic resonance imaging is rarely indicated or needed to make the diagnosis of lateral epicondylitis.

Operative Indications

Although most patients respond favorably to nonoperative treatment and time, recurrence of symptoms is not uncommon. Surgical intervention is indicated when symptoms persist or recur despite therapeutic attempts, such as activity modification, bracing, cortisone injections, and four to six months of physical therapy. One exception is in those instances when a patient has sustained a direct trauma, causing a partial tear of the ECRB; surgery may be indicated sooner in these patients.

Contraindications

Although there are very few absolute contraindications to surgical intervention, an active infection of the elbow would prohibit surgery in a patient with lateral epicondylitis. A relative contraindication is severe ankylosis of the elbow, although a clinical diagnosis of lateral epicondylitis would be less likely in these patients.

ARTHROSCOPIC TREATMENT

A thorough preoperative history and physical examination is necessary to determine whether the patient has had previous surgical procedures about the elbow, such as an ulnar nerve transposition, which may alter surgical planning. Generally, the arthroscopic release procedure for lateral epicondylitis is performed on an outpatient basis. A regional anesthetic can be used, but a general anesthetic is preferred in the author's center because it allows prone positioning of the patient and objective assessment of neurovascular status after the procedure is complete.

AUTHOR'S PREFERRED TECHNIQUE

With the patient in the prone position, a tourniquet is applied to the upper arm, which is placed in a commercial arm holder or on a pillow of soft foam (Fig. 1). Positioning in this manner allows full extension and flexion of the elbow to 120°. The arm is prepared and draped in a standard fashion, and the anatomic landmarks are outlined. For safe location of the portals, the following anatomic landmarks are outlined on the skin: the medial epicondyle and intermuscular septum, the ulnar nerve, the olecranon, and, laterally, the lateral epicondyle and the radial head. The forearm is wrapped with a compressive dressing that helps to prevent leakage of fluid distally into the soft tissues. The arm is exsanguinated, and the tourniquet is inflated. Using an 18-gauge needle, the joint is distended with 20 to 30 mL of fluid injected via the posterolateral soft-spot portal (Fig. 2). Distention of the joint pushes the neurovascular structures anteriorly and protects them from instruments (Fig. 3).

First, the proximal medial portal is created through a 2 to 3 mm skin incision using a #11 blade scalpel. The subcutaneous tissue is spread with a hemostat (Fig. 4). This portal is located approximately 2 cm proximal to the medial epicondyle and 1 cm anterior to the intermuscular septum. Next, a blunt trocar and cannula are introduced into the joint while maintaining direct contact with the anterior edge of the humerus. Backflow of saline confirms accurate placement within the joint. A 4-mm, 30° angled arthroscope is introduced, and a systematic evaluation is carried out.

Initially, the radiocapitellar joint can be visualized. Pronation and supination of the forearm allows full examination of the radial head. The undersurface of the capsule should be examined for tears or abnormalities. These lesions can be classified as type I (normal appearance of the capsule), type II (a horizontal rent in the capsule), or type III (complete rupture of the capsule) (Fig. 5) (9). Chondromalacia of the radiocapitellar joint is sometimes present, and, often, thickening of the synovium or a plica can be identified in this area. This thickening is often a source of irritation to the patient and can cause symptoms that mimic lateral epicondylitis. As the arthroscope is retracted medially, the coronoid can be seen.

The lateral portal is established by one of two methods—outside-in or inside-out. Using the inside-out technique, the arthroscope is pushed against the desired entry point on the lateral capsule. The arthroscope is removed from the medial portal, and a Wissinger rod is inserted through the cannula and passed out through the lateral skin portal when the skin is incised. Next, a larger cannula is threaded over the rod and the cannula is introduced. With the outside-in technique, an 18-gauge needle is used to localize the proximal lateral portal. This portal is typically located 2 cm proximal to the lateral epicondyle and 1 cm anterior to the intermuscular septum. Again, the nick-and-spread technique is used prior to introducing the cannula and trocar into the joint. When the arthroscope is inserted into this lateral portal, initially, the surgeon views medially and completes a systematic diagnostic examination. This examination also includes evaluation of the articular surface of the distal humerus. Associated disorders or other abnormal findings are dealt with at this time.

Next, with the arthroscope placed back into the proximal medial portal, a small shaver is introduced through the lateral portal cannula and the capsule is removed to expose a portion of the common extensor tendon. The ECRB tendon lies between this tendon and the capsule, which has been removed (Fig. 6). A radiofrequency probe is inserted to debride the tendon, and the remaining tissue can be ablated with the probe (Fig. 7). If scissors or a shaver is preferred, the tendon is debrided before it is released. The aim is to release the tendon from its origin on the lateral epicondyle. Dissection is begun proximally and is extended distally. Care is taken to stay above the equator of the radial head to avoid damage to the lateral collateral ulnar ligament, which can potentially destabilize the elbow. Once the tendon has been fully released, the elbow is extended and the wrist is volar-flexed to ensure that the entire tendinous attachment has been released.

To complete a full arthroscopic evaluation of the elbow, the direct lateral portal and posterolateral portal (placed in the lateral soft spot) can be used to evaluate the posterior compartment. Often, there is diseased tissue in the posterior aspect of the radiocapitellar region that can be excised with the arthroscope in the posterolateral portal and the shaver in the direct lateral portal.

The portals are closed with interrupted nylon sutures. A local anesthetic can be injected into the subcutaneous tissue around the portal sites for postoperative pain relief. Be aware that, because of its proximity to the ulnar nerve, anesthetic placed around the proximal medial portal could lead to confusion when the patient's postoperative neurovascular status is checked. Sterile dressings are applied, and the patient's arm is placed in a sling. The patient is awakened and discharged when appropriate.

PEARLS AND PITFALLS

1. Outline the surface anatomy and rule out ulnar nerve subluxation.
2. Avoid impingement from the arm holder that could prevent appropriate portal placement and reduce working room for completion of the procedure.
3. Look for associated synovitis, as well as capsular tearing, and remove the inflammatory synovitis concurrently.
4. Understand the related anatomy of the lateral ulnar collateral ligament to prevent inadvertent release and the development of postoperative iatrogenic posterolateral instability.

POSTOPERATIVE REGIMEN

Patients are encouraged to begin active and passive range of motion of the elbow in the first 24 to 48 hours after surgery. Depending on the amount of swelling, which may or may not be present, full extension can usually be achieved within three to five days. Patients usually return within a week for removal of stitches and, at that time, if they have difficulty regaining motion, they are sent to a therapist for instruction. Simple stretching and strengthening exercises, such as those included in the preoperative regimen, are begun as the patient's symptoms permit. Patients are advised against dorsiflexion and volar flexion of the wrist, with the elbow in extension until the soft tissue inflammation has subsided. Patients can return to light activities as tolerated. Return-to-work status in these patients ranges from one day to a few months.

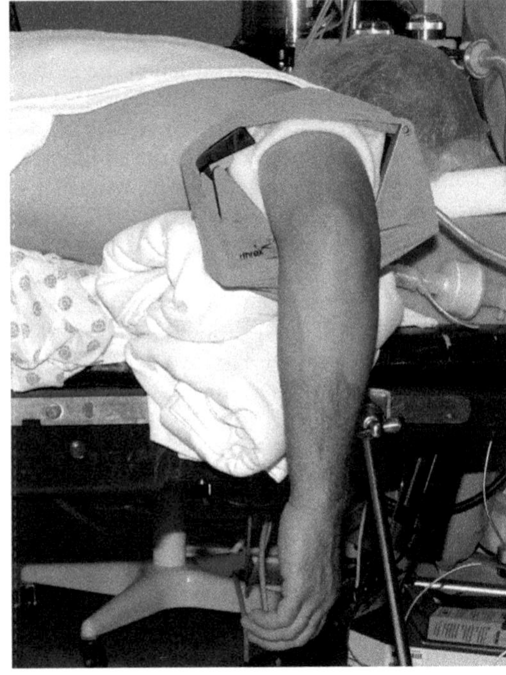

FIGURE 1 The affected extremity is positioned, with the shoulder abducted to 90° and the arm supported in a commercial arm holder. The elbow is flexed to 90°, with the forearm hanging freely over the edge of the table.

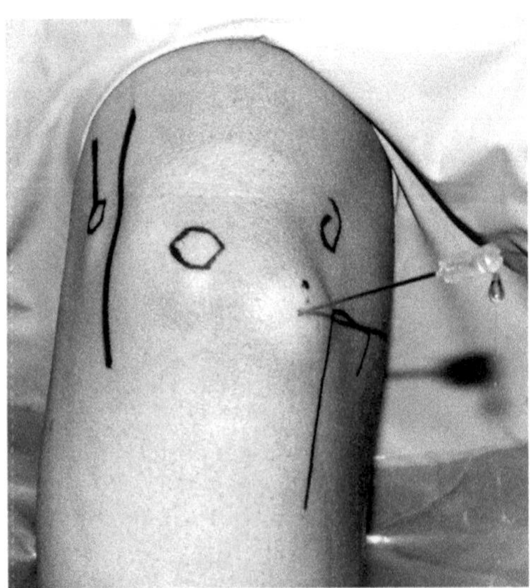

FIGURE 2 The anatomic landmarks are identified and marked, and the joint is distended through an 18-gauge needle introduced into the posterolateral soft spot.

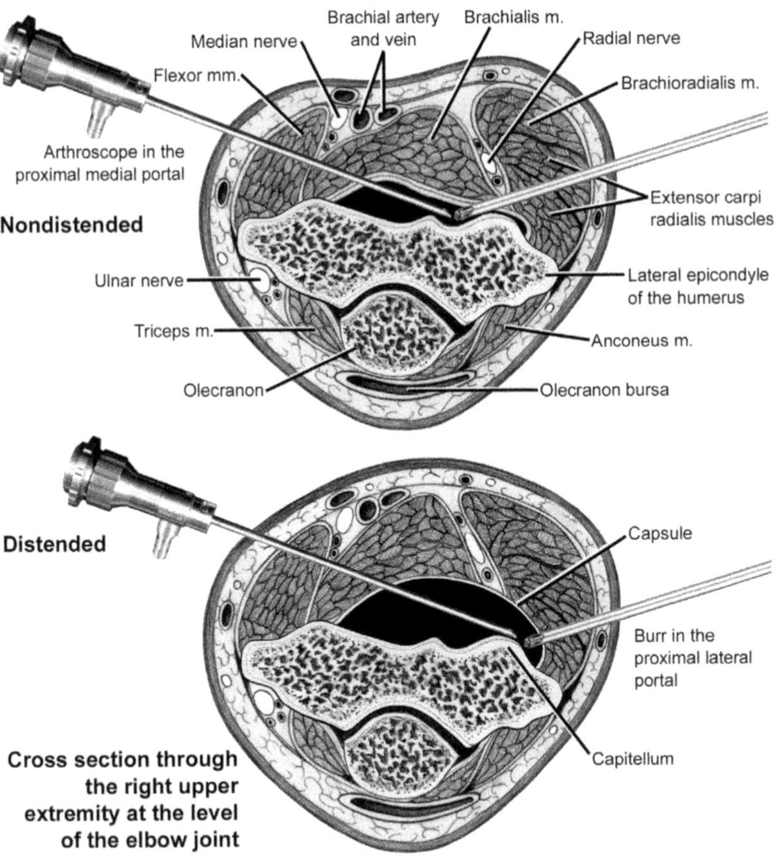

FIGURE 3 Cross-section through the right upper extremity at the level of the elbow joint. Distention of the joint pushes the neurovascular structures anteriorly and protects them from instruments.

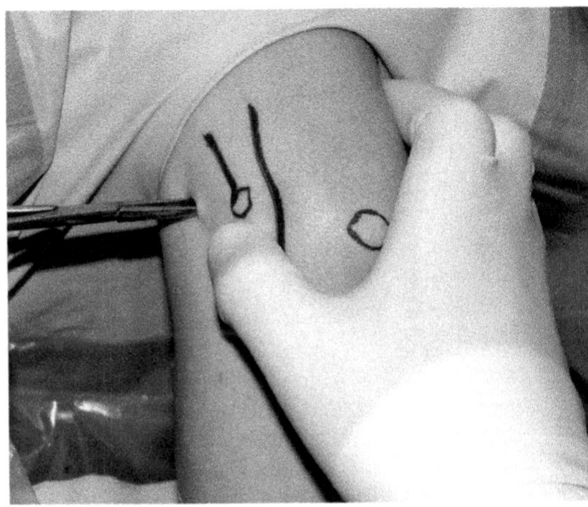

FIGURE 4 A hemostat is used to spread the tissues and establish the proximal medial portal.

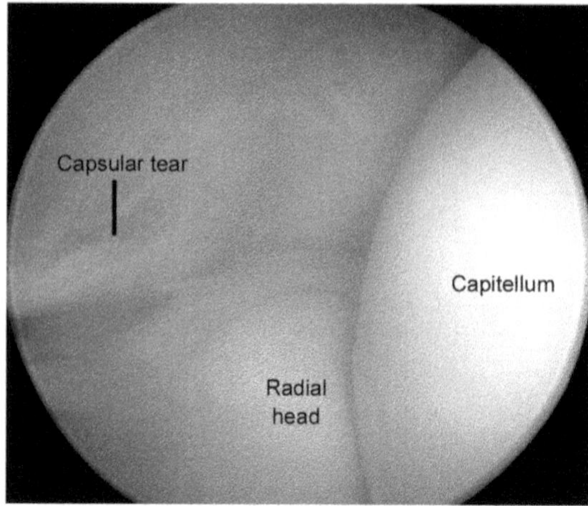

FIGURE 5 With the arthroscope in the proximal medial portal, the capitellum, radial head, and capsular tear can be seen.

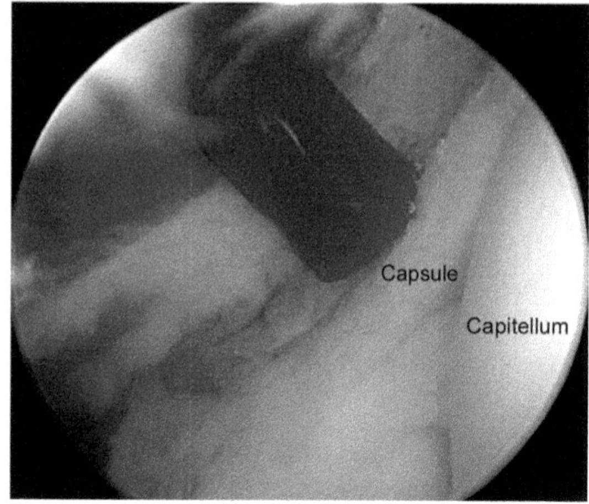

FIGURE 6 After the torn capsule is debrided, the deep layer of the extensor digitorum communis tendon and the origin of the extensor carpi radialis brevis tendon can be seen.

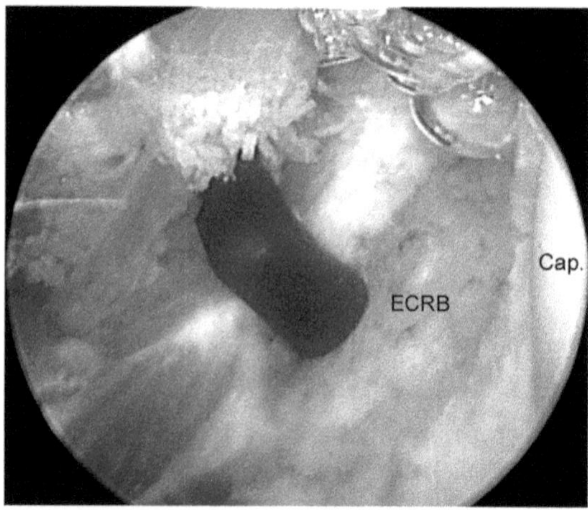

FIGURE 7 After removal of the torn capsule with the monopolar radiofrequency probe, the extensor carpi radialis brevis tendon is released. *Abbreviations*: Cap, capitellum; ECRB, extensor carpi radialis brevis.

REFERENCES

1. Morris H. The rider's sprain. Lancet 1882; II:133–134.
2. Kraushaar BS, Nirschl RP. Tendinosis of the elbow (tennis elbow). Clinical features and findings of histological, immunohistochemical, and electron microscopy studies. J Bone Joint Surg Am 1999; 81(2):259–278.
3. Baker CL, Nirschl RP. Lateral tendon injury: open and arthroscopic treatment. In: Altchek DW, Andrews JR, eds. The Athlete's Elbow. Philadelphia: Lippincott Williams & Wilkins, 2001:91–103.
4. Nirschl RP. Muscle and tendon trauma: tennis elbow. In: Morrey BF, ed. The Elbow and Its Disorders. 1st ed. Philadelphia: WB Saunders, 1985:537–552.
5. Fairbank SM, Corlett RJ. The role of the extensor digitorum communis muscle in lateral epicondylitis. J Hand Surg (Br) 2002; 27(5):405–409.
6. Greenbaum B, Itamura J, Vangsness CT, et al. Extensor carpi radialis brevis. An anatomical analysis of its origin. J Bone Joint Surg Br 1999; 81(5):926–929.
7. Nirschl RP. Elbow tendinosis/tennis elbow. Clin Sports Med 1992; 11(4):851–870.
8. Nirschl RP, Pettrone FA. Tennis elbow. The surgical treatment of lateral epicondylitis. J Bone Joint Surg Am 1979; 61(6):832–839.
9. Baker CL, Murphy KP, Gottlob CA, et al. Arthroscopic classification and treatment of lateral epicondylitis: two-year clinical results. J Shoulder Elbow Surg 2000; 9(6):475–482.

31 Elbow Arthroscopy: Loose Body Removal and Synovial Plicae Debridement

Gabriel D. Brown, Hari Ankem, John-Erik Bell, and Theodore A. Blaine
Center for Shoulder, Elbow, and Sports Medicine, Department of Orthopedic Surgery, Columbia Presbyterian Medical Center, New York, New York, U.S.A.

LOOSE BODIES

Loose bodies occur most commonly in the knee (90% of cases), followed by the elbow, and in rare cases the hip and shoulder (1). Milgram et al. classified loose bodies by clinical etiology into osteochondral fractures, degenerative disease of the articular cartilage, and synovial chondromatosis (2–6).

While osteochondral fractures may lead to acute formation of loose bodies in the elbow, loose bodies may also occur as a result of osteochondritis dissecans (7). Osteochondritis dissecans of the elbow typically occurs in adolescents and young adults between the ages of 12 and 14 (7–9). The mechanism of injury is usually overuse, with repeated microtrauma being the most common factor. The most frequently affected site is the capitellum (Fig. 1), but osteochondritis dessicans (OCD) has been reported in the trochlea, radial head, and olecranon (10,11).

Degenerative disease of the articular cartilage may lead to the formation of loose bodies through fragmentation of the articular surface, fracture of osteophytes, or de novo formation of chondral or osteochondral nodules in the synovium of degenerative joints. Shearing forces may lead to subtle osteochondral fragments that become a nidus for the formation of loose bodies, which then grow with nutritional support from the synovial fluid. While a degenerative mechanism for loose body formation may be more common in older patients, it can also occur in throwing athletes with valgus extension overload syndrome (12,13).

PATIENT EVALUATION

Patients with loose bodies typically present with mechanical symptoms such as pain, catching, clicking, and locking (14–17). Loss of extension occurs in many patients, and intermittent pain is experienced with locking of the loose body between articular surfaces. Patients often recall a specific inciting event or history of trauma. An overuse mechanism may be the etiology in manual laborers and in athletes such as baseball pitchers and gymnasts, in whom osteochondritis dissecans could be suspected (12,18–21).

Radiographic examination includes standard anterioposterior (AP), lateral, and axial views (15) (Fig. 2A and B). The AP view is taken in full extension, the lateral in 90° of flexion and the axial in maximal flexion. Ward et al. (21) found plain radiographs to be 69% specific and 79% sensitive for the detection of loose bodies in the elbow joint. CT and MRI may be more useful in the identification of loose bodies not easily visualized on plain radiographs. (Figs. 3 and 4) The same authors found CT arthrography to be 71% specific and 100% sensitive for loose body detection. Dubberley et al. (22) showed that neither CT arthrography nor MRI were more accurate than plain radiographs for the detection of loose bodies in the elbow joint. They found that MRI and CT arthrography had excellent sensitivity (92% to 100%) but low to moderate specificity (15% to 77%) in the detection of posterior loose bodies. Neither MRI nor CT arthrography were consistently sensitive (46% to 91%) or specific (13% to 73%) for the detection of anterior loose bodies. The overall sensitivity for either compartment was 88% to 100% and the overall specificity

---

Please refer to pages 334–338 for the figures in this chapter.

was 20% to 70%. Arthroscopy is the gold standard for diagnosis of loose bodies against which radiographs, CT arthography, and MRI were measured in these studies.

INDICATIONS

The initial therapies for patients with symptoms consistent with loose bodies are rest, ice, non-steroidal anti-inflammatory medications, and activity modification (16). When conservative measures fail, arthroscopic or open removal of loose bodies is inidcated. Loose body removal from the elbow joint is the most fundamental indication for elbow arthroscopy (23,8,15,17,24–26).

SYNOVIAL PLICAE

The presence of synovial folds or plicae, has been well documented in the knee (27–29). In 1988, Commandre et al. (30) published a single case and Clarke (31) published a case series of three patients with synovial plicae of the elbow joint. Antuna et al. (32) reported on 14 patients treated arthroscopically for "snapping elbow" who were noted to have hypertrophic synovial folds intraoperatively. Kim et al. (33) published a case series of 12 patients with lateral elbow pain noted arthroscopically to have hypertrophic synovial plicae. Several authors have suggested a relationship between these lateral synovial folds and lateral epicondylitis (34,35).

Synovial plicae of the elbow that are symptomatic can be broadly categorized into anterior and posterior varieties. The symptomatic lateral synovial fringe can be further subdivided into anterolateral and posterolateral types, depending on the clinical signs and arthroscopy findings (30,31). Of these synovial plica, the posterolateral is the most rare.

The anterior synovial plicae are predominantly localized to anterolateral aspect of the radiocapitellar joint, in relation to annular ligament complex. These lesions usually present as mechanical symptoms such as snapping, popping or clicking within the flexion arc, especially along the anterolateral aspect of the elbow joint and are clinically detectable by the flexion pronation test (32,36).

PATIENT EVALUATION AND INDICATIONS

Symptoms of synovial plicae of the elbow are similar to those of patients with loose bodies. Symptoms include aching, stiffness, intermittent loss of motion, clicking, and catching (16,31–33). Pain occurs with flexion and extension of the elbow in some degree of pronation. O'Driscoll (32) described the flexion–pronation test in which passive flexion and extension of the pronated arm in the range of 90° to 110° reproduces the snapping sensation suggestive of radiocapitellar plicae. Unlike patients with loose bodies, those with synovial plicae do not typically recall any antecedent trauma (33).

Diagnostic imaging proposed to detect synovial plica include dynamic pneumatic arthrography (36) and MRI (37). (Fig. 5) Currently, MRI arthrogram is the author's preferred imaging technique, although the sensitivity and specificity in detecting synovial plica has not been reported. Awaya et al. correlated anatomy with clinical symptoms in patients with elbow synovial folds and determined that plicae greater than 3 mm thick were associated with clinical symptoms. Kim et al. (33) used two criteria to determine whether synovial tissue was abnormal: thickness greater than 3 mm and an irregular or nodular appearance as visualized on MRI. MRI arthrography is useful in this study, particularly in the absence of a significant effusion.

The indications for arthroscopic synovial plica debridement include pain or mechanical symptoms that are refractory to nonoperative treatment. Typically, a three-month course of physical therapy, anti-inflammatories, and corticosteroid injections is required before surgical treatment is considered (31–33).

CONTRAINDICATIONS

Contraindications to both arthroscopic loose body removal and plica debridement may include potential altered neurovascular anatomy. A subluxating ulnar nerve may place the nerve at increased risk and therefore obviates against an arthroscopic procedure. Surgeon inexperience with elbow arthroscopy is a relative contraindication; in general, if the procedure time exceeds two hours, soft tissue swelling will prevent the completion of the arthroscopic procedure, and thus an open technique has to be performed. This should always be discussed with the patient prior to surgery.

SURGICAL TECHNIQUE

Elbow arthroscopy may be performed under general or regional anesthesia (Fig. 6), both having their own advantages and disadvantages. Regional anesthesia minimizes postoperative pain and morbidity, however it may not allow immediate postoperative neurologic examination, which can be useful in early identification of nerve injury. The patient is positioned in the lateral decubitus position, as described by O'Driscoll and Morrey, with the affected extremity placed on an arm support (35) (Fig. 7). A nonsterile tourniquet is placed high on the arm, and the arm is prepped and draped. The arm is exsanguinated and the tourniquet inflated to 250 mmHg, leaving the forearm wrapped in elastic bandage to minimize postoperative swelling.

Landmarks are outlined, including the olecranon tip, the medial and lateral epicondyles, the radial head, and the ulnar nerve (Fig. 8). The flexed elbow joint is distended with 25 to 30 mL of sterile saline from the "soft spot," which is found in the center of a triangle formed by the olecranon tip, the radial head, and the lateral epicondyle. With the elbow flexed and distended, the distance between the neurovascular structures and the portals is increased significantly (38).

The arthroscope is inserted through the "soft spot" portal initially to examine the posterior aspect of the joint. The proximal posterolateral portal is then established approximately 2 cm proximal to the tip of the olecranon along the lateral border of the triceps tendon, and a space is created. This portal is utilized for removal of loose bodies, debridement of synovium, and debridement of osteophytes. This allows thorough inspection of the olecranon fossa, as well as the medial and lateral gutters. Care should be taken while debriding the medial gutter as the ulnar nerve is adjacent to capsule at the medial gutter.

Since multiple loose bodies are frequently encountered (and the number of loose bodies found during arthroscopy frequently is greater than those observed radiographically), it is essential to completely inspect both the anterior and posterior compartments of the elbow in all cases of loose body removal (38,39). The anterolateral portal is placed first at the anterior aspect of the radiocapitellar joint. The proximal anteromedial portal is then created under direct visualization using a spinal needle, and is typically located approximately 2 cm proximal to the medial epicondyle and just anterior to the medial intermuscular septum. It is important to preoperatively assess the mobility of the ulnar nerve to ensure that it does not subluxate anteriorly, which would increase the likelihood of injury during creation of anteromedial portals. The arthroscope is alternated between the proximal anteromedial and anterolateral portals to inspect the lateral and medial sides of the anterior elbow, respectively. As loose bodies are removed, their extraction is documented with the arthroscope both in and out of the joint to demonstrate to the patient postoperatively (Fig. 9).

Typically, synovial plicae will be found in the anterior radiocapitellar joint, and can be debrided with arthroscopic cautery or shaver from the anterolateral portal while viewing from the proximal anteromedial portal. (Fig. 10) However, in some cases the plica may be present in the posterior radiocapitellar joint and will not be visualized from the anterior portals. Therefore, it is important to examine the posterior fossa and posterior radiocapitellar joint to identify these plica and perform complete debridement. (Fig. 11)

Once debridement of plicae and/or loose body removal is performed, the joint is irrigated and wounds are closed with nonabsorbable interrupted sutures. An intra-articular drain is left. Closure of portals is important to prevent fistula formation since the soft tissue envelope is very thin in the elbow. Local anesthetic is not typically used if an immediate postoperative neurologic examination is planned.

REHABILITATION

Patients who undergo loose body removal or plica debridement without associated procedures should be encouraged to start moving the elbow in the immediate postoperative period without restriction, in order to prevent postoperative stiffness. Typically, this is done with a physical therapist for the first four to six weeks and through a home program, thereafter. Typically, these procedures do not result in any appreciable loss of motion.

RESULTS (LOOSE BODY REMOVAL)

O'Driscoll et al. (24) evaluated 23 patients (24 elbows) treated with arthroscopic removal of loose bodies. Hundred percent of those patients found intraoperatively to have an isolated diagnosis of loose bodies improved as a result of the procedure, whereas 75% of those with additional pathology benefited from the procedure. Ogilvie-Harris et al. (26) reported on 33 patients treated arthroscopically for loose body removal. Pain was improved in 85% of patients, locking in 92%, and swelling in 71% of patients. Overall, 89% of patients had significant improvement following the arthroscopic procedure.

RESULTS (SYNOVIAL PLICA DEBRIDEMENT)

Clarke et al. (31) reported resolution of symptoms in all of their three patients where debridement of synovial plica was performed. Additionally, they described "kissing lesions" of chondromalacia on the radial head which corresponded to the area of contact of the synovial folds in all three patients. Antuna et al. (32) reported complete relief in 12 of the 14 patients following arthroscopic debridement. One of the patients who failed surgery had an associated posterolateral rotatory elbow instability. Thirteen of their patients had "kissing lesions" of chondromalacia on the radial head, and three patients had chondromalacia of the capitellum. Kim (33) reported excellent results in 11 of 12 patients treated with arthroscopic debridement. They found associated chondromalacia involving the capitellum and posterolateral distal humerus in five patients; the radial head was involved in two patients. Their results were not affected by the presence of chondromalacia in any of these seven patients.

PEARLS AND PITFALLS

Intra-articular retractors have been popularized by O'Driscoll and can be particularly useful during elbow arthroscopy. Retractors are typically placed from accessory portals, and would enter the joint from the same side as the arthroscope. When are typically place a posterior retractor through the posterocentral portal and the anterior retractor through an anterolateral or anteromedial portal, it dramatically improves the viewing space and helps to reduce the risk to the adjacent neurovascular structures associated with synovectomy or capsulectomy.

For loose bodies that are highly mobile and difficult to grasp, a needle can be used to skewer it, holding it in place while it is grasped. For loose bodies that are attached to capsule or synovium, detachment can be performed by obtaining a strong grasp of the fragment, then rolling the instrument until the stalk of tissue to which it is adhered tears. If the loose body is too large to be extracted through the portal incision, it can be excised in a piecemeal fashion.

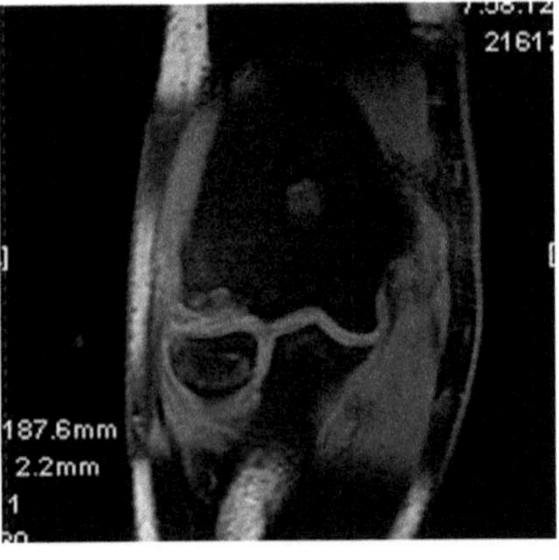

FIGURE 1 Coronal view MRI scan of the right elbow in a 14-year-old male patient with osteochondritis dissecans of the elbow.

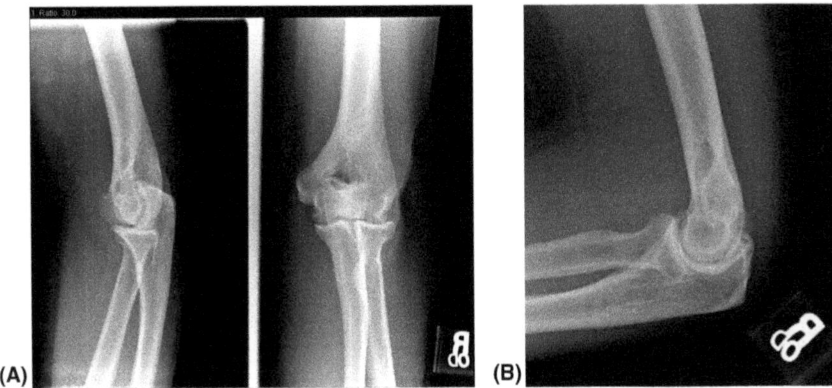

FIGURE 2 Anterioposterior, oblique (**A**) and lateral (**B**) radiographs of the right elbow in a patient with osteoarthritis and loose bodies.

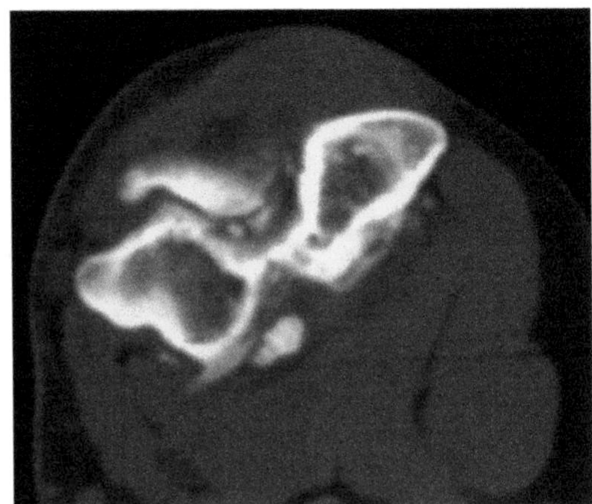

FIGURE 3 Axial view CT scan of an elbow with loose bodies present in the olecranon fossa.

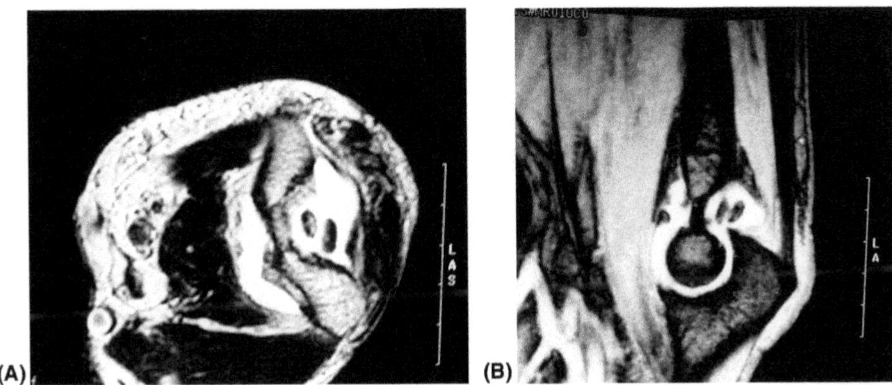

FIGURE 4 Axial and lateral view MRI scans of an elbow with osteoarthritis and loose bodies. Loose bodies are seen on the axial view in the posterior olecranon fossa (**A**) and both anteriorly and posteriorly on the lateral view (**B**).

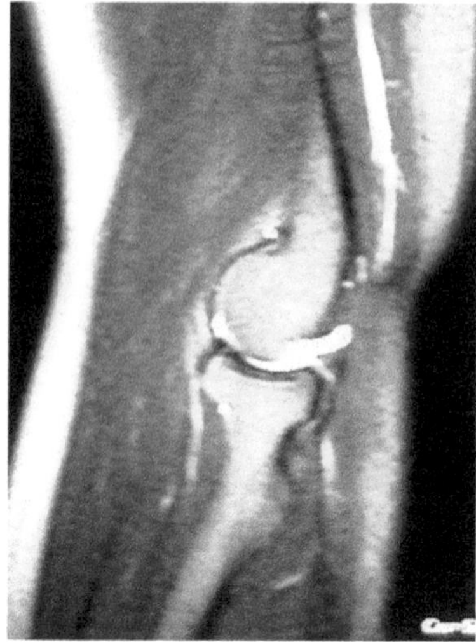

FIGURE 5 Lateral view MRI scan demonstrating an impinging posterolateral synovial plica.

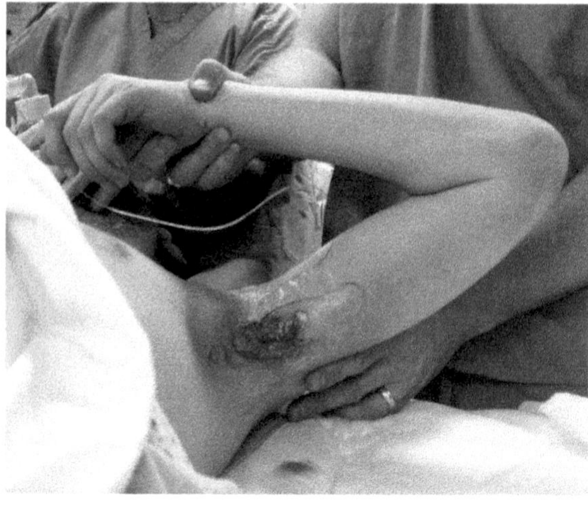

FIGURE 6 An axillary catheter is placed in some patients for regional anesthesia and postoperative pain control.

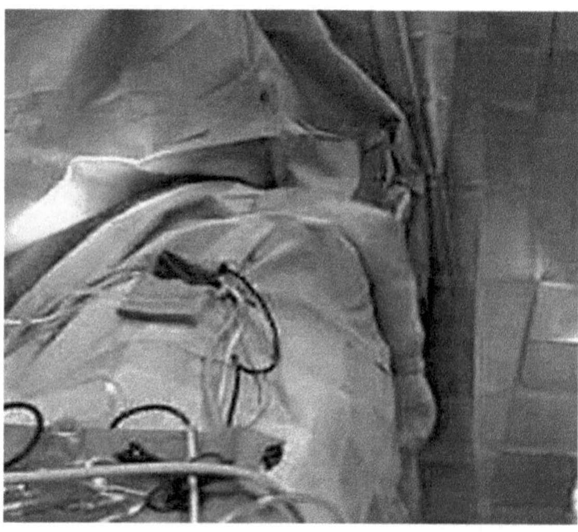

FIGURE 7 The patient is placed in the lateral decubitus position with the arm draped over an arm support.

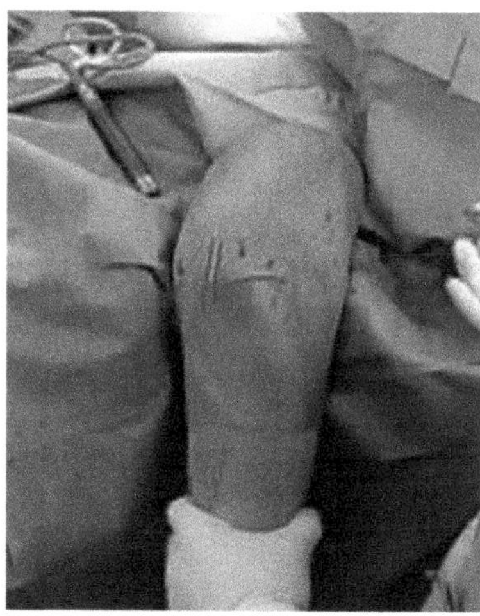

FIGURE 8 The anatomic landmarks including the ulnar nerve are marked before making incisions, as are the locations of the arthroscopic portals.

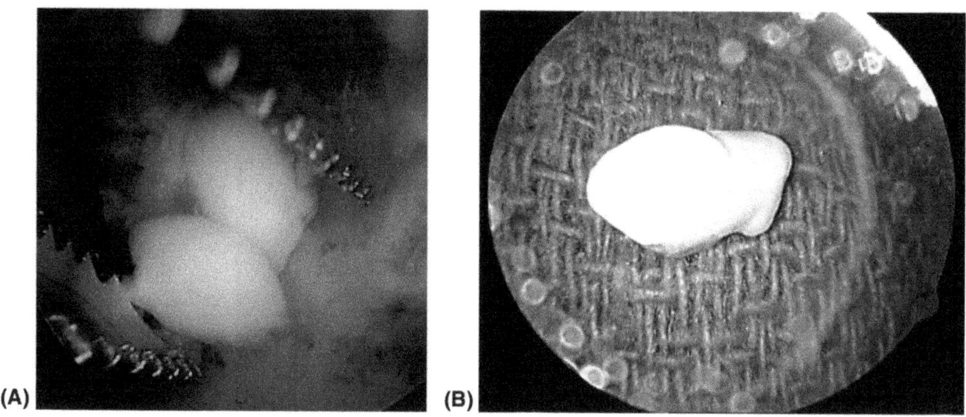

FIGURE 9 A loose body is identified and removed with a large serrated grasper (**A**). Its complete removal from the joint is documented with the arthroscope on a blue towel (**B**).

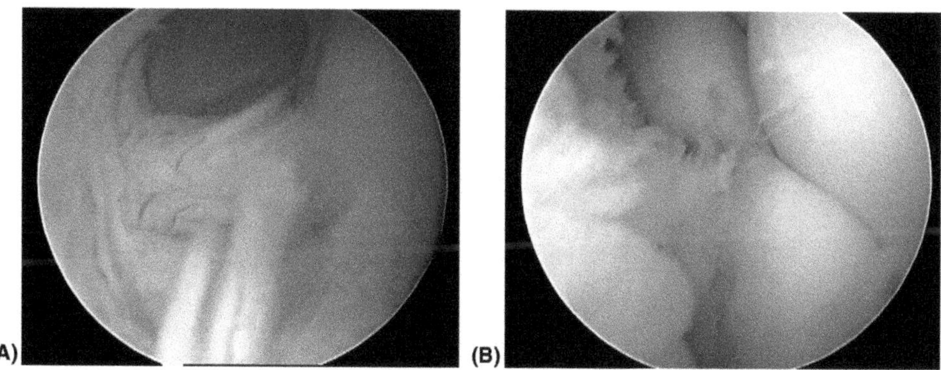

FIGURE 10 An arthroscopic view of the anterior radiocapitellar joint where an anterior radiocapitellar synovial plica is identified (**A**) and debrided (**B**).

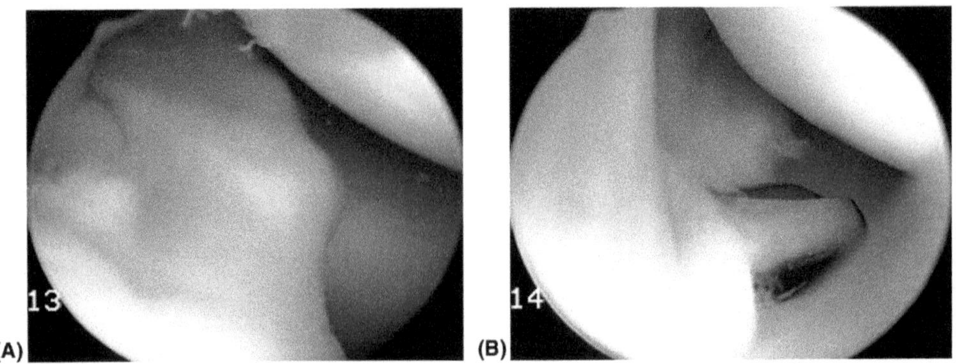

FIGURE 11 An arthroscopic view of the posterior radiocapitellar joint where a posterior radiocapitellar synovial plica is identified (**A**) and debrided (**B**).

REFERENCES

1. Phemister, DB. The causes of and changes in loose bodies arising from the articular surface of the joint. Journal of Bone and Joint Disease 1924; 6:278–315.
2. Kamineni S, O'Driscoll SW, Morrey BF. Synovial osteochondromatosis of the elbow. J Bone Joint Surg Br 2002; 84(7):961–966.
3. Milgram JW. The classification of loose bodies in human joints. Clin Orthop Relat Res 1977; (124): 282–291.
4. Milgram JW. The development of loose bodies in human joints. Clin Orthop Relat Res 1977; (124): 292–303.
5. Milgram JW. Synovial osteochondromatosis: a histopathological study of thirty cases. J Bone Joint Surg Am 1977; 59(6):792–801.
6. Mueller T, Barthel T, Cramer A, Werner A, Gohlke F. Primary synovial chondromatosis of the elbow. J Shoulder Elbow Surg 2000; 9(4):319–322.
7. Baumgarten TE, Andrews JR, Satterwhite, YE. The arthroscopic classification and treatment of osteochondritis dissecans of the capitellum. Am J Sports Med 1998; 26(4):520–523.
8. Bradley JP, Petrie RS. Osteochondritis dissecans of the humeral capitellum. Diagnosis and treatment. Clin Sports Med 2001; 20(3):565–590.
9. Schenck RC Jr, Goodnight JM. Osteochondritis dissecans. J Bone Joint Surg Am 1996; 78(3):439–456.
10. Bednarz PA, Paletta GA Jr, Stanitski CL. Bilateral osteochondritis dissecans of the knee and elbow. Orthopedics 1998; 21(6):716–719.
11. Vanthournout I, Rudelli A, Valenti P, Montagne JP. Osteochondritis dissecans of the trochlea of the humerus. Pediatr Radiol 1991; 21(8):600–601.
12. Ahmad CS, ElAttrache NS. Valgus extension overload syndrome and stress injury of the olecranon. Clin Sports Med 2004; 23(4):665–676, x.
13. Wilson FD, Andrews JR, Blackburn TA, McCluskey G. Valgus extension overload in the pitching elbow. Am J Sports Med 1983; 11(2):83–88.
14. Bell MS. Loose bodies in the elbow. Br J Surg 1975; 62(11):921–924.
15. Greis PE, Halbrecht J, Plancher KD. Arthroscopic removal of loose bodies of the elbow. Orthop Clin North Am 1995; 26(4):679–689.
16. McFarland EG, Gill HS, Laporte DM, Streiff, M. Miscellaneous conditions about the elbow in athletes. Clin Sports Med 2004; 23(4):743–763, xi–xii.
17. McGinty JB. Arthroscopic removal of loose bodies. Orthop Clin North Am 1982; 13(2):313–328.
18. Andrews JR, Craven WM. Lesions of the posterior compartment of the elbow. Clin Sports Med 1991; 10(3):637–652.
19. Grana WA, Rashkin A. Pitcher's elbow in adolescents. Am J Sports Med 1980; 8(5):333–336.
20. Jackson DW, Silvino N, Reiman P. Osteochondritis in the female gymnast's elbow. Arthroscopy 1989; 5(2):129–136.
21. Ward WG, Belhobek GH, Anderson TE. Arthroscopic elbow findings: correlation with preoperative radiographic studies. Arthroscopy 1992; 8(4):498–502.
22. Dubberley JH, Faber KJ, Patterson SD, et al. The detection of loose bodies in the elbow: the value of MRI and CT arthrography. J Bone Joint Surg Br 2005; 87(5):684–686.
23. Andrews JR, St. Pierre RK, Carson WG Jr. Arthroscopy of the elbow. Clin Sports Med 1986; 5(4): 653–662.
24. O'Driscoll SW. Elbow arthroscopy for loose bodies. Orthopedics 1992; 15(7):855–859.
25. O'Driscoll SW, Morrey BF. Arthroscopy of the elbow. Diagnostic and therapeutic benefits and hazards. J Bone Joint Surg Am 1992; 74(1):84–94.
26. Ogilvie-Harris DJ, Schemitsch E. Arthroscopy of the elbow for removal of loose bodies. Arthroscopy 1993; 9(1):5–8.
27. Broom MJ, Fulkerson JP. The plica syndrome: a new perspective. Orthop Clin North Am 1986; 17(2):279–281.
28. Nottage WM, Sprague, NF, 3rd Auerbach, BJ Shahriaree H. The medial patellar plica syndrome. Am J Sports Med 1983; 11(4):211–214.
29. Patel D. Arthroscopy of the plicae–synovial folds and their significance. Am J Sports Med 1978; 6(5):217–225.
30. Commandre FA, Taillan B, Benezis C, Follacci FM, Hammou JC. Plica synovialis (synovial fold) of the elbow. Report on one case. J Sports Med Phys Fitness 1988; 28(2):209–210.
31. Clarke RP. Symptomatic, lateral synovial fringe (plica) of the elbow joint. Arthroscopy 1988; 4(2): 112–116.
32. Antuna SA, O'Driscoll SW. Snapping plicae associated with radiocapitellar chondromalacia. Arthroscopy 2001; 17(5):491–495.
33. Kim DH, Gambardella RA, Elattrache NS, Yocum LA, Jobe FW. Arthroscopic treatment of posterolateral elbow impingement from lateral synovial plicae in throwing athletes and golfers. Am J Sports Med 2006; 34(3):438–444.
34. Boyd HB, McLeod AC Jr. Tennis elbow. J Bone Joint Surg Am 1973; 55(6):1183–1187.

35. Mullett H, Sprague M, Brown G, Hausman M. Arthroscopic treatment of lateral epicondylitis: clinical and cadaveric studies. Clin Orthop Relat Res 2005; 439:123–128.
36. Akagi M, Nakamura T. Snapping elbow caused by the synovial fold in the radiohumeral joint. J Shoulder Elbow Surg 1998; 7(4):427–429.
37. Awaya H, Schweitzer ME, Feng SA, et al. Elbow synovial fold syndrome: MR imaging findings. AJR Am J Roentgenol 2001; 177(6):1377–1381.
38. Lynch GJ, Meyers JF, Whipple TL, Caspari RB. Neurovascular anatomy and elbow arthroscopy: inherent risks. Arthroscopy 1986; 2(3):190–197.
39. O'Driscoll SW, Morrey BF. Arthroscopy of the elbow: a critical review. Orthopaedic Transactions 1990; 14:258–259.

32 Arthroscopic Management of Valgus Extension Overload

Christopher S. Ahmad
Center for Shoulder, Elbow, and Sports Medicine, Department of Orthopedic Surgery, Columbia Presbyterian Medical Center, New York, New York, U.S.A.

INDICATIONS FOR SURGERY

Valgus extension overload most commonly affects overhead athletes. The repetitive forces on the elbow cause chondromalacia, osteophytes, and possible loose bodies localized to the posteromedial aspect of the olecranon. For isolated posteromedial impingement, elbow pain is localized to the medial aspect of the olecranon and is present in both the acceleration and deceleration phases of throwing. Patients may report limited extension, which is caused by impinging posterior osteophytes or locking and catching from loose bodies. Pain localized to the posterior compartment may be elicited by the examiner by manipulating the elbow in pronation, valgus, and forced extension.

Anterior-posterior, lateral, oblique, and axillary views of the elbow may reveal posteromedial olecranon osteophytes and loose bodies within the articulation, as shown in Figures 1 and 2. Computed tomography and magnetic resonance imaging may further define loose bodies and osteophytes, as shown in Figure 3. Nonoperative treatment consists of a period of rest, anti-inflammatory medication, improvement in pitching or throwing mechanics, and flexor pronator muscle strengthening. Surgical treatment is indicated for those patients who maintain symptoms of valgus extension overload despite nonoperative management.

CONTRAINDICATIONS

An important contraindication to performing isolated olecranon debridement is the presence of combined medial collateral ligament (MCL) insufficiency. Basic science studies have demonstrated that excessive olecranon resection increases the strain on the MCL during valgus stress and increases valgus instability (1,2). In addition, MCL insufficiency causes contact alterations in the posteromedial compartment that may be the initial cause of chondrosis and osteophyte formation that causes symptomatic valgus extension overload (3). Therefore, careful history, physical examination, and advanced imaging should be performed to avoid missed MCL injuries. If MCL insufficiency exists and isolated posteromedial decompression procedure is performed, the athlete is at risk of developing symptomatic MCL instability when returning to throwing.

TECHNIQUES

Patients may be positioned in a supine, prone, or lateral decubitus position. The author prefers lateral decubitus with a nonsterile tourniquet and an arm support. If concomitant MCL reconstruction following the arthroscopy is anticipated, the supine position may be preferred so that repositioning is avoided. Alternatively, the arthroscopy may be performed in the lateral decubitus position, followed by repositioning and repeat prepping and draping for the MCL reconstruction.

Routine diagnostic arthroscopy is performed initially in the anterior compartment with standard portals. The posteromedial decompression is then performed in the posterior compartment. Evaluation of the posterior compartment requires creation of direct posterior and

---

Please refer to pages 343–345 for the figures in this chapter.

posterior lateral portals (Fig. 4). The posterolateral portal is placed just lateral to the triceps tendon and 1 cm proximal to the olecranon tip. The elbow is held in 30° of flexion to relax the triceps while establishing the portal and is used initially for visualization. The direct posterior portal splits the triceps in its midline, 3 cm proximal to the olecranon tip. Posterior compartment diagnostic arthroscopy evaluates the presence of osteophytes on the posteromedial aspect of the olecranon, loose bodies, and any evidence of chondromalacia. Figure 5 illustrates proper placement of instruments and the desired olecranon resection. A small osteotome is inserted through the direct posterior portal to remove the osteophytes, as shown in Figures 6 and 7. The olecranon may be further contoured with a burr (Fig. 8). Care is taken to limit olecranon resection to the osteophytes present, since overaggressive resection leads to increased stress on the MCL during throwing. Often, osteophytes may exist in the olecranon fossa, which are also debrided. When olecranon contouring is complete, a lateral radiograph may be obtained intraoperatively to assess adequate bone removal and to ensure that no bone debris remains in the soft tissues surrounding the elbow. Care should be taken to avoid injury to the ulnar nerve, which lies in the cubital tunnel. When using motorized instruments near the medial gutter, suction should be avoided.

PITFALLS AND COMPLICATIONS

The ulnar nerve is adjacent to the medial gutter soft tissues and is at risk if aggressive debridement is performed in this area. Suction should therefore be avoided in this area. If concern exists for ulnar nerve injury, the nerve should be explored through an open incision and protected during the debridement. Ulnar nerve irritation may be caused by medial osteophytes and should be assessed with Tinel's sign in the cubital tunnel preoperatively. Ulnar nerve subluxation should be noted when symptoms exist or elbow arthroscopy is being planned. If ulnar nerve subluxation exists, the medial arthroscopy portal should be made with direct open visualization and protection of the nerve. If ulnar neuritis exists preoperatively, then ulnar nerve transposition should be considered.

Unrecognized MCL injuries not addressed during arthroscopy for valgus extension overload may result in painful inability to throw due to the MCL insufficiency. Therefore, great emphasis is placed on assessing the MCL prior to planned posteromedial decompression surgery and, if injured, the patient must be appropriately counciled. Combined posteromedial olecranon debridement with MCL reconstruction should be considered, with the patient aware of the increased recovery time required for MCL reconstruction.

REHABILITATION

Postoperative rehabilitation consists of active elbow flexion and extension exercises initiated immediately following surgery. Emphasis is also placed on restoring flexor-pronator strength. It is also important to continue to strengthen the rotator cuff and peri-scapular muscles to avoid shoulder injures upon return to throwing. At six weeks, a progressive throwing program is initiated and plyometric exercises and neuromuscular training is enhanced. Endurance exercises are progressed and return to competition is typically allowed at three to four months postoperatively.

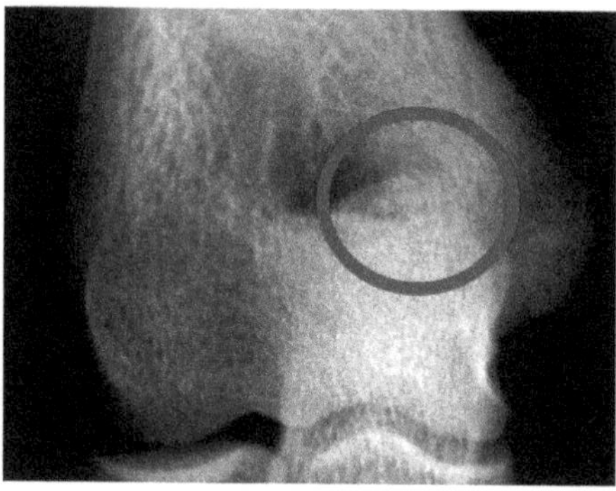

FIGURE 1 An AP X-ray demonstrating osteophyte on posteromedial aspect of olecranon.

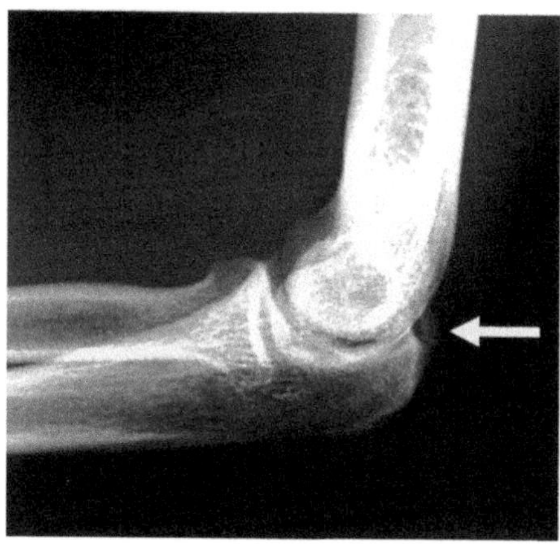

FIGURE 2 Lateral X-ray demonstrating osteophyte on olecranon tip.

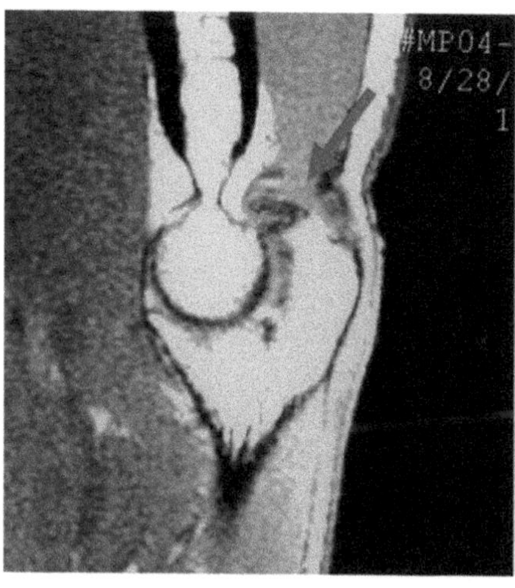

FIGURE 3 Sagittal magnetic resonance imaging demonstrating osteophyte on olecranon tip and loose body in posterior compartment.

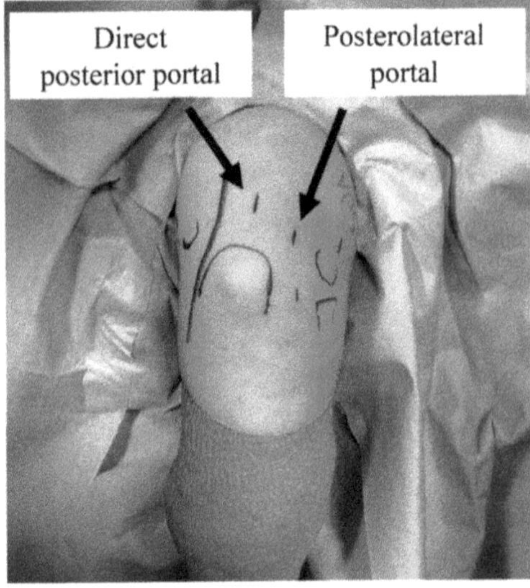

FIGURE 4 Arthroscopy set-up with direct posterior and posterolateral portals indicated.

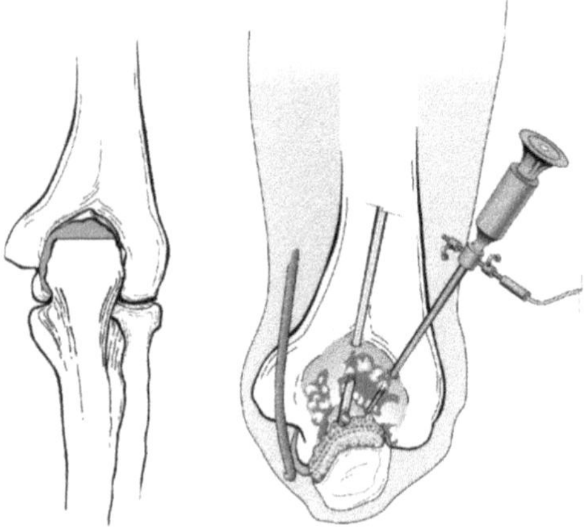

FIGURE 5 Illustration depicting instrument positioning and olecranon resection. *Source*: Adapted from Ref. 4.

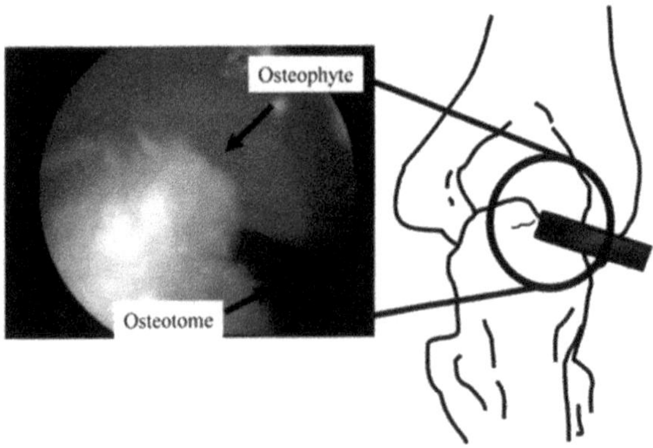

FIGURE 6 Osteophyte on olecranon tip with osteotome in position. *Source*: Adapted from Ref. 5.

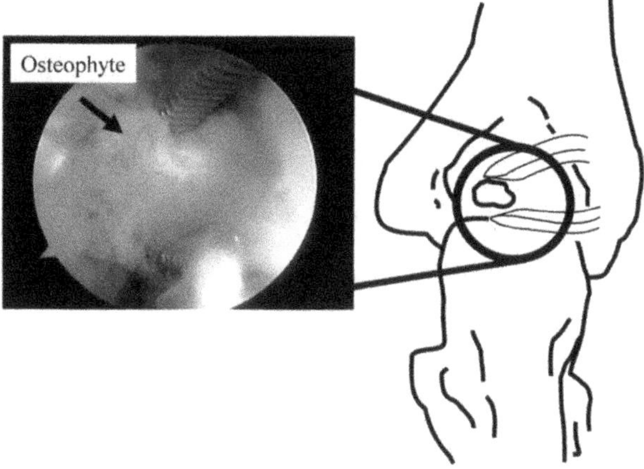

FIGURE 7 Removal of osteophyte. *Source*: Adapted from Ref. 5.

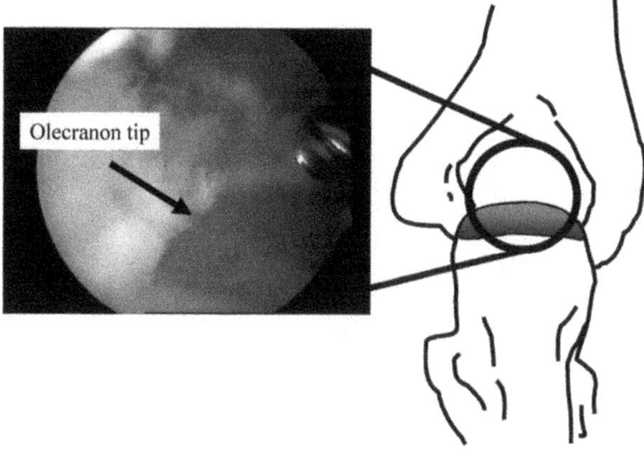

FIGURE 8 Olecranon tip, following contouring with a burr. *Source*: Adapted from Ref. 5.

REFERENCES

1. Kamineni S, ElAttrache NS, O'Driscoll SW, et al. Medial collateral ligament strain with partial posteromedial olecranon resection. A biomechanical study. J Bone Joint Surg Am 2004; 86-A(11):2424–2430.
2. Kamineni S, Hirahara H, Pomianowski S, et al. Partial posteromedial olecranon resection: a kinematic study. American Shoulder and Elbow Surgeons Open Annual Meeting 2002; Dallas.
3. Ahmad CS, Park MC, Elattrache NS. Elbow medial ulnar collateral ligament insufficiency alters posteromedial olecranon contact. Am J Sports Med 2004; 32(7):1607–1612.
4. ElAttrache NS, Ahmad CS. Valgus extension overload and olecranon stress fractures. Sports Med Arthrosc Rev 2003; 11:25–29.
5. Ahmad CS, ElAttrache NS. Posteromedial decompression of valgus extension overload. Advanced Reconstruction Elbow, AAOS in print.

33 Arthroscopic Capsular Release of the Elbow

Robert Z. Tashjian, Ryan Chen, and Leesa M. Galatz
Department of Orthopedic Surgery, Washington University School of Medicine, Barnes-Jewish Hospital, St. Louis, Missouri, U.S.A.

INTRODUCTION

Elbow arthroscopy has been used to manage loose bodies, symptomatic plicae, osteochondral defects (OCDs), lateral epicondylitis, and elbow contractures. Its utilization in the treatment of elbow contractures has increased in recent years due to distinct advantages compared to open procedures. In addition to the lower morbidity from less soft tissue dissection, arthroscopy allows uncompromised visualization of the complex elbow articulation. The primary indications for arthroscopic capsular release in the setting of elbow stiffness are osteoarthritis, post-traumatic contracture, and rheumatoid arthritis.

INDICATIONS

Osteoarthritis

Osteoarthritis of the elbow is characterized by relative joint space preservation, the presence of loose bodies, capsular contracture, and hypertrophic osteophyte formation. Patients present clinically with restricted range of motion and pain at the extremes of motion secondary to impingement on osteophytes. Capsular contracture develops subsequent to loss of motion. Surgical indications for the management of the osteoarthritic elbow include functional limitation, painful stiffness, and mechanical symptoms. Patients must have failed nonoperative management. Whether the approach is open or arthroscopic, the primary goals of surgical management in the osteoarthritic elbow are removal of impinging osteophytes, release of the contracted capsule, and removal of loose bodies (1). Ulnohumeral arthroplasty has been used to describe this comprehensive approach to open joint debridement, with satisfactory results in the long-term (2,3).

Improvement in pain and range of motion has been reported with arthroscopic debridement and capsular release of the osteoarthritic elbow. Cohen et al. (4) reported more improvement in pain than range of motion with arthroscopic debridement and olecranon fossa fenestration in 26 patients at a mean follow-up of 35.3 months. Ogilvie-Harris et al. (5) managed 21 patients who had elbow osteoarthritis and posterior impingement with arthroscopic debridement, removal of loose bodies, and osteophyte excision of the olecranon and olecranon fossa. Fourteen patients achieved excellent and seven achieved good results at a mean follow-up of 35 months. Savoie et al. (6) showed decreased pain and improvement in total range of motion of 81° after arthroscopic synovectomy, osteophyte excision, and olecrenon fossa fenestration in 24 patients. Radial head excision was performed in 18 of the 24 patients in this series.

Rheumatoid Arthritis

Pathologic deterioration in the rheumatoid elbow results from synovitis, capsular contracture, symmetric joint space destruction, periarticular erosions, and late bony deformity. Indications for arthroscopic intervention include functional limitation, synovitis, contracture, and pain refractory to disease modification or age that precludes consideration for total elbow arthroplasty. Ideal candidates for arthroscopic intervention should demonstrate radiographic preservation of cartilage and have no major bony deformity (7). Arthroscopic intervention for the rheumatoid elbow includes synovectomy, osteophyte excision, and capsular release.

Please refer to pages 353–355 for the figures in this chapter.

There has been controversy with regard to the longevity of both open as well as arthroscopic synovectomy in the rheumatoid patient (7–11). Arthroscopy may result in less complete synovectomy as compared to the open approach (7). Despite this skepticism, several studies have demonstrated pain relief from arthroscopic synovectomy. Nemoto et al. (12) reported pain relief and improved function in 10 patients who underwent arthroscopic synovectomy at a mean follow-up of 37 months. Horiuchi et al. (13) showed that improved outcome with arthroscopic synovectomy has been associated with elbows that have remaining cartilage and less deformity. In their series, arthroscopic synovectomy resulted in better improvement when the patient was managed with disease modification. This underscores the importance of concomitant medical management of the systemic arthritis.

Post-Traumatic Contracture

Loss of motion of the elbow may result from capsular contracture, intra-articular adhesions, loose bodies, and impinging osteophytes or articular incongruity, following fracture or dislocation. Indications for arthroscopic management of contracture include limitation of activities of daily living and painful stiffness. Surgical candidates must have failed nonoperative measures, such as aggressive therapy and static-progressive splinting. Patients must also demonstrate willingness to comply with postoperative rehabilitation.

Arthroscopic capsular release of post-traumatic elbow contracture results in improved range of motion and outcome. Phillips and Strasburger (14) reported the results of 25 patients who underwent arthroscopic release of an elbow contracture. The contracture was post-traumatic in 15 patients, and these improved in total arc of motion from 80° preoperatively to 130° postoperatively. Kim and Shin (15) reported improvement in elbow range of motion from 73° to 123° in 15 patients who underwent arthroscopic treatment of post-traumatic elbow arthrofibrosis. The patients in the studies by Kim and Phillips (14,15), with a post-traumatic etiology as opposed to an arthritic etiology, had a more severe preoperative restriction in motion, but no significant difference in the total postoperative arc of motion between the groups postoperatively. Ball et al. (16) reported an improved arc of motion from 82° to 124° in 14 patients who underwent arthroscopic capsular release. The postoperative functional score from the American Shoulder and Elbow Surgeons Elbow Assessment Form was 28.3 out of 30, and all patients reported that they would undergo the surgery again.

CONTRAINDICATIONS

A contraindication to arthroscopic surgery of the elbow is the presence of local infection in proximity to portal sites. Ankylosis secondary to heterotopic ossification with the inability to enter the joint and distend the capsule is a contraindication to arthroscopic management. Because the location of the ulnar nerve is less predictable, a subcutaneous ulnar nerve transposition is a relative contraindication to arthroscopy and a submuscular transposition is a strict contraindication.

COMPLICATIONS

Neurologic

Because of the proximity to neurovascular structures, arthroscopy of the elbow has a higher rate of iatrogenic neurologic complications than knee or shoulder arthroscopy. Despite an historical incidence of 1% to 14%, a recent review of 473 cases reported a 2% incidence of neurologic complication (17,18). Less soft tissue is present between the capsule and major nerves around the elbow. Injuries to the radial, posterior interosseous, medial antebrachial, median, anterior interosseous, and ulnar nerves have been described (19–22). Most are transient nerve palsies, which resolve with observation alone.

Preoperative capsular contracture is a risk factor for perioperative nerve injury (17). Capsular distention with saline increases the distance between the articular surface and the capsule/neurovascular structures, increasing the safety zone for establishing portals. Diminished distension in patients with contractures places these structures at increased risk. The normal capsule will reach maximal distention at 20 mL of fluid. An elbow with significant contracture may only reach a maximal distention of 10 to 15 mL. Rheumatoid patients are also at increased risk. The anterior capsule and brachialis may be thin in these patients, providing less of a barrier to surrounding nerves. Bony landmarks for nerves may be significantly altered, as a result of arthritic deformity. Finally, traction neuritis has been reported with open capsular release and must be considered with arthroscopic release as well (23).

Infection

The incidence of infection or prolonged drainage from portals after elbow arthroscopy is 8% (17). Prolonged drainage was the most common complication reported by Kelly et al (17). This occurred most commonly at the lateral portal sites, given the thin tissue plane between the skin and the joint. Less drainage was appreciated with suture repair of portal sites instead of steri-strips. Superficial infection may be prevented by early recognition of portal site drainage. Deep infection (a joint space infection) occurred in 0.8% of patients, all of whom received intra-articular steroids at the conclusion of the procedure (17).

Contracture

Although contracture is usually improved with intervention of the stiff elbow, it may not improve or may increase slightly. Postoperative contracture greater than 20° is uncommon (17).

Compartment Syndrome

Compartment syndrome from fluid extravasation is a potential complication of elbow arthroscopy. While there are no reported cases of compartment syndrome in the literature, significant swelling can occur during elbow arthroscopy, especially after capsular release through a midlateral portal. Intraoperative swelling warrants close monitoring during surgery.

SURGICAL TECHNIQUE

Most surgeons prefer general anesthesia for elbow arthroscopy. General anesthesia without a regional block allows immediate postoperative neurologic assessment. A block may also be utilized postoperatively for pain control, once a neurologic exam has been performed, but this precludes further evaluations to monitor for excessive swelling or possible compartment syndrome. General anesthesia also provides complete muscle relaxation that is required during arthroscopy along with versatility in patient positioning. Finally, increased tourniquet pressures are often better tolerated under general anesthesia.

No special camera equipment or instrumentation is required, in order to perform elbow arthroscopy. A standard 4.0 mm, 30° large-joint arthroscope is routinely utilized. Low-flow cannulas for the arthroscope should be used to decrease fluid extravasation into the soft tissues. Blunt trocars are used to gain access to the joint to avoid possible nerve injury. An upper arm tourniquet is routinely used. Gravity or pump can be used for fluid administration. The authors prefer a pump because of the greater control it allows. Pressure is set at 30 mmHg, but appropriate pressure settings may vary between pumps and between manufacturers. To protect soft tissue from entrapment and potential neurovascular injury, 4.5 mm cannulas and 3.5 mm hooded shavers and burrs are routinely used.

Several specialized instruments have been developed to make elbow arthroscopy easier and to avoid iatrogenic nerve injury. A guidewire and set of cannulated dilators allow precise localization of joint entry for portals under direct visualization, once the initial portal is established. The guidewire is placed in the joint in the desired location. Cannulated dilators (Arthrex, Inc.; Naples, Florida, U.S.A.) are then passed over the guidewire to expand the portal tract. Specially designed capsular biters with a longer blunt limb, which are part of the Elbow Arthroscopy Instrumentation Set (Arthrex, Inc.; Naples, Florida, U.S.A.), can be used during anterior capsule release. The longer blunt limb facilitates the elevation of the capsule from the overlying brachialis and neurologic structures, thereby potentially limiting nerve injury. Blunt-tipped switching sticks can be placed inside the joint through an accessory proximal lateral portal. They are used to retract or push anterior soft tissue away from the bone to increase the working space inside the joint (1).

Patient Positioning

Patients can be in a supine, prone, or lateral decubitus position for arthroscopic capsular release. The authors prefer the lateral decubitus position for all of their elbow arthroscopy (Fig. 1).

Arthroscopic Portals

Several different portals, anterior and posterior, are required to access the elbow joint. Portal positions are divided into anterior and posterior. Anterior-lateral portals include the anterolateral, midanterolateral, and proximal anterolateral. The anterolateral portal, originally described by Andrews and Carson (24), is located 3 cm distal and 1 cm anterior to the lateral epicondyle. The radial nerve lies within 0 to 2 mm of this portal, depending on elbow position; therefore, its use has fallen out of favor. A more proximal lateral portal is preferred by most surgeons (25). The proximal anterolateral portal is located 2 cm proximal and 1 cm anterior to the lateral epicondyle (26). A large anterior ridge osteophyte, common in elbow osteoarthritis, often blocks entrance using the proximal anterolateral portal. If this is the case, a midanterolateral portal at the level of the radiocapitellar joint can improve access to the joint.

The anteromedial and proximal anteromedial portals are the most commonly used medial portals. The proximal anteromedial portal, described by Poehling (27), is 2 cm proximal to the medial epicondyle just anterior to the intermuscular septum. This portal is safer than the anteromedial portal, as described by Andrews (24), because it enters the joint more parallel to the median nerve. The authors use the proximal anteromedial portal to initially enter the joint.

Three posterior portals are commonly used: the direct posterior, the posterolateral, and the midlateral (soft spot) portal. The direct posterior is 2 cm proximal to the tip of the olecranon. The posterolateral portal is lateral to the triceps at the level of the tip of the olecranon. These portals serve as the working and viewing portals for the posterior compartment. The midlateral portal (soft spot) lies in the lateral soft spot, which is defined as the triangle between the radial head, olecranon tip, and the lateral epicondyle on the lateral aspect of the elbow. This portal provides good access to the posterior capitellum, inferior radial head, and the radioulnar joint.

Preferred Setup and Technique

Patients are placed in the lateral decubitus position after induction of general anesthesia. A nonsterile tourniquet is placed high on the arm, and the arm is positioned in a well-padded arm holder. After sterile prepping and draping, landmarks are drawn on the elbow (medial and lateral epicondyles, radial head, capitellum, ulnar nerve, and olecranon) along with portal sites, as described earlier. The ulnar nerve should be palpated to confirm its location to make sure it does not subluxate. An 18-gauge spinal needle is placed through the soft spot to insufflate the elbow with approximately 20 cc of saline. Joint insufflation increases the distance between neurovascular structures and the bone, expanding the safety margin in establishing the initial viewing portal. Importantly, insufflation does not increase the distance between the capsule and the neurovascular structures. Safety is improved during portal placement, but nerves are still at risk during capsular release. The arm is exsanguinated, and the tourniquet inflated to a 250 or 300 mmHg.

The proximal anteromedial portal or proximal anterolateral portal is created first. The authors use the proximal anteromedial portal as their initial viewing portal. A #11 blade is used to incise the skin only to protect the cutaneous nerves. The blunt arthroscopic trocar is introduced into the joint, keeping the trocar against the anterior humeral cortex in the direction of the radiocapitellar joint. A mid- or proximal anterolateral portal is established next using a guidewire and cannulated dilator. This portal should be placed at the level of the radiocapitellar joint or proximal, but not distal. Anterior displacement of this portal may compromise the radial nerve.

In the setting of degenerative arthritis, all obvious loose bodies in the anterior compartment should be removed. The space in the anterior compartment is increased by elevating the anterior capsule bluntly from the anterior humeral cortex, proximally exposing the radial head and coronoid fossae. All bony work in the anterior compartment should be completed prior to capsular release to limit soft tissue swelling. A shaver and burr can be introduced through the lateral portal to remove osteophytes on the distal humerus and deepen the radial head and coronoid fossae (Figs. 2 and 3). The tip of the coronoid should be removed with a burr such that, with full elbow flexion, there is no impingement on the distal humerus (Figs. 3 and 4). The camera is moved to the lateral side using switching sticks to maintain portal access. The working instruments are placed through the medial portal to remove any remaining osteophyte not previously visualized.

Once all osteophytes have been removed, the anterior capsule can be released (Fig. 5). Capsular release should be started laterally, while there is still significant distention in the joint. A biter with a longer blunt arm can be used to dissect between the anterior capsule and brachialis (Fig. 6). The radial nerve is directly anterior to the radial head just outside the capsule and is at risk with anterior capsule resection. Staying proximal to the radial head can help avoid injury to the radial nerve during capsular release. Medially, the brachialis protects the overlying median nerve and brachial artery (Fig. 7).

The posterolateral portal is the initial viewing portal for the posterior compartment. A #11 blade is used to incise the skin, triceps fascia, and the deep joint capsule. This is a safe area in terms of neurovascular structures. A blunt arthroscopic trocar is advanced towards the olecranon fossae and into the posterior joint. The trocar is swept medially and laterally to develop a working space and release the posterior capsule. Slight extension of the elbow can often aid entry into the posterior compartment. A central posterior portal is created as an initial working portal. An 18-gauge needle is used to localize this portal. A shaver is introduced first to remove adhesions in the posterior compartment. A shaver and burr are then used to remove osteophytes both medially and laterally along the edge of the distal humeral articular surface. Removal of osteophytes at the olecranon tip and along the medial and lateral aspects of the ulna is performed. Switching the camera to the central posterior portal may aid in the removal of humeral osteophytes in the lateral gutter, using the posterolateral portal as a working portal. Extreme caution should be taken with removal of medial gutter osteophytes, as the ulnar nerve is directly adjacent to the posterior bundle of the medial collateral ligament and is at risk for injury.

With the camera in the posterolateral portal, a soft-spot portal can be created using a spinal needle for portal localization. A #11 blade should be used to incise the skin and deep capsule to aid entry into the joint. A shaver and burr can be used to remove any significant scar tissue, loose bodies, or osteophytes in the lateral gutter around the posterior aspect of the capitellum and radial head.

In the setting of extreme extension contractures with less than 90° of flexion preoperatively, a release of the posterior bundle of the medial collateral ligament will be required to significantly improve flexion. Release can be easily and safely performed through a small open incision at the level of the cubital tunnel. Ulnar nerve transposition or decompression may also be considered at this time, given the predisposition for ulnar neuropathy after correction of severe flexion limitations (23).

Special Considerations

Large osteophytes are not always present in the setting of post-traumatic contracture. Capsular resection may be all that is required. This is evident based on preoperative radiographic studies and intraoperative visualization. In patients with rheumatoid arthritis, the risk for nerve injury is increased if a synovectomy is performed. Arthroscopic synovectomy should only be considered by surgeons who have significant experience with elbow arthroscopy. Osteophyte removal and capsular release can also be performed with synovectomy to improve motion, if necessary. Radial head excision can be concomitantly performed in patients with articular deformity of the radial head, limiting rotation in the presence of a competent medial collateral ligament. Radial head resection is initiated anteriorly, but completion of the excision is accomplished by viewing from the posterolateral portal with instruments placed through a lateral soft-spot portal.

PEARLS AND PITFALLS

Proper patient positioning is important. Unencumbered medial and lateral access to the elbow is required during surgery. The elbow must be positioned such that the torso does not restrict access. This is critical when using the lateral position where medial access can be compromised if the arm is not positioned perpendicular to the torso in the arm holder.

Neurologic injury during elbow arthroscopy is one of the most concerning associated complications. A number of measures can be utilized to lower the risk for neurologic injury. Joint insufflation prior to portal placement significantly increases the distance between the bony and the capsule/neurologic structures (28). Guidewire localization of portals under direct visualization limits the risk of errant portal placement and potential nerve injury. Finally, retractors may be placed through accessory portals (for instance, using both a mid and proximal anterolateral portal), which can help enlarge and maintain a working space in the anterior compartment. An accessory posterior portal can be made 2 cm proximal to the central posterior portal through which a retractor (switching stick) may be used to enhance posterior visualization.

In the setting of previous ulnar nerve transposition, extreme care must be utilized with development of a medial portal. A small open incision can be made to safely establish this portal. A prior subcutaneous ulnar nerve transposition is considered a relative contraindication to elbow arthroscopy. A submuscular ulnar nerve transposition is an absolute contraindication.

Infection is a potentially devastating complication, following arthroscopic elbow surgery. Persistent drainage from arthroscopy portals has been reported after up to 5% of elbow arthroscopies (17). Drainage most often occurred from lateral portal sites because they are more superficial. Recommendations for limiting drainage include closing all portal sites with nylon sutures in a locked horizontal mattress stitch. An elbow with persistently draining portals should be immobilized in a splint and placed on oral antibiotics until the drainage stops. Sutures are generally removed between 10 days and 2 weeks.

REHABILITATION AND POSTOPERATIVE CARE

Postoperative care for patients after arthroscopic osteocapsular arthroplasty is focused on minimizing elbow swelling, infection prophylaxis, and preservation of motion gains achieved during surgery. All patients are splinted for 24 hours in extension for edema control and pain relief. Soft dressings are applied under the splint and are left intact after splint removal, allowing motion exercises but maintaining a sterile environment until the initial postoperative visit at one to two weeks.

Patients begin a home physical therapy program after the anterior extension splint is removed on the second postoperative day. Active-assisted elbow flexion/extension and forearm supination/pronation exercises are performed several times per day. Activities of daily living are encouraged. If motion loss occurs within the first two to three weeks, it is possible to perform a gentle manipulation under anesthesia to release any early adhesions.

Physical therapy is not routinely prescribed for patients after arthroscopic treatment of elbow arthritis, if a patient is doing well with home exercises. If limitations in motion and strength are recognized, a formal therapy program is instituted usually at three to six weeks postoperatively. Also, static progressive splinting may be utilized in the setting of motion loss after surgery. Finally, the authors have rarely utilized continuous passive motion after arthroscopic release in the setting of a primary arthroscopic procedure. In patients who have already failed a release and require further surgery, continuous passive motion has been prescribed starting immediately postoperative. There is little evidence confirming whether therapy versus splinting versus continuous passive motion provides better maintenance of motion.

CONCLUSIONS

With the advancement of arthroscopic techniques, arthroscopic tools, and surgeon skill levels, disorders, including primary osteoarthritis, rheumatoid arthritis, and post-traumatic contractures, can now be effectively treated utilizing arthroscopy. Benefits of arthroscopic treatment include limited surgical morbidity because of limited exposure and decreased soft-tissue dissection. While the potential benefits are high, the risks are potentially even higher in inexperienced hands. A thorough knowledge of elbow anatomy and a significant elbow arthroscopic experience is required for extensive procedures, including synovectomy and capsular release in rheumatoid arthritis or debridement and release for osteoarthritis. While the procedures still remain technically difficult, elbow arthroscopy for arthritic disorders will be performed more frequently, as surgical experience with these techniques improves.

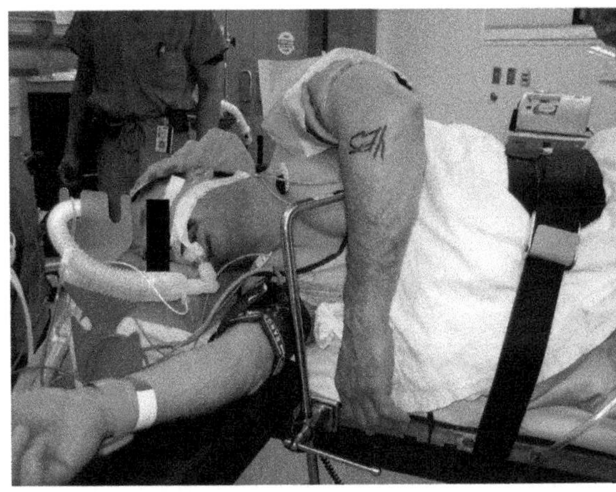

FIGURE 1 Patient in the lateral decubitus position with an unsterile tourniquet and the arm positioned in a bolstered arm holder.

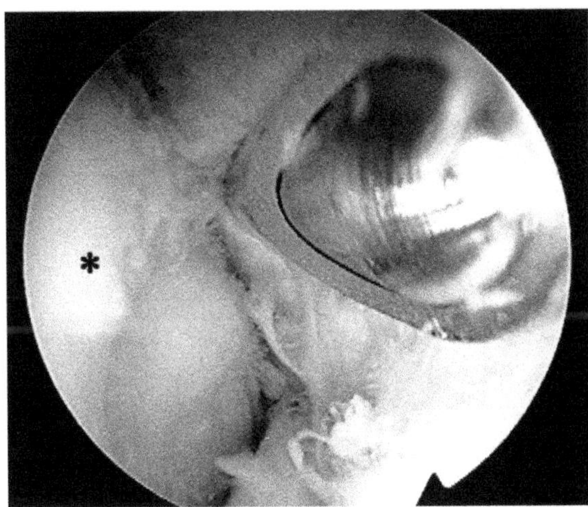

FIGURE 2 Anterior compartment of the elbow in setting of osteoarthritis with large anterior humeral osteophyte (*) on left along with a shaver in the proximal anterolateral portal.

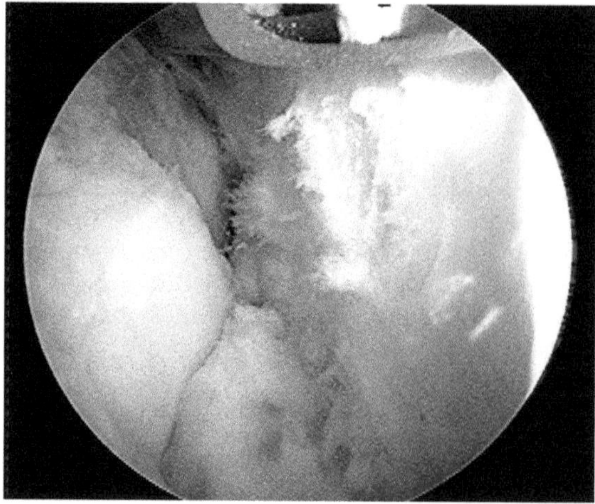

FIGURE 3 View of anterior joint prior to release from proximal anteromedial portal with resected coronoid and anterior humeral osteophytes.

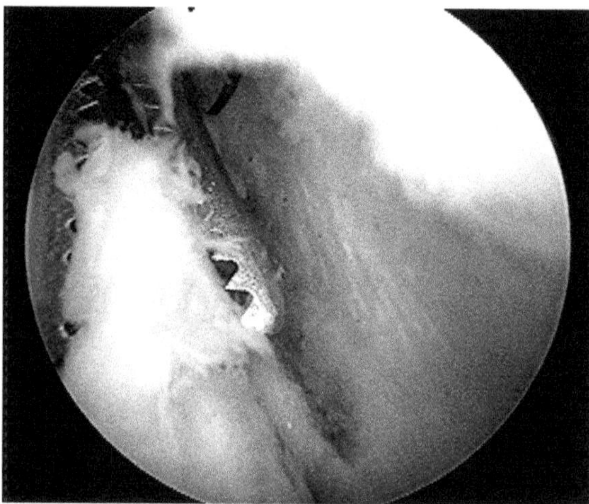

FIGURE 4 Grasper in proximal anterolateral portal removing a large coronoid osteophyte.

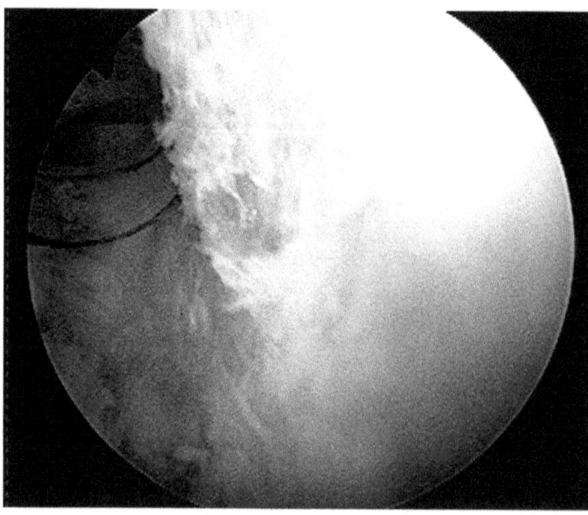

FIGURE 5 Thickened anterior joint capsule with cannula in the proximal anterolateral portal (note the relatively small anterior joint space).

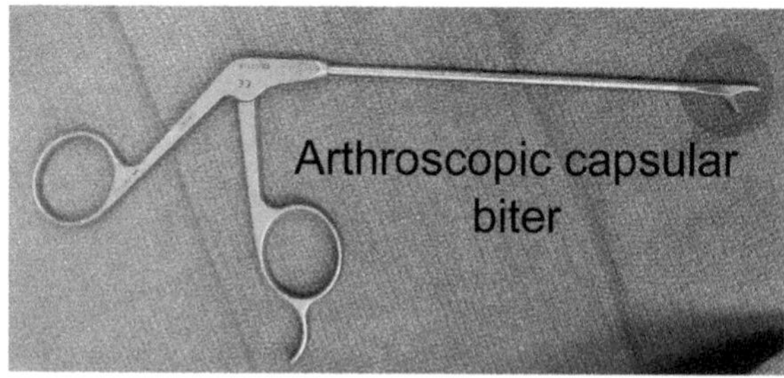

FIGURE 6 Arthroscopic biter with long blunt limb for anterior capsule release.

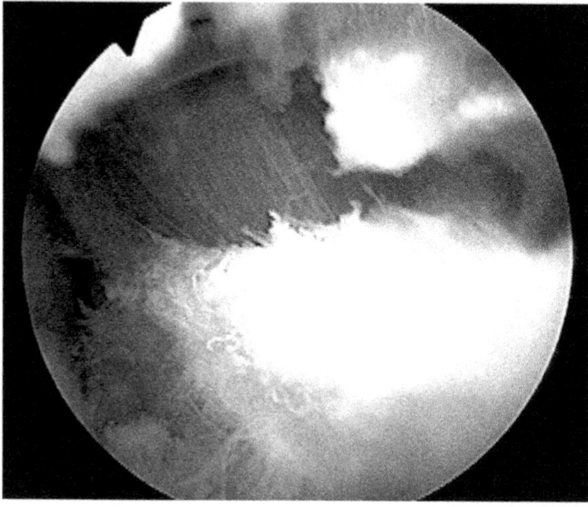

FIGURE 7 Released anterior joint capsule with underlying brachialis protecting the median nerve and brachial artery.

REFERENCES

1. O'Driscoll SW. Arthroscopic treatment for osteoarthritis of the elbow. Orthop Clin 1995; 26(4): 691–706.
2. Antuna SA, Morrey BF, Adams RA, et al. Ulnohumeral arthroplasty for primary degenerative arthritis of the elbow: long-term outcome and complications. J Bone Joint Surg Am 2002; 84(12):2168–2173.
3. Phillips NJ, Ali A, Stanley D. Treatment of primary degenerative arthritis of the elbow by ulnohumeral arthroplasty. A long-term follow-up. J Bone Joint Surg Br 2003; 85(3):347–350.
4. Cohen AP, Redden JF, Stanley D. Treatment of osteoarthritis of the elbow: a comparison of open and arthroscopic debridement. Arthroscopy 2000; 16(7):701–707.
5. Ogilvie-Harris DJ, Gordon R, MacKay M. Arthroscopic treatment for posterior impingement in degenerative arthritis of the elbow. Arthroscopy 1995; 11(4):437–443.
6. Savoie FH III, Nunley PD, Field LD. Arthroscopic management of the arthritic elbow: indications, technique, and results. J Shoulder Elbow Surg 1999; 8(3):214–219.
7. Lee BP, Morrey BF. Arthroscopic synovectomy of the elbow for rheumatoid arthritis. A prospective study. J Bone Joint Surg Br 1997; 79(5):770–772.
8. Gendi NS, Axon JM, Carr AJ, et al. Synovectomy of the elbow and radial head excision in rheumatoid arthritis. Predictive factors and long-term outcome. J Bone Joint Surg Br 1997; 79(6):918–923.
9. Lonner JH, Stuchin SA. Synovectomy, radial head excision, and anterior capsular release in stage III inflammatory arthritis of the elbow. J Hand Surg Am 1997; 22(2):279–285.
10. Maenpaa HM, Kuusela PP, Kaarela K, et al. Reoperation rate after elbow synovectomy in rheumatoid arthritis. J Shoulder Elbow Surg 2003; 12(5):480–483.
11. Tulp NJ, Winia WP. Synovectomy of the elbow in rheumatoid arthritis. Long-term results. J Bone Joint Surg Br 1989; 71(4):664–666.
12. Nemoto K, Arino H, Yoshihara Y, et al. Arthroscopic synovectomy for the rheumatoid elbow: a short-term outcome. J Shoulder Elbow Surg 2004; 13(6):652–655.
13. Horiuchi K, Momohara S, Tomatsu T, et al. Arthroscopic synovectomy of the elbow in rheumatoid arthritis. J Bone Joint Surg Am 2002; 84(3):342–347.
14. Phillips BB, Strasburger S. Arthroscopic treatment of arthrofibrosis of the elbow joint. Arthroscopy 1998; 14(1):38–44.
15. Kim SJ, Shin SJ. Arthroscopic treatment for limitation of motion of the elbow. Clin Orthop Rel Res 2000; 375:140–148.
16. Ball CM, Meunier M, Galatz LM, et al. Arthroscopic treatment of post-traumatic elbow contracture. J Shoulder Elbow Surg 2002; 11(6):624–629.
17. Kelly EW, Morrey BF, O'Driscoll SW. Complications of elbow arthroscopy. J Bone Joint Surg Am 2001; 83(1):25–34.
18. O'Driscoll SW, Morrey BF. Arthroscopy of the elbow: diagnostic and therapeutic benefits and hazards. J Bone Joint Surg Am 1992; 74(1):84–94.
19. Haapaniemi T, Berggren M, Adolfsson L. Complete transaction of the median and radial nerves during arthroscopic release of post-traumatic elbow contracture. Arthroscopy 1999; 15(7):784–787.
20. Hahn M, Grossman JA. Ulnar nerve laceration as a result of elbow arthroscopy. J Hand Surg Br 1998; 23(1):109.
21. Jones GS, Savoie FH III. Arthroscopic capsular release of flexion contractures (arthrofibrosis) of the elbow. Arthroscopy 1993; 9(3):277–283.
22. Ruch DS, Poehling GG. Anterior interosseus nerve injury following elbow arthroscopy. Arthroscopy 1997; 13(6):756–758.
23. Aldridge JM III, Atkins TA, Gunneson EE, et al. Anterior release of the elbow for extension loss. J Bone Joint Surg Am 2004; 86(9):1955–1960.
24. Andrews JR, Carson WG. Arthroscopy of the elbow. Arthroscopy 1985; 1:97–107.
25. Stothers K, Day B, Regan WR. Arthroscopy of the elbow: anatomy, portal sites, and a description of the proximal lateral portal. Arthroscopy 1995; 11:449–457.
26. Field LD, Altchek DW, Warren RF, et al. Arthroscopic anatomy of the lateral elbow: a comparison of three portals. Arthroscopy 1994; 10:602–607.
27. Poehling GG, Whipple TL, Sisco L. Elbow arthroscopy: a new technique. Arthroscopy 1989; 5: 222–224.
28. Lynch GJ, Meyers JF, Whipple TL, Caspari RB. Neurovascular anatomy and elbow arthroscopy: inherent risks. Arthroscopy 1986; 2:190–197.

34 Arthroscopic Osteocapsular Arthroplasty

Joaquin Sanchez-Sotelo
Department of Orthopedic Surgery, Mayo Clinic Rochester, Rochester, Minnesota, U.S.A.

INTRODUCTION

Elbow arthritis is relatively common and debilitating. Successful treatment of this condition requires a thorough understanding of the underlying pathology. Depending on the etiology and severity of the condition, the articular surface may need to be addressed to obtain a successful outcome after surgery. Interestingly, the symptoms of most patients with elbow osteoarthritis may be improved by surgical debridement of abnormal bone and capsule (1,2).

Pain and loss of motion are the two main complaints of patients with elbow arthritis. The preoperative evaluation of these patients should be directed to determine the source of symptoms. Pain originated at the articular surface is reproduced usually by resisted flexion or extension in the mid-arc of motion, which increases the load through the joint. Oftentimes, pain in osteoarthritic elbows will only be reproduced by impingement of capsule and osteophytes in terminal flexion or extension. This type of pain is eliminated by debridement of the structures that impinge against each other. Similarly, osteophyte debridement and capsular release may restore motion in a large proportion of patients with elbow osteoarthritis. Elbow replacement or interposition arthroplasty are required for patients with symptomatic involvement of the articular surface, which is more common in post-traumatic osteoarthritis and exceptional in primary osteoarthritis (1,2).

The term "osteocapsular arthroplasty" describes a surgical procedure directed to eliminate impingement between osteophytes in different locations of the joint (including the olecranon, coronoid, and radial head and their respective humeral fossae) (*osteo-*), resect contracted capsular tissue (*-capsular*), and trim flaps of fibrous tissue or delaminated cartilage in order to improve pain and motion. The concept of eliminating the sources of impingement by accurate recontouring of the articular prominences and their correspondent fossae is not new. Combined with capsular release, this has been the basic strategy underlying standard open procedures used to treat extrinsic elbow stiffness (such as the lateral column procedure). Advancements in the field of elbow arthroscopy have allowed the development of a safe and effective arthroscopic technique to perform osteocapsular arthroplasty of the elbow (3–6). The indications, contraindications, and technique of this procedure are reviewed in this chapter.

INDICATIONS

Arthroscopic osteocapsular arthroplasty is indicated to improve pain and/or motion in patients with symptoms secondary to capsular contracture and impingement (Table 1). The typical candidate is a male patient with a long-standing history of heavy weight use (e.g., construction workers and weight-lifters), stiffness, pain at the extremes of motion, and hypertrophic osteophytes (Fig. 1). Patients with post-traumatic osteoarthritis may also benefit from this procedure, provided the articular surface does not need to be addressed. Selected patients with inflammatory arthritis may improve with synovectomy, capsular release, and articular debridement, but most of the times they exhibit less hypertrophic bony changes and more advanced involvement of the articular surface.

Please refer to pages 362–363 for the figures in this chapter.

TABLE 1 Arthroscopic Osteocapsular Arthroplasty: Indications and Contraindications

Indications	
Main indication	Primary hypertrophic osteoarthritis
Other	Post-traumatic osteoarthritis (minimal joint surface involvement) Inflammatory arthritis (selected cases)
Contraindications	
Absolute	Need to address the articular surface to improve pain/motion Instability Lack of experience with elbow arthroscopy Unwillingness to comply with postoperative program
Relative	Need to remove hardware or address associated nerve problems Prior ulnar nerve transposition

CONTRAINDICATIONS

Osteocapsular arthroplasty is contraindicated in cases where pain, motion, and/or function will not improve unless the articular surface is addressed in patients with severe articular cartilage damage, bone loss, or deformity (Table 1). Patients with post-traumatic arthritis and associated instability who require reconstruction of ligaments or bone will not improve completely with isolated osteocapsular arthroplasty.

The main neurovascular structures of the arm are very close to the elbow joint. Nerve transection is a well-known complication of arthroscopic elbow surgery (7). In addition, adequate visualization inside the elbow joint may be difficult, especially when contracture limits capsular distention and mobility. For all these reasons, unfamiliarity with elbow arthroscopy should be considered a contraindication for this procedure. Prior ulnar nerve transposition should also be considered a relative contraindication, unless the ulnar nerve can be identified and protected. Compliance with postoperative instructions is critical after this procedure, especially to maintain the increased motion achieved in surgery. Unwillingness to comply with the postoperative program is also considered a contraindication for this procedure.

Mild-to-moderate involvement of the articular surface is a relative contraindication for this procedure, as it may improve symptoms only partially. However, interposition arthroplasty and elbow replacement are not associated with successful long-term outcomes in young patients with elbow osteoarthritis, and osteocapsular arthroplasty may be offered to patients with articular involvement, provided they understand that their pain will not be resolved completely. Finally, the need for hardware removal or nerve decompression may mandate open surgery, unless the surgeon is extremely experienced in arthroscopic elbow surgery.

TECHNIQUE

Principles

The basic principles of elbow arthroscopy and other arthroscopic procedures have been described in previous chapters of this book (Chapters 28, 29). The author focuses on the specific technical aspects of arthroscopic osteocapsular arthroplasty. Some general principles should be taken

TABLE 2 Surgical Principles of Arthroscopic Osteocapsular Arthroplasty

- Establish a good view before removing any bone or soft tissue
  - Use an arthroscopic pump or alternative system
  - Release the capsule from the humerus from the very beginning
  - Use retractors
- Complete bone recontouring before resecting the capsule
- Perform a complete and accurate three-dimensional bone recontouring
- Perform as complete a capsulectomy as possible
- Avoid neurovascular injury
  - Decompress neurovascular structures as needed (ulnar nerve)
  - Always work under good visualization
  - Avoid suction connected to shavers or burrs
  - Avoid motorized instruments close to the location of neurovascular structures

into consideration to improve the safety and efficacy of arthroscopic osteocapsular arthroplasty (Table 2).

1. *Establish a good view before removing any bone or soft tissue.* Adequate visualization is paramount in order to perform a complete osteocapsular arthroplasty without damage to the articular cartilage or adjacent neurovascular structures. Visualization is difficult to obtain in osteoarthritis due to the hypertrophic osteophytes, nonelastic capsule, and limited motion. It may be improved by capsular stripping of the humerus at the beginning of the procedure, as well as the use or an arthroscopic pump and retractors inside the joint.
2. *Complete bone recontouring before resecting the capsule.* Maintenance of the integrity of the capsule until the end of the procedure provides several advantages, including maintenance of capsular distention with fluid to aid in joint visualization, decreased extravasation of fluid into the adjacent musculature, and protection of neurovascular structures in close proximity to the capsule.
3. *Perform a complete and accurate three-dimensional bone recontouring.* In primary hypertrophic osteoarthritis of the elbow, osteophytes proliferate in a predictable manner. The success of osteocapsular arthroplasty partly depends on a complete three-dimensional recontouring of the elbow joint bones. Failure to identify and remove all sources of impingement may translate in persistent discomfort or suboptimal motion after surgery (Fig. 2).
4. *Perform a complete capsulectomy.* Failure to remove enough capsular tissue will limit elbow motion and facilitate recurrence of stiffness (Fig. 3). The anterior band of the medial collateral ligament and the lateral collateral ligament complex should be preserved to avoid instability, but the posterior band of the medial collateral ligament oftentimes needs to be released in order to obtain full flexion.
5. *Avoid neurovascular injury.* Nerve injury is one of the most feared reported complications of arthroscopic elbow surgery. The close proximity of all three main nerve trunks (ulnar, radial, and median nerves) to the joint places them at risk, especially when motorized instruments are used. The risk of iatrogenic nerve injury is decreased by a sound knowledge of the anatomic location of the nerves, working under good visualization, avoidance of suction connected to motorized instruments, and avoidance of motorized instruments close to the location of the nerves.

The Ulnar Nerve

It is currently recognized that the ulnar nerve plays a major role in the pathology and outcome of elbow stiffness (8). Patients with preoperative ulnar nerve symptoms and/or less than 90° of flexion have an increased risk of symptomatic ulnar nerve compression with progressive elbow flexion, which may manifest as a sensory or mixed ulnar neuropathy or as medial-sided elbow pain that will limit maintenance of elbow flexion during physical therapy.

Several factors may explain the propensity of the ulnar nerve to become compromised in elbow stiffness: (*i*) the nerve may be encased in fibrous tissue or surrounded by prominent osteophytes, (*ii*) its location posterior to the axis of elbow flexion places this nerve at risk of compression behind the medial epicondyle with progressive elbow flexion, and (*iii*) the limited amount of preoperative nerve excursion may make the nerve less prone to tolerate full excursion with increased motion. In addition, the combination of postoperative swelling and aggressive physical therapy [especially, continuous passive motion (CPM)] may further jeopardize the ulnar nerve.

When the ulnar nerve needs to be addressed, the author's preference is to do so at the beginning of the procedure. The ulnar nerve is transposed in an anterior subcutaneous position using a posterior midline skin incision (Fig. 4); the medial skin flap not only allows nerve transposition, but also placement of instruments in the anterior and posterior compartments from the medial side and less subcutaneous edema secondary to fluid extravasation. The transposition should include nerve dissection from the distal third of the arm to the proximal third of the forearm, preservation of the nerve vasculature, ample release of the superficial and deep fascias of the flexor carpi ulnaris, and resection of the prominent medial intermuscular septum. Once the ulnar nerve is completely dissected, it should be protected throughout the procedure. Currently, some surgeons favor ulnar nerve decompression without transposition. The indications of ulnar nerve decompression and transposition are not firmly established.

Osteocapsular Arthroplasty

The arthroscopic part of the procedure may start on the anterior or the posterior compartment, based on surgeon preferences (9,10). The author's preference is to start anteriorly, unless the pathology is much more severe in the posterior compartment. An anteromedial portal is created 1 to 2 cm proximal to the medial epicondyle and immediately anterior to the intermuscular septum. Care should be taken to avoid injury to the ulnar nerve when this portal is created, especially if the ulnar nerve subluxes anteriorly. The arthroscope is inserted through the anteromedial portal, and an anterolateral portal is created under direct vision 1 to 2 cm proximal to the lateral epicondyle. A blunt instrument may then be used from the lateral side to strip the capsule off the distal humerus in order to create a working space and obtain adequate visualization. Additional instruments may be inserted through proximal anteromedial and proximal anterolateral portals (2–3 cm proximal to the other two portals) to be used as retractors, placing the anterior capsule and soft tissue structures under tension.

A light synovectomy and capsular debridement may be performed early in order to improve visualization, but as mentioned earlier, the capsule should be preserved largely intact until the bone recontouring has been completed. Intra-articular osteocartilaginous bodies are removed from the joint; although occasionally these are loose bodies, most of the times they are attached to the elbow capsule cartilage or bone. Progressive elbow flexion is then used to bring the coronoid and its osteophytes into view, allowing resection of coronoid osteophytes. The coronoid and radial fossas are recreated by removal of abnormal bone. Care should be taken to recreate the depth, height, and width of these fossas to fully accommodate the coronoid and radial head in full flexion (Fig. 2). The lateral and medial columns should not be violated to decrease the risk of postoperative fracture. Osteophytes in other locations of the anterior compartment whose impingement limits motion and may be painful are also removed. Areas of cartilage degeneration and soft-tissue flaps may also be débrided as needed.

The anterior capsulectomy is started, once the areas of anterior bone impingement have been cleared (Fig. 3). It is safer to start the capsulectomy on the medial side, as the radial nerve lies extremely close to the anterior capsule on the lateral side of the joint. A shaver may be used to remove a very limited amount of capsule on the medial side until muscular fibers are visualized. Then, a manual arthroscopic instrument is used to progressively dissect and resect a strip of capsule on a medial direction. Once this capsulotomy has been completed from a medial to a lateral direction, a shaver may be applied to the free edges of the capsule to complete the capsulectomy, taking care to prevent injury to the median and radial nerves.

The posterior compartment is then addressed in a similar way. The joint may be initially visualized from the direct lateral portal just above the radial head. A shaver inserted through a posterior midline portal may be used to remove the abundant soft tissue usually present in the olecranon fossa. The osteophytes in the olecranon fossa, olecranon, and other locations may then be removed with a burr. The posterior capsulectomy is then completed. Care should be taken on the posteromedial aspect of the joint, as the ulnar nerve lies in close proximity at risk to be injured. However, failure to release the posterior bundle of the medial collateral ligament in this location may limit elbow flexion. The range of motion obtained at the end of the procedure should be documented, once the tourniquet has been released.

PEARLS AND PITFALLS

Arthroscopic osteocapsular arthroplasty is a challenging operation. The keys for success after this procedure include good patient selection, careful assessment and management of the ulnar nerve, proficiency in arthroscopic elbow surgery, complete and accurate removal of extra bone and contracted capsule, avoidance of iatrogenic nerve injury, and compliance with the postoperative rehabilitation program. Failures are most of the times explained by inadequate patient selection and failure to perform a complete debridement due to poor visualization or lack of experience.

REHABILITATION

The main goal of the rehabilitation program after elbow osteocapsular arthroplasty is to preserve the motion achieved during surgery. Patients with worse preoperative motion usually require more intensive and prolonged rehabilitation in order to preserve motion. Most patients benefit from a combination of CPM and bracing.

CPM can be extremely helpful to maintain motion early after surgery. Once the integrity of the neurovascular structures has been verified, an interscalenic or axillary block may be used to help control pain. Ideally, patients should use the CPM machine most of the day. The machine is initially used to work on terminal extension and terminal flexion. Once the desired end-points of motion have been achieved, the elbow is ranged throughout the arc of motion. Continuous motion displaces fluid from the elbow region and has other beneficial effects on the joint. Depending on the severity of preoperative stiffness, inflammatory response to surgery, and compliance, passive motion may be used for just a few days or up to three or four weeks. Selected patients benefit from a more extended period of CPM treatment.

In most cases, bracing is instituted after a period of CPM, although some patients may be treated with an elbow brace immediately after surgery. The main goal of bracing is to stretch the soft tissues that limit terminal flexion and terminal extension (Fig. 5). There is little data in the literature to determine the ideal bracing program. Generally, terminal extension is better tolerated than terminal flexion. For that reason, the author recommends patients to sleep with the elbow in as much extension as possible. During the day, they alternate two-hour periods of flexion and extension with breaks of 30 minutes to one hour in between. Patients with substantial preoperative stiffness require bracing for 6 to 12 weeks. When bracing is discontinued, patients should monitor their motion and resume the bracing program if they experience recurrence of stiffness.

Inhibitors of prostaglandin synthesis are known to decrease ectopic bone formation. Although there is no published data to strongly support their use after joint debridement, the author recommends his patients to take indomethacin (25 mg three times a day) during the first six weeks after surgery, in an effort to decrease the inflammatory response and hopefully the risk of ectopic bone formation or recurrence.

SUMMARY

Arthroscopic osteocapsular arthroplasty has emerged as an extremely successful minimally invasive procedure for the treatment of most patients with primary hypertrophic osteoarthritis and selected cases of post-traumatic and inflammatory arthritis. This procedure involves removal of osteophytes to recreate the three-dimensional anatomy of the distal humerus and proximal ulna and radius, resection of contracted capsule, removal of loose bodies, and debridement of areas of cartilage degeneration. The need to address the articular surface in order to obtain pain relief or functional motion is a contraindication for this procedure.

The success of arthroscopic osteocapsular arthroplasty depends on the ability of the surgeon to perform a complete and accurate debridement while protecting the neurovascular structures in close proximity to the joint. The ulnar nerve should be evaluated carefully and either decompressed or transposed at the time of surgery in patients with preoperative symptoms or less than 90° of flexion. The CPM and bracing are used to maintain the range of motion achieved in surgery.

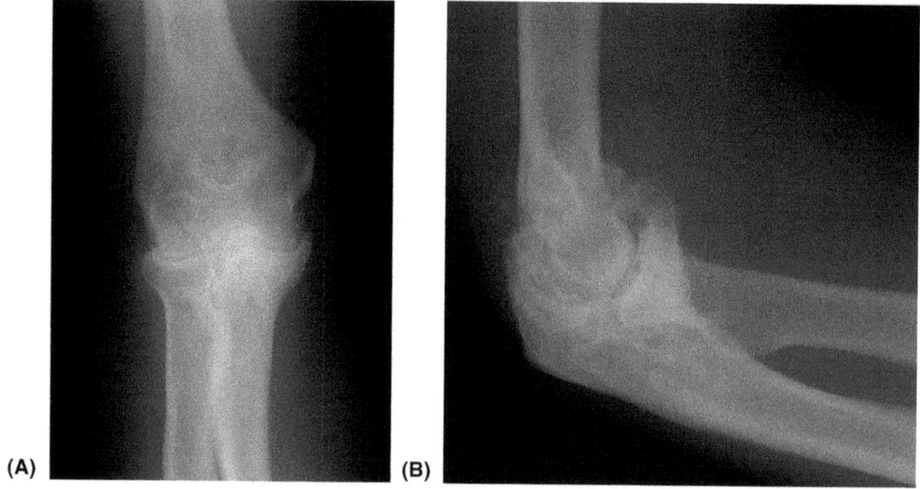

FIGURE 1 (**A** and **B**) Typical radiographic changes in primary elbow osteoarthritis. The articular joint line is largely preserved, and there are prominent osteophytes at the olecranon, the coronoid and the humeral fossae, as well as other locations.

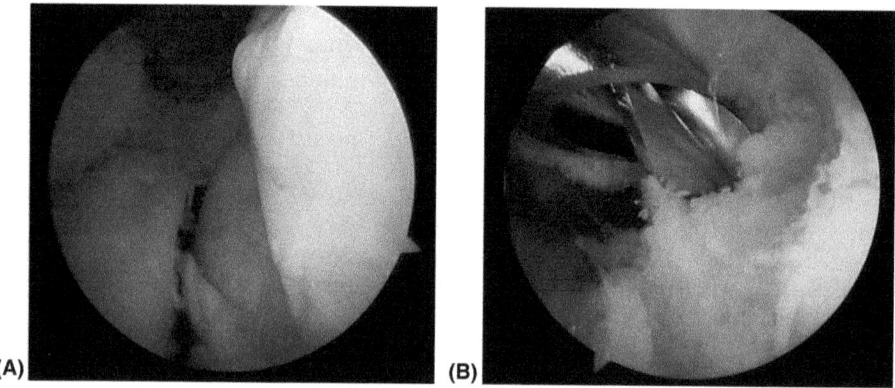

FIGURE 2 (**A**) Arthroscopic view of the anterior compartment of an osteoarthritic elbow prior to removal of loose bodies and debridement of osteophytes. (**B**) An arthroscopic burr may be used to recreate the three-dimensional anatomy of the elbow joint.

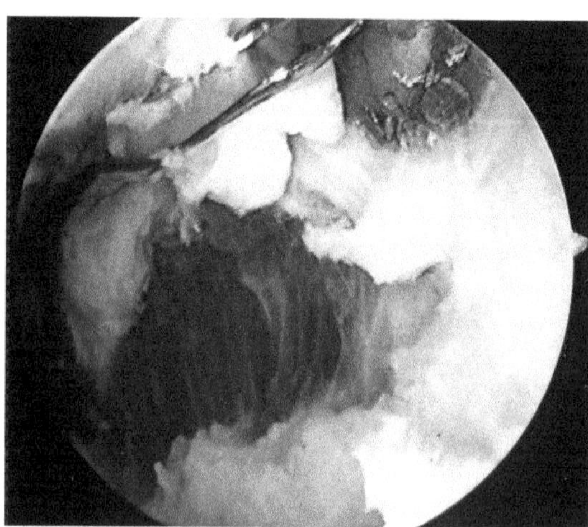

FIGURE 3 The capsulectomy should be as complete as possible in order to maximize motion. The muscular fibers of the brachialis are seen behind the resected anterior capsule.

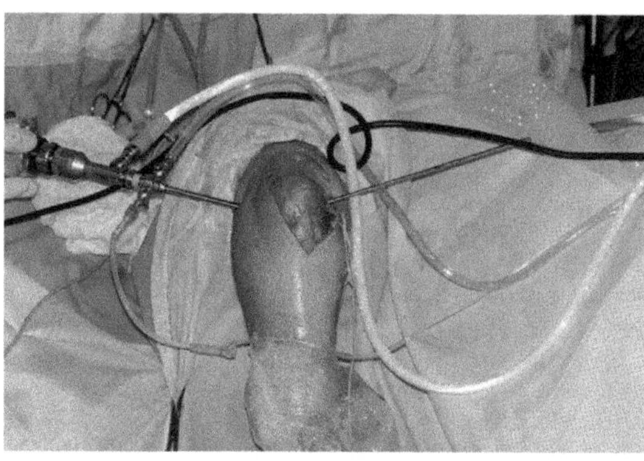

FIGURE 4 In patients with preoperative symptoms or less than 90° of flexion, the ulnar nerve needs to be transposed or decompressed. This illustration shows subcutaneous ulnar nerve transposition through elevation of a medial skin flap, which is then used for insertion of arthroscopic instruments.

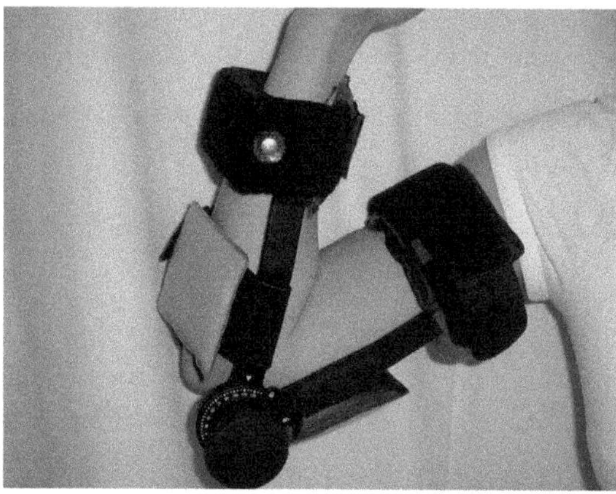

FIGURE 5 Elbow bracing is commonly used in the postoperative rehabilitation after osteocapsular arthroplasty.

REFERENCES

1. Gramstad, GD, Galatz, LM. Management of elbow osteoarthritis. J Bone Joint Surg Am 2006; 88: 421–430.
2. Steinmann SP, King GJ, Savoie FH III. Arthroscopic treatment of the arthritic elbow. J Bone Joint Surg Am 2005; 87:2114–2121.
3. Ogilvie-Harris DJ, Gordon R, MacKay M. Arthroscopic treatment for posterior impingement in degenerative arthritis of the elbow. Arthroscopy 1995; 11:437–443.
4. Cohen AP, Redden JF, Stanley D. Treatment of osteoarthritis of the elbow: a comparison of open and arthroscopic debridement. Arthroscopy 2000; 16:701–706.
5. Savoie FH III, Nunley PD, Field LD. Arthroscopic management of the arthritic elbow: indications, technique, and results. J Shoulder Elbow Surg 1999; 8:214–219.
6. Ball CM, Meunier M, Galatz LM, Calfee R, Yamaguchi K. Arthroscopic treatment of post-traumatic elbow contracture. J Shoulder Elbow Surg 2002; 11:624–629.
7. Haapaniemi T, Berggren M, Adolfsson L. Complete transection of the median and radial nerves during arthroscopic release of post-traumatic elbow contracture. Arthroscopy 1999; 15:784–787.
8. Antuna SA, Morrey BF, Adams RA, O'Driscoll SW. Ulnohumeral arthroplasty for primary degenerative arthritis of the elbow: long-term outcome and complications. J Bone Joint Surg Am 2002; 84-A:2168–2173.
9. O'Driscoll SW. Arthroscopic treatment for osteoarthritis of the elbow. Orthop Clin North Am 1995; 26:691–706.
10. Ramsey ML. Elbow arthroscopy: basic setup and treatment of arthritis. Instr Course Lect 2002; 51:69–72.

35 Arthroscopic Medial Epicondylectomy

Hyun-Min Kim, Robert Z. Tashjian, and Ken Yamaguchi
Department of Orthopedic Surgery, Washington University School of Medicine, Barnes-Jewish Hospital, St. Louis, Missouri, U.S.A.

INTRODUCTION

Cubital tunnel syndrome is the second most common nerve entrapment neuropathy of the upper extremity after carpal tunnel syndrome. Five possible locations of nerve entrapment include the arcade of Struthers, medial intermuscular septum, medial epicondyle, cubital tunnel itself with the arcade of Osborne, and deep flexor pronator aponeurosis. In addition to compression of the ulnar nerve at these locations, traction-related deformation of the ulnar nerve during elbow flexion is also thought to be a causative factor. This deformation results in increased intraneural pressure, whereas the cross-sectional areas of the cubital tunnel and the ulnar nerve at the elbow decrease (1). Ulnar nerve strain is greatest with maximum elbow flexion directly behind the medial epicondyle (2). In the normal cubital tunnel, the ulnar nerve strain that occurs with elbow flexion does not cause any symptoms or signs, whereas in the pathologic condition, symptoms and signs of ulnar neuropathy occur with elbow flexion. Another source of nerve compression occurs at the posterior bundle of the medial collateral ligament (PMCL), which forms the floor of the cubital tunnel. The posterior bundle tightens in elbow flexion and thus compresses the ulnar nerve (3).

There are many surgical procedures for ulnar nerve release at the elbow. These fall under three categories: (*i*) simple decompression, (*ii*) decompression with anterior transposition (submuscular, intramuscular, and subcutaneous), and (*iii*) medial epicondylectomy. These all have their advantages and drawbacks, but no single technique is suitable for all types of cubital tunnel syndrome. Open medial epicondylectomy has been reported frequently in the literature because of its potential advantages of preservation of the ulnar nerve blood supply and gliding tissues surrounding the nerve. However, various problems may occur after open medial epicondylectomy, which include medial instability of the elbow due to injury of the anterior bundle of the medial collateral ligament, loss of the protective prominence of the medial epicondyle, postoperative tenderness of the operative site, nerve subluxation, flexion contracture of the elbow, and weakness related to detachment of the common flexor pronator origin. To minimize these potential disadvantages, Le Viet (4) and Popa and Dubert (5) modified the original technique described by King and Morgan (6) by introducing an open frontal, partial medial epicondylectomy. In the modified procedure, only the posterior part of the medial epicondyle was resected in the coronal plane, allowing some anterior translation of the ulnar nerve. They reported that this partial medial epicondylectomy is a safe and effective method for treating patients with cubital tunnel syndrome, regardless of the preoperative grade of nerve compression. This chapter describes an arthroscopic method for achieving the same goals of open medial epicondylectomy for treating cubital tunnel syndrome.

INDICATIONS

Arthroscopic medial epicondylectomy can be potentially used for the treatment of all cases of cubital tunnel syndrome in which deepening of the cubital tunnel and removal of encroaching

---

Please refer to pages 369–372 for the figures in this chapter.

soft tissue (e.g., the PMCL) are thought to be beneficial; and, it can also be used for prophylactic ulnar nerve decompression. Specific examples of such cases are as follows.

1. Primary osteoarthritis of the elbow accompanied by cubital tunnel syndrome: Osteoarthritis usually results in loose bodies, osteophytes, ossification of the olecranon fossa, and loss of motion, all of which may be successfully treated by arthroscopic procedures (e.g., osteocapsular arthroplasty). Osteophytes or loose bodies at the medial epicondyle or olecranon tip can compress the ulnar nerve. Along with the removal of osteophytes and loose bodies, medial epicondylectomy can be concomitantly performed.
2. Primary osteoarthritis of the elbow without cubital tunnel syndrome, but with severe joint stiffness: Patients with preoperative flexion less than 90° to 100° have a tendency to develop postoperative ulnar nerve symptoms after a capsular release procedure. This is thought to be because of excessive nerve stretching and narrowing of cubital tunnel when the elbow is flexed further. Therefore, prophylactic decompression of the ulnar nerve should be considered in patients with preoperative flexion less than 90° to 100°.
3. Severe post-traumatic elbow stiffness regardless of the presence of cubital tunnel syndrome: Prophylactic medial epicondylectomy may be considered for the same reason as indicated above.
4. Post-traumatic elbow stiffness with cubital tunnel syndrome.
5. Cubital tunnel syndrome in the elbow of throwing athletes: The elbow of throwing athletes is often complicated by various abnormalities, such as ulnar collateral ligament tears, ulnar neuritis, flexor-pronator muscle strain or tendinitis, medial epicondyle apophysitis or avulsion, valgus extension overload syndrome with olecranon osteophytes, olecranon stress fractures, osteochondritis dissecans of the capitellum, and loose bodies. Arthroscopic procedures can be helpful in treating most of these abnormalities except ulnar collateral ligament tears.

RELATIVE CONTRAINDICATIONS

Arthroscopic medial epicondylectomy for the treatment of ulnar nerve neuropathy is an extremely difficult, potentially hazardous operation. Only the most experienced elbow arthroscopy surgeons should be performing it at this time. In the future, specific instrumentation will hopefully be developed to make the procedure safer. In the absence of such instrumentation, extreme caution should be employed before performing this operation.

Another relative contraindication could be severity of the ulnar neuropathy. Significant sensory or motor deficiency of the ulnar nerve (e.g., intrinsic muscle atrophy in the hand, or severe hypoesthesia or anesthesia in the ulnar) could be considered a relative contraindication, given the relative newness of this technique. The efficacy of this procedure for more severe cases of ulnar nerve neuropathy has not been demonstrated. Generally, these more severe cases, especially early in the process, should be treated with more established techniques.

CONTRAINDICATIONS

1. Failed previous anterior ulnar nerve transposition: An open exploration should be considered to locate the site of recurrent nerve entrapment.
2. Tardy ulnar nerve palsy due to cubitus valgus deformity: A correction osteotomy with or without ulnar nerve transposition should be sought.
3. Ganglions or tumors compressing the ulnar nerve from outside of the joint: An open approach should be used to identify and remove the source of nerve compression.
4. Ulnar nerve compression by fascial constrictions (e.g., compression at the arcade of Struthers, the medial intermuscular septum, and the deep flexor pronator aponeurosis): An open approach should be employed to address these compression sites.
5. Ulnar neuropathy due to ulnar nerve subluxation or dislocation: An open approach should be used to address the cause.
6. Failed previous open ulnar nerve decompression or medial epicondylectomy procedures: An open approach is preferred in these situations.

7. Ulnar neuropathy in the elbow with medial instability: Medial instability should be addressed prior to the treatment of ulnar neuropathy.
8. Recurrent ulnar neuropathy symptoms after arthroscopic medial epicondylectomy: An open approach is preferred in these recurrent situations.

SURGICAL TECHNIQUE

Anesthesia, Positioning, and Equipment

Elbow arthroscopy can be performed under either general or regional anesthesia. Benefits of general anesthesia include complete muscle relaxation, improved airway protection, and maintenance of a postoperative neurological examination. A regional anesthetic can be administered after arthroscopy, once a neurological examination has been performed. A postoperative block precludes future neurologic assessments, which may be problematic especially in the setting of significant swelling where there may be concern for compartment syndrome. Maintenance of a neurologic examination is even more critical when performing an arthroscopic medial epicondylectomy since there is a significant potential risk for ulnar nerve injury. General anesthesia without a postoperative regional block is the authors' preferred anesthesia method for arthroscopic medial epicondylectomy.

The authors' preferred positioning is lateral decubitus, which provides excellent access to the posterior compartment that is critical in performing an arthroscopic medial epicondylectomy. While the prone position also provides excellent posterior access, there are a number of drawbacks including difficult airway management and poorer pulmonary ventilation.

Arthroscopy is performed utilizing a standard 4.0-mm 30° large-joint arthroscope. Low-flow cannulas and blunt trocars are utilized to limit soft tissue fluid extravasation and iatrogenic neurovascular or chondral injury. A pump is utilized for fluid administration with pressure set at 35 mmHg also limiting soft tissue swelling. Arthroscopy is performed under tourniquet with pressure set at 300 mmHg. In order to safely perform a medial epicondylectomy, 4.0 hooded shavers and burrs along with an arthroscopic cautery device is required. The authors utilize an Arthrocare Wand (ArthroCare; Austin, Texas, U.S.A.) cautery at a lower intensity level (setting of 4).

Portal Placement

Arthroscopic portals required for medial epicondylectomy include the posterolateral and direct posterior portal. The posterolateral portal can be established anywhere along the lateral border of the triceps and is very safe. The authors routinely place this portal slightly proximal to the level of the tip of the olecranon. The direct posterior portal is located 3 cm proximal to the tip of the olecranon and penetrates the triceps tendon. During medial epicondylectomy, the direct posterior portal is the working portal, and the posterolateral portal is the viewing portal (Fig. 1).

Surgical Technique

The patient is placed under general anesthesia and then positioned in the lateral decubitus position. A nonsterile tourniquet is placed high on the arm, and a padded arm bolster is used to position the elbow in 90° of flexion. The tourniquet is raised to 300 mmHg after preoperative intravenous antibiotics are administered. All surface landmarks are outlined on the elbow, including the radial head, capitellum, lateral and medial epicondyles, and the ulnar nerve. The authors routinely perform an arthroscopic medial epicondylectomy as part of a procedure, which often includes either concomitant capsular release or osteocapsular arthroplasty. Consequently, posterior portal sites (midlateral, posterolateral, and direct posterior) are marked along with anterior portal sites (proximal anteromedial and proximal anterolateral), which are used for the anterior compartment procedures.

Anterior compartment arthroscopy is first performed, if necessary, for the treatment of contractures or arthritis. Once the anterior compartment procedures have been completed, posterior compartment arthroscopy along with medial epicondylectomy is performed. The posterolateral portal is established utilizing a #11 blade incising from skin through to the joint capsule. The arthroscope cannula with the blunt trocar is inserted and swept medially and laterally to release the posterior capsule and develop a working space. A camera is then inserted into cannula in the posterolateral portal. A direct posterior portal is localized under direct visualization 3 cm proximal to the tip of the olecranon using an 18 gauge spinal needle. Using a #11 blade, the direct posterior portal is created by incising the skin, triceps, and posterior capsule. A 4.0-mm shaver is introduced posteriorly into the olecranon fossa, and debridement of adhesions and capsule further exposes the posterior compartment.

If osteocapsular arthroplasty is being concomitantly performed, removal of posterior humeral osteophytes in both the medial and lateral gutters along with loose body removal and olecranon tip resection is completed using a hooded 4.0-mm shaver and burr. A cone-tipped burr removes humeral and olecranon osteophytes with precision. A round-tipped burr is used to deepen the olecranon fossa.

With the camera in the posterolateral portal, an Arthrocare cautery device is inserted in the direct posterior portal to initiate medial epicondylectomy. In order to perform the epicondylectomy, the PMCL must be released off the medial epicondyle. The Arthrocare is used to progressively release the capsule and humeral origin of the posterior bundle off the medial epicondyle, working in a posterior-to-anterior direction (Figs. 2–5). Forearm muscle contraction should be monitored to limit inadvertent injury to the ulnar nerve. Release should be continued anteriorly for approximately 0.5 to 1 cm in order to release the entire posterior bundle (Fig. 6).

The posterior bundle forms the anatomic floor of the cubital tunnel, therefore release of the ligament from the humerus and subsequent removal of bone from the ligament's origin effectively deepens the cubital tunnel. Also, release of the posterior bundle can significantly improve flexion deficits if elbow release is being performed. Posterior bundle release is required in the setting of severe flexion deficits (<100°), otherwise full flexion cannot be restored.

After release of the posterior bundle, a 4.0-mm hooded cone-tipped burr is placed in the direct posterior portal. Several millimeters of bone are then removed from the insertion site of the posterior bundle (Figs. 7 and 8). Use of the burr in this location is obviously hazardous. There is certainly a possibility of soft tissue entrapment within the burr, which can effectively pull the ulnar nerve in towards the structures. Because of this, the surgeon should burr only small amounts of bone at the time and practice stopping the blades. Additionally, until a good space is obtained, the burr is placed in the oscillating mode. Oscillating mode can effectively remove medial epicondyle bone while limiting the chances of "sucking in" surrounding soft tissue. The effect is analog to that of an oscillating saw used to remove cast. Additionally, it is very important to maintain the floor of the cubital tunnel as an intact structure protecting the ulnar nerve from the burr. The floor of the cubital tunnel, in addition to the hood of the burr, adds a measure of safety for the ulnar nerve. The released posterior bundle and capsule lie between the nerve and burr during bone removal, improving the safety. Suction should be limited during burring to avoid soft tissue entrapment. The result is an "epicondyloplasty" with deepening of the cubital tunnel, as opposed to an "epicondylectomy" with complete or partial en-block removal of the medial epicondyle as described for an open procedure (Figs. 9 and 10).

PEARLS AND PITFALLS

Nerve injury is a primary concern when performing an arthroscopic medial epicondylectomy. Posterior compartment work can be difficult in the supine position, therefore prone or lateral decubitus positioning is recommended. In the setting of a very tight posterior compartment with limited working space, an accessory portal can be established 1 to 2 cm proximal to the direct posterior portal for retractor placement. A switching stick can be placed through this accessory portal to improve visualization and increase the space between the articular surface and surrounding joint capsule and structures.

Cautery devices should be placed on a lower setting to avoid potential thermal injury to the ulnar nerve. Cautery is extremely useful in performing the posterior bundle release since stimulation of the ulnar nerve can warn the surgeon of its proximity. Hooded shavers and burrs are required in the procedure to prevent potential soft tissue entrapment and iatrogenic nerve injury. Finally, there should be a low threshold in converting to an open release at any point in the procedure. The surgeon should have significant knowledge of elbow anatomy along with elbow arthroscopic experience prior to attempting an arthroscopic medial epicondylectomy.

POSTOPERATIVE CARE AND REHABILITATION

Portal sites are closed with interrupted locking figure-of-eight nylon sutures to limit drainage. Elbows are splinted for 24 hours after arthroscopic medial epicondylectomy with an anterior splint in full extension. A second layer of sterile dressings is placed under the splint in the operating room, which will remain on the elbow until follow-up at one week postoperatively. The sterile soft dressings allow patient-directed elbow exercises several times per day, starting on the second postoperative day working on elbow flexion/extension/supination/pronation along with wrist and hand range of motion exercises. Oral antibiotics are continued for two weeks until skin incisions have completely healed. Sutures are removed and adhesive skin closures are applied at two weeks postoperatively. Patients are allowed to return to light everyday activities after dressings are removed although they are advised to limit strenuous activities for up to six to eight weeks.

CONCLUSION

Arthroscopic medial epicondylectomy has a number of attractive features in managing cubital tunnel syndrome. It is a minimally invasive procedure, which preserves the blood supply to the ulnar nerve. It directly addresses the causative factors of nerve compression and traction without insulting normal structures. It is an arthroscopic procedure, which can be conveniently adopted as an extension of elbow arthroscopic work when it is needed, without the need of converting to an open procedure. It should be emphasized, however, that the ulnar nerve is just one tissue plane away from where the arthroscopic work takes place and demands special precautions from the performing surgeon.

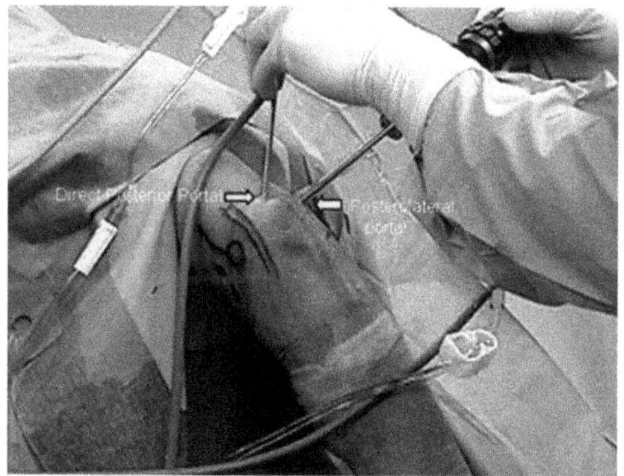

FIGURE 1 In an arthroscopic medial epicondylectomy, the posterolateral portal is used as the viewing portal, and the direct posterior portal as the working portal. The arthroscope is inserted through the posterolateral portal and directed toward the medial epicondyle. An Arthrocare cautery device is inserted through the direct posterior portal for releasing the posterior bundle of the medial collateral ligament.

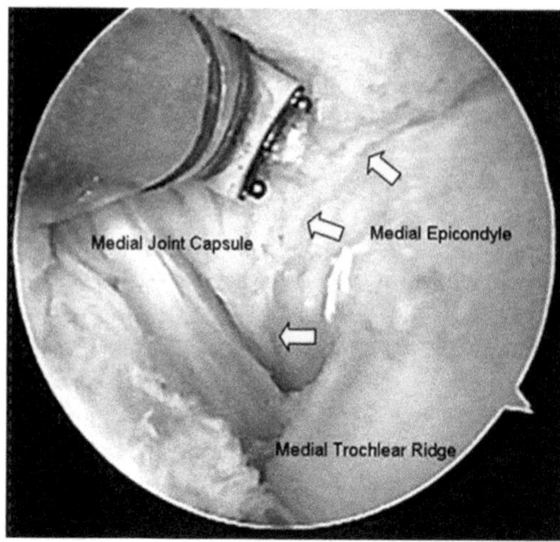

FIGURE 2 Once soft tissue is debrided at the posteromedial corner with an arthroscopic shaver, the insertion of the medial joint capsule on the posterior surface of the medial epicondyle is readily visible (*yellow arrows*). The capsule on the posterior surface of medial epicondyle is released first with Arthrocare. Then the Arthrocare is moved gradually downward to release the capsule on the posteroinferior surface of the medial epicondyle.

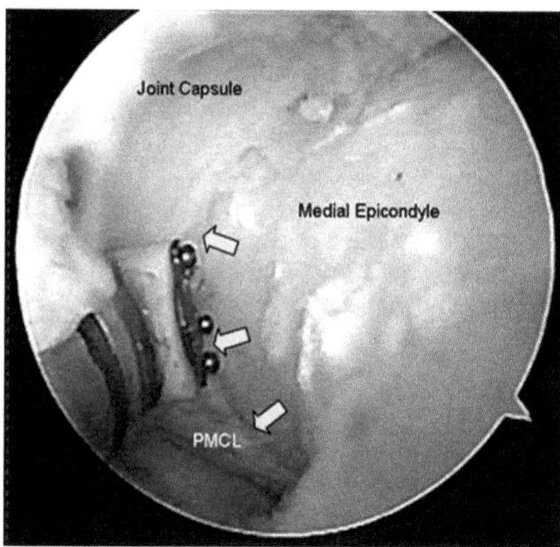

FIGURE 3 The Arthrocare is now placed at the posteroinferior surface of the medial epicondyle, releasing the insertion of the medial joint capsule and posterior bundle of the medial collateral ligament (*blue arrows*). *Abbreviation*: PMCL, posterior bundle of the medial collateral ligament.

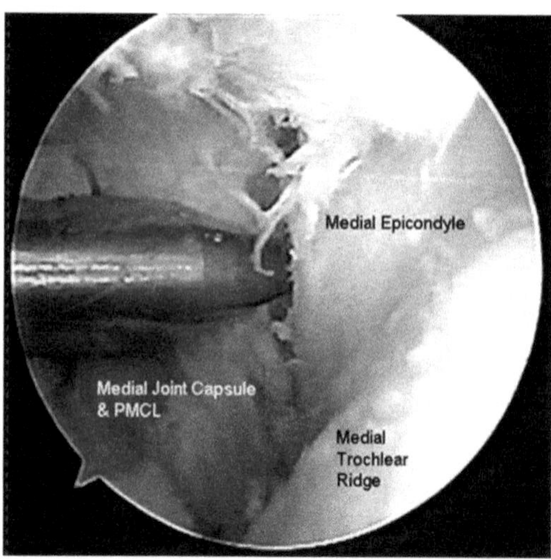

FIGURE 4 A blunt trocar can be used to confirm the right tissue plane or the extent of capsular release. *Abbreviation*: PMCL, posterior bundle of the medial collateral ligament.

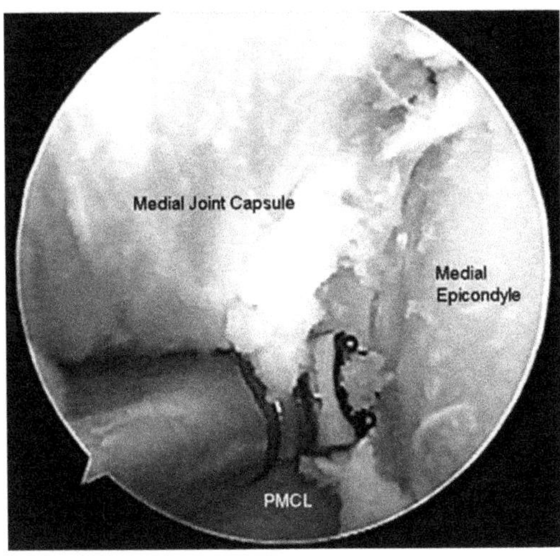

FIGURE 5 The medial joint capsule and posterior bundle of the medial collateral ligament are being released on the posteroinferior surface of the medial epicondyle. *Abbreviation*: PMCL, posterior bundle of the medial collateral ligament.

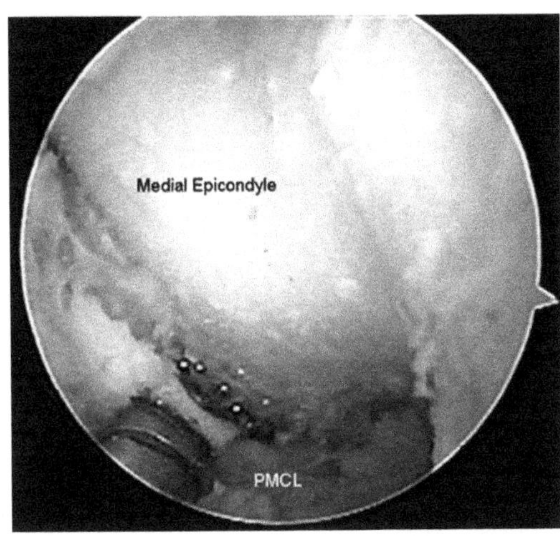

FIGURE 6 Once the posteroinferior surface of the medial epicondyle is cleared, release is continued anteriorly for approximately 0.5 to 1 cm in order to release the entire posterior bundle of the medial collateral ligament. It should be noted that right beneath the released posterior bundle is the ulnar nerve, and a lower setting of the Arthrocare Wand should be used. *Abbreviation*: PMCL, posterior bundle of the medial collateral ligament.

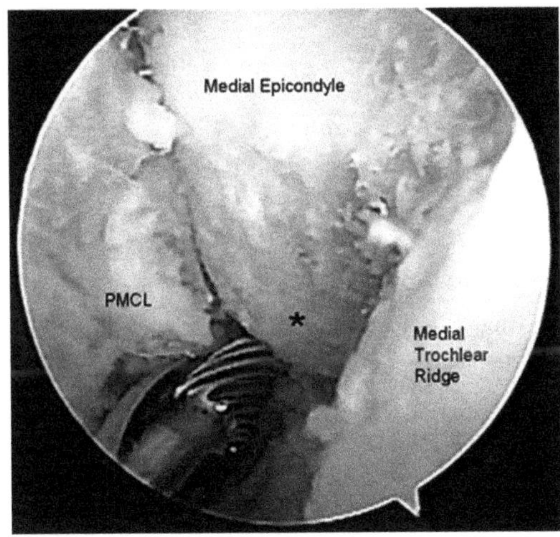

FIGURE 7 After the release of the posterior bundle of the medial collateral ligament, a 4.0-mm hooded cone-tipped burr is employed for bone resection. Bone resection starts with removing several millimeters of bone from the posteroinferior corner of the medial epicondyle. Then the remaining inferior bone of the medial epicondyle is readily visible (*), facilitating the subsequent inferior bone resection. The hood side of the burr should be directed toward the posterior bundle of the medial collateral ligament, and suction should be turned off during burring in order to minimize the risk of ulnar nerve injury. *Abbreviation*: PMCL, posterior bundle of the medial collateral ligament.

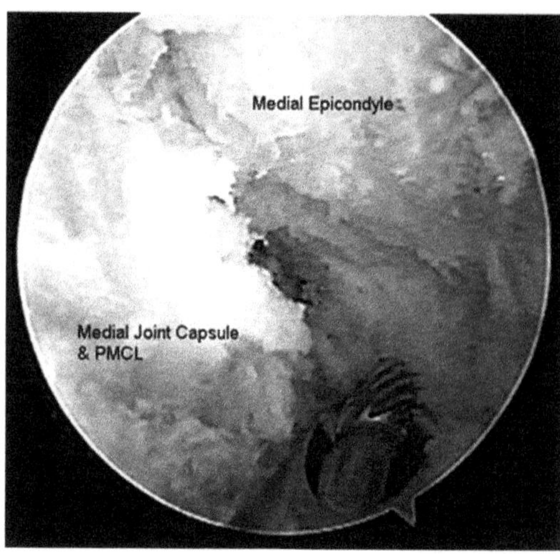

FIGURE 8 Several millimeters of bone have been removed from the inferior aspect of the medial epicondyle, completing the medial epicondylectomy procedure. *Abbreviation*: PMCL, posterior bundle of the medial collateral ligament.

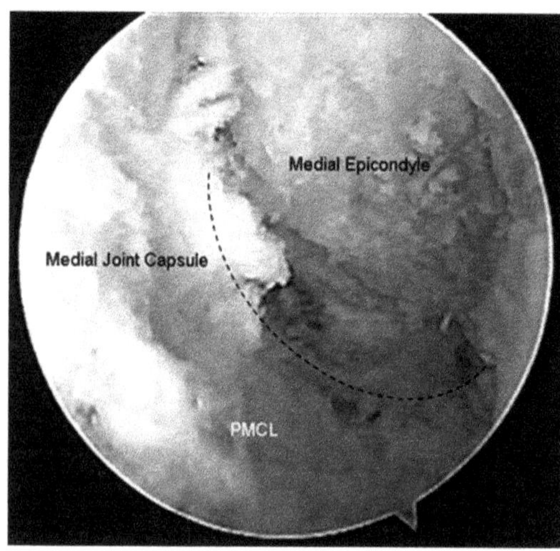

FIGURE 9 The dotted line shows the outline of the original medial epicondyle before bone resection, demonstrating the amount of bone resected. Usually, several millimeters of bone is removed from the posterior and inferior aspect of the medial epicondyle, but the amount of resection varies in individual cases. *Abbreviation*: PMCL, posterior bundle of the medial collateral ligament.

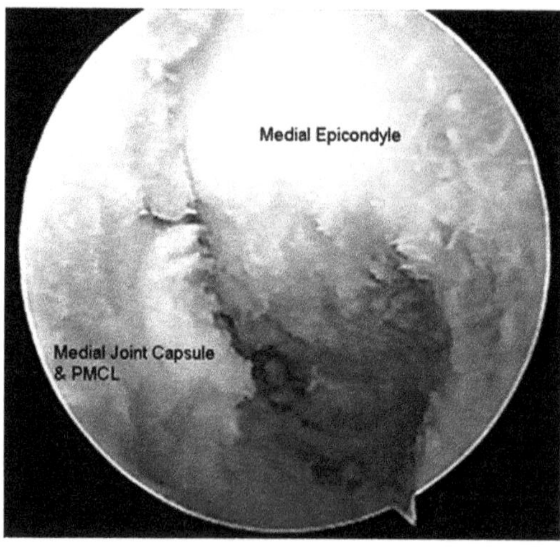

FIGURE 10 Completed medial epicondylectomy. The release of the posterior bundle of the medial collateral ligament and bone resection at the posterior and inferior aspect of the medial epicondyle result in deepening of the cubital tunnel, allow slight anterior translation of the ulnar nerve, and thus reduce strain in the ulnar nerve. *Abbreviation*: PMCL, posterior bundle of the medial collateral ligament.

REFERENCES

1. Gelberman RH, Yamaguchi K, Hollstien SB, et al. Changes in interstitial pressure and cross-sectional area of the cubital tunnel and of the ulnar nerve with flexion of the elbow. An experimental study in human cadavera. J Bone Joint Surg Am 1998; 80(4):492–501.
2. Toby EB, Hanesworth D. Ulnar nerve strains at the elbow. J Hand Surg (Am) 1998; 23(6):992–997.
3. Callaway GH, Field LD, Deng XH, et al. Biomechanical evaluation of the medial collateral ligament of the elbow. J Bone Joint Surg Am 1997; 79(8):1223–1231.
4. Le Viet D. Frontal partial epicondylectomy for release of the ulnar nerve at the elbow. Chirurgie 1991; 117(10):868–873.
5. Popa M, Dubert T. Treatment of cubital tunnel syndrome by frontal partial medial epicondylectomy. A retrospective series of 55 cases. J Hand Surg (Br) 2004; 29(6):563–567.
6. King T, Morgan FP. The treatment of traumatic ulnar neuritis. Mobilisation of the ulnar nerve at the elbow by removal of the medial epicondyle and adjacent bone. Aust NZ J Surg 1950; (20):33–45.

36 Arthroscopic Reduction Internal Fixation of Elbow Fractures

Taylor D. Brown and John P. Peden
Mississippi Sports Medicine and Orthopedic Center, Jackson, Mississippi, U.S.A.

Felix H. Savoie and Larry D. Field
Upper Extremity Service, Mississippi Sports Medicine and Orthopedic Center, and Department of Orthopedic Surgery, University of Mississippi School of Medicine, Jackson, Mississippi, U.S.A.

INDICATIONS

The indications for elbow arthroscopy continue to expand. In 1984, Caspari (1) greatly increased the indications for arthroscopy of the knee when he reported on 20 cases of arthroscopic visualization during the reduction of tibial plateau fractures. Intra-articular fractures pose an increased degree of difficulty for the orthopedic surgeon to treat and an increased morbidity to the patient with regard to long-term function and pain. When treating intra-articular fractures, arthroscopic assistance not only facilitates a more anatomic articular reduction, but it also allows identification of other associated injuries. The benefit of arthroscopic reduction is further enhanced when fracture fragments can be stabilized with percutaneous fixation techniques, limiting exposure and soft tissue dissection. Arthroscopic reduction internal fixation (ARIF) is now an accepted technique in the treatment of certain fractures about the knee, ankle, elbow, and wrist.

Leaders of elbow arthroscopy have reported scattered cases of arthroscopic treatment of elbow fractures. This chapter describes which fracture patterns are amenable to ARIF and details our techniques to treat these elbow injuries. ARIF is indicated for fractures with intra-articular extension which can he adequately stabilized with percutaneous fixation techniques.

CONTRAINDICATIONS

The contraindications for ARIF include the same contraindications to elbow arthroscopy, including inability to palpate the bony landmarks about the elbow, preoperative neurologic injury, as well as limitations of fracture patterns. Extra-articular fractures and fractures requiring more extensive exposure for more extensive fixation are not amenable to ARIF.

TECHNIQUES

Surgical Set Up and Positioning

Following induction of general anesthesia, the patient is positioned in a prone position with the operative side brought to the edge of the table. An arm board parallel to the table is centered at the shoulder. A padded block, matching the thickness of the chest roll, rests on the arm board and supports the arm parallel with the floor. Alternatively, the lateral decubitus position can be used. A tourniquet is applied high on the arm. The hand and forearm are placed in an impervious stockinette and wrapped with an elastic gauze to limit swelling and extravasation of arthroscopy fluid (Fig. 1).

The surgeon stands at the side of the bed with the operative limb directly in front of him. The arthroscopy tower and monitor are located on the opposite side of the bed and surgeon. A sterile Mayo standing beside the arthroscopy tower and positioned over the draped patient,

---

Please refer to pages 379–382 for the figures in this chapter.

serves as a base for equipment from the tower to be used within the operative field. A second sterile mayo tray and scrubbed surgical assistant stand on the same side of the patient as the surgeon. A sterile draped fluoroscopy machine is positioned parallel to the table at the head or foot of the patient and is brought into the operative field as needed. Although the reduction of fracture fragments are confirmed arthroscopically, the placement of hardware must be confirmed with fluoroscopy.

The elbow joint is distended with an injection of 30 to 40 cc of sterile saline, directed through the triceps tendon toward the olecranon fossa or through the area of the soft spot portal. The elbow is brought into a position of 90° to 95° of flexion. The location of a proximal anteromedial portal 2 cm proximal to the medial epicondyle and 2 cm anterior to the intermuscular septum is marked, and the path is confirmed with a spinal needle that pierces the capsule and returns a few drops of saline. The path for the portal is created using a hemostat to spread the tissues and palpate the intermuscular septum. A small blunt metal trocar and cannula are inserted to formalize the proximal anteromedial portal. The standard 30° arthroscope is inserted through the cannula and diagnostic arthroscopy is carried out with gravity flow epinephrine laden irrigation. A proximal anterolateral portal is established 2 cm proximal and 1 cm anterior to the lateral epicondyle using an outside-in technique localized with a spinal needle and created with a hemostat to spread the tissues. Another small blunt metal trocar and cannula is inserted under arthroscopic visualization. This second portal is useful not only to identify and manipulate fragments within the anterior compartment of the elbow but also to establish a separate inflow and outflow to clear the hemarthrosis and fibrinous debris associated with an acute, intra-articular fracture.

After completing all necessary work in the anterior elbow joint, the proximal anteromedial small cannula is exchanged for a large cannula over a switching stick and inflow is established there. Our first posterior portal is a proximal posterocentral portal established 2 cm proximal to the olecranon tip, passing through the triceps tendon. A complete diagnostic arthroscopy of the medial and lateral gutters, the olecranon fossa, the olecranon tip, and posterior radiocapitellar joint can be visualized with the arthroscope in this portal. Additional portals can be created and percutaneous hardware can be placed, as directed by the fracture orientation anywhere from this posterocentral portal to the lateral epicondyle. Any other portals needed as well as the specific details of each fracture pattern are discussed individually. Wound care and dressings are placed in standard fashion. Application of a long arm posterior splint is applied depending on fracture pattern and stability.

Distal Humerus Fractures

Capitellum

Numerous authors have reported the successful arthroscopic treatment of osteochondritis dessicans (OCD) and fractures of the capitellum (2–6). Our technique for treating capitellar fractures involves visualization through a proximal anteriomedial portal. A shaver is introduced through a proximal anterolateral portal to remove the fibrinous debris and hemarthrosis. A cannula is used to maintain the portal, and the backside of the shaver is directed toward the anterior capsule at all times to protect the overlying posterior interosseous nerve. Reduction of the fragment is accomplished with a Kirschner wire passed through the lateral cannula, which is used as a joystick, or a second lateral incision can be made 2 cm proximal to the lateral epicondyle, just anterior to the intermuscular septum, and a freer elevator can be brought down into the joint, just anterior to the humeral cortex, and used as both a capsular retractor and reduction tool. In some cases, a portion of the lateral collateral ligament will need to be released with the motorized shaver or percutaneously with a blade, to facilitate reduction of the fragment. The arthroscope is used to magnify and precisely confirm the articular reduction. The lateral Kirschner wire is advanced across the fracture line to provisionally hold the fragment. A type I fracture has enough bone to be fixed with a headless cannulated screw. This screw can be placed over the already placed guide wire, or any number of additional guide wires can be placed from posterior to anterior percutaneously through the posterolateral portion of the elbow. These fractures usually occur in a coronal plane and are frequently amenable to fixation perpendicular to the fracture plane, directly posterior to anterior or directly anterior to posterior. Position can be confirmed with fluoroscopy, and the anteromedial arthroscope can be used to observe and prevent any anterior capsular penetration.

Fluoroscopy is used to identify final reduction and hardware position (Figs. 2–4). An attempt can be made to fix a type II fracture with some bone attached with a bioabsorbable implant; otherwise, the fragment can be excised as described earlier with a motorized shaver. Diagnostic arthroscopy of the posterior elbow is completed, and the patient is placed in a posterior splint for a week prior to initiating a motion program.

Unicondylar Fractures

Milch classified unicondylar fractures as type I and type II based upon the size of the fragment. Type II fractures cross from one column across to the articular portion of the other column, which are inherently unstable, and require operative reduction and fixation. Nondisplaced type I fractures can be treated with immobilization, but this can lead to stiffness, and most type I fractures, both displaced and nondisplaced, are usually treated with operative reduction and fixation (7). These fractures are amenable to ARIF, as they have an intra-articular portion that can be anatomically reduced with arthroscopic visualization and stability can be achieved with percutaneous lag screw fixation.

We use our standard positioning and create our first portal on the side of the elbow least affected by trauma. For lateral column injuries, our standard proximal anteromedial portal is created and the arthroscope is inserted. We create our standard anterolateral portal and use this to clear the debris from the fracture site, as well as direct the reduction of the fragment, and align the articular surfaces. We create a proximal posterocentral portal to visualize the posterior fracture reduction. A separate posterolateral portal is also useful to clear debris from the posterior portion of the fracture. A separate incision is made over the lateral epicondyle, and a guide wire is inserted into the lateral epicondyle and directed up the lateral column toward the distal humeral shaft. The guide wire is advanced and position is confirmed on fluoroscopic images. A second guidewire is placed parallel to the first to control rotation. Care must be taken not to penetrate the coronoid or olecranon fossa with this hardware and this can be confirmed by viewing both the anterior and posterior joint sequentially. A single, self-drilling and self-tapping cannulated partially threaded small fragment cancellous screw is passed over the guide wire and compresses and stabilizes the lateral column fragment.

For a medial column injury, our first portal is a proximal anterolateral portal, and a proximal anteromedial is created as a working portal after a small incision is made centered over the medial epicondyle to confirm location of the ulnar nerve within the ulnar groove. In a manner analogous to that just described for lateral column injuries, a medial column injury can be reduced and fixed with a single self-drilling and self-tapping cannulated partially threaded small fragment cancellous screw passed over the guide wire to compresses and stabilize the medial column fragment. Diagnostic arthroscopy of the posterior elbow is completed, and the patient is placed in a posterior splint for a week prior to initiating a motion program (Figs. 5–7).

Supracondylar and Intercondylar Fractures

Many of these fractures are too comminuted to achieve adequate, stable fixation with percutaneous screws and require open reduction and internal fixation with plates and screws. The arthroscope can be useful to visualize articular reduction even during these open procedures and confirm intraosseous guide wire and screw placement.

Noncomminuted supracondylar and intercondylar fractures classified as A2.3 and C1 may be amenable to ARIF in limited situations with low demand patients with adequate bone density. In manner as described earlier for unicondylar injury, a combined fixation including partially threaded lag screws directed up each column into the distal humeral shaft will sometimes achieve adequate stabilization. For intercondylar fractures, a third screw can be directed from medial to lateral, over a guide wire, to achieve compression between the two condylar fragments. Again, both anterior and posterior views are required to confirm no penetration of the coronoid or olecranon fossa.

As with all elbow fractures treated with ARIF, failure to achieve adequate stabilization is an indication to proceed to open reduction internal fixation of the fracture. Our prone positioning facilitates the posterior exposure most commonly used to treat complex fractures of the distal humerus. We place an arm board parallel to the table and this arm board can be used to support the upper extremity in an internally or externally rotated position, with the elbow flexed to approach fractures as dictated.

Medial Epicondyle

Minimally displaced fractures can be treated with a period of immobilization for 7 to 14 days. Displaced fractures in adults or young throwing athletes require reduction and fixation. Although this is an extracapsular injury, the arthroscope is useful to confirm adequate reduction and medial stability after fixation, as well as extra-articular hardware placement.

A small longitudinal incision is made centered over the subcutaneous portion of the medial epicondyle, and the ulnar nerve is confirmed to lie posterior to the epicondyle in the ulnar groove. A retractor can be placed posterior to the epicondyle to protect the nerve and keep it located. Standard anterior portals are created and arthroscopy of the anterior elbow is carried out. Any other associated injuries are noted. Medial instability on valgus stress is confirmed when viewed through either portal.

A fluoroscope is used to direct hardware placement and reduction. Kirschner wires are used to joystick the epicondylar fragment as needed and are then directed across the fracture into the medial column of the distal humerus. Usually two parallel wires are placed. A single self-drilling and self-tapping cannulated partially threaded small fragment cancellous screw is passed over the guide wire and compresses and stabilizes the medial epicondylar fragment. While viewing through the anterolateral portal, medial stability on valgus stress testing can be confirmed. The instruments are removed from the joint and the medial incision is closed. The patient is placed in a posterior long arm splint for two weeks, at which time a motion program is initiated.

Proximal Ulna Fractures

Coronoid Process

Coronoid fractures are usually associated with an elbow dislocation or radial head fracture. Type I fractures involve just a fleck of the tip of the coronoid, and the treatment is directed by the associated pathology. Liu (8) has reported two cases of type I coronoid fractures which went on to cause loss of motion and loose body formation which were successfully treated with arthroscopic debridement.

Type II coronoid fractures can be treated with early motion if the elbow remains stable. Unstable type II and type III fractures require operative intervention. If the fracture fragments are comminuted, a hinged external fixator is useful to maintain a congruent joint while the soft tissue supports of the elbow heal. Larger cornoid fragments can be fixed with partially threaded screws to restore joint stability (9).

We use our standard prone position and anterior diagnostic arthroscopy portals. The size of the coronoid fragment is assessed and the fracture bed is cleared, using instruments passed through the anterolateral portal. If the fragment is large enough for screw threads to obtain purchase, we proceed with screw fixation of the fragment. The arthroscope is transferred to the lateral portal. An anterior cruciate ligament tibial tunnel targeting device is inserted through the proximal anteromedial portal and used to maintain the fragment in a reduced position. A guide wire is then drilled posterior to anterior through the proximal ulna, across the fracture, and into the coronoid fragment. This guide wire is then exchanged with a single self-drilling and self-tapping cannulated partially threaded small fragment cancellous screw. If the fragment is small, we will pass a suture through small fragment and then retrieve the limbs of the suture with a suture retriever through two targeted tunnels drilled as described for cannulated screw placement. The limbs of the suture are then tied together over the posterior border of the ulna. Associated injuries are treated appropriately and the arm is placed in a long arm posterior splint or hinged external fixator if needed.

Proximal Radius

Radial Head

Nondisplaced Mason type I radial head fractures are best treated with early motion. Comminuted Mason type III radial head fractures are treated with open reduction internal fixation, radial head replacement, or radial head excision. Displaced type II fractures of the radial head frequently block motion and require reduction and fixation (10). ARIF of this injury pattern is analogous to ARIF of Schatzker type I split tibial plateau fractures. A percutaneous lag screw compresses the fracture, and the concave surface of the radial head is even similar to the concave lateral tibial plateau. Arthroscopic reduction and percutaneous fixation of a radial neck fracture in a child has been reported (11).

Our standard prone position and proximal anterior portals are used to begin the diagnostic arthroscopy. Frequently, the displaced fragment of a type II radial head fracture is best visualized from a proximal posterocentral portal. Inflow is maintained through the anteromedial cannula. Rotation of the forearm allows complete visualization of the fracture anatomy. Instruments are introduced through a soft spot portal created in an outside-in fashion, and the fragment is reduced with the use of a motorized shaver and freer elevator. A Kirschner wire is placed percutaneously near the site of a posterior soft spot portal to pierce the fragment and joystick it into position. A magnified view of the articular surface directs the reduction. The forearm is rotated so that the Kirschner wire is oriented perpendicular to the fracture plane. The wire is advanced and then a headless cannulated self-compressing screw is placed over the wire. A headless screw prevents injury to the surrounding annular ligament and proximal radioulnar joint. The patient is placed in a posterior splint for a week prior to initiating a motion program (Figs. 8–10).

PEARLS AND PITFALLS

Caspari stated that arthroscopic reduction of fractures is technique-dependent and difficult, limiting its use to experienced arthroscopists. Critical to successful arthroscopic techniques is a thorough evaluation of the fracture. When fracture stability is a concern do to comminution or quality of bone, standard open reduction with rigid fixation should be performed to avoid postoperative loss of fixation or stiffness from necessary limited rehabilitation.

REHABILITATION

Intra-articular fractures are best managed with fixation that allows early motion. Therefore, after wound healing, passive elbow ROM is initiated. When bone healing has progressed, typically at four to six weeks, active motion is begun. Strengthening is initiated at 10 to 12 weeks.

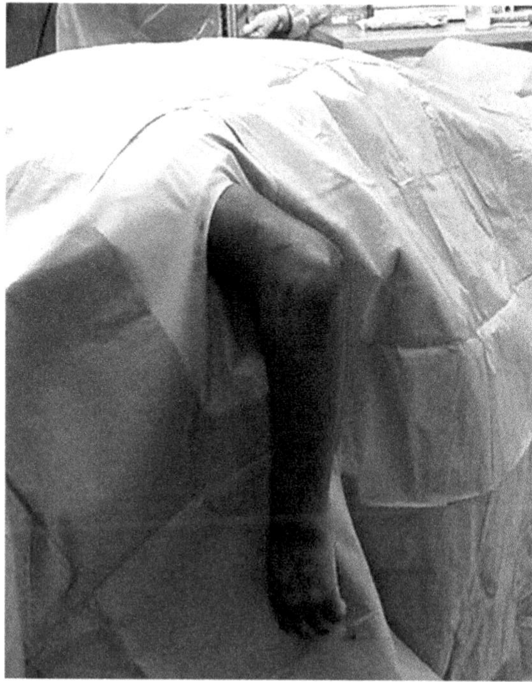

FIGURE 1 Photograph of a patient in our standard prone position.

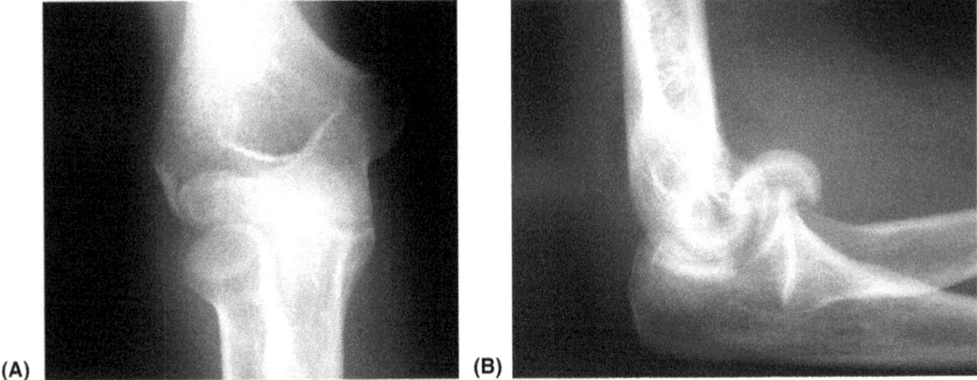

FIGURE 2 Radiographs of type 1 capitellar fracture: (**A**) anteroposterior image and (**B**) lateral image.

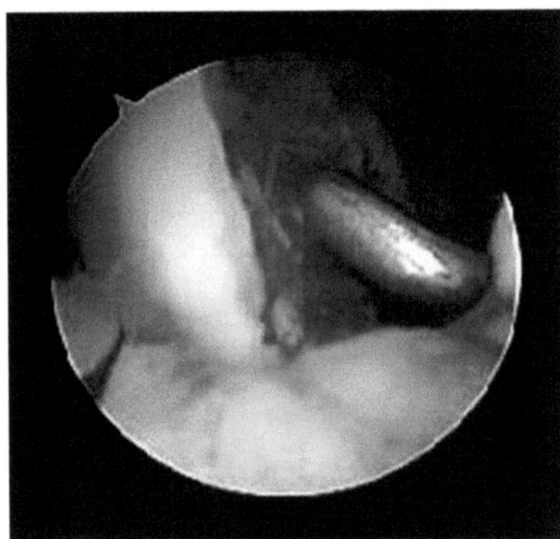

FIGURE 3 Arthroscopic image of type 1 capitellar fracture being reduced.

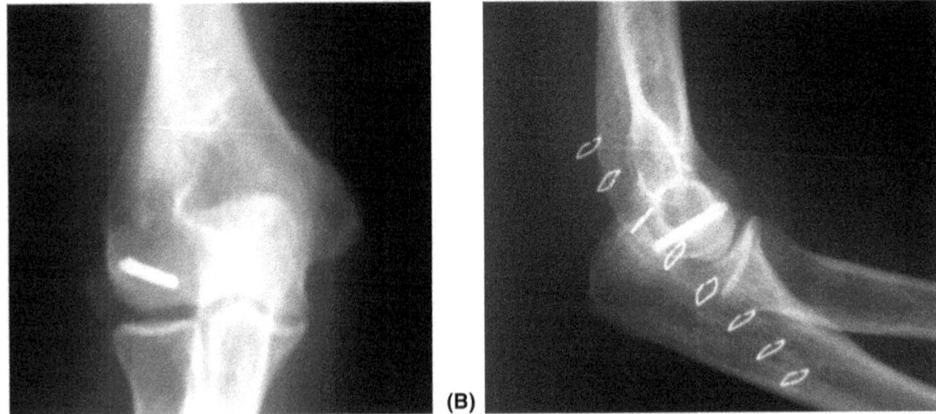

FIGURE 4 Radiographs of screw fixation of type1 capitellar fracture: (**A**) anteroposterior image and (**B**) lateral image.

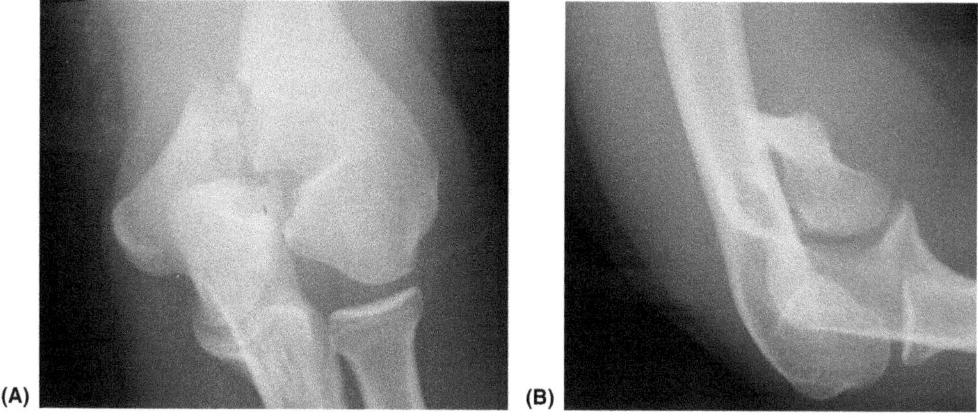

FIGURE 5 Radiographs of medial condyle fracture: (**A**) anteroposterior image and (**B**) lateral image.

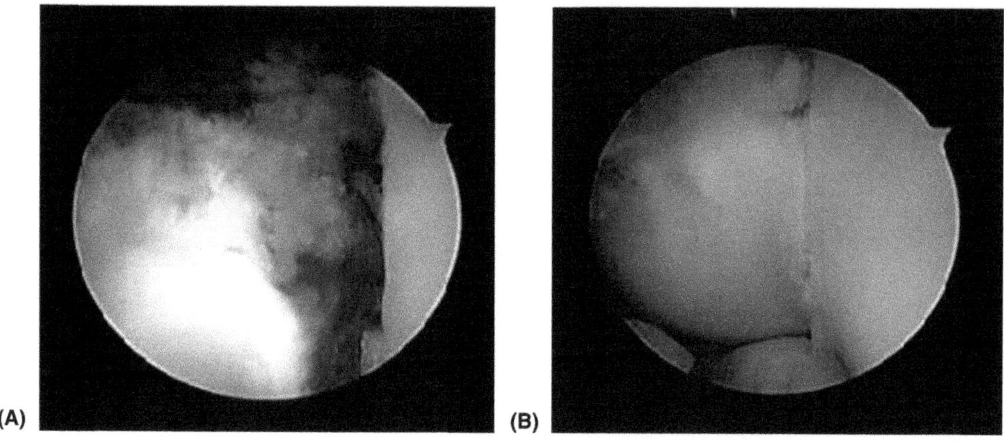

FIGURE 6 Arthroscopic image of medial condyle fracture: (**A**) before reduction and (**B**) following reduction.

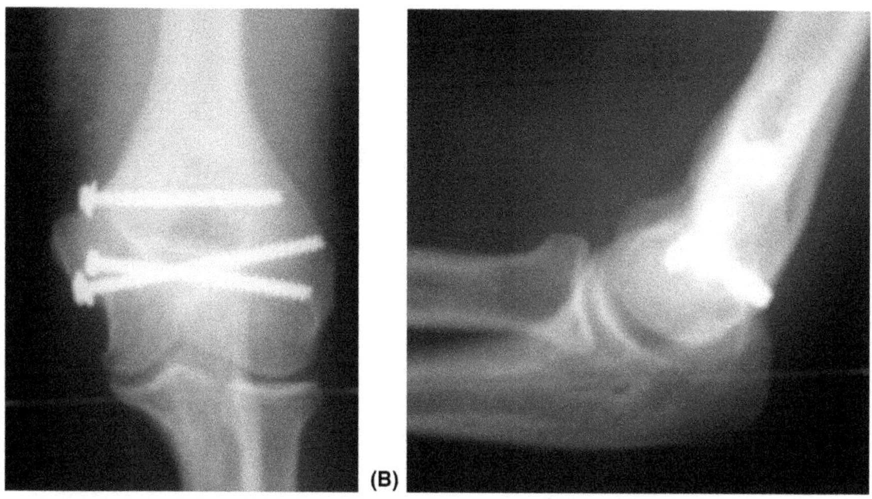

FIGURE 7 Radiographs of screw fixation of medial condyle fracture: (**A**) anteroposterior image and (**B**) lateral image.

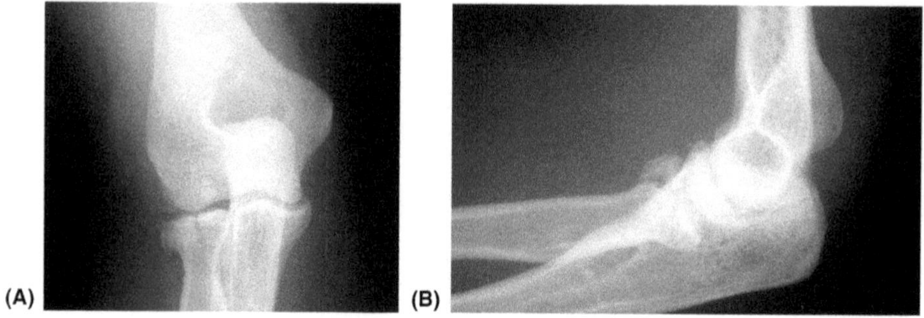

FIGURE 8 Radiographs of a radial head fracture: (**A**) anteroposterior image and (**B**) lateral image.

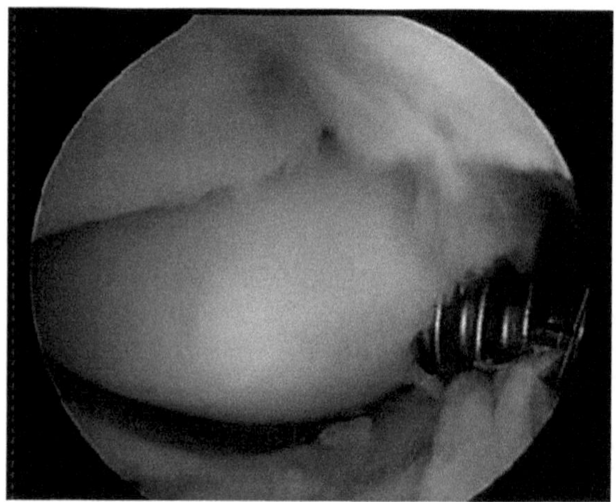

FIGURE 9 Arthroscopic image of radial head fracture.

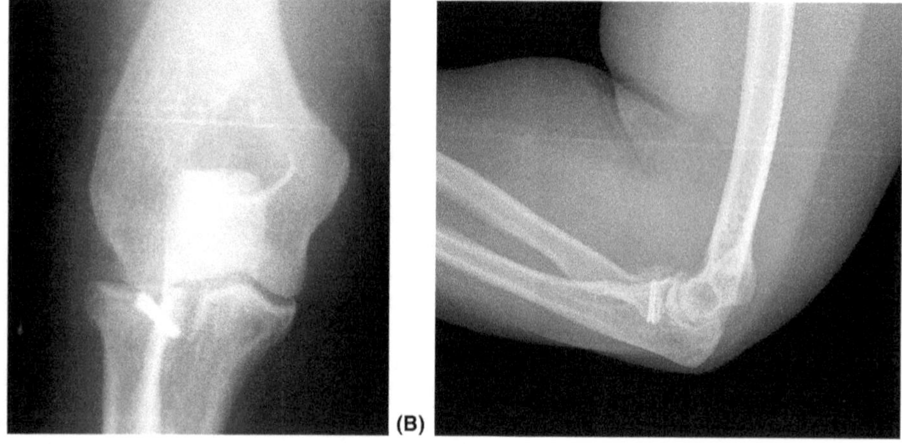

FIGURE 10 Radiographs of screw fixation of radial head fracture: (**A**) anteroposterior image and (**B**) lateral image.

REFERENCES

1. Caspari RB, Hutton PMJ, Whipple TL, et al. The role of arthroscopy in the management of tibial plateau fractures. Arthroscopy 1985; 1(2):76–82.
2. Krijnen MR, Lim L, Willems WJ. Arthroscopic treatment of osteochondritis dissecans of the capitellum: Report of 5 female athletes. Arthroscopy 2003; 19(2):210–214.
3. Pill SG, Ganley TJ, Flynn JM. Osteochondritis dissecans of the capitellum: Arthroscopic-assisted treatment of large, full-thickness defects in young patients. Arthroscopy 2003; 19(2):222–225.
4. Cain EL, Dugas JR, Wolf RS, et al. Elbow injuries in throwing athletes: a current concepts review. Am J Sports Med 2003; 31(4):621–635.
5. Feldman MD. Arthroscopic excision of type II capitellar fractures. Arthroscopy 1997; 13(6):743–748.
6. Hardy P, Menguy F, Guillot S. Arthroscopic treatment of capitellum fracture of the humerus. Arthroscopy 2002; 18(4):422–426.
7. Jupiter JB. Fractures of the distal humerus in adults. In: Morrey BF, ed. The Elbow and Its Disorders. 3rd ed. Philadelphia: Saunders, 2000:293–330.
8. Liu SH, Henry M, Bowen R. Complications of type 1 coronoid fractures in competitive athletes: Report of two cases and review of the literature. J Shoulder Elbow Surg 1996; 5:223–227.
9. Regan WD. Coronoid process and monteggia fractues. In: Morrey BF, ed. The Elbow and Its Disorders. 3rd ed. Philadelphia: Saunders, 2000:396–408.
10. Morrey BF. Radial head fractures. In Morrey BF, ed. The Elbow and Its Disorders. 3rd ed Philadelphia: Saunders, 2000:341–364.
11. Dawson FA, Inostroza F. Arthroscopic reduction and percutaneous fixation of a radial neck fracture in a child. Arthroscopy 2004; 20(6):90–93.

Index

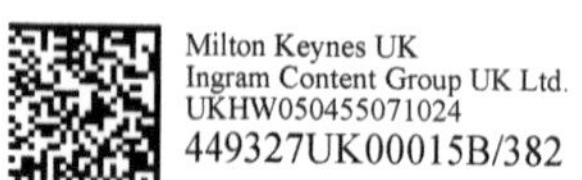

Milton Keynes UK
Ingram Content Group UK Ltd.
UKHW050455071024
449327UK00015B/382

9 780367 389482